CALCIFIC AORTIC VALVE DISEASE

Edited by **Elena Aikawa**

Calcific Aortic Valve Disease
http://dx.doi.org/10.5772/46239
Edited by Elena Aikawa

Contributors

Kaan Kirali, Fahrettin Oz, Fatih Tufan, Ahmet Ekmekcı, Omer A. Sayin, Huseyin Oflaz, Hideaki Senzaki, Hirofumi Saiki, Mehmet Demir, Lazar Velicki, Stamenko S. Šušak, Marijan Majin, Dušan Popović, Ivana Burazor, Robert B Hinton, Claudia Goettsch, Ioan Tilea, Horatiu Suciu, Brindusa Tilea, Cristina Maria Tatar, Razvan Constantin Serban, Mihaela Ispas, Juan Bustamante, Sergio Juan Cánovas López, Ángel G. Pinto, Omer Leal, Ibrahim Akin, Gino Gerosa, Laura Iop, Maria G. Barderas, Carlijn V Bouten, Saskia Van Loon, Anthal Smits, Anita Driessen-Mol, Frank Baaijens, Dena Wiltz, Alicia Blancas, Liezl Balaoing, Alex Arevalos, Matthew Sapp, Xing Zhang, K. Jane Grande-Allen, Katherine Yutzey, Elaine Wirrig, Orihashi, George Tokmaji, Berto Bouma, Dave Koolbergen, Bas De Mol, Masanori Aikawa

Published by InTech

Janeza Trdine 9, 51000 Rijeka, Croatia

Publishing Process Manager Ana Pantar
Technical Editor InTech DTP team
Cover InTech Design team

Additional hard copies can be obtained from orders@intechopen.com

Calcific Aortic Valve Disease, Edited by Elena Aikawa
p. cm.
ISBN 978-953-51-1150-4

For EU product safety concerns:
IN TECH d.o.o., Prolaz Marije Krucifikse Kozulić 3, 51000 Rijeka, Croatia,
info@intechopen.com or visit our website at intechopen.com.

Meet the editor

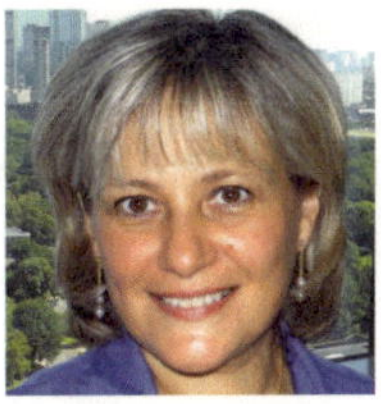

Dr. Elena Aikawa received her medical degree from the First Moscow Medical Institute, Moscow, Russia in 1984, and obtained a Ph.D. degree in pathology from Institute of Biophysics, Moscow in 1989. She joined Brigham and Women's Hospital (BWH), Boston in 1991. She is currently an Assistant Professor of Medicine at BWH and Harvard Medical School. She also is a Director of Vascular Biology Program at the Center for Interdisciplinary Sciences and a Principal Investigator at the Center for Excellence in Cardiovascular Research at BWH. Her research focuses on the pathogenesis of valvular heart disease and the mechanisms of cardiovascular calcification. She is a member of the National Institutes of Health (NIH) Working Group on Calcific Aortic Valve Stenosis and of the editorial boards of PLoS ONE, Journal of Extracellular Vesicles, and Arteriosclerosis, Thrombosis, and Vascular Biology. Her work in cardiovascular research is recognized worldwide, as reflected by numerous invited lectures and publications.

Contents

Preface

Valvular heart diseases represent an underappreciated yet serious and growing problem. Due to population aging, calcific aortic valve disease (CAVD) has become the most common heart valve disease in developed and rapidly developing regions of the world, affecting approximately 25% of adults over 65 years of age. No therapies exist to slow this disease progression, and surgical valve replacement is the only effective treatment. More than 275,000 aortic valve replacements are performed annually worldwide, and this number is expected to triple by 2050. Although rheumatic heart disease continues to be an important problem in developing countries, its prevalence has generally declined. This book will address CAVD as a common heart valve disease, focusing predominantly on the underlying mechanisms and current treatment approaches. We hope that this book will enable readers to grasp the current knowledge and focus on the possibility of preventing disease progression in the near future.

The book is divided into six sections and comprised of 18 chapters written by well-recognized investigators from United States, Europe, and Asia. Section I focuses on the biology and function of the normal aortic valve. Chapter 1 is written by a research group lead by Dr. K. Jane Grande-Allen, a renowned investigator in the field of cardiac valve extracellular matrix and valve biology. It describes the role of major and minor matrices in normal valves, focusing on extracellular matrix function and biomechanical properties. Chapter 2, written by Prof. Tilea Ioan, deals with the anatomy and function of normal aortic valve components. Section II provides current insight into the mechanisms of CAVD. It begins with Chapter 3, written by Prof. Katherine Yutzey, a prominent scholar in valve developmental biology, who provides an overview of signaling pathways involved in valve development and their reactivation during CAVD progression. This chapter also describes osteogenic-related molecular pathways involved in CAVD, and provides an outlook on developing therapeutics to treat CAVD. The next two chapters (Chapter 4, written by Dr. Erik Fung, and Chapter 5, written by Dr. Claudia Goettsch) offer evolving insights into the mechanisms of CAVD, including NOTCH signaling and microRNA dysregulation. Topics covered in Section III include proteomics and metabolomics in Chapter 6, written by Dr. Maria Barderas; and genetics in Chapter 7, written by Dr. Robert Hinton. Both chapters represent innovative technology platforms recently developed to identify DNA, RNA, proteins, and peptides in different biological compartments, which could serve as biomarkers for various diseases. Section IV reviews advances in the field of heart valve tissue engineering and is comprised of two chapters written by leaders in the field (Chapter 8, written by Prof. Carlijn Bouten, and Chapter 9, written by Prof. Gino Gerosa). New cutting-edge approaches, including heart valve tissue engineering and tissue-guided regeneration, have been proposed to overcome the limitations of current valve substitutes. These chapters describe the foreign body response to implantation of biomaterials, preclinical and clinical models, principles of tissue engineering, and strategies to improve viable and functional aortic valve substitutes. Section V provides comprehensive information on bicuspid aortic valve (BAV) disease, in Chapter 10, written by Dr. George Tokmaji, and Chapter 11, written by Dr. Mehmed Demir. This section covers the diagnosis, treatment, and complications of BAV disease, and is particularly important because BAV is a common congenital cardiac abnormality affecting 2% of the population, and presenting in 50% of adults undergoing valve replacement for severe CAVD. Finally, Section VI is comprised of seven chapters written by an international team, including Drs. Velicki Lazar, Oz Fahrettin, Karali Kaan, Juan Bustamate, Akin Ibrahim, and Kazumasa Orihashi, and covers different aspects of CAVD treatment options, including the recently developed transcatheter aortic valve implantation. Chapter 18, written by Hideaki Senzaki on congenital aortic stenosis in pediatric patients, closes this section.

This book will provide the most up-to-date knowledge in the fast-growing and ever-changing field of aortic valve pathobiology. We hope that it will be useful for cardiologists, cardiovascular surgeons, fellows, and scientists who, we believe, should always be searching for updates in diagnosis, treatment, and research advancement. This open-access book will provide the most current information on CAVD.

I acknowledge my mentors — Dr. Frederick J. Schoen, for introducing me to the exciting biology of cardiac valve disease, and Dr. Peter Libby, for his continuous support and inspiration. And I can never thank my family enough — especially my husband, Dr. Masanori Aikawa, for believing in me and encouraging me throughout my career.

Elena Aikawa, MD, PhD
Associate Professor of Medicine
Harvard Medical School
Director, Vascular Biology Program
Center for Interdisciplinary Cardiovascular Sciences
Brigham and Women's Hospital
Boston, USA

Section 1

Biology and Function of Normal Aortic Valve

Chapter 1

Extracellular Matrix Organization, Structure, and Function

Dena Wiltz, C. Alexander Arevalos, Liezl R. Balaoing, Alicia A. Blancas, Matthew C. Sapp, Xing Zhang and K. Jane Grande-Allen

Additional information is available at the end of the chapter

http://dx.doi.org/10.5772/52842

1. Introduction

Heart valves are thin, complex, layered connective tissues that direct blood flow in one direction through the heart. There are four valves in the heart, located at the entrance to and exit from the ventricular chambers. The normal function of the heart valves is essential to cardiovascular and cardiopulmonary physiology. The opening and closing of valve leaflets at precise times during the cardiac cycles contributes to the generation of sufficiently high pressure to eject blood from the ventricles, and also prevents blood from flowing backwards into the heart instead of forward towards the systemic circulation and the lungs.

The ability of heart valves to open and close repeatedly, as well as the maintenance of the phenotypes of valvular cells, is made possible by their tissue microstructure, specifically the composition and orientation of extracellular matrix (ECM). The ECM within heart valves is primarily comprised of collagen, elastic fibers, and proteoglycans and glycosaminoglycans, although other ECM components are present as well. Taken together, the ECM performs several roles in heart valves. First, the ECM plays a biomechanical role: it is responsible for the unique mechanical behavior of the valve tissue and thus the overall valve function. Second, the valvular cells are bound to and surrounded by the ECM that is located within the immediate vicinity of the cell; this ECM is specifically known as the pericellular matrix (PCM). The PCM influences cell function by serving as a source of ligands for cell surface receptors, which transfers mechanical strains (experienced by the leaflet tissues) to the cells and initiates intracellular signaling pathways. Third, the various types of ECM have different innate mechanical behaviors, for example with collagen being stiffer than elastic fibers, and a growing body of research has demonstrated that the phenotype and function of cells, including valve cells, are influenced by the stiffness of the substrate to which they are adhered [1]. These two latter functions of the ECM are considered to be mechanobiological as opposed to merely biomechanical since they affect cell behavior. Fourth, ECM has binding sites for growth factors and other soluble molecules found in the extracellular space, and thus the ECM serves as a reservoir for numerous bioactive factors than can affect cell behavior if they are released (such as when the ECM is degraded) or if a cell migrates close to this ECM reservoir.

Overall, the heart valve field is beginning to appreciate that there are numerous interactions between the ECM, valve cells, and valve mechanics. Given the complicated relationships that are being demonstrated, it is not surprising that alterations to the normal arrangement or composition of ECM, which frequently occur in valve disease, significantly and detrimentally impact valve function in a rather vicious cycle. For this reason, there has been an increasing effort to characterize the ECM within normal heart valves not only to elucidate valve biomechanics and mechanobiology, but also to obtain a solid basis for comparison with diseased valves.

This chapter will provide an overview of the ECM within heart valves, focusing on the aortic valve. After detailing the layered structure of the valve leaflets, each type of ECM component will be described and discussed in relation to its role in valve function and, in some instances, valve dysfunction.

2. The aortic valve leaflets are layered structures

Aortic valve leaflets consist of three main layers: the fibrosa, spongiosa, and ventricularis. Each layer has a distinct composition that aids in the normal mechanical and biochemical behavior of the valve. In diseased states, however, the composition of the layered structures can be altered compared to healthy tissues.

The fibrosa layer, close to the outflow surface, is mainly composed of collagen fibers with a small amount of elastic fibers, which are the major stress-bearing components and provide strength to maintain coaptation during diastole [2]. The circumferential alignment and orientation of collagen fibers contribute to the biological stress-strain relationship for aortic valve leaflets (Figure 1). This bilinear stress-strain curve represents the high extension with a low load and high elastic modulus with a high load applied [3]. Moreover, the particular architecture of collagen fibers contributes to the anisotropic mechanical behavior of the fibrosa layer. It has been found that the fibrosa is 4-6 times stiffer in the circumferential direction than in the radial direction [4].

The middle spongiosa layer of the leaflet predominantly consists of glycosaminoglycans and proteoglycans, particularly hyaluronan, which form a foam-like structure and bind a large amount of water. The spongiosa layer absorbs energy during compression, and facilitates the arrangement of collagen fibrils in the fibrosa and elastin in the ventricularis during the cardiac cycles [5].

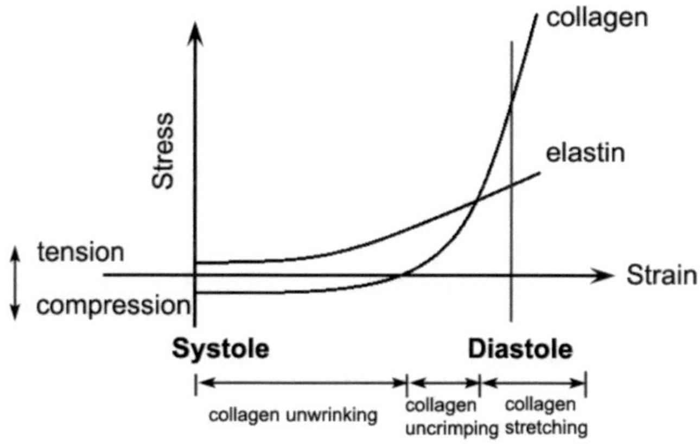

Figure 1. Schematic drawing of stress-strain relationships for collagen and elastin fibers during valve motion, reproduced with permission [3]

The ventricularis layer, close to the inflow surface, is rich in elastin with a moderate amount of collagen, which extends in diastole and recoils during systole [6]. The recoil of elastin restores the crimp of collagen fibrils and decreases the surface area of the stretched tissue from the closing phase [5]. The thickness of the three layers varies from the base to the free edge of the cusp [7].

It is worth noting that elastic fibers were found to span the whole leaflet, and connect or anchor three discrete layers together [6,8]. In addition, elastin provides intrafibrillar connections between collagen bundles in the fibrosa layer, whereas it forms a three-dimensional interconnected network in the spongiosa layer [8]. During unloading, the intrafiber elastin, which has high extensibility, helps the collagen fibers return to their wavy and crimped state [6]. These interconnected structures of elastic fibers anchor the discrete layers together, and prevent delamination, which therefore improves the continuity of material behavior of the whole leaflet. Table 1 summarizes the key ECM components in the layers and their major functions.

Location	Main Component(s)	Major Function(s)
Fibrosa	Collagen	Stress bearing
Spongiosa	Glycosaminoglycans and proteoglycans	Conferring flexibility, dampening vibrations from closing, and resisting delamination
Ventricularis	Elastin	Restoration of the wavy and crimped state of collagen fibers

Table 1. The key ECM components in each layer of the leaflet and their major functions

The structures of the leaflets described above provide the following critical functions [6,9–11]: 1) anisotropic mechanical behavior withstanding circumferential stress and extending radially; 2) bilinear biological stress-strain behavior allowing the leaflet to extend before bearing load in the closed phase; 3) elastic recoil to fully open the valve and restore the layer structures for the next cycle. The particular shape of the leaflets and their unique macro- and micro-structures cause the anisotropic mechanical behavior along the circumferential and radial directions of the leaflets [9–11].

During the closed phase (diastole), the leaflets experience the maximum load. Collagen bundles in the fibrosa layer are the major stress-bearing component withstanding approximately 80 mm Hg pressure while the valve is closed and bulging back towards the ventricle [3]. Collagen fibrils are assembled into parallel collagen fiber bundles oriented along the circumferential direction in the leaflet, which are able to withstand such high tensile forces. However, collagen fibers cannot be compressed, making the alignment of collagen (waviness and crimping) important for decreasing the area of the stretched fibrosa layer. Although the collagen fibrils have limited extensibility (approximately 1-2% yield strain), the waviness and crimping allows the fibrosa to withstand roughly 40% strain under loading. Straightening of wavy fibers provides approximately 17% strain, whereas the crimping allows additional approximately 23% strain [6]. In addition, the strains of the cusps in the closed phase are anisotropic, i.e., the strains differ in the radial and circumferential directions [11].

During valve opening, cusps become relaxed through recoil of the elongated, taut elastin. This restores the wavy and crimped state of collagen fibers while decreasing the surface area of the cusps. The GAG-rich spongiosa layer facilitates the rearrangements of the collagen and elastic fibers during the cardiac cycle, dampens vibration from closing, and resists delamination between layers [6,8].

It is evident that normal aortic valve function is maintained, in part, by not only the composition but also the arrangement and orientation of ECM components, particularly collagen, elastin, and GAGs, in the leaflets. Furthermore, it is important to note that alteration of the composition [12] and mechanics [13] of ECM in the aortic valve leaflets was found in diseased conditions. In calcific aortic valve disease (CAVD), collagen bundles and elastin fibers in the fibrosa layer were disrupted and disorganized [14]; meanwhile, there was increased proteoglycan deposition [12]. Matrix metalloproteinases (MMPs) [14,15] and the potent elastase cathepsin S [16], which are produced by macrophages, contribute to this ECM remodeling. Moreover, ECM proteins related to bone, i.e., osteocalcin and osteonectin, were present in the calcified fibrosa layer [17]. These proteins promote mineralization, and their presence suggests the osteoblastic differentiation of valve interstitial cells (VICs).

In addition, excessive myofibroblast differentiation from VICs, leading to ECM accumulation and fibrosis, was influenced by remodeling of ECM in the fibrosa and facilitated by elastin degradation [18]. Furthermore, myofibroblast differentiation from VICs and calcification *in vitro* have been shown to be dependent on ECM composition [19].

Taken together, the macroscopic layered structure and the microscopic structure in each layer of the leaflets impart pronounced anisotropic mechanical behavior that allows the valve to open and close during a great number of cardiac cycles throughout life. These structures are tailored to fulfill the normal functions and maintain the homeostasis of the leaflets in a healthy condition. However, abnormal alteration of composition and mechanics of ECM in these structures may lead to calcific heart valve disease.

3. Collagen comprises a significant portion of the aortic valve leaflet fibrosa

Collagen is an essential component of the aortic valve's layered structure and is vital for maintaining the tissue's mechanical integrity. Mainly responsible for tensile strength, collagen is a strong load-bearing protein created and regulated by VICs. Although present throughout the entire valve, collagen is largely located in the fibrosa where it reduces high tensile stresses. In addition to its central role in valve mechanics, collagen acts as a regulator of VIC phenotype and calcification. Insight into the structure of collagen reveals its unique mechanical properties that support aortic valve function.

Fibrillar collagens are high strength fibers that comprise nearly all of the valve's collagen content. Fibrillar collagens are groups of 3 coiled polypeptide chains that assemble together in tightly packed parallel arrangements. These coils are approximately 300 nm long and join together in a staggered banding pattern with a periodicity of 67 nm [20]. The aortic valve is mainly composed of fibrillar collagen types I, III, and V. Each of these collagens is constructed from different types of alpha chains that govern the overall function of the collagen molecule. Together, these three collagen types work to provide the aortic valve with unique mechanical properties suited for maintaining unidirectional blood flow.

Synthesis of fibrillar collagen is an essential mechanism for maintaining the valve's mechanical integrity. This complex process originates within VICs and is completed in the valve ECM. Production of collagen begins with the intracellular creation of polypeptide alpha chains. There exist ten distinct polypeptide chains that consist of approximately 300 consecutive Gly-X-Y amino acid sequences flanked by small terminal domains. The secondary structure of collagen is created by folding alpha chains into a right-handed alpha helix with the peptide bonds localized at the backbone of the helix and the amino acid side chains facing outward. With slightly less than three residues per turn and a pitch of approximately 8.6 nm, glycine residues are positioned in such a way that the side chains of these residues allow for the formation of the helix. The single hydrogen side chains of these glycine residues allows for the formation of a triple helix structure [21].

The tertiary structure of collagen involves the formation of a left-handed triple helix constructed in the C to N direction. These triple helices exist as both homotrimers and heterotrimers of alpha chains. Collagen type III is a homotrimer of $\alpha1$(III) while collagen type I is a heterotrimer of $\alpha1$(I) and $\alpha2$(I). Additionally, collagen type V is a heterotrimer of $\alpha1$(V) and $\alpha2$(V). Known as procollagen, the tertiary structure molecule is approximately 1.5 nm wide and longer than 300 nm. For creation of the final supramolecular structure, the procollagen molecule is transported into the ECM for crosslinking and fibril formation. After modification in the extracellular space, procollagen is converted into tropocollagen, which undergoes fibrillogenesis where the triple helices are packed together into bundles. Crosslinking of the fibrils ensures the stability of the complex [21].

The arrangement of collagen fiber bundles is crucial to the proper functioning of the aortic valve. Collagen fibers are organized into multilayer structures linked by thin membranes containing variably aligned collagen. Ranging from 10 to 50 μm in size, these membranes are believed to be much more extensible than the collagen fiber bundles they connect. These multilayer structures can easily slide past one another during valve movement, providing the combination of flexibility and tensile strength necessary for the required mechanics during valve opening and closing [22].

Collagen constitutes approximately 90% of the protein content of the valve insoluble matrix [23]. The vast majority of the valve's content is composed of collagens type I, III, and V. Together, these fibrillar collagens account for 60% of the valve's dry weight [24]. There is approximately 74% collagen type I, 24% collagen type III, and 2% collagen type V distributed throughout the valve [25–27]. Whereas collagen type I mainly exists in the fibrosa, collagen type III is expressed ubiquitously throughout all three layers [25].

Collagen fibers mainly function to reduce stress on the leaflets during systole and diastole. While elastin controls initial valve opening and closing, collagen fibers reduce peak stresses in the leaflet matrix by an estimated 60%. These fibers have an important role in stabilizing leaflet motion [28]. Throughout leaflet movement, collagen fibers adjust position to resist tensile forces. As transvalvular pressure increases, the ventricularis expands in the circumferential direction, causing collagen fibers to become highly aligned. This is believed to increase the cuspal stiffness of the valve during diastole and prevent overextension of the valve [29].

The heterogeneous distribution of collagen throughout the aortic valve provides high strength in areas of greater stress while also allowing the valve to achieve a large degree of flexibility. Within the fibrosa, the primary tensile load-bearing layer, collagen fibers are highly aligned in the circumferential direction, resulting in tissue anisotropy. The arrangement of these fibers corresponds to the direction of highest tensile stress. In contrast, the ventricularis endures smaller tensile forces involved with initial opening and closing of the valve [30]. In addition to circumferentially oriented collagen, the largest and strongest collagen fiber bundles are localized in the areas of greatest tensile stress along the lower part of the commissure and coapting regions [22]. This unique arrangement and positioning of collagen reduces high tensile loads on the valve while allowing flexibility to open and close.

Comparisons between the fibrosa and ventricularis indicate that the fibrosa has a greater elastic modulus in the circumferential direction but a similar elastic modulus in the radial direction. These mechanical differences are largely the result of the number of aligned collagen fibers in each direction. With fewer collagen fibers, the ventricularis is approximately half as stiff as the fibrosa in the circumferential direction. In the radial direction, however, each layer contains approximately the same amount of collagen fibers and has similar elastic moduli [31]. Taken together, the multilayer valve structure causes aortic valves to be less stiff and more extensible radially than circumferentially [32].

Collagen achieves high strength and extensibility with the aid of additional mechanisms that contribute to the valve's mechanical properties. These include collagen cross-links, collagen crimp, and layer corrugations. Collagen cross-links function to increase the strength of aligned collagen. In the circumferential direction, the number of collagen cross-links per collagen molecule directly corresponds to the elastic modulus. However, this relationship does not apply to the radial direction, possibly due to the presence of elastin [31]. When there is no mechanical stress on the leaflet, the fibrosa exists as a number of folds in the radial direction known as corrugations. Large extensibility is achieved through these collagen corrugations in combination with collagen crimp. When stress is applied to the leaflet, initial extension is accomplished by straightening of the collagen crimp. Further stress causes the corrugations to unfold in the radial direction [30]. Together, collagen crimp and corrugations allow the fibrosa to extend further in the radial direction when compared to the circumferential direction.

Throughout the lifetime of the aortic valve, collagen synthesis and degradation are responsible for maintaining adequate valve strength and extensibility. Constant turnover of collagen allows the valve to adapt to regional changes in tensile strength. *In vitro* studies show that VICs respond to cyclic mechanical loading as a way to balance collagen synthesis and degradation. Cyclic stretch of valve leaflets stimulates VIC collagen type III production. In particular, the amount and duration of the stretching can have an effect on the amount of collagen produced [27]. Additionally, VICs in culture express collagen type I and collagen type III mRNA for new matrix synthesis [33]. New collagen production is localized to specific regions of the valve depending on the collagen type that is produced. Collagen type I synthesis occurs in the fibrosa around, but not within, areas of mature collagen. Collagen type III synthesis, however, mainly occurs outside of the fibrosa [34]. Collagen degradation is also an important function of VICs and acts as an essential control to collagen production. Studies have shown that VICs seeded into collagen scaffolds express MMPs that degrade the scaffold in a heterogeneous manner [33]. Thus, VICs continuously regulate the mechanical properties of the surrounding ECM through collagen synthesis and degradation.

Aside from its mechanical functions, collagen has been shown to regulate VIC phenotype and calcification potential. *In vitro* studies were unable to induce calcification in VICs cultured on collagen proteins in standard media. It is believed that collagen actively inhibits VIC calcification [19]. Other studies have shown that scaffold collagen content also affects VIC proliferation. Specifically, one study reported that VICs adhered and spread on collagen surfaces but were not able to proliferate [35]. Another study showed that VIC proliferation decreased on scaffolds containing higher collagen content [36]. An *in vitro* study indicated that matrix stiffness regulates VIC differentiation to myofibrogenic or osteogenic phenotypes in calcific conditions [37].

4. Elastic fibers comprise a significant portion of the ventricularis layer of the aortic valve leaflets

Elastic fibers are macromolecular assemblies of several different molecules. The majority of the elastic fiber consists of elastin, an insoluble protein generated by lysyl oxidase crosslinking of soluble tropoelastin monomers (approximately 70 kDa). The elastin tends to be located in the inner core of the elastic fiber and is surrounded by a fine mesh of microfibrils.

These microfibrils are predominantly fibrillin-1, but to a lesser extent Fibrillin-2. Microfibril associated glycoproteins (MAGPs), fibulins, and other proteins are also present in the microfibrillar sheath [38]. At the light microscope level, one can observe the fine elastic fibers by histological staining with Voerhoff's stain or related methods, but when tissue sections are viewed with transmission electron microscopy, there is a clear distinction between the electron-dense elastin core and the microfibrillar sheath [39].

The unique mechanical behavior of the elastic fiber is conferred primarily by the mechanical function of elastin and fibrillin. Crosslinked elastin is remarkable for its ability to undergo high amounts of deformation when subjected to small amounts of load, as well as to recoil back to its original dimensions, when the load is removed, with very little loss of energy. Fibrillin-1, the most widely studied of the microfibrillar components, is also highly extensible. Fibrillin and the other microfibrillar components also coordinate, in a complicated manner still under investigation [38], to aid in the cross-linking of tropoelastin and assemble the final elastic fiber. Interestingly, fibrillin is not always associated with elastic fibers. Fibrillin can often be found by itself, in which it may independently function as a mechanical, load-bearing but highly extensible scaffold [40]. Numerous domains in fibrillin exist for binding integrins, heparan sulafate proteoglycans, and growth factors, which point to substantial roles for alone fibrillin and mature elastic fibers in mediating cell signaling and adhesion [41].

In semilunar heart valves, elastin is found primarily within the ventricularis layer on the inflow side of the leaflet, but is also abundant in the middle spongiosa layer. A thin, frequently imperceptible layer of elastic fibers, the aterialis, is found atop the collagen-rich fibrosa layer. These elastic fibers merge with the intima of the adjacent arterial well, but the overall function of the arterialis has not been well characterized [42].

In the ventricularis, elastic fibers are present in dense and continuous sheets across the whole of the leaflet. These fiber sheets are the most significant contributor to the mechanical properties of the ventricularis [6,30], which can be demonstrated when all ECM components but elastin are removed when using NaOH digestion. After this treatment, the digested ventricularis matches the mechanical behavior of the undigested ventricularis radially, indicating a strong presence of elastin in the radial direction [30]. The elastic fibers within the ventricularis undergo considerable, continual stretch from the initial stage of closure, when blood flow vortices are starting to push the leaflets towards the valve orifice, to the final coapted position of the leaflets. The extension of these elastic fibers accommodates the unfolding of the fibrosa layer, which is normally corrugated in the unloaded position. During this unfolding process, the elastic fibers are bearing the loading of the entire leaflet [43]. Even at high strains, when the collagen in the fibrosa is considered to dominate mechanical properties, the elastin in the ventricularis still plays a significant role. This effect was shown when separated ventricularis was preloaded to mimic its intact configuration; the separated ventricularis was shown to bear load before the separated fibrosa [44]. It has been speculated that this response acts as a safety mechanism to prevent radial overextension of the aortic valve leaflet. Then, when the pressure across the valve is reduced, the elastic fiber sheet in the ventricularis recoils and retracts the leaflets back toward the annular attachment to the arterial wall, a process that involves the re-folding of the corrugations in of the fibrosa. This action restores the original shape and orientation of collagen quickly and consistently to prepare for the next cycle of valve closing. Although the elastic sheet in the ventricularis has fibers that are also oriented circumferentially as well as radially, elastin does not appear to play an important role in the mechanical behavior of the leaflet in the circumferential direction. Valve leaflets exposed to cyclic circumferential stretch and cultured under flow for 48 hours maintained a constant concentration of elastic, suggesting that elastogenesis was not activated during the duration of stretch [45]. However, it is speculated that connections between the elastic fiber and collagen networks facilitate the radial extensibility of the ventricularis layer and the overall leaflet [43]. There are also some elastic fibers in the fibrosa, which surround and connect the collagen fibers, thus preserving collagen crimp and the characteristic corrugated nature of the fibrosa [6,46,47].

The elastic fiber structure in the spongiosa has been characterized much less than in the ventricularis, partly due to the difficulty in isolating its structure from the rest of the leaflet [30]. This elastic structure, however, has been observed during microdissection separating the leaflet [30,48], with scanning electron microscopy (SEM) [6,46], micro-computed tomography (micro-CT) [6], immunohistochemistry (IHC) [25], and autofluorescence imaging [49,50], which all have shown a fine elastic fiber network emanating from the ventricularis and connecting to the fibrosa. We have recently reported that the thickness of this elastic fiber network in the spongiosa is significantly thicker in the hinge and coaptation region than in the belly region of the aortic valve leaflet [8]. We also found two distinct patterns of spongiosa elastic fibers within the leaflet: (i) a rectilinear pattern in the hinge and coaptation region; and (ii) a radially oriented stripe pattern in the belly. Overall, it is believed that the elastic fibers in the spongiosa contribute to valve function in three ways. First, they connect the elastic fibers in the ventricularis to collagen in the fibrosa, which allows coupling of the mechanics of the two layers and matrix components, while using elastic recoil to exert preload on the fibrosa. Second, they distribute stress between collagen and elastic fibers, particularly at low strains. Third, they passively allow relative movement and shear between the outer layers [5,6,48].

Given the presence of a thick, rectilinearly-arranged structure of elastic fibers in the spongiosa of the hinge and coaptation regions, it is speculated that this elastin structure plays a role in leaflet flexure [5,30]. Flexure of the leaflet towards the outflow direction compresses the fibrosa and applies tension to the ventricularis. Rather than undergoing compression, however, the fibrosa may attempt to buckle separately from the leaflet, thereby exaggerating its corrugated configuration. The leaflet would subsequently bend at the troughs of this corrugation, where the second moment of inertia would be locally reduced, albeit temporarily. Buckling would only occur with shearing between the fibrosa and ventricularis, which is allowed by both the compliant elastic fibers in the spongiosa connecting the two outer layers as well as by GAGs in the spongiosa lubricating the outer layer movement [5,30,51,52]. Recoil from the elastic fibers in the spongiosa would then return the fibrosa to its original configuration so it could undergo the next cycle of loading [5,30]. At the hinge, where bending occurs in the opposite direction, it is speculated that the elastic fiber-rich ventricularis compresses readily without buckling, most likely due to the tensile preload already exerted on the ventricularis, but that leaflet deflection may be limited by the stiff fibrosa, which would not allow the leaflet to bend [4,53]. Limited flexure at the hinge would allow the leaflet to absorb pressure from reverse blood flow in diastole, but prevents distention of the leaflet. Thus, our finding of a thicker spongiosa and elastic fiber structure in flexural regions provides evidence of a significant role for elastin in flexure [8]. In addition, the thick network of elastic fibers that we have observed in the spongiosa of the coaptation region may play a role in dampening vibrations that result from valve closing [5].

5. The middle layer, the spongiosa, is comprised mainly of glycosaminoglycans and proteoglycans

Glycosaminoglycans and proteoglycans (GAGs and PGs, respectively) comprise a significant part of the aortic valve leaflets. PGs and GAGs are mainly found in the spongiosa layer of the valve, located between the ventricularis and fibrosa, where they play a vital role in maintaining normal valve function. Previous work has shown that GAGs and PGs serve to not only provide mechanical support to the tissue but also aid in the normal biological functions of the valve [54]. Therefore, it is crucial to fully understand the function of GAGs and PGs in both the normal and possible diseased states of tissues.

GAGs are composed of long and unbranched chains of repeating disaccharides, which consist of a hexosamine and either, depending on the GAG type, uronic acid or galactose. There exist the following families of GAGs with each group being defined by its composition: hyaluronan (HA), heparin, heparan sulfate (HS), chondroitin sulfate (CS), dermatan sulfate (DS), and keratan sulfate (KS) (Table 2) [55–58].

GAGs are primarily formed in the lumen of the Golgi apparatus. The formation process occurs, except in the case of HA, with glycosyltransferases alternatively adding a uronic acid or galactose with a hexosamine to a protein core. The attachment to the protein core varies based on the GAG type. Heparin, HS, CS, and DS are attached to a serine residue, connected to the protein core, via xylose. KS can attach to the protein core either by an asparagine residue at the N-terminus or linked to serine or threonine at the O-terminus. HA does not attach to a protein core. It is synthesized by the addition of sugars to the non-reducing termini of the forming polysaccharide by HA synthase, without a protein backbone. In all cases, modifications can be made to the resulting polysaccharides. Two noteworthy changes include sulfation of the chains and epimerization of the uronic acid. These changes do not occur, however, with HA. Sulfation and epimerization modifications can give a more distinct characteristic to the GAG chains. The epimerization of the uronic acid of CS leads to the production of DS. Epimerization also occurs on heparin and HS. Sulfation can occur in CS, DS, heparin, HS, and KS. N-sulfation takes place in heparin and HS; whereas, O-sulfation can take place in heparin, HS, CS, and DS. In addition to epimerization and sulfation, phosphorylation of the xylose linkage—occurring among CS, DS, heparin, and HS to their respective protein cores—can take place [54,58,59]. Through gel electrophoresis, it has been found that

HA comprises approximately half of the total GAG content in aortic valves [60]. It is important to note that all GAGs, with the exception of HA, exist *in vivo* as components of PGs.

Glycosaminoglycan	Uronic acid	Galactose	Hexosamine
Hyaluronan	Glucuronic	-	N-acetylglucosamine
Heparin	Glucuronic Iduronic	-	N-acetylglucosamine
Heparan sulfate	Glucuronic Iduronic	-	N-acetylglucosamine
Chondroitin sulfate	Glucuronic	-	N-acetylgalactosamine
Dermatan sulfate	Glucuronic Iduronic	-	N-acetylgalactosamine
Keratan sulfate	-	+	N-acetylglucosamine

Table 2. List of glycosaminoglycans and their composition [59]

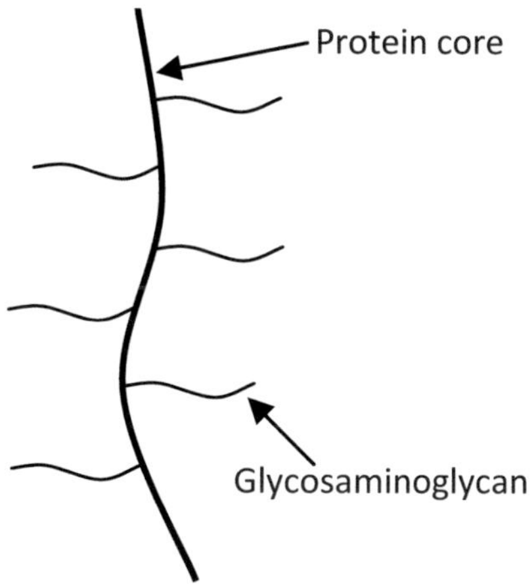

Figure 2. Proteoglycan structure

PGs are formed when GAGs are added to a protein core through a covalent linkage (Figure 2). During PG synthesis, a protein core moves from the endoplasmic reticulum of a cell to the Golgi apparatus, where GAGs are then added to the protein core [55]. PGs can be found in intracellular organelles, on the cell surface, and in the extracellular matrix (ECM) [59]. PGs found in the ECM can be divided into three categories: PGs found within the basement membrane, hyalectans or PGs that interact with HA and lectins, and small leucine-rich PGs (SLRPs) or PGs that contain a leucine motif and have considerably low molecular weights. These PGs can be further classified by the type of protein backbone they contain, as well as the amount, type, and sulfation pattern of the GAGs that are attached to the backbone. More than thirty PGs have been characterized [61]. For example, well-characterized PGs that exist in cardiovascular tissue include decorin, biglycan, and versican. Decorin and biglycan have a core protein size of 40 kDa and are a part of the SLRP family of PGs. They contain CS and DS GAG chains [61]. Versican is a large, chondroitin sulfate proteoglycan. It interacts with HA, and therefore is a hyalectan PG [62]. Other significant PGs in mammalian tissues include perlecan—a basement membrane protein that contains HS and CS, aggrecan—a hyalectan containing CS, and syndecans—a family of cell surface heparan sulfate proteoglycans containing HS and CS [61].

GAGs, and in turn PGs, have a significant role in aortic valve tissue behavior. GAGs have been shown to enhance the viscoelastic properties of the valve leaflets through binding of water molecules [63]. The sulfation and carboxylation on the GAGs make them highly negatively-charged polysaccharides. This negative charge draws in water molecules. Once the tissue becomes hydrated, it acts like a sponge for the valve leaflets. As noted previously, GAGs and PGs are highly abundant in the middle layer of the aortic valve leaflet. One of the main functions of this cushioned layer, the spongiosa, is to provide a barrier between two other layers, the ventricularis and fibrosa, of the valve. This barrier allows for proper shearing between the layers as well as compressibility of the leaflet without compromising the leaflet's overall structural or biological integrity when mechanical stimuli are applied to aortic valve leaflets [63,64]. The mechanical competency that GAGs provide is crucial to the aortic valve leaflets. The aortic valve leaflets serve to ensure unidirectional blood flow from the left ventricle to the aorta. In order to guarantee normal blood flow, the leaflets must open and close properly. Therefore, the flexibility that GAGs provide to the leaflet is crucial to the normal valve's function. In addition, the space that GAGs occupy and form in the matrix serve to organize other molecules within the structure. The structure and hydration that GAGs provide also allow for biological cues to occur within the valve. Moreover, GAGs are known to aid in cell migration, proliferation, act as receptors for signaling molecules, bind growth factors, and serve in the recruitment of various cell types [54].

It is believed that GAGs/PGs likely play an active role in aortic valve tissue disease. Research has shown regional variation of decorin, biglycan, versican and HA in, near, and distal to regions of calcification in diseased aortic valves, suggesting the occurrence of remodeling in the tissue during an unhealthy state [65]. In addition, although the exact causation of calcific aortic valve disease is unknown, it is speculated that it may be due, at least in part, to an inflammatory process [17]. Interestingly, GAGs are thought to play an active role, quite often in the case of cellular injury, in many inflammatory processes for a variety of cell types and have shown to alter in structure and localization in these processes [66]. In addition, some researchers believe that lipid binding due to the unique structure of GAGs may be critical to the accumulation of lipids in calcified aortic valves, a characteristic that is hypothesized to aid in valvular calcification [67]. Although the specific mechanisms underlying calcific aortic valve disease are not quite understood, the complex nature and distinguishable differences of GAGs in both healthy and diseased tissue give rise to the possibility of GAGs being a key factor in valve calcification.

GAGs are very complex disaccharides that highly dictate the behavior of PGs. These polysaccharides are vital in maintaining mechanical, structural, and biological integrity of the aortic valve. Although there is growing interest in further elucidating the role of GAGs in healthy tissues, the exact role of GAGs in diseased aortic valves needs further investigation, as well.

6. Minor ECM components in heart valves also play significant roles in normal valve function and in pathological states

The extracellular matrix of heart valves contain a number of minor components that perform a variety of functions. They are important in valve development, function, and pathology. The study and further characterization of these minor ECM components not only facilitates the development of targeted therapies but would also aid in the microenvironmental mimicry needed for potential tissue engineering applications.

Vitronectin is a glycoprotein that is approximately 75 kDa in size and is present in both serum and the ECM as an adhesive substrate [68]. It is involved in the inhibition of the complement system [68] and is associated with the regulation of hemostasis [69]. Vitronectin also promotes cellular attachment to ECM and is involved in cellular migration [68]. This glycoprotein, along with fibronectin, is found in moderate amounts in aortic, pulmonary, and mitral valves, localizing around valve endothelial cells (VEC) on the inflow layer [25]. In addition, both fibronectin and vitronectin have been shown to associate with collagen fibers in chordae tendinae [70].

Fibronectin is a dimer glycoprotein which consists of two ~250 kDa subunits and is a component of the extracellular matrix [71]. There are many various isoforms of fibronectin, which is the result of alternative mRNA splicing [71]. In addition to being an insoluble ECM component secreted primarily by fibroblasts, soluble fibronectin is also found in the plasma [71]. Fibronectin acts by binding to integrins, collagens, fibrin, and heparin sulfate proteoglycans [71], which allows it to participate in wound healing [72,73] and act as a critical player in embryogenesis [74]. Although not a major ECM component in heart valves, valve interstitial cells (VIC) secrete fibronectin in response to valve damage, providing a means for cell migration [75].

Additionally, fibronectin, along with osteonectin and periostin, confers stiffness to the fibrosa layer [76]. Periostin is a component of the ECM that acts as a ligand for α-V/β-3 and α-V/β-5 integrins and is known to support adhesion and epithelial migration [77]. It is present in the extracellular matrix of several types of tissues and is upregulated in several types of cancers [78]. Recombinant periostin has been shown to promote cardiomyocyte proliferation and angiogenesis after a myocardial infarction [79]. It has been shown previously that periostin plays a role in murine embryonic valve development and remains present in the valves throughout the lifespan even when there is no pathological calcification [80]. A recent study involving chick cardiac development suggests that the presence of periostin in the developing heart may provide a means of organizing other ECM molecules in order to facilitate early epithelial-mesenchymal transition (EMT) [81]. However, the overexpression of periostin and osteopontin can lead to valve calcification.

Osteopontin is a phosphoprotein, meaning that it contains chemically bound phosphoric acid. Originally found in bone, it also contains the arginine-glycine-aspartate (RGD) motif more commonly attributed to fibronectin and is also a constituent of ECM in other tissues [82]. It is secreted by various tissues such as fibroblasts [82] and immune cells, including dendritic cells, macrophages, and neutrophils [83]. Osteopontin is known to interact with various surface receptors that make it a crucial player in bone remodeling [84], wound healing, inflammation, and immune responses [83]. It is also known to be involved in vascular remodeling during endothelial injury [82]. Osteopontin is present in valves calcified as a result of disease as well as in calcified bioprosthetic heart valves [85]. The calcification process of aortic valves closely resembles osteoblast differentiation in regards to expression of genes characteristic of bone formation, such as osteopontin and osteocalcin [86].

Osteocalcin is a small, non-collagenous protein that is considered a late-stage marker for bone formation and is one of a small group of proteins that are osteoblast-specific [87,88]. It is present in general circulation [87] and its capacity for binding hydroxyapatite and calcium suggests that it is largely involved in mineral deposition [88], but it also has recently been shown to act in a hormone-like manner by enhancing insulin secretion [87]. Its traditional role as a product of bone indicates that valve calcification may actually be a result of active bone formation in the valve tissue [86]. This bone formation may be the result of VEGF secretion by endothelial cells during neoangiogenesis occurring in response to inflammation, as seen in rheumatic valve calcification [89]. Additionally, increased serum levels of osteocalcin were shown to be indicative of aortic valve disease in patients [90].

In addition to the matrix proteins, matrix metalloproteinases (MMPs) and their inhibitors (TIMPs) are also found in heart valves. They assist in tissue development and remodeling and can be used as indicators of disease. It is also believed that the ECM degradation resulting from MMP activity serves to release growth factors bound to ECM components and thus alter the microenvironment chemically, as well as structurally [91]. Calcified leaflets from stenotic valves have been shown to express levels of MMP-2 that are similar to those of normal valves but express higher levels of MMP-3, MMP-9, and TIMP-1 [14]. MMP-1, produced by activated myofibroblasts and macrophages, is also prevalent in calcific aortic valve stenosis and may be related to high TNF-α levels resulting from inflammation [92].

7. The basement membrane supports valve endothelial cells and acts as a barrier between circulating blood and subendothelial components

The basement membrane is a myriad of proteins, proteoglycans, and glycoproteins that not only supply a substrate to anchor the valve endothelial cells, but also has a large array of biological activities that regulate spatial organization, sequester growth factors, modulate angiogenesis and migration, and regulate the diffusion of nutrients through it towards the underlying valve interstitial cells [93]. The major constituents of the basement membrane are laminin, perlecan, collagen type IV and VIII, nidogen, and the glycoprotein SPARC (secreted protein, acidic and rich in cysteine). Each of these constituents play a role in the overall function of the basement membrane. In addition, MMPs contribute to the biological activity that occurs within the basement membrane. Understanding basement membrane composition and behavior, during both healthy and diseased states of the aortic valve, may lead to a better understanding of calcific aortic valve disease.

Laminins belong to a family of heterotrimeric glycoproteins composed of combinations of α, β, and γ chains that form a cross-like structure averaging between 400-900 kDa in size [94,95]. Laminins play an integral role in the formation of the supportive ECM network. The unique cross-like shape allows laminin molecules to bind with neighboring laminins and ECM via the three short chains, and use the long alpha chain as a cell anchoring site [96]. In addition to their structural contributions to the basement membrane, laminins are essential for proper biological activity. These glycoproteins have been shown to promote cell adhesion, migration, differentiation, and maintenance of cellular phenotype [94,97,98]. Dysfunction in laminin expression has been linked to diseases with improper tissue formation such as muscular dystrophy, epidermolysis bullosa, and various nephritic syndromes [94,99].

Although laminin is not as ubiquitous as collagen, this basement membrane component has been highly investigated as an ECM substrate for *in vitro* cultures. However, this glycoprotein may influence valve cell types differently. *In vivo* and *in vitro* studies have shown that laminin interacts with endothelial and epithelial cells, and can help maintain physiological functionality of the cells [97,100,101]. However, VICs cultured on laminin have been found to support high quantities of calcific nodule formation in the presence of TGF-β, when compared to subendothelial ECM components collagen type I and fibronectin [19,102]. The various regions of laminin protein have been reported to mediate specific cell responses. The G-domains of laminin α chains are associated with heparin binding and cell adhesion, whereas regions along the laminin β chains promote cell differentiation [98,100,101]. The peptide sequence YIGSR from the laminin β-1 chain has been shown to promote endothelial cell adhesion and proliferation, however, it also influences other cell types including smooth muscle and tumor cells [98,101]. VICs cultured on YIGSR were also shown to promote calcific nodule formation, although less than those seeded on fibronectin derived RGDS peptides. However, when the 67-kDa laminin cell receptor was blocked, the YIGSR seeded VIC cultures significantly increased in nodule formation and gene expression for various myogenic and osteogenic markers, suggesting that disruption in laminin binding may be linked to valve calcification [103]. IKVAV, another peptide sequence derived from the laminin α1-chain, has been linked to promoting angiogenesis, cell migration and spreading [97,98,104]. Though most work with this peptide has been done with endothelial and tumor cells, its ability to promote angiogenesis may also be a future area of interest in studying how angiogenesis mediates valve tissue calcification. Furthermore, laminin influence on cell activity varies between cell types, and may promote VIC activation and tissue calcification in diseased states.

Perlecan (Pln) is one of the more abundant heparan sulfate proteoglycans and is found in several tissues including in the endochondral barrier in bones [105]; however, it is primarily localized in vascular basement membranes. It has a major role in regulating the development of blood vessels, the heart, cartilage, and the nervous system. Physiologically, perlecan plays a prominent role in regulating cellular proliferation, differentiation, organization, and mediating inflammation [106]. Perlecan derives its functionality from five protein subdomains which share their sequence homology with several other proteins [107]. Domain 1 contains an SEA (Sperm protein, Enteokinase, Agrin) module and three SGD (Ser-Gly-Asp) tripeptide sequences to which three heparan sulfate (HS) glycosaminoglycans attach. These HS can bind and sequester several important growth factors for determining endothelial quiescence in a process known as matricrine signaling. The SEA section is unique to perlecan, and it has no known function other than to influence the O-linked glycosylation of the SGD domain. Interestingly, it has been shown that several factors that determine the activity of these sugar chains vary greatly by the cell source that is producing them [108]. These factors can include the ratio of heparan sulfate to chondroitin sulfate, the length of the chains, and the sulfation level of the chains which all affect how the chains modulate the bioactivity of nearby growth factors. Domain II contains 4 low-density lipoprotein receptor sequences and one immunoglobulin-like repeat. Domain III contains three laminin-like domain modules and eight epidermal growth factor-like repeats. Domain IV, the largest domain, contains many N-CAM-like Ig repeats. Domain V has been demonstrated to be the major cell-binding domain of perlecan due to the laminin and agrin homologies that it contains. Domain V can also be glyocosylated, which can contribute along with domain I to the matricrine signaling capabilities of perlecan, which could potentially contribute to the development of CAVD [109].

Matricrine signaling occurs when the ECM modulates cell behavior by controlling the local levels of growth factor concentrations by sequestering or releasing them when the underlying matrix is intact or degraded, respectively [109]. Proteoglycans, like perlecan, and their GAG chains are the major sites for matricrine signaling due to their heparan sulfate and chondroitin sulfate chains electrostatically binding free growth factors. Their role in the pathology of CAVD is widely unexplored despite their presence in normal valves and their increased production in diseased valves [67]. It is known that PGs and GAGs play an integral role in the progression of atherosclerosis via sequestering of inflammatory molecules and lipids [110–113] and mediating angiogenesis into the vessel supplying an entry way for additional inflammatory entities. Both of these factors are seen histologically in CAVD, but their role is merely speculative at this moment.

Collagens in the basement membrane can form lateral, axial, and linear connections with surrounding ECM. Of the basement membrane collagens, collagen IV (COL IV) is the most abundant and essential for network formation. Only found in basement membrane tissues, COL IV molecules are approximately 400 kDa, and composed of two α_1, and one α_2 [115–117]. COL IV proteins have many biologically active domains that can influence specific cellular responses, as well as have specific affinities to other molecules such as BMP-4, fibronectin, Von Hippel Lindau protein, and factor IX [115,117]. Mapping of COL IV protein reveals 3 major integrin motifs that are located in strategic regions to promote cell activity or protein degradation when activated [115]. During angiogenesis and tumor invasion, COL IV is degraded by MMP-2 and MMP-9 enzymes to allow for cell migration and infiltration into the matrix. Studies have found that the cleavage sites also overlap with many integrin binding domains such as $\alpha_1\beta_1$, resulting in the availability of $\alpha_v\beta_3$ integrin binding sites known to promote neutrophil binding [115,118]. Collagen IV networks are highly adhesive to all cells types except erythrocytes [115,119]. Furthermore, cell binding has been found to be enhanced in the presence of various ECM molecules such as perlecan, SPARC, and von Willebrand factor (vWF) [115,118,119]. Interestingly, COL IV also has numerous anti-angiogenic domains that are activated after MMP degradation at the non-collagenous (NC) 1 domain, thereby limiting angiogenesis or migration of endothelial and tumor cells [115]. The changes in COL IV bioactivity depending on the domain region and cleavage state can greatly affect the functionality of surrounding cells. Dysfunctional COL IV expression or mutations in the heterotrimer formation have been found to be extremely detrimental and cause matrix disorders such as Goodpasture's syndrome or Alport syndrome [94,115]. Therefore, additional studies should be done to investigate how the highly bioactive COL IV meshworks may promote the onset of calcification in valve tissues.

COL VIII has also been found to play a network forming role, maintaining the sheet-like structure ECM, while sequestering various integrin binding sites and growth factors. COL VIII is smaller than COL IV, and can form tetrahedral and hexagonal assemblies [117,118]. Though work on COL VIII in regards to valve tissues has been limited, vascular basement membrane studies have found that COL VIII plays a large role in interacting with subendothelial cells such as smooth muscle cells and fibroblasts. In vitro, COL VIII promotes fibroblast proliferation and migration [114]. Furthermore, COL VIII may be linked to atherogenesis, a pathology similar to CAVD, as its expression in cells is upregulated during vessel injury [114,120]. This collagen has even been found to interact with elastic fibers in liver tissues, suggesting it may have a bridging function between the basement membrane components and subendothelial ECM [118]. Therefore, COL VIII could play an integral role in mediating valve interstitial and endothelial cell communication. Recent studies have found after enzyme cleavage at the NC1 domain, the resulting C-terminal fragment known as vastatin will prevent endothelial cell proliferation and induce cell apoptosis [120]. While some work has investigated using vastatin as an anti-angiogenic agent, further studies are needed to elucidate how it may affect the functionality of surrounding cells and ECM, especially in older valve tissue.

Similar to perlecan, nidogen is a 150 kDa glycoprotein that has sequence homologies with other basement membrane proteins. It consists of two amino (G1, G2) and one carboxyl (G3) terminal globular domains that are connected by a rod domain composed primarily of endothelial growth factor repeats [121]. Nidogen binds collagen type IV, perlecan, and laminin. This binding contributes to the hypothesis that nidogen is important in basement membrane assembly; although some recent animal studies have demonstrated that nidogen may not be necessary for basement membrane formation [121]. The role of nidogen in CAVD is unexplored, but it may play a role in maintaining valvular basement membrane functionality by regulating infiltration of inflammatory agents [93].

SPARC positive neovascularisation is a documented histological change in CAVD [122]. Secreted protein acidic and rich in cysteine (SPARC), also known as osteonectin, is a small basement membrane protein. It interacts with cells, binds to other members of the basement membrane, growth factors, various proteases, and is found in newly developing neovessels.

Intact SPARC protein inhibits cellular proliferation and has anti-angiogenic activity in vitro [123]. However, enzymatic degradation of SPARC can release matricryptic fragments with the KGHK motif that may induce angiogenic activity both *in vitro* and *in vivo* [124]. SPARC has been observed lining blood vessels in early to mid stage calcified valves suggesting the presence of a fully formed basement membrane lining these vessels [125]. However, the presence of the other constituents of the basement membrane is merely speculative at this point as the studies investigating their presence during CAVD have not been completed.

8. Summary

In conclusion, the last several years have witnessed significant acceleration in the number of studies characterizing specific types of extracellular matrix in heart valves, although there is still much to be learned. The basement membrane of heart valves, and its role in regulating valvular endothelial cell function, are particularly understudied. The broad scope of cell-matrix and matrix-matrix interactions within heart valves, and how these are regulated by the local, dynamic signaling environment, is another subject that merits further investigation. We expect that insights gained from these research endeavors will lead to novel treatments for valve diseases in the future.

Author details

Dena Wiltz, C. Alexander Arevalos, Liezl R. Balaoing, Alicia A. Blancas, Matthew C. Sapp, Xing Zhang and K. Jane Grande-Allen

Department of Bioengineering, Rice University, Houston, TX, USA

References

[1] Nemir S, West JL. Synthetic materials in the study of cell response to substrate rigidity. *Annals of Biomedical Engineering*. 2010 Jan;38(1):2–20.

[2] Sacks MS, Schoen FJ, Mayer, Jr. JE. Bioengineering challenges for heart valve tissue engineering. *Annual Review of Biomedical Engineering*. 2009 Jan;11:289–313.

[3] Schoen FJ, Levy RJ. Founder's Award, 25th Annual Meeting of the Society for Biomaterials, perspectives. Providence, RI, April 28-May 2, 1999. Tissue heart valves: current challenges and future research perspectives. *Journal of Biomedical Materials Research*. 1999 Dec 15;47(4):439–65.

[4] Vesely I, Lozon A. Natural preload of aortic valve leaflet components during glutaraldehyde fixation: effects on tissue mechanics. *Journal of Biomechanics*. 1993 Feb;26(2): 121–31.

[5] Schoen FJ. Aortic valve structure-function correlations: role of elastic fibers no longer a stretch of the imagination. *Journal of Heart Valve Disease*. 1997 Jan;6(1):1–6.

[6] Scott MJ, Vesely I. Aortic valve cusp microstructure: the role of elastin. *Annals of Thoracic Surgery*. 1995;60(Fig 2):S391–S394.

[7] Filion RJ, Ellis CG. A finite difference model of O2 transport in aortic valve cusps: importance of intrinsic microcirculation. *American Journal of Physiology. Heart and Circulatory Physiology*. 2003 Nov;285(5):H2099–104.

[8] Tseng H, Grande-Allen KJ. Elastic fibers in the aortic valve spongiosa: A fresh perspective on its structure and role in overall tissue function. *Acta Biomaterialia*. 2011 Jan 19;7(5):2101–8.

[9] Missirlis YF, Chong M. Aortic valve mechanics–Part I: material properties of natural porcine aortic valves. *Journal of Bioengineering*. 1978;2(3-4):287.

[10] Sauren AAHJ, van Hout MC, van Steenhoven AA, Veldpaus FE, Janssen JD. The mechanical properties of porcine aortic valve tissues. *Journal of Biomechanics*. 1983 Jan; 16(5):327–37.

[11] Lee JM, Courtman DW, Boughner DR. The glutaraldehyde-stabilized porcine aortic valve xenograft. I. Tensile viscoelastic properties of the fresh leaflet material. *Journal of Biomedical Materials Research*. 1984 Jan;18(1):61–77.

[12] Hinton RB, Lincoln J, Deutsch GH, Osinska H, Manning PB, Benson DW, et al. Extracellular matrix remodeling and organization in developing and diseased aortic valves. *Circulation Research*. 2006 Jun 9;98(11):1431–8.

[13] Chen WLK, Simmons CA. Lessons from (patho)physiological tissue stiffness and their implications for drug screening, drug delivery and regenerative medicine. *Advanced Drug Delivery Reviews*. 2011 Apr 30;63(4-5):269–76.

[14] Fondard O, Detaint D, Iung B, Choqueux C, Adle-Biassette H, Jarraya M, et al. Extracellular matrix remodelling in human aortic valve disease: the role of matrix metalloproteinases and their tissue inhibitors. *European Heart Journal*. 2005 Jul;26(13): 1333–41.

[15] Edep ME, Shirani J, Wolf P, Brown DL. Matrix metalloproteinase expression in nonrheumatic aortic stenosis. *Cardiovascular Pathology*. 9(5):281–6.

[16] Aikawa E, Aikawa M, Libby P, Figueiredo J-L, Rusanescu G, Iwamoto Y, et al. Arterial and aortic valve calcification abolished by elastolytic cathepsin S deficiency in chronic renal disease. *Circulation*. 2009 Apr 7;119(13):1785–94.

[17] Mohler, III ER, Gannon FH, Reynolds C, Zimmerman R, Keane MG, Kaplan FS. Bone formation and inflammation in cardiac valves. *Circulation*. 2001 Mar 20;103(11):1522–8.

[18] Simionescu A, Simionescu DT, Vyavahare NR. Osteogenic responses in fibroblasts activated by elastin degradation products and transforming growth factor-beta1: role of myofibroblasts in vascular calcification. *American Journal of Pathology*. 2007 Jul; 171(1):116–23.

[19] Rodriguez KJ, Masters KS. Regulation of valvular interstitial cell calcification by components of the extracellular matrix. *Journal of Biomedical Materials Research. Part A*. 2009 Sep 15;90(4):1043–53.

[20] Bailey AJ, Paul RG, Knott L. Mechanisms of maturation and ageing of collagen. *Mechanisms of Ageing and Development*. 1998 Dec 1;106(1-2):1–56.

[21] Ottani V, Martini D, Franchi M, Ruggeri A, Raspanti M. Hierarchical structures in fibrillar collagens. *Micron*. 2002 Jan;33(7-8):587–96.

[22] Doehring TC, Kahelin M, Vesely I. Mesostructures of the aortic valve. *Journal of Heart Valve Disease*. 2005 Sep;14(5):679–86.

[23] Eriksen HA, Satta J, Risteli J, Veijola M, Väre P, Soini Y. Type I and type III collagen synthesis and composition in the valve matrix in aortic valve stenosis. *Atherosclerosis*. 2006 Nov;189(1):91–8.

[24] Kunzelman KS, Cochran RP, Murphree SS, Ring WS, Verrier ED, Eberhart RC. Differential collagen distribution in the mitral valve and its influence on biomechanical behaviour. *Journal of Heart Valve Disease*. 1993 Mar;2(2):236–44.

[25] Latif N, Sarathchandra P, Taylor PM, Antoniw J, Yacoub MH. Localization and pattern of expression of extracellular matrix components in human heart valves. *Journal of Heart Valve Disease*. 2005 Mar;14(2):218–27.

[26] Cole WG, Chan D, Hickey AJ, Wilcken DEL. Collagen composition of normal and myxomatous human mitral heart valves. *Biochemical Journal*. 1984 Apr 15;219(2):451–60.

[27] Ku C-H, Johnson PH, Batten P, Sarathchandra P, Chambers RC, Taylor PM, et al. Collagen synthesis by mesenchymal stem cells and aortic valve interstitial cells in response to mechanical stretch. *Cardiovascular Research*. 2006 Aug 1;71(3):548–56.

[28] de Hart J, Peters GWM, Schreurs PJG, Baaijens FPT. Collagen fibers reduce stresses and stabilize motion of aortic valve leaflets during systole. *Journal of Biomechanics*. 2004 Mar;37(3):303–11.

[29] Sacks MS, Smith DB, Hiester ED. The aortic valve microstructure: effects of transvalvular pressure. *Journal of Biomedical Materials Research*. 1998 Jul;41(1):131–41.

[30] Vesely I, Noseworthy R. Micromechanics of the fibrosa and the ventricularis in aortic valve leaflets. *Journal of Biomechanics*. 1992 Jan;25(1):101–13.

[31] Balguid A, Rubbens MP, Mol A, Bank RA, Bogers AJJC, van Kats JP, et al. The role of collagen cross-links in biomechanical behavior of human aortic heart valve leaflets--relevance for tissue engineering. *Tissue Engineering*. 2007 Jul;13(7):1501–11.

[32] Stephens EH, de Jonge N, McNeill MP, Durst CA, Grande-Allen KJ. Age-related changes in material behavior of porcine mitral and aortic valves and correlation to matrix composition. *Tissue Engineering. Part A*. 2010 Mar;16(3):867–78.

[33] Dreger SA, Thomas PS, Sachlos E, Chester AH, Czernuszka JT, Taylor PM, et al. Potential for synthesis and degradation of extracellular matrix proteins by valve interstitial cells seeded onto collagen scaffolds. *Tissue Engineering*. 2006 Sep;12(9):2533–40.

[34] Stephens EH, Grande-Allen KJ. Age-related changes in collagen synthesis and turnover in porcine heart valves. *Journal of Heart Valve Disease*. 2007 Nov;16(6):672–82.

[35] Masters KS, Shah DN, Walker GA, Leinwand LA, Anseth KS. Designing scaffolds for valvular interstitial cells: cell adhesion and function on naturally derived materials. *Journal of Biomedical Materials Research. Part A*. 2004 Oct 1;71(1):172–80.

[36] Taylor PM, Sachlos E, Dreger SA, Chester AH, Czernuszka JT, Yacoub MH. Interaction of human valve interstitial cells with collagen matrices manufactured using rapid prototyping. *Biomaterials*. 2006 May;27(13):2733–7.

[37] Yip CYY, Chen J-H, Zhao R, Simmons CA. Calcification by valve interstitial cells is regulated by the stiffness of the extracellular matrix. *Arteriosclerosis, Thrombosis, and Vascular Biology*. 2009 Jun;29(6):936–42.

[38] Wagenseil JE, Mecham RP. New insights into elastic fiber assembly. *Birth Defects Research Part C: Embryo Today: Reviews*. 2007 Dec;81(4):229–40.

[39] Mecham RP, Davis EC. Elastic fiber structure and assembly. In: Yurchenco PD, Birk DE, Mecham RP, editors. *Extracellular Matrix Assembly and Structure*. 1994. p. 281–314.

[40] Haston JL, Engelsen SB, Roessle M, Clarkson J, Blanch EW, Baldock C, et al. Raman microscopy and X-ray diffraction, a combined study of fibrillin-rich microfibrillar elasticity. *Journal of Biological Chemistry*. 2003 Oct 17;278(42):41189–97.

[41] Bax DV, Mahalingam Y, Cain S, Mellody K, Freeman L, Younger K, et al. Cell adhesion to fibrillin-1: identification of an Arg-Gly-Asp-dependent synergy region and a heparin-binding site that regulates focal adhesion formation. *Journal of Cell Science*. 2007 Apr 15;120(Pt 8):1383–92.

[42] Stephens EH, Kearney DL, Grande-Allen KJ. Insight into pathologic abnormalities in congenital semilunar valve disease based on advances in understanding normal valve microstructure and extracellular matrix. *Cardiovascular Pathology*. 2011 Feb 22.

[43] Schoen FJ. Cardiac valve prostheses: pathological and bioengineering considerations. *Journal of Cardiac Surgery*. 1987 Mar;2(1):65–108.

[44] Klövekorn WP, Meisner H, Paek SU, Sebening F. Long-term results after right ventricular outflow tract reconstruction with porcine and allograft conduits. *Thoracic and Cardiovascular Surgeon*. 1991 Dec;39 Suppl 3:225–7.

[45] Misfeld M, Sievers H-H. Heart valve macro- and microstructure. *Philosophical Transactions of the Royal Society of London. Series B, Biological Sciences*. 2007 Aug 29;362(1484):1421–36.

[46] Scott MJ, Vesely I. Morphology of porcine aortic valve cusp elastin. *Journal of Heart Valve Disease*. 1996 Sep;5(5):464–71.

[47] Vesely I. The role of elastin in aortic valve mechanics. *Journal of Biomechanics*. 1998 Feb;31(2):115–23.

[48] Stella JA, Sacks MS. On the biaxial mechanical properties of the layers of the aortic valve leaflet. *Journal of Biomechanical Engineering*. 2007 Oct;129(5):757–66.

[49] Konig K, Schenke-Layland K, Riemann I, Stock UA. Multiphoton autofluorescence imaging of intratissue elastic fibers. *Biomaterials*. 2005;26(5):495–500.

[50] Christov AM, Liu L, Lowe S, Icton C, Dunmore-Buyze J, Boughner DR, et al. Laser-induced fluorescence (LIF) recognition of the structural composition of porcine heart valves. *Photochemistry and Photobiology*. 1999 Mar;69(3):382–9.

[51] Talman EA, Boughner DR. Glutaraldehyde fixation alters the internal shear properties of porcine aortic heart valve tissue. *Annals of Thoracic Surgery*. 1995 Aug;60(2 Suppl):S369–73.

[52] Talman EA, Boughner DR. Effect of altered hydration on the internal shear properties of porcine aortic valve cusps. *Annals of Thoracic Surgery*. 2001 May;71(5 Suppl):S375–8.

[53] Vesely I, Boughner DR, Song T. Tissue buckling as a mechanism of bioprosthetic valve failure. *Annals of Thoracic Surgery*. 1988;46(3):302–8.

[54] Esko JD, Kimata K, Lindahl U. Proteoglycans and Sulfated Glycosaminoglycans. In: Varki A, Cummings RD, Esko JD, editors. *Essentials of Glycobiology*. 2nd editio. 2009.

[55] Silbert JE, Sugumaran G. Biosynthesis of chondroitin/dermatan sulfate. *IUBMB Life*. 2002 Oct;54(4):177–86.

[56] Bodevin-Authelet S, Kusche-Gullberg M, Pummill PE, DeAngelis PL, Lindahl U. Biosynthesis of hyaluronan: direction of chain elongation. *Journal of Biological Chemistry*. 2005 Mar 11;280(10):8813–8.

[57] Sasisekharan R, Venkataraman G. Heparin and heparan sulfate: biosynthesis, structure and function. *Current Opinion in Chemical Biology*. 2000 Dec;4(6):626–31.

[58] Funderburgh JL. Keratan sulfate: structure, biosynthesis, and function. *Glycobiology*. 2000 Oct;10(10):951–8.

[59] Prydz K, Dalen KT. Synthesis and sorting of proteoglycans. *Journal of Cell Science*. 2000 Jan;113 Pt 2:193–205.

[60] Murata K. Acidic glycosaminoglycans in human heart valves. *Journal of Molecular and Cellular Cardiology*. 1981 Mar;13(3):281–92.

[61] Iozzo RV. Matrix proteoglycans: from molecular design to cellular function. *Annual Review of Biochemistry*. 1998 Jan;67:609–52.

[62] Wight TN. Versican: a versatile extracellular matrix proteoglycan in cell biology. *Current Opinion in Cell Biology*. 2002 Oct;14(5):617–23.

[63] Bhatia A, Vesely I. The effect of glycosaminoglycans and hydration on the viscoelastic properties of aortic valve cusps. *Conference Proceedings: Annual International Conference of the IEEE Engineering in Medicine and Biology Society*. 2005 Jan;3:2979–80.

[64] Lincoln J, Lange AW, Yutzey KE. Hearts and bones: shared regulatory mechanisms in heart valve, cartilage, tendon, and bone development. *Developmental Biology*. 2006 Jun 15;294(2):292–302.

[65] Stephens EH, Saltarrelli JG, Baggett LS, Nandi I, Kuo JJ, Davis AR, et al. Differential proteoglycan and hyaluronan distribution in calcified aortic valves. *Cardiovascular Pathology*. 2010 Dec 23;

[66] Taylor KR, Gallo RL. Glycosaminoglycans and their proteoglycans: host-associated molecular patterns for initiation and modulation of inflammation. *FASEB Journal*. 2006 Jan;20(1):9–22.

[67] Grande-Allen KJ, Osman N, Ballinger ML, Dadlani HM, Marasco S, Little PJ. Glycosaminoglycan synthesis and structure as targets for the prevention of calcific aortic valve disease. *Cardiovascular Research*. 2007 Oct 1;76(1):19–28.

[68] Felding-Habermann B, Cheresh DA. Vitronectin and its receptors. *Current Opinion in Cell Biology*. 1993 Oct;5(5):864–8.

[69] Preissner KT, Seiffert D. Role of vitronectin and its receptors in haemostasis and vascular remodeling. *Thrombosis Research*. 1998 Jan 1;89(1):1–21.

[70] Akhtar S, Meek KM, James V. Immunolocalization of elastin, collagen type I and type III, fibronectin, and vitronectin in extracellular matrix components of normal and myxomatous mitral heart valve chordae tendineae. *Cardiovascular Pathology*. 1999;8(4):203–11.

[71] Pankov R, Yamada KM. Fibronectin at a glance. *Journal of Cell Science*. 2002 Oct 15;115(Pt 20):3861–3.

[72] Valenick LV, Hsia HC, Schwarzbauer JE. Fibronectin fragmentation promotes alpha4beta1 integrin-mediated contraction of a fibrin-fibronectin provisional matrix. *Experimental Cell Research*. 2005 Sep;309(1):48–55.

[73] Ffrench-Constant C, Van de Water L, Dvorak HF, Hynes RO. Reappearance of an embryonic pattern of fibronectin splicing during wound healing in the adult rat. *The Journal of Cell Biology*. 1989 Aug;109(2):903–14.

[74] George EL, Georges-Labouesse EN, Patel-King RS, Rayburn H, Hynes RO. Defects in mesoderm, neural tube and vascular development in mouse embryos lacking fibronectin. *Development*. 1993 Dec;119(4):1079–91.

[75] Fayet C, Bendeck MP, Gotlieb AI. Cardiac valve interstitial cells secrete fibronectin and form fibrillar adhesions in response to injury. *Cardiovascular Pathology*. 2007;16(4):203–11.

[76] Combs MD, Yutzey KE. Heart valve development: regulatory networks in development and disease. *Circulation Research*. 2009 Aug 28;105(5):408–21.

[77] Gillan L, Matei D, Fishman DA, Gerbin CS, Karlan BY, Chang DD. Periostin secreted by epithelial ovarian carcinoma is a ligand for alpha(V)beta(3) and alpha(V)beta(5) integrins and promotes cell motility. *Cancer Research*. 2002 Sep 15;62(18):5358–64.

[78] Tilman G, Mattiussi M, Brasseur F, van Baren N, Decottignies A. Human periostin gene expression in normal tissues, tumors and melanoma: evidences for periostin production by both stromal and melanoma cells. *Molecular Cancer*. 2007 Jan;6:80.

[79] Polizzotti BD, Arab S, Kühn B. Intrapericardial delivery of gelfoam enables the targeted delivery of Periostin peptide after myocardial infarction by inducing fibrin clot formation. *PloS One*. 2012 Jan;7(5):e36788.

[80] Kruzynska-Frejtag A, Machnicki M, Rogers R, Markwald RR, Conway SJ. Periostin (an osteoblast-specific factor) is expressed within the embryonic mouse heart during valve formation. *Mechanisms of Development*. 2001 May;103(1-2):183–8.

[81] Kern CB, Hoffman S, Moreno R, Damon BJ, Norris RA, Krug EL, et al. Immunolocalization of chick periostin protein in the developing heart. *The Anatomical Record. Part A, Discoveries in Molecular, Cellular, and Evolutionary Biology*. 2005 May;284(1):415–23.

[82] Ashizawa N, Graf K, Do YS, Nunohiro T, Giachelli CM, Meehan WP, et al. Osteopontin is produced by rat cardiac fibroblasts and mediates A(II)-induced DNA synthesis and collagen gel contraction. *Journal of Clinical Investigation*. 1996 Nov;98(10):2218–27.

[83] Wang KX, Denhardt DT. Osteopontin: role in immune regulation and stress responses. *Cytokine & Growth Factor Reviews*. 2008;19(5-6):333–45.

[84] Choi ST, Kim JH, Kang E-J, Lee S-W, Park M-C, Park Y-B, et al. Osteopontin might be involved in bone remodelling rather than in inflammation in ankylosing spondylitis. *Rheumatology*. 2008 Dec;47(12):1775–9.

[85] Srivatsa SS, Harrity PJ, Maercklein PB, Kleppe L, Veinot J, Edwards W, et al. Increased cellular expression of matrix proteins that regulate mineralization is associated with calcification of native human and porcine xenograft bioprosthetic heart valves. *Journal of Clinical Investigation*. 1997 Mar 1;99(5):996–1009.

[86] Rajamannan NM, Subramaniam M, Rickard D, Stock SR, Donovan J, Springett M, et al. Human aortic valve calcification is associated with an osteoblast phenotype. *Circulation*. 2003 May 6;107(17):2181–4.

[87] Lee NK, Sowa H, Hinoi E, Ferron M, Ahn JD, Confavreux C, et al. Endocrine regulation of energy metabolism by the skeleton. *Cell*. 2007 Aug 10;130(3):456–69.

[88] Gundberg CM, Hauschka PV, Lian JB, Gallop PM. Osteocalcin: isolation, characterization, and detection. *Methods in Enzymology*. 1984 Jan;107(1975):516–44.

[89] Rajamannan NM, Nealis TB, Subramaniam M, Pandya S, Stock SR, Ignatiev CI, et al. Calcified rheumatic valve neoangiogenesis is associated with vascular endothelial growth factor expression and osteoblast-like bone formation. *Circulation*. 2005 Jun 21;111(24):3296–301.

[90] Levy RJ, Zenker JA, Lian JB. Vitamin K-dependent calcium binding proteins in aortic valve calcification. *Journal of Clinical Investigation*. 1980 Feb;65(2):563–6.

[91] Nagase H, Visse R, Murphy G. Structure and function of matrix metalloproteinases and TIMPs. *Cardiovascular Research*. 2006 Feb;69(3):562–73.

[92] Kaden JJ, Dempfle C-E, Grobholz R, Fischer CS, Vocke DC, Kiliç R, et al. Inflammatory regulation of extracellular matrix remodeling in calcific aortic valve stenosis. *Cardiovascular Pathology*. 2005;14(2):80–7.

[93] Yip CYY, Simmons CA. The aortic valve microenvironment and its role in calcific aortic valve disease. *Cardiovascular Pathology*. 2011;20(3):177–82.

[94] Kreis T, Vale R. Guidebook to the Extracellular Matrix, Anchor, and Adhesion Proteins. 2nd ed. Kreis T, Vale R, editors. 1999.

[95] Timpl R, Rohde H, Robey PG, Rennard SI, Foidart J-M, Martin GR. Laminin--a glycoprotein from basement membranes. *Journal of Biological Chemistry*. 1979 Oct 10;254(19):9933–7.

[96] Durbeej M. Laminins. *Cell and Tissue Research*. 2010 Jan;339(1):259–68.

[97] Okazaki I, Suzuki N, Nishi N, Utani A, Matsuura H, Shinkai H, et al. Identification of biologically active sequences in the laminin alpha 4 chain G domain. *Journal of Biological Chemistry*. 2002 Oct;277(40):37070–8.

[98] Pradhan S, Farach-Carson MC. Mining the extracellular matrix for tissue engineering applications. *Regenerative Medicine*. 2010 Nov;5(6):961–70.

[99] McGowan KA, Marinkovich MP. Laminins and human disease. *Microscopy Research and Technique*. 2000 Nov 1;51(3):262–79.

[100] Hozumi K, Suzuki N, Nielsen PK, Nomizu M, Yamada Y. Laminin alpha1 chain LG4 module promotes cell attachment through syndecans and cell spreading through integrin alpha2beta1. *Journal of Biological Chemistry*. 2006 Oct;281(43):32929–40.

[101] Ponce ML, Nomizu M, Delgado MC, Kuratomi Y, Hoffman MP, Powell S, et al. Identification of endothelial cell binding sites on the laminin gamma 1 chain. *Circulation Research*. 1999 Apr;84(6):688–94.

[102] Gwanmesia P, Ziegler H, Eurich R, Barth M, Kamiya H, Karck M, et al. Opposite effects of transforming growth factor-β1 and vascular endothelial growth factor on the degeneration of aortic valvular interstitial cell are modified by the extracellular matrix protein fibronectin: implications for heart valve engineering. *Tissue Engineering. Part A*. 2010 Dec;16(12):3737–46.

[103] Gu X, Masters KS. Regulation of valvular interstitial cell calcification by adhesive peptide sequences. *Journal of Biomedical Materials Research. Part A*. 2010 Jun 15;93(4): 1620–30.

[104] Genové E, Shen C, Zhang S, Semino CE. The effect of functionalized self-assembling peptide scaffolds on human aortic endothelial cell function. *Biomaterials*. 2005 Jun; 26(16):3341–51.

[105] Ishijima M, Suzuki N, Hozumi K, Matsunobu T, Kosaki K, Kaneko H, et al. Perlecan modulates VEGF signaling and is essential for vascularization in endochondral bone formation. *Matrix Biology*. 2012 May;31(4):234–45.

[106] Knox SM, Whitelock JM. Perlecan: how does one molecule do so many things? *Cellular and Molecular Life Sciences*. 2006 Nov;63(21):2435–45.

[107] Farach-Carson MC, Carson DD. Perlecan--a multifunctional extracellular proteoglycan scaffold. *Glycobiology*. 2007 Sep;17(9):897–905.

[108] Ellis AL, Pan W, Yang G, Jones K, Chuang C, Whitelock JM, et al. Similarity of recombinant human perlecan domain 1 by alternative expression systems bioactive heterogenous recombinant human perlecan D1. *BMC Biotechnology*. 2010 Jan;10:66.

[109] Chen J-H, Simmons CA. Cell-matrix interactions in the pathobiology of calcific aortic valve disease: critical roles for matricellular, matricrine, and matrix mechanics cues. *Circulation Research*. 2011 Jun;108(12):1510–24.

[110] Wilkinson TS, Bressler SL, Evanko SP, Braun KR, Wight TN. Overexpression of hyaluronan synthases alters vascular smooth muscle cell phenotype and promotes monocyte adhesion. *Journal of Cellular Physiology*. 2006 Feb;206(2):378–85.

[111] Nakashima Y, Fujii H, Sumiyoshi S, Wight TN, Sueishi K. Early human atherosclerosis: accumulation of lipid and proteoglycans in intimal thickenings followed by mac-

rophage infiltration. *Arteriosclerosis, Thrombosis, and Vascular Biology*. 2007 May;27(5): 1159–65.

[112] Wight TN. Cell biology of arterial proteoglycans. *Arteriosclerosis*. 1989;9(1):1–20.

[113] Yan J, Stringer SE, Hamilton A, Charlton-Menys V, Götting C, Müller B, et al. Decorin GAG synthesis and TGF-β signaling mediate Ox-LDL-induced mineralization of human vascular smooth muscle cells. *Arteriosclerosis, Thrombosis, and Vascular Biology*. 2011 Mar;31(3):608–15.

[114] Plenz GAM, Deng MC, Robenek H, Völker W. Vascular collagens: spotlight on the role of type VIII collagen in atherogenesis. *Atherosclerosis*. 2003 Jan;166(1):1–11.

[115] Parkin JD, San Antonio JD, Pedchenko V, Hudson B, Jensen ST, Savige J. Mapping structural landmarks, ligand binding sites, and missense mutations to the collagen IV heterotrimers predicts major functional domains, novel interactions, and variation in phenotypes in inherited diseases affecting basement membranes. *Human Mutation*. 2011 Feb;32(2):127–43.

[116] Soininen R, Haka-Risku T, Prockop DJ, Tryggvason K. Complete primary structure of the alpha 1-chain of human basement membrane (type IV) collagen. *FEBS Letters*. 1987 Dec;225(1-2):188–94.

[117] Shuttleworth CA. Type VIII collagen. *International Journal of Biochemistry & Cell Biology*. 1997 Oct;29(10):1145–8.

[118] Wells RG. Function and metabolism of collagen and other extracellular matrix proteins. In: Rodés J, Benhamou J-P, Blei A, Reichen J, Rizzetto M, editors. *Textbook of Hepatology*. 3rd ed. 2002. p. 264–73.

[119] Tsilibary EC, Reger LA, Vogel AM, Koliakos GG, Anderson SS, Charonis AS, et al. Identification of a multifunctional, cell-binding peptide sequence from the a1(NC1) of type IV collagen. *Journal of Cell Biology*. 1990 Oct;111(4):1583–91.

[120] Xu R, Yao Z-Y, Xin L, Zhang Q, Li T-P, Gan R-B. NC1 domain of human type VIII collagen (alpha 1) inhibits bovine aortic endothelial cell proliferation and causes cell apoptosis. *Biochemical and Biophysical Research Communications*. 2001 Nov 23;289(1): 264–8.

[121] Kang SH, Kramer JM. Nidogen is nonessential and not required for normal type IV collagen localization in Caenorhabditis elegans. *Molecular Biology of the Cell*. 2000 Nov;11(11):3911–23.

[122] Charest A, Pépin A, Shetty R, Côté C, Voisine P, Dagenais F, et al. Distribution of SPARC during neovascularisation of degenerative aortic stenosis. *Heart*. 2006 Dec; 92(12):1844–9.

[123] Chlenski A, Liu S, Crawford SE, Volpert OV, DeVries GH, Evangelista A, et al. SPARC is a key Schwannian-derived inhibitor controlling neuroblastoma tumor angiogenesis. *Cancer Research*. 2002 Dec 15;62(24):7357–63.

[124] Sage H. Pieces of eight: bioactive fragments of extracellular proteins as regulators of angiogenesis. *Trends in Cell Biology*. 1997 May;7(5):182–6.

[125] Kalluri R, Zeisberg E. Controlling angiogenesis in heart valves. *Nature Medicine*. 2006 Oct;12(10):1118–9.

Chapter 2

Anatomy and Function of Normal Aortic Valvular Complex

Ioan Tilea, Horatiu Suciu, Brindusa Tilea, Cristina Maria Tatar, Mihaela Ispas and Razvan Constantin Serban

Additional information is available at the end of the chapter

http://dx.doi.org/10.5772/53403

1. Introduction

Recently, the interest in the anatomy of the normal aortic valve complex has augmented, mostly because of the increasing use of conservative surgical techniques for repairing or replacing cardiac valves. The knowledge of the anatomy also has important implications in the manufacture of prostheses that must conform to this anatomical configuration.

1.1. Historical perspective

The earliest documented interest in the anatomy of the aortic valvular complex stems from the Renaissance, with the description and drawings by Leonardo da Vinci. [1]

Leonardo da Vinci had an almost perfect understanding of the physiology of the human heart. But he had no inkling of the circulation of the blood, and the existence of one-way valves was incompatible with the ancient belief that the heart simply churned blood in and out of the ventricles, thus generating heat and 'vital spirit'. Unable to reconcile what he had observed with what he believed to be true, Leonardo reached an impasse. He became trapped in describing the motion of the blood through the valves in even more detail. And there, it seems, his anatomical work came to an end. [2]

The next anatomist to study the aortic valve was Andreas Vesalius. Then, for almost 400 years the study of the human heart was very sporadic and limited.

The 19th century brought in the era of anatomic dissection and the knowledge on the aortic valve grew wider. Henle was the first to introduce the term "arterial root". During the first half of the 20th century the rise in autopsy rates in Europe and North America facilitated the study of cardiac anatomy. [3]

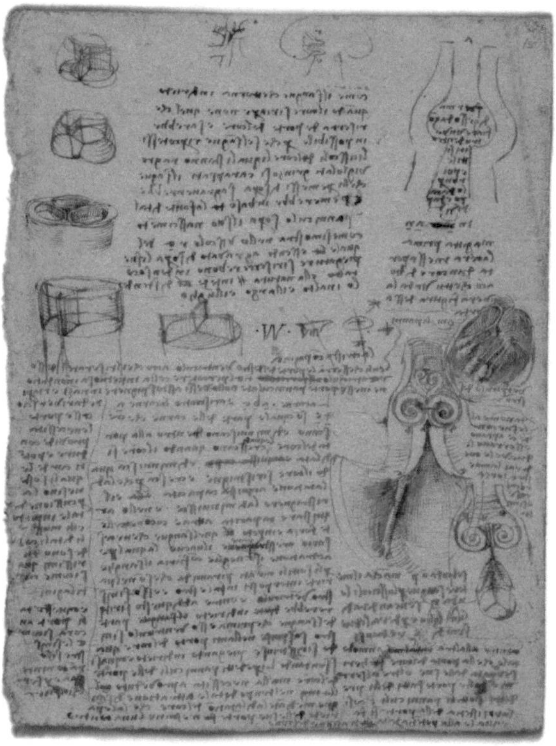

Figure 1. Leonardo da Vinci - The aortic valve, from the Royal Collection © Her Majesty Queen Elizabeth II - http://www.royalcollection.org.uk/collection/919082/the-aortic-valve

Nowadays the need to understand the anatomy of the aortic valve is crucial, therefore the books and articles devoted to this topic are numerous.

1.2. Definitions

There is still no consensus on the best way to describe the anatomy of the aortic root [4].

The term "aortic root" refers to the aortic valve from its position at the left ventricular outlet to its junction with the ascending portion of the aorta. [5] It is the direct continuation of the left ventricular outflow tract.

Aorto-ventricular junction refers to the junction between the left ventricular structures and the aortic valvular sinuses, this representing the anatomic junction, or the semilunar lines of attachment of the arterial valvular leaflets, this locus representing the haemodynamic ventriculo-arterial junction [4].

http://dx.doi.org/10.5772/53403

Annulus is conventionally described as the virtual ring, formed by joining the basal attachment points of the leaflets within the left ventricle.

Nodule of Arantius is the small fibrous mound that forms at the center of each leaflet when the closing edge meets the free edge.

Between the free and closing edges, to each side of the nodule are two crescent-shaped areas known as the lunulae, which represent the sites of cusp apposition during valve closure. [6]

1.3. Embryology

The development of the aortic valve complex is extremely complicated and not yet fully understood.

The heart begins as a single tube that separates into two tubes and begins to twist rightward onto itself, called "d" looping.

Cells from the primary cardiac crescent, formed bilaterally within the embryonic disc, migrate into the cervical region of the developing embryo to form the primary heart tube. With further growth, cells from a second cardiogenic area, located posterior to the dorsal wall of the developing pericardial cavity, migrate into the cardiac region. The cells from this secondary heart field populate the outflow tract and the aortic arches. [7]

The heart tube is composed of an outer layer of myocardium and an inner lining of endocardial cells, separated by an extensive extracellular matrix referred to as the cardiac jelly. After rightward looping of the heart, the cardiac jelly overlying the future atrioventricular canal and outflow tract expands into swellings known as cardiac cushions. [8]

Subsequent to looping, the outflow tract possesses a characteristic dog-leg bend which divides the outflow tract into proximal and distal portions.

The cushions contained within the myocardial wall go through significant changes. In addition to the cushions that have fused to separate the proximal outflow tract into prospective aortic and pulmonary components, two further intercalated cushions have grown in the opposite quadrants of the common outflow tract. Formation of cavities in the fused distal parts of the proximal cushions, along with similar cavitation in the intercalated cushions, now produces the primordiums of the arterial valvular leaflets and sinuses. These structures, therefore, are formed in the most distal part of the proximal outflow tract, immediately upstream relative to the developing sinotubular junction. The cavitation of the cushions leaves the central luminal part of each cushion to form the arterial valvular leaflets, with the peripheral part arterialising to form the wall of the supporting valvular sinuses. The rightward and inferior of the intercalated cushions forms one sinus of the aortic valve, while the opposite leftward and superior intercalated cushion forms the non-adjacent sinus of the pulmonary valve. The adjacent sinuses and valvular leaflets, in contrast, are excavated from the fused distal parts of the proximal cushions, with each of the two fused cushions forming one sinus and leaflet of the aortic valve, together with the adjacent sinus and leaflet of the pulmonary valve. [7]

The definitive fetal cardiac structure is developed by 8 weeks.

2. Histological structure

Function of normal heart valves is based on their properties of ensuring unidirectional blood flow without regurgitation. They open and close 40 million times a year and 3 billion times over a lifetime. This property depends on the mobility, pliability, and structural integrity of their leaflets. The competency of the aortic valvular complex depends on the stretching and molding of its 3 cusps to fill the orifice during the closed phase of the cardiac cycle. [9]

2.1. Dynamic relations between the aortic valvular complex and its histological structure

The substantial changes in size and shape of the valve cusps and leaflets that occur during the cardiac cycle are facilitated by a highly complex internal microarchitecture. The layered structure of the aortic valve is formed by: a dense collagenous layer close to the outflow surface, which provides the primary strength component, a central core of loose connective tissue, and an elastin layer below the inflow surface. The essential functional components of the heart valves comprises the valvular endothelial cells (VECs), the valvular interstitial cells (VICs), and extracellular matrix (ECM), including collagen, elastin and glycosaminoglycans. [9]

The major component of valve cusps is collagen, 43% to 55% (predominantly type I but also some type III) [10] and 11% elastin. The quantity, quality, and architecture of the valvular ECM, particularly collagen, elastin, and glycosaminoglycans, are the major determinants of not only the cyclical functional mechanics over the second-to-second periodicity of the cardiac cycle, but also the lifetime durability of a valve. The cells of the heart valves through complex cell-ECM interactions, transduce forces into molecular changes that mediate normal valve function and pathobiology. Through such mechanisms, healthy heart valves are able to maintain homeostasis, adapt to an altered stress state, and repair injury via connective tissue remodeling mediated by the synthesis, repair, and remodeling of the several ECM components. [9]

The most abundant cell type in the aortic valve are VICs. They are distributed throughout all of its layers, are crucial for valvular function [11] and synthesize the ECM. VICs mediate matrix remodeling and continuously repair functional damage to collagen and the other ECM components. As a response to injury VICs may translate from one phenotypic state to another during valvular homeostasis. The 5 distinct VIC phenotypes include embryonic progenitor endothelial/mesenchymal cells (eVICs), quiescent VICs (qVICs), activated VICs (aVICs), postdevelopmental/adult progenitor VICs (pVICs), and osteoblastic VICs (ob-VICs). [12] Adult heart valve VICs have characteristics of resting fibroblasts, are quiescent, without synthetic or destructive activity for extracellular matrix. They are activated by abrupt changes in the mechanical stress during intrauterine maturation.Once activated VICs can differentiate into a variety of other cell types, including myofibroblasts and osteoblasts. [11]

The blood-contacting surfaces of the aortic valve are lined by endothelial cells. VECs resemble to endothelial cells but evidence is increasing that VECs are phenotypically different from vascular endothelial cells elsewhere in the circulation, which is consistent with the increasing recognition of more widespread endothelial heterogeneity across circulatory sites,

http://dx.doi.org/10.5772/53403

[13] and the possibility that VECs may interact with VICs to maintain the integrity of valve tissues. [14] Evidence indicates that different transcriptional profiles are expressed by VECs on the opposite faces of a normal adult pig aortic valve and these may contribute to localization of early pathological aortic valve calcification [15]. Abnormal hemodynamic forces can cause tissue remodeling and inflammation which may lead to aortic valve diseases. [11]

2.2. Normal aortic valve development

An understanding of valve architecture and cellular changes that occur in cardiac valves during fetal development, maturation, and aging would provide mechanistic insights into the pathogenesis of congenital and acquired valve abnormalities and aid assessment of therapeutic strategies for valve disease. A study which performed quantitative histological assessment of 91 human semilunar valves obtained from second and third trimester fetus, neonates, children and normal adults found very interesting results. [16]

Valves must accommodate to substantial hemodynamic changes throughout lifetime. Large populations of VICs undergo phenotypic modulation to become activated myofibroblasts and return to quiescent fibroblasts during adaptive remodeling in response to changing environmental conditions. [17-19] VICs and VECs functions likely influence ECM synthesis and remodeling. Fetal valves possess a dynamic/adaptive structure and contain cells with an activated/immature phenotype. During postnatal life, activated cells gradually become quiescent, whereas collagen matures through increased fiber thickness and alignment. Fetal second-trimester semilunar (aortic and pulmonary) valves lack distinguishable layers, are composed primarily of proteoglycans, have no detectable elastin, small amounts of disorganized collagen, and are histologically identical. [20] Fetal valves structure differs, even late in gestation, from that of adult valves, which have a trilayered architecture with a highly specialized and functionally adapted ECM. The study demonstrated that fetal valves have much higher cellular densities than adult valves, associated with an increased cell proliferation-to-apoptosis ratio. VICs density was highest in the second trimester and decreased progressively throughout gestation and postnatally. Fetal VICs proliferation indices were likewise greater than those of adult valves. Valvular cell turnover is high during fetal development and continues at a low rate postnatally. [16]

They also demonstrated physiological activation of endothelial cells that consistently expressed high levels of SMemb, MMP-1, MMP-13, ICAM-1, and VCAM-1 in fetal and children's valves in contrast to adult valves. Valvular cells that are activated in utero undergo phenotypic changes at birth and gradually become quiescent, whereas collagen matures through increased fiber thickness and alignment. This suggests a progressive adaptation to the prevailing hemodynamic environment. [16]

3. Structure and anatomy of the aortic root

The aortic valve is the cardiac centerpiece and forms the bridge between the left ventricle and the ascending aorta. Its components are the sinuses of Valsalva, the fibrous interleaflet triangles, and the valvular leaflets themselves. [1]

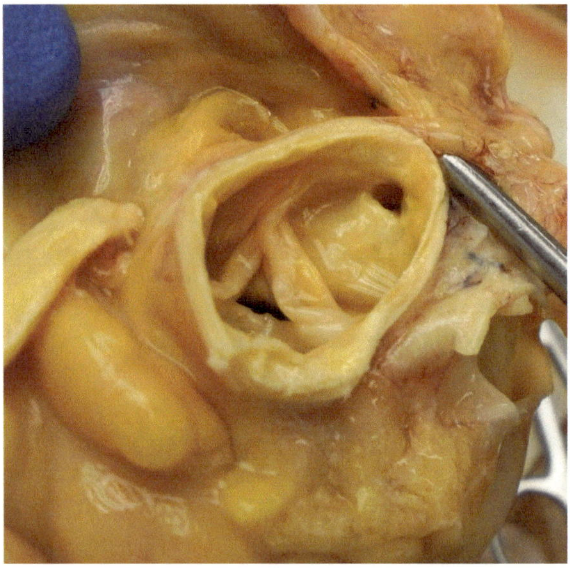

Figure 2. View of a dissected heart (the atrial chambers and the arterial trunks are removed). The heart is photographed from above. [4]

3.1. The "Annulus" controversy

When defined literally "annulus" refers to a little ring. The aortic root contains at least 3 circular rings and 1 crown-like ring. [21] The valvular leaflets are attached throughout the length of the root. Therefore, seen in 3 dimensions, the leaflets take the form of a 3-pronged coronet, with the hinges from the supporting ventricular structures forming the crown-like ring (Figure 1). The base of the crown is a virtual ring, commonly known as "annulus". This plane represents the inlet from the left ventricular outflow tract into the aortic root and is the diameter that is typically analysed by the echocardiographer when providing measurements of the diameter of the annulus.

The controversy arises from the fact that on one hand there are multiple rings described and on the other hand, the term "annulus" appears to describe a circle, a fibrous ring on which the leaflets are inserted, but such a structure does not exist in the anatomy of the aortic valve. No consensus has been found yet.

http://dx.doi.org/10.5772/53403

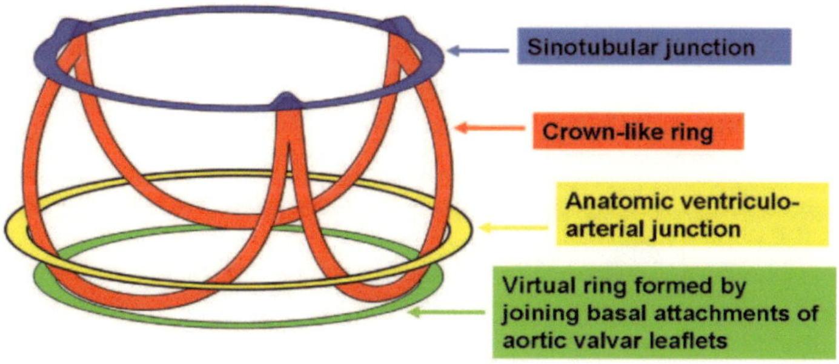

Figure 3. The "rings" of the aortic root [1]

3.2. Anatomic versus hemodynamic ventriculo-arterial junction

As we have shown in figure 3, there is a marked discrepancy between the circular anatomic junction and the semilunar hemodynamic junction. [22] The hemodynamic junction separates the root into those compartments exposed to aortic as opposed to left ventricular pressures. By virtue of the semilunar attachments of the leaflets, portions of the fibrous aortic root are exposed to ventricular pressures, these being the superior portions of the interleaflet triangles, whereas portions of the left ventricle are exposed to aortic pressures, these being the most basal portions within the sinus of Valsalva. [1]

3.3. Aortic sinuses, location of the coronary arteries and sinotubular junction

The spaces between the luminal surface of the three bulges on the aortic root and their respective valvular leaflets are known as the aortic sinuses of Valsalva. [5] The sinuses are named according to the arteries arising from within them (right, left, and noncoronary). The right sinus structures have the greatest dimensions followed by the non coronary sinus, and finally the left coronary sinus. [23]

Distance between the ostium and Valsalva's sinus		Sex	
		Male	Female
Left commissure	left coronary	9.7	9.3
	right coronary	11.2	10.7
Right commissure	left coronary	10.9	10.8
	right coronary	11.3	9.9
Bottom of the Valsalva's sinus	left coronary	13.4	13.0
	right coronary	15.0	13.8

Table 1. Mean values of the distances of the ostium and its relation to the corresponding Valsalva's sinus (in mm) in both sexes (adapted from [24])

In the majority of cases, the orifices of the coronary arteries arise within the 2 anterior sinuses of Valsalva, usually positioned just below the sinotubular junction, but are rarely centrally located. It is not unusual, however, for the arteries to be positioned superior relative to the sinotubular junction. Accessory coronary arterial orifices are found in the majority of the anterior aortic sinuses. [25]

Several studies emphasize on the importance of large variations of coronary ostia origins. Also, there are significant differences between in vivo and ex vivo measurements regarding the right coronary ostium. [26,27]

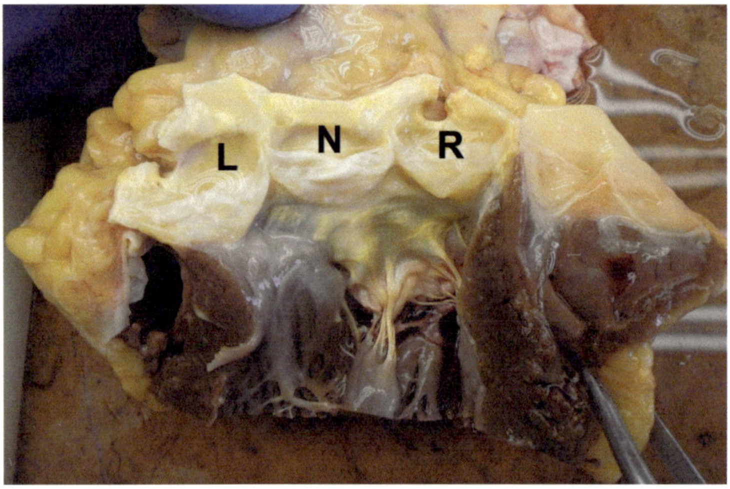

Figure 4. Left (L) and right (R) aortic sinuses that give origin to the main coronary arteries and the non-coronary (N) sinus. [5]

The superior border of the sinuses is the sinotubular junction (also known as the supra-aortic ridge). On the outside, the sinotubular junction is where the tubular portion of the aorta joins onto the sinusal portion. Inside, there is usually a slightly raised ridge of thickened aortic wall. But the sinotubular junction is not perfectly circular. It takes on the contour of the three sinuses, giving it a mildly trefoil or scalloped outline. [5]

A comparison between the circumferences measured at the level of the sinotubular junction and at the level of the aortic root base shows that the circumference of the sinotubular junction is 95% of the circumference measured at the aortic root base. [23]

3.4. Aortic valvular leaflets

The normal aortic valve has three leaflets. Each of the three leaflets has a free margin and a margin where it is attached in semilunar fashion to the aortic root. The maximal height of each leaflet is considerably less than that of its sinus on account of its scoop-shaped free margin. When the valve opens, the leaflets fall back into their sinuses without the potential of occluding any coronary orifice. The semilunar hingelines of adjacent leaflets meet at the level of the sinotubu-

http://dx.doi.org/10.5772/53403

lar junction, forming the commissures. The body of the leaflets are pliable and thin in the young, although its thickness is not uniform. With age, the leaflets become thicker and stiffer.

Each leaflet has a somewhat crimped surface facing the aorta and a smoother surface facing the ventricle. The leaflet is slightly thicker towards its free margin. On its ventricular surface is the zone of apposition, known as the lunulae, occupying the full width along the free margin and spanning approximately one-third of the depth of the leaflet. This is where the leaflet meets the adjacent leaflets during valvular closure. At the midportion of the lunulae, the ventricular surface is thickened to form the nodule of Arantius that extends along 60% of the inferior margin of the lunulae. When the valve is in closed position, the inferior margin of the lunulaes meet together, separating blood in the left ventricular cavity from blood in the aorta. Fenestrations in the lunulaes are common, especially in the elderly, but the valve remains competent because they are above the closure line. [5]

The leaflets have a core of fibrous tissue, with endothelial linings on their arterial and ventricular aspects. Their origin from the supporting left ventricular structures, where the ventricular components give rise to the fibroelastic walls of the aortic valvular sinuses, marks the anatomic ventriculo-arterial junction. Significantly, in those areas where the leaflets arise from the ventricular myocardium, their basal attachments are well below the level of the anatomic ventriculo-arterial junction. [1]

Leaflet	**Measure**	**Sex**	
		Male	**Female**
Left coronary	Leaflet height	15.2	14.9
	Lunulae width	4.6	4.3
	Lunulae length	30.7	29.3
	External intercommissural distance	25.4	23.5
	Internal Intercommissural distance	20.0	18.5
Right coronary	Leaflet height	15.2	14.5
	Lunulae width	4.4	4.2
	Lunulae length	30.4	27.9
	External intercommissural distance	24.5	23.8
	Internal Intercommissural distance	19.2	18.7
Noncoronary	Leaflet height	15.0	14.6
	Lunulae width	4.3	4.2
	Lunulae length	30.3	28.2
	External intercommissural distance	24.4	22.1
	Internal Intercommissural distance	20.1	19.1

Table 2. Mean values of the height of the leaflets and size of the lunulae (width and length) and internal intercommissural distances in mm in both sexes (adapted from [24])

Variations exist among individuals in the dimensions of the root, but in the same individual, there can be marked variations in all aspects of the dimensions of the individual leaflets, including the height, width, surface area and volume of each of the supporting sinuses of Valsalva. [28, 29, 30] A study of 200 normal hearts revealed that the average width, measured between the peripheral zones of attachment along the sinus ridge, for the right, the noncoronary, and the left coronary leaflets was 25.9, 25.5, and 25.0 mm, respectively. [28]

3.5. Interleaflet fibrous triangles

As a result of the semilunar attachment of the aortic valvular leaflets, there are 3 triangular extensions of the left ventricular outflow tract that reach to the level of the sinotubular junction. [31] These triangles, however, are formed not of ventricular myocardium but of the thinned fibrous walls of the aorta between the expanded sinuses of Valsalva. Their most apical regions represent areas of potential communication with the pericardial space or, in the case of the triangle between the right and left coronary aortic leaflets, with the plane of tissue interposed between the aorta and anteriorly located sleeve-like subpulmonary infundibulum. [1]

The triangles are thinner and less collagenous than the hingelines or the sinusal walls. These areas are potential sites of aneurysmal formation. [32]

3.6. The relationships of the aortic root

The aortic root is positioned to the right and posterior relative to the subpulmonary infundibulum. The leaflets of the aortic valve are attached only in part to the muscular walls of the left ventricle, since so as to fit the orifices of both aortic and mitral valves within the circular profile of the left ventricle, there is no muscle between them in the ventricular roof. The aortic root, furthermore, is wedged between the orifices of the two atrioventricular valves. The root is related to all four cardiac chambers. [4]

The plane of the aortic valve tilts inferiorly at an angle to the pulmonary valve. The nadirs of the aortic sinuses lie in a plane at an angle of 30º from the horizontal. [32] Thus, the arterial surface of the closed leaflets of the aortic valve is directed not only upwards but also rightward at an angle of at least 45º to the median plane. [33]

3.6.1. Relationship between the left ventricular outflow tract and the aortic root

The left ventricular outflow tract is composed of a muscular component and a more extensive fibrous component. The orientation of the outflow tract is known to change with aging. In individuals aged under 20 years, the angle varies between 135 and 180 degrees and the left ventricular outflow tract represents a more direct and straight extension into the aortic root. In hearts from individuals aged over 60 years, the angle varies between 90 and 120 degrees and the left ventricular outflow tract may not extend in straight fashion into the aortic root but rather in a rightward "dog leg". [1]

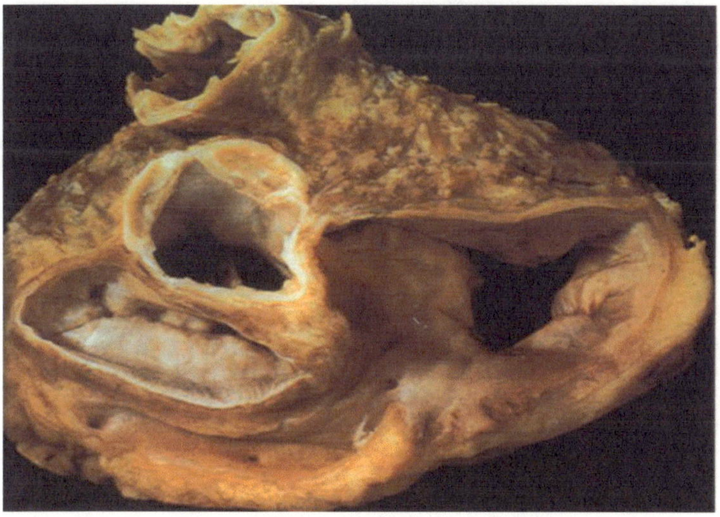

Figure 5. A dissected atrioventricular junction viewed from above showing how the aortic valve wedges itself between the mitral and tricuspid valves (reproduced from http://www.rjmatthewsmd.com)

3.6.2. Interleaflet triangles and their relationship to the mitral valve and membranous septum

Guarding the left ventricular outflow tract, the aortic root also has an intimate relationship with the ventricular septum and the mitral valve. In attitudinal orientation, it is apparent that the aortic root leans rightward slightly, over the ventricular septum, to overly the right ventricle. In the elderly, the relationship between septal crest and aortic root changes to give a sigmoid-shaped ventricular septum. [4]

Relative to the aorta, the mitral valve is located posterior and to the left, the tricuspid valve is located inferiorly and to the right.

The ends of the area of fibrous continuity are thickened to form the left and right fibrous trigones. The interleaflet triangle between the noncoronary and left coronary leaflet is part of the area of fibrous continuity because the aortic-mitral curtain seen from within the left ventricular outflow tract represents the equivalent of the anterior mitral valvular annulus. The interleaflet triangle located between the right coronary and noncoronary aortic leaflets is confluent with the membranous septum. Together, the membranous septum and the right fibrous trigone form the central fibrous body of the heart. This is the area within the heart where the membranous septum, the atrioventricular valves and the aortic valve join in fibrous continuity. [1]

3.6.3. Relationship between the aortic valve and the conduction system

The atrioventricular node, located in the wall of the right atrium at the apex of the triangle of Koch, is relatively distant from the root. As the conduction axis, penetrates to the left, through the central fibrous body, however, it is positioned at the base of the interleaflet triangle between the non- and right coronary aortic sinuses. Having penetrated through the fibrous plane providing atrioventricular insulation, the bundle then branches on the crest of the muscular ventricular septum, the left bundle branch fanning out on the smooth left ventricular side, while the cord-like right bundle branch penetrates back through the muscular septum, emerging on the septal surface in the environment of the medial papillary muscle (figure 6). [4]

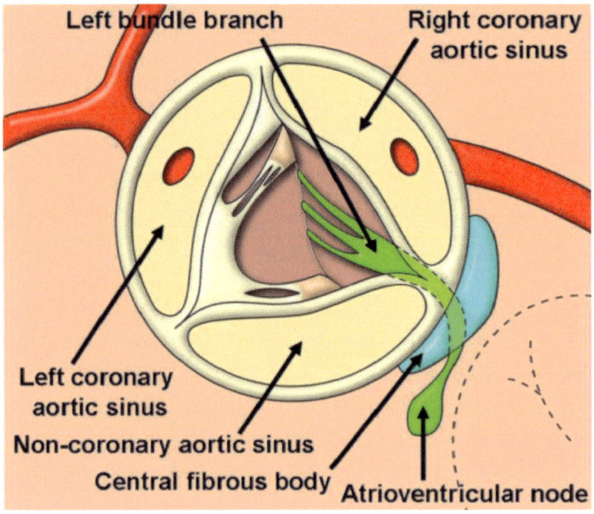

Figure 6. Aortic sinuses, coronary arteries and the the location of the atrioventricular conduction axis, as seen by looking down through the aortic root (schematic from [4])

4. Microscopic anatomy

The aortic valve is composed of different structures, each one with its own histological profile. The histology of the aortic root is characterized by a gradual shift from the primarily elastic aorta to the muscular ventricle. [31]

The annulus is a dense collagenous meshwork, in which elastic and collagenous fibrils and also neuronal structures are present. At the commissure level originate the collagen fibres of the intermediate layer, which are orientated in a radial fashion. Here, they do not only infiltrate the intima layer of the aortic root, but they also radiate into the media layer where they are anchored. The endothelial cells are separated by the basal layer from the elastic fibres and collagenous fibrils. The endothelial cells show microvilli at their surface, which increase the overall surface area for an increased exchange of substances.

The interleaflet triangles are different in their microscopic structure. The triangle between the left-coronary and non-coronary sinus forms part of the aortic–mitral valvular curtain, is histologically fibrous and equivalent to the mitral valve leaflet structure. The triangle between the non-coronary and the right-coronary aortic sinus is incorporated within the membranous part of the septum and is also made of fibrous tissue. In contrast, the triangle between the right-coronary and left-coronary sinus in the area of the subpulmonary infundibulum is supported by muscular tissue and only fibrous at its apex.

The sinuses are arranged with very different components, but the largest part of all the three sinuses is composed in a similar manner to the three layers of the aortic wall: tunica intima, tunica media and tunica externa (adventitia). The inner layer of the intima is composed of endothelial cells arranged in the direction of the vessel. The subendothelial connective tissue is arranged in the same manner as the endothelial cells. This layer is divided from the intima by the membrana elastica interna. The media is composed of circular arranged structures: smooth muscle cells, elastic fibres, collagen fibres type II and III and proteoglycans. The adventitia is the external layer. It is separated from the intima by the membrana elastica externa. Similar to the intima, the elements of the adventitia are arranged in a longitudinal fashion and composed of collagen fibres of type I. The sinotubular junction shows the same principal arrangement of tissue elements compared with the sinuses and the ascending aorta, but the diameter of the wall is thicker. [34]

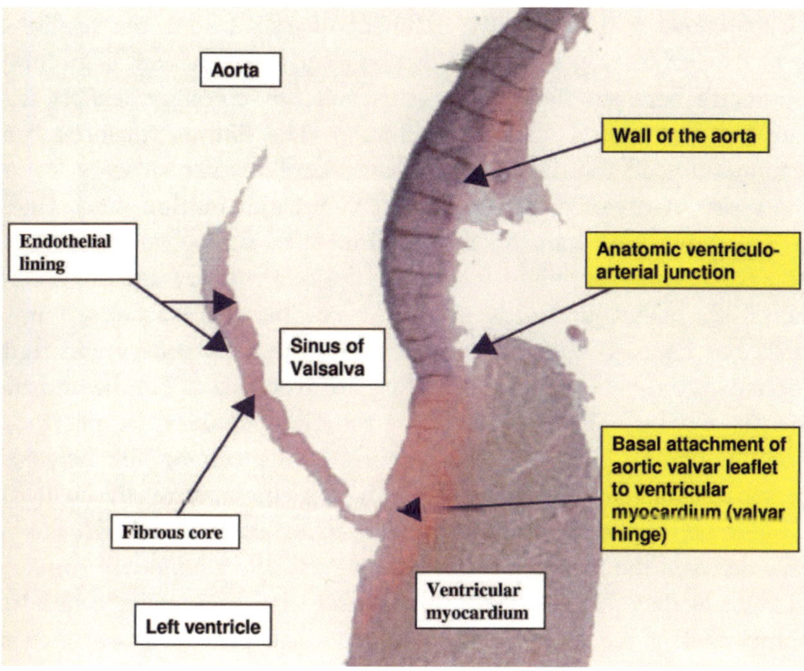

Figure 7. Histology of the aortic valvular complex [1]

The aortic valve leaflet is a three-layered structure (lamina ventricularis, lamina spongiosa and lamina fibrosa) composed of differing amounts of collagen, elastin, and glycosaminoglycans, that form a well-defined honeycomb or spongelike structure, suggesting that elastin forms a matrix that surrounds and links the collagen fiber bundles. [35] The leaflets are covered by a continuous layer of endothelial cells with a smooth surface on the ventricular side and numerous ridges on the arterial side. The arrangement of the endothelial cells is across, not in line with the direction of flow. [36]

5. Surgical anatomy

A thorough knowledge of the anatomy of the aortic valve and its relations to the surrounding cardiac structures is a prerequisite for the successful completion of the repair or replacement performed by the surgeon.

Surgical descriptions of the aortic root are not always similar with the anatomical descriptions, leading to a series of confusional data. Also the in vivo measurement of the valve components don't always correspond to the ex vivo measurements, in part due to the movement of the heart and its structures during the cardiac cycle.

By sequentially following the line of attachment of each leaflet, the relationship of the aortic valve to its surrounding structures can be clearly understood. Beginning posteriorly, the commissure between the noncoronary and left coronary leaflets is positioned along the area of aorto-mitral valvular continuity. The fibrous subaortic curtain is beneath this commissure. To the right of this commissure, the noncoronary leaflet is attached above the posterior diverticulum of the left ventricular outflow tract. Here the valve is related to the right atrial wall. As the attachment of the noncoronary leaflet ascends from its nadir toward the commissure between the noncoronary and right coronary leaflets, the line of attachment is directly above the portion of the atrial septum containing the atrioventricular node. The commissure between the noncoronary and right coronary leaflets is located directly above the penetrating atrioventricular bundle and the membranous ventricular septum. The attachment of the right coronary leaflet then descends across the central fibrous body before ascending to the commissure between the right and left coronary leaflets. Immediately beneath this commissure, the wall of the aorta forms the uppermost part of the subaortic outflow. An incision through this area passes into the space between the facing surfaces of the aorta and pulmonary trunk. As the facing left and right leaflets descend from this commissure, they are attached to the outlet muscular component of the left ventricle. Only a small part of this area in the normal heart is a true outlet septum, since both pulmonary and aortic valves are supported on their own sleeves of myocardium. Thus, although the outlet components of the right and left ventricle face each other, an incision below the aortic valve enters low into the infundibulum of the right ventricle. As the lateral part of the left coronary leaflet descends from the facing commissure to the base of the sinus, it becomes the only part of the aortic valve that is not intimately related to another cardiac chamber. [37]

6. Ecocardiographic anatomy

The ability to record high-quality echocardiographic images and obtain accurate Doppler flow recordings are essential determinants of the overall value of the echocardiographic examination. As such, echocardiography is highly operator dependent. It is difficult to overemphasize the critical role of the person who performs the imaging. To obtain a comprehensive and accurate echocardiogram, the echocardiographer must understand the anatomy and physiology of the aortic valve and have a thorough knowledge of the ultrasound equipment to optimize the quality of the recording. [38]

6.1. Transthoracic Echocardiography (TTE)

Anatomic evaluation of the aortic valve is based on a combination of short- and long-axis images to identify the number of leaflets, and to describe leaflet mobility, thickness, and calcification.

Two-dimensional imaging of the normal aortic valve in the parasternal long axis view demonstrates two leaflets (right and noncoronary), while the parasternal short axis demonstrates a symmetrical structure with three uniformly thin leaflets that open equally, forming a circular orifice during most of systole. During diastole, the normal leaflets form a three pointed star with a slight thickening or prominence at the central closing point formed by the aortic leaflet nodules, known as the nodules of Arantius. The three aortic valve leaflets may also be visualized in a subcostal view.

The aortic valve leaflets appear thin and delicate and may be difficult to visualize. In the long-axis view, the leaflets open rapidly in systole and appear as linear parallel lines close to the walls of the aorta. With the onset of diastole, they come together and are recorded as a faint linear density within the plane of the aortic annulus. Because the velocity of valve motion during opening and closing is high relative to the frame rate of most echocardiographic systems, the normal aortic valve is usually visualized either fully opened or closed but rarely in any intermediate position. In the basal short-axis view, the three aortic leaflets can be visualized within the annulus during diastole. The three lines of coaptation can be recorded, normally forming a Y (sometimes referred to as an inverted Mercedes-Benz sign). With the onset of systole, the leaflets open out of the imaging plane, providing a view of the aortic annulus. The short-axis perspective is most helpful to determine the number of leaflets and whether fusion of one or more commissures is present. In patients who are difficult to image, normal leaflets are so delicate that they are hard to visualize, generally an indication that they are morphologically normal. [38]

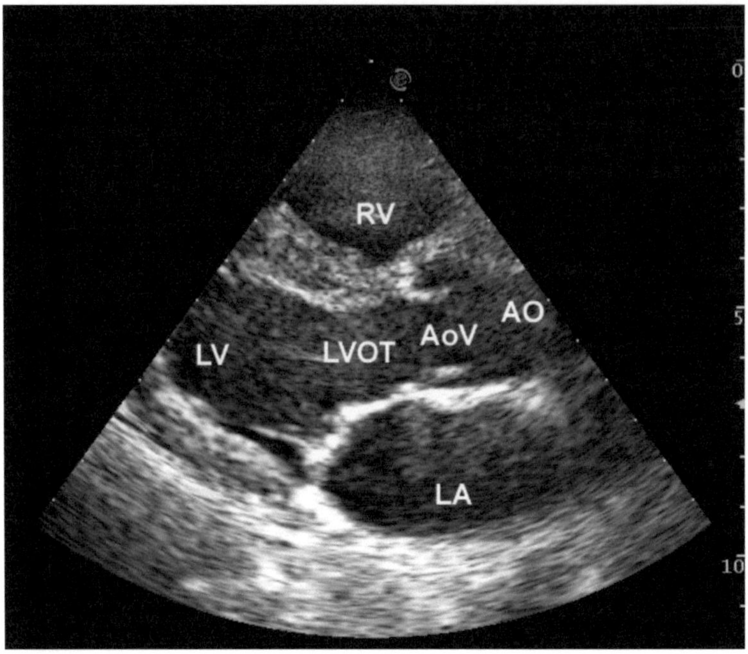

Figure 8. Transthoracic echocardiogram, parasternal long axis view. Aortic valve is open (author's collection).

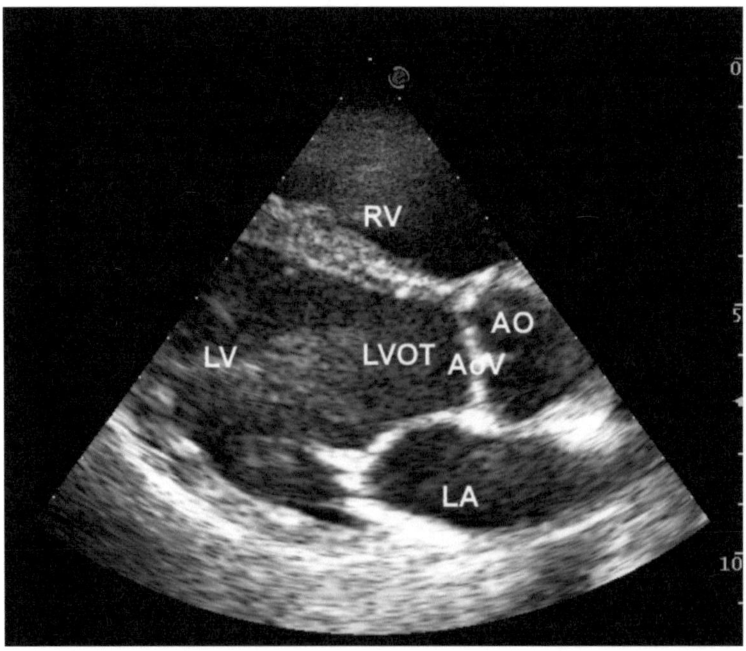

Figure 9. Transthoracic echocardiogram, parasternal long axis view. Aortic valve is closed (author's collection).

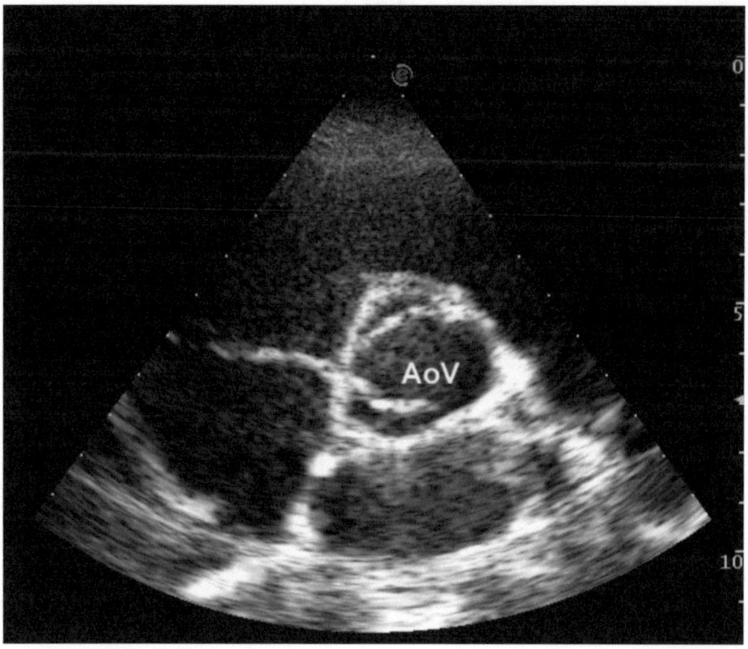

Figure 10. Transthoracic echocardiogram, suprasternal view. Aortic valve is open (author's collection).

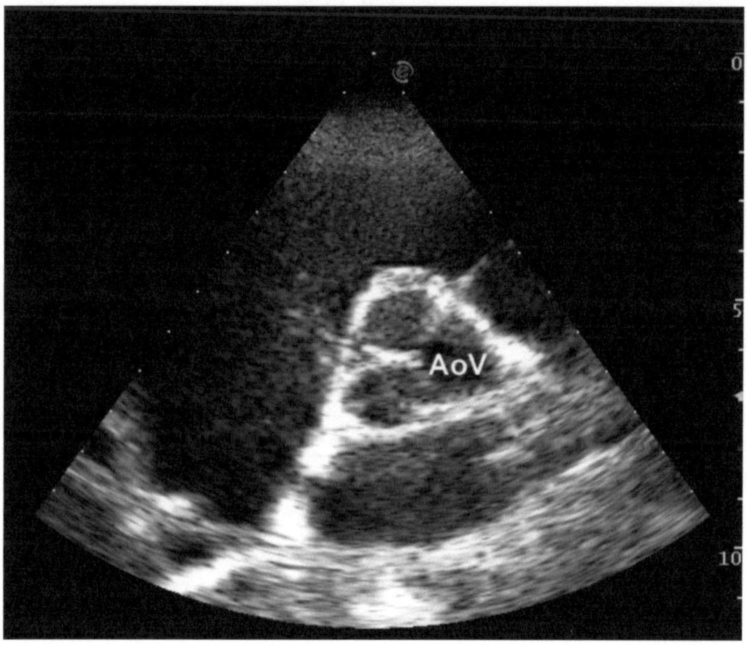

Figure 11. Transthoracic echocardiogram, suprasternal view. Aortic valve is closed (author's collection).

6.2. Transesophageal Echocardiography (TEE)

Transthoracic imaging usually is adequate, although TEE may be helpful when image quality is suboptimal.

To characterize the aortic valve using TEE, the valve should be imaged in short-axis view (the aortic valve can generally be visualized in a plane between 30 to 60º from the transverse 0º) and long-axis view (typically at 120 to 160° from transverse 0º).

The short-axis view is the only view that provides a simultaneous image of all three leaflets. The leaflet adjacent to the atrial septum is the noncoronary leaflet, the most anterior is the right coronary leaflet, and the other is the left coronary leaflet. The probe is withdrawn or anteflexed slightly to move the imaging plane superiorly through the sinuses of Valsalva to bring the right and left coronary ostia and then the sinotubular junction into view. The probe is then advanced to move the imaging plane through and then proximal to the AV annulus to produce a short axis view of the left ventricular outflow tract. The mid esophageal short-axis view at the level of the leaflets is used to measure the length of the free edges of the leaflets and the area of the aortic valve orifice by planimetry.

In the long axis view, the left ventricular outflow tract appears toward the left of the display and the proximal ascending aorta toward the right. The leaflet that appears anteriorly or toward the bottom of the display is always the right coronary, but the leaflet that appears posteriorly in this cross-section may be the left or the noncoronary, depending on the exact location of the imaging plane as it passes through the valve. The mid esophageal long-axis view is the best cross-section for assessing the size of the aortic root by measuring the diameters of the annulus, sinuses of Valsalva, sinotubular junction and proximal ascending aorta, adjusting the probe to maximize the internal diameter of these structures. The diameter of the annulus is measured during systole at the points of attachment of the aortic valve leaflets to the annulus and is normally between 1.8 and 2.5 cm.

The deep transgastric view is obtained by advancing the probe deep into the stomach and positioning the probe adjacent to the left ventricular apex. The exact position of the probe and transducer is more difficult to determine and control deep in the stomach, but some trial and error flexing, turning, advancing, withdrawing, and rotating of the probe develops this view in most patients. In the deep transgastric long-axis view, the aortic valve is located in the far field at the bottom of the display with the left ventricular outflow tract directed away from the transducer. Detailed assessment of valve anatomy is difficult in this view because the left ventricular outflow tract and aortic valve are so far from the transducer, but Doppler quantification of flow velocities through these structures is usually possible. [39]

The TEE examination is also performed intraoperative to refine and confirm preoperative diagnosis, to assess the etiology and severity of aortic valve disease, to measure the annulus and to prepare the surgeon for other alternatives.

6.3. Three-Dimensional Echocardiography (3DE)

3DE represents a major innovation in cardiovascular ultrasound. Advancements in computer and transducer technologies permit real-time 3DE acquisition and presentation of cardiac structures from any spatial point of view.

A complete 3D TTE exam requires multiple acquisitions from the parasternal, apical, subcostal, and suprasternal transducer positions. Because the volume-rendered 3D data set can be cropped to display a variety of intracardiac structures by choosing different cut planes as an alternative to "view" (referred to heart's orientation to the body axis), "anatomic planes" (referred to the heart itself) can be used to describe image orientation. [40]

For the visualization of the aortic valve the 3DE TTE protocol is the parasternal long-axis view with and without color (narrow angle and zoomed acquisitions) and the 3DE TEE protocol is the 60º mid-esophageal, short-axis view with and without color (zoomed or full-volume acquisition) and the 120º mid-esophageal, long-axis view with and without color (zoomed or full-volume acquisition).

The common approaches for imaging the aortic valve by 3D TTE are from the parasternal and apical views. Three-dimensional data sets including the aortic root can be cropped and rotated for a dynamic 3D rendering of the aortic valve, which can be visualized from both the aortic and ventricular perspectives, as well as sliced in any desired longitudinal or oblique plane.

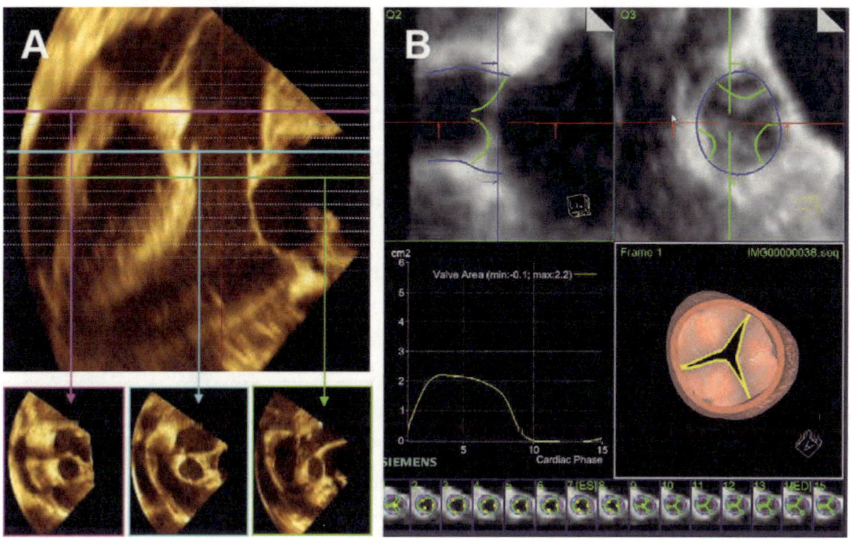

Figure 12. Three-dimensional TEE data set cropped to demonstrate the aorta in long axis (A, top). Using this image, in face views of the sinotubular junction (A, bottom left), sinus of Valsalva (A, bottom middle), and aortic annulus (A, bottom right) can be obtained for assessment. Dynamic, automatic tracking of the aortic valve leaflets (B, top left) and annulus (B, top right) can be performed, providing aortic valve area throughout the cardiac cycle (B, middle left and bottom strip). A model derived from the automated tracking is also produced (middle right). [41]

Real-Time 3D can be realized by obtaining a TEE 2D image of the aortic valve at either the 60º midesophageal, short-axis view or the 120º midesophageal, long-axis view. After the 2D image is optimized, narrow-angled acquisitions can be used to optimize the 3D image and to examine aortic valve and root anatomy. After acquisition, the aortic valve should be oriented with the right coronary cusp located inferiorly, regardless of whether the aortic or the left ventricular outflow tract perspective is presented.

Color Doppler 3D TEE imaging should also be performed to detect the initial appearance of flow at the onset of systole. [41]

7. Functional anatomy

The aortic root is a complex structure that requires analysis part by part but always remembering that all the parts contribute to form one functional unit, a three-dimensional structure adjoining distally to the aorta and proximally to the ventricle.

The aortic valve, like the pulmonary valve, has no tensor apparatus (i.e., chordae tendineae or papillary muscles). The commissures form tall, peaked spaces between the attachments of adjacent leaflets and attain the level of the aortic sinotubular junction, the ridge that separates the sinus and tubular portions of the ascending aorta. The functional aortic valve orifice can be at the sinotubular junction or proximal to it. [42]

The three half moon-shaped leaflets form pocket-like tissue flaps that are avascular. Just below the free edge of each leaflet is a ridgelike closing edge. At the center of each leaflet, the closing edge meets the free edge and forms the nodule of Arantius. Between the free and closing edges, to each side of the nodule are two crescent-shaped areas known as the lunulae, which represent the sites of leaflet apposition during valve closure. Lunular fenestrations, near the commissures are common and increase in size and incidence with age. [43] However, owing to their position distal to the closing edge, they rarely produce valvular incompetence. [42] When viewed from above, the linear distance along the closing edge of a leaflet is much greater than the straight-line distance between its two commissures. This extra length of leaflet tissue is necessary for nonstenotic opening and nonregurgitant closure of the valve. [6] Normally, the diameter of the aortic annulus at the hinge points of the aortic valve is about equal to the diameter of the ascending aorta at the sinotubular junction. [44] When the valve opens, the leaflets fall back into their sinuses without the potential of occluding any coronary orifice. The semilunar hingelines of adjacent leaflets meet at the level of the sinotubular junction, forming the commissures. The body of the leaflets are pliable and thin in the young, although its thickness is not uniform.

The commissure between the right and posterior aortic leaflets overlies the membranous septum and contacts the commissure between the anterior and septal leaflets of the tricuspid valve. The commissure between the right and left aortic leaflets contacts its corresponding pulmonary commissure and overlies the infundibular septum. The intervalvular fibrosa, at the commissure between the left and posterior aortic cusps, fuses the aortic valve to the anterior mitral leaflet. [6, 42]

A study of 100 formalin-fixed hearts from adult patients with normally functioning aortic valves found that the luminal area of the aorta at the sinotubular junction increased with age and with heart weight, where increased heart weight was attributed to systemic hypertension. [45] Volume-wise, the sinuses are largest when the valve closes, serving as reservoirs during ventricular diastole and allow filling of the coronary arteries.

When left ventricular pressure exceeds that in the aortic root, the valvular leaflets are pushed apart and fall back into their respective sinuses, allowing unimpeded ejection of blood. The orifices of the coronary arteries are commonly found close to the level of the sinotubular junction. [25]

8. Conclusion

In the new era of cardiac surgery, now more then ever, the need to further study the aortic valve complex anatomy and function is greater.

A thorough knowledge of the anatomy of the aortic valve and its relationships is essential to understanding aortic valve pathology and many congenital cardiac malformations. Also it is crucial for the diagnosis and treatment (both surgical and conservatory) of aortic valve pathology.

Accurate understanding of the anatomy of interest is of cardinal importance for the development of devices and treatment protocols. We emphasize the importance of considering anatomic variations in the development of treatments, an understanding of the intraindividual and interindividual variations that may exist can lead to refinements in current designs of valvular prostheses.

Although the aortic valve is the most intensely studied cardiac valve, there is still no consensus on how to describe its components and a universal terminology is yet to be found. The multidisciplinary approach will continue to be crucial in working through these challenges.

Author details

Ioan Tilea[1], Horatiu Suciu[3], Brindusa Tilea[2], Cristina Maria Tatar[1], Mihaela Ispas[3] and Razvan Constantin Serban[3]

1 Internal Medicine Clinic, Division of Cardiology, University of Medicine and Pharmacy Tirgu Mures, Romania

2 Infectious Disease Clinic, University of Medicine and Pharmacy Tirgu Mures, Romania

3 Cardiology Clinic, Emergency Clinical County Hospital Tirgu Mures, Romania

References

[1] Piazza N, de Jaegere P, Schultz C, Becker AE, Serruys PW, Anderson RH. Anatomy of the aortic valvular complex and its implications for transcatheter implantation of the aortic valve. Circ Cardiovasc Interv. 2008; 1:74–81. DOI: 10.1161/CIRCINTERVENTIONS.108. 780858

[2] Clayton M, Nature 484, 19 April 2012, 314–316, doi:10.1038/484314a

[3] Hurst WJ, King SB, Walter PF, Freisinger GC, Edward JE. Atherosclerotic coronary heart disease: angina pectoris, myocardial infarction, and other manifestations of myocardial ischemia. In: Hurst's the Heart. 6th ed. New York: McGraw-Hill; 1986:882–1008.

[4] Anderson RH. The surgical anatomy of the aortic root, in: Multimedia Manual of Cardiothoracic Surgery, doi:10.1510/ mmcts. 2006.002527

[5] Siew YH, Structure and anatomy of the aortic root, European Journal of Echocardiography (2009) 10, i3–i10 doi:10.1093/ejechocard/jen243

[6] Edwards WD., Anatomy of the Cardiovascular System: Clinical Medicine. Vol 6. Philadelphia: Harper & Row; 1984:1–24.

[7] Anderson RH, Webb S, Brown NA, Lamers W, Moorman A. Development of the heart: (3) Formation of the ventricular outflow tracts, arterial valves, and intrapericardial arterial trunks, September 2003;89:1110–18.

[8] Anderson RH, Webb S, Brown NA, Lamers W, Moorman A. Development of the heart (1): septation of the atriums and ventricles. Heart. 2003; 89: 949–958.

[9] Schoen FJ. Evolving Concepts of Cardiac Valve Dynamics: The Continuum of Development, Functional Structure, Pathobiology, and Tissue Engineering. Circulation 2008;118:1864-1880.

[10] Bashey RI, Bashey HM, Jimenez SA. Characterization of pepsinsolubilized bovine heart-valve collagen. Biochem J. 1978;173:203–208.

[11] Rajamannan NM, Evans FJ, Aikawa E, Grande-Alen KJ, Demer LL, Heistad DD at al. Calcific aortic valve disease: not simply a degenerative process. Review and Agenda for Research From the National Heart and Lung and Blood Institute Aortic Stenosis Working Group. Circulation. 2011;124:1783-1791.

[12] Liu AC, Joag VR, Gotlieb AI. The emerging role of valve interstitial cell phenotypes in regulating heart valve pathobiology. Am J Pathol. 2007; 171:1407–1418.

[13] Aird WC. Phenotype heterogeneity of the endothelium, I: Structure, function, and mechanisms. II. Representative vascular beds. Circ Res. 2007;100:158 –173, 174–190.

[14] Butcher JT, Nerem RM. Valvular endothelial cells regulate the phenotype of interstitial cells in co-culture: effects of steady shear stress. Tissue Eng. 2006;12:905–915.

[15] Simmons CA, Grant GR, Manduchi E, Davies PF. Spatial heterogeneity of endothelial phenotypes correlates with side-specific vulnerability to calcification in normal porcine aortic valves. Circ Res. 2005;96:792-799.

[16] Aikawa E, Whittaker P, Farber M, Mendelson K, Padera RF, Aikawa M at al. Human semilunar cardiac valve remodeling by activated cells from fetus to adult: implications for postnatal adaptation, pathology, and tissue engineering. Circulation. 2006;113:1344-1352

[17] Rabkin-Aikawa E, Aikawa M, Farber M, Kratz JR, Garcia-Cardena G, Kouchoukos NT, Mitchell MB, Jonas RA, Schoen FJ. Clinical pulmonary autograft valves: pathologic evidence of adaptive remodeling in the aortic site. J Thorac Cardiovasc Surg. 2004;128:552–561.

[18] Rabkin-Aikawa E, Farber M, Aikawa M, Schoen FJ. Dynamic and reversible changes of interstitial cell phenotype during remodeling of cardiac valves. J Heart Valve Dis. 2004;13:841–847.

[19] Rabkin E, Hoerstrup SP, Aikawa M, Schoen FJ. Evolution of cell phenotype and extracellular matrix in tissue-engineered heart valves during in-vitro maturation and in-vivo remodeling. J Heart Valve Dis. 2002;11:308–314.

[20] Maron BJ, Hutchins GM. The development of the semilunar valves in the human heart. Am J Pathol. 1974;74:331–344.

[21] Anderson RH. Clinical anatomy of the aortic root. Heart. 2000;84:670–673

[22] Davies MJ. Pathology of Cardiac Valves. London: Butterworths & Co; 1980. p1–61.

[23] Berdajs D, Lajos P, Turina M. The anatomy of the aortic root. Cardiovasc Surg 2002. 10(4):320–327

[24] Jatene MB, Monteiro R, Guimarães MH, Veronezi SC, Koike MK, Jatene FB et al. Aortic valve assessment. Anatomical study of 100 healthy human hearts. Arq. Bras. Cardiol. 1999; 73(1):81-86.

[25] Muriago M, Sheppard MN, Ho SY, Anderson RH. Location of the coronary arterial orifices in the normal heart. Clin Anat. 1997;10: 297–302.

[26] Cavalcanti JS, de Melo NC, de Vasconcelos RS. Morphometric and topographic study of coronary ostia. Arq Bras Cardiol 81(4).2003; 359–362, 355-358

[27] Knight J, Kurtcuoglu V, Muffly K, Marshall W Jr, Stolzmann P, Desbiolles L et al, Ex vivo and in vivo coronary ostial locations in humans, Surgical and Radiologic Anatomy October 2009, Volume 31, Issue 8, pp 597-604

[28] Vollebergh FE, Becker AE. Minor congenital variations of cusp size in tricuspid aortic valves: possible link with isolated aortic stenosis. Br Heart J. 1977; 39:1006 –1011.

[29] Silver MA, Roberts WC. Detailed anatomy of the normally functioning aortic valve in hearts of normal and increased weight. Am J Cardiol. 1985; 55:454–461.

[30] [30]. Roberts WC. The structure of the aortic valve in clinically isolated aortic stenosis: an autopsy study of 162 patients over 15 years of age. Circulation. 1970; 42:91–97.

[31] Sutton JP III, Ho SY, Anderson RH. The forgotten interleaflet triangles: a review of the surgical anatomy of the aortic valve. Ann Thorac Surg. 1995; 59:419–427.

[32] McAlpine WA. Heart and Coronary Arteries. Berlin: Springer-Verlag. 1975. p9–26.

[33] Walmsley R. Anatomy of left ventricular outflow tract. Br Heart J. 1979; 41:263–7.

[34] Misfeld M, Sievers H-H. Heart valve macro and micro structure. Phil. Trans. R. Soc. B. 2007; 362:1421–1436. doi:10.1098/rstb.2007.2125

[35] Scott M, Vesely I. Aortic valve cusp microstructure: the role of elastin. Ann Thorac Surg. Aug 1995; 60(2 Suppl):S391-4

[36] Deck J.D. Endothelial cell orientation on aortic valve leaflets. Cardiovasc. Res. 1986; 20: 760–767.

[37] Mill MR, Wilcox BR, Anderson RH. Surgical Anatomy of the Heart. Cohn LH, Edmunds LH Jr, eds. Cardiac Surgery in the Adult. New York: McGraw-Hill, 2003:31-52.

[38] Feigenbaum H, Armstrong WF and Ryan T. Feigenbaum's Echocardiography, 6th edn. (2004). Lippincott Williams & Wilkins, Philadelphia, USA. ISBN 0-7817-3198-4

[39] Shanewise JS, Cheung AT, Aronson S, Stewart WJ, Weiss RL, Mark JB et al. ASE/SCA guidelines for performing a comprehensive intraoperative multiplane transesophageal echocardiography examination: recommendations of the American Society of Echocardiography Council for Intraoperative Echocardiography and the Society of Cardiovascular Anesthesiologists Task Force for Certification in Perioperative Transesophageal Echocardiography. J Am Soc Echocardiogr 1999; 12:884.

[40] Muraru D, Cardillo M, Livi U, Badano LP. 3-dimensional transesophageal echocardiographic assessment of papillary muscle rupture complicating acute myocardial infarction. J Am Coll Cardiol. 2010; 56:e45.

[41] Lang RM, Badano LP, Tsang W, Adams DH, Agricola E, Buck T, et al, EAE/ASE Recommendations for Image Acquisition and Display Using Three-Dimensional Echocardiography, J Am Soc Echocardiogr 2012; 25:3-46.

[42] Edwards WD. Applied anatomy of the heart. In: Giuliani ER, Fuster V, Gersh BJ, et al, eds. Cardiology Fundamentals and Practice. Vol 1. 2nd ed. St Louis: Mosby-Year Book; 1991: 47–112.

[43] Malouf JF, Edwards WD, Tajik AJ, Seward JB. Functional anatomy of the heart. In: Fuster V, Alexander RW, O'Rourke RA, et al, eds. The heart. 11th ed. New York, NY: McGraw-Hill, 2004; 75–83.

[44] Stewart W. Intraoperative echocardiography. In: Topol EJ, ed. Textbook of Cardiovascular Medicine. Philadelphia: Lippincott-Raven; 1998:1497–1525.

http://dx.doi.org/10.5772/53403

[45] Sliver MA, Roberts WC. Detailed anatomy of the normally functioning aortic valve in hearts of normal and increased weight. Am J Cardiol. 1985; 55:454–61.

Section 2

Mechanisms of Calcific Aortic Valve Disease

Chapter 3

Developmental Pathways in CAVD

Elaine E. Wirrig and Katherine E. Yutzey

Additional information is available at the end of the chapter

http://dx.doi.org/10.5772/54356

1. Introduction

Calcific Aortic Valve Disease (CAVD) occurs in >2% of the population over 65 years of age and often leads to valvular stenosis that necessitates valve replacement [1]. CAVD is a progressive disease, often manifesting first as aortic valve sclerosis and later developing into stenosis and valve dysfunction [2]. The specific molecular and cellular mechanisms of CAVD initiation and advancement are not well defined, and inhibitors of CAVD progression have not been identified. The current standard of treatment for CAVD is aortic valve replacement [3]. Presently, there are no pharmacologic-based treatments for CAVD, and new therapeutic approaches for CAVD are needed. The majority of aortic valves that are replaced have congenital malformations, such as bicuspid aortic valve (BAV), establishing a link between valve development and disease mechanisms [4].

The molecular mechanisms of CAVD include activation of signaling pathways implicated in both heart valve development (valvulogenesis) and bone development (osteogenesis) [5-8]. These include activation of regulators of progenitor specification, cell proliferation, and differentiation. Heart valves and bone are complex connective tissues with compartmentalized ECM produced by specialized cell types. Over the past several years, extensive progress has been made in defining molecular regulatory mechanisms in heart valve and bone development (Reviewed in [8-10]). Strikingly, regulatory pathways that control development of cartilage, tendon and bone also are active in developing valves [8, 11]. In addition, recent studies have reported induction of molecular regulators of valvulogenesis and osteogenesis in CAVD [7, 12-14]. However, it is not known if these developmental mechanisms have reparative functions or contribute to the progression of CAVD.

Here we review molecular mechanisms of valve and bone development as they relate to molecular mechanisms of CAVD. Recent studies have provided evidence for the involvement of specific regulatory pathways in CAVD as activators or inhibitors of disease progression.

Additional research in animal models and human patient specimens is necessary to determine the detrimental molecular regulatory pathways that promote CAVD progression and also beneficial pathways that potentially inhibit CAVD. In the future, manipulation of these pathways could be exploited therapeutically in the treatment of patients with CAVD or with aortic valve sclerosis that precedes calcification.

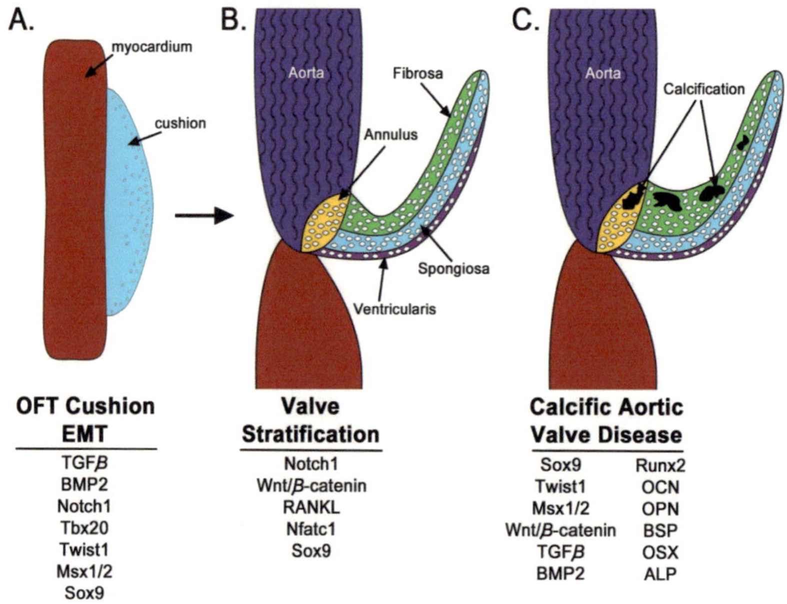

Figure 1. Molecular pathways active during endocardial cushion development and valve stratification are reactivated in CAVD. (A) Early stages of OFT cushion development are marked by ECM deposition, EMT, and neural crest cell infiltration. Factors necessary for EMT and mesenchymal cell function are expressed. (B) During late embryonic development and early postnatal development, the aortic valve becomes stratified and possesses three ECM layers. Factors necessary for ECM remodeling are active at this stage. (C) In CAVD, the ECM remodels and the valve becomes thickened. Calcification (black nodules) is typically observed in the collagen-rich fibrosa layer. Many factors expressed during OFT cushion development and valve stratification are reactivated during disease. Furthermore, osteogenic factors involved in bone development are also observed in CAVD. Please see text for details and references. OFT = outflow tract, EMT = epithelial-to-mesenchymal transition, ECM = extracellular matrix, CAVD = calcific aortic valve disease.

2. The cellular and molecular regulation of valve development

2.1. Overview of valve development

Valve development begins with the formation of endocardial cushions in the atrioventricular (AV) canal and outflow tract (OFT) of the primitive heart tube, which occurs at embryonic day (E)9-10 in mice, E3 in chickens, and E31-35 in humans [8]. The first evidence of endocardial cushion formation is the separation of the endocardium and overlying myocardium in the AV canal by expansion of the cardiac jelly through increased expression of hyaluronan (Figure 1) [15]. These swellings are invested with mesenchymal cells that arise from endothelial-to-mesenchymal transformation (EMT) of the endocardium [16]. Similar swelling and induction of EMT occur approximately a day later in the cardiac OFT cushions that will contribute to the semilunar valves [17]. Endocardial EMT is induced by signaling molecules, including bone morphogenetic proteins (BMPs), emanating from the adjacent myocardium in the AVC and OFT [8, 18-20]. Once established, the endocardial cushions expand through increased extracellular matrix (ECM) production and cell proliferation of mesenchymal and endothelial cells. The AV cushions subsequently fuse to separate right and left cardiac channels. In addition, lateral cushions are induced in the AV sulcus that will give rise to the mural leaflets of the mitral and tricuspid valves [21]. Neural crest cells (NCCs) migrate into the cushions of the cardiac OFT, contributing to the septum between the aortic and pulmonic roots and also to the morphogenesis of individual semilunar valve leaflets [21, 22]. At this point, distinct primordia of individual valve leaflets become apparent and proliferation of valve interstitial cells (VICs) is reduced [23]. Valve morphogenesis occurs with elongation and thinning of the valve primordia, in addition to ECM remodeling and stratification. In general, the development of the AV and semilunar (SL) valves is similar, but there are some differences in the sources of cells and structure of the resulting leaflets [8, 10, 11, 24]. In mature SL and AV valves, the ECM is stratified into collagen-rich fibrosa, proteoglycan-rich spongiosa, and elastin-rich (atrialis-ventricularis) layers oriented relative to blood flow [24].

2.2. Embryonic origins of valve cell lineages

The primary embryonic source of adult semilunar valve interstitial cells is the endothelial-derived cells of the endocardial cushions, that arise as a result of EMT as determined by Tie2-Cre lineage tracing in mice [23, 25]. Since the cardiac OFT is derived from the secondary heart field (SHF), semilunar VICs derived from OFT endocardium also are SHF-derived [20, 26]. NCC-derived cells are present in adult mouse semilunar valve leaflets as demonstrated by cell lineage tracing with Wnt1-Cre [27]. These cells are predominant throughout the aortic and pulmonic valve leaflets, but are enriched in the leaflets adjacent to the aorticopulmonary septum, which also is derived from NCCs [21, 28]. NCCs are required for semilunar valve morphogenesis and remodeling, likely by providing signals necessary for cell lineage differentiation and leaflet maturation [29, 30]. Another potential source of VICs is the epicardium, which contributes cells to the parietal leaflets of AV valves [31]. However, epicardial-derived cells (EPDCs) have not been not reported to contribute to the semilunar valves, based on Wt1 Cre fatemapping studies [31, 32]. Recent studies have reported that bone marrow-derived stem cells (BMSCs) are present in the developing and mature semilunar valves [33, 34]. Additional work is necessary to determine if these cells have lineages and functions distinct from the predominant endocardial cushion-derived or neural crest-derived VICs. It is possible that valve cell lineages derived from different developmental sources have distinct functions in normal and diseased aortic valves, but this has not yet been demonstrated. The sources of increased proliferative cells in diseased valves are relatively unknown, but could be any of these embryonic sources or, alternatively, an infiltrating cell type.

2.3. Transcription factors involved in valve development

Several transcription factors have been implicated in various processes of endocardial cushion formation and EMT (reviewed in [8, 35]). Notch pathway function in EMT is dependent on the transcription factor RBPJ, which activates expression of the bHLH transcription factor *snail1* (Snail) in endothelial cells [36]. Snail represses *ve-cadherin* gene expression, and loss of Snail in endothelial cells inhibits endocardial cushion formation [36, 37]. The mesenchymal valve progenitor cells of the endocardial cushions express several transcription factors characteristic of a variety of embryonic mesenchymal progenitor populations. These factors include, Twist1, Msx1/2, Tbx20, and Sox9 [18, 38-41]. Gain and loss of function studies have demonstrated critical roles for Tbx20, Twist1, and Sox9 in endocardial cushion mesenchymal cell proliferation [38-40]. Twist1 promotes *tbx20* expression directly and also regulates several genes associated with cell proliferation and migration [38, 42]. After endocardial cushion fusion and formation of valve primordia, mesenchymal genes, notably *twist1* [43], are down-regulated and cell proliferation is decreased [23, 24, 44]. In normal adult valves, there is little to no cell proliferation [24, 44], and expression of valve developmental transcription factors including Twist1, Sox9, and Msx2 is not detectable [13]. However, all of these factors are predominantly expressed in adult human CAVD (see below).

Additional regulatory pathways control heart valve ECM remodeling and compartmentalization. Loss of NFATc1 results in defective remodeling of the AV and SL valves in mice, with embryonic lethality by E14.5 [45, 46]. EMT occurs with loss of NFATc1, but valve primordia fail to remodel and mature ECM molecules are not expressed in null mice or in cultured VICs with inhibition of receptor activator of nuclear factor κ-B ligand (RANKL) or calcineurin signaling upstream of NFATc1 activation [45, 47]. In addition to being required for endocardial cushion mesenchymal proliferation, Sox9 also promotes cartilage-like ECM gene expression in valve progenitor cells [48]. In late stage mouse embryos, loss of Sox9 in remodeling valves results in reduced proteoglycan expression, and Sox9 haploinsufficiency in adults leads to valve calcification [40, 49]. Conversely, the bHLH transcription factor Scleraxis, critical for tendon development, promotes expression of elastic/tendon-like matrix genes in cultured valve progenitor cells [48]. Loss of Scleraxis in mice is not lethal, but heart valve defects similar to myxomatous valve disease occur in these animals [50]. Little is known of the transcriptional regulatory mechanisms that control the development of the valve fibrosa layer, which is most critically involved in CAVD.

2.4. Signaling pathways in valve development

Several essential embryonic signaling pathways have been implicated in endocardial cushion formation and EMT (Table 1) (reviewed in [8]). Transforming growth factor (TGF)β signaling was the first pathway implicated in endocardial cushion formation and is required for EMT in chicken and mouse embryonic systems (reviewed in [16]). BMP signaling from the myocardium is required in endothelial cells for the initiation of EMT in the AV canal, and BMP2 and 4 are the predominant ligands involved in endocardial cushion development [18-20]. Notch signaling also is required for EMT as described above. Moreover, Notch signaling is required for expression of TGFβ ligands and receptors, in addition to activating

http://dx.doi.org/10.5772/54356

BMP signaling, which promotes mesenchymal cell invasion [36, 51]. Likewise, vascular endothelial growth factor (VEGF) signaling promotes endocardial cushion endothelial cell proliferation and EMT [47, 52]. Furthermore, targeted mutagenesis of β-catenin has implicated Wnt/β-catenin signaling in endocardial cushion EMT and mesenchymal proliferation [53, 54]. Thus multiple pathways are involved in endocardial cushion EMT and mesenchymal cell proliferation. However, the intersection and specific cellular functions of these pathways have not been fully determined.

A. Signaling pathways			
	Role in valvulogenesis	Role in osteogenesis	Role in CAVD
VEGF	EMT, endothelial proliferation	angiogenesis	angiogenesis
Notch	EMT	Inhibit OB differentiation	represses calcification
TGFβ	EMT	bone homeostasis	promotes VIC calcification
FGF	promotes tenascin expression	OB proliferation, differentiation	blocks VIC calcification
BMP	EMT, PG expression	promotes OB specification	active in CAVD
Wnt/β-catenin	EMT, fibrosa expression	promotes OB differentiation	active in CAVD
RANKL	ECM remodeling	OC differentiation	promotes VIC calcification
B. Transcription factors			
	Role in valvulogenesis	Role in osteogenesis	Role in CAVD
Twist1	ECC proliferation, migration	represses differentiation	active in CAVD
Msx2	EMT, proliferation	present in progenitors, OB	active in CAVD
Sox9	proliferation, PG expression	progenitor proliferation, cartilage differentiation	active in CAVD inhibits calcification
NFATc1	endothelial proliferation, ECM remodeling	promotes OC differentiation promotes OB differentiation	reported in CAVD
Runx2	not present	promotes OB differentiation	active in CAVD
Osterix	not present	promotes OB differentiation	reported in CAVD

[a]Please see text for details and references. [b]Abbreviations used: CAVD=calcific aortic valve disease; ECM=extracellular matrix; EMT=endothelial to mesenchymal transition; OB=osteoblast; OC=osteoclast; PG=proteoglycan; VIC=valve interstitial cell.

Table 1. Signaling pathways and transcription factors involved in valvulogenesis, osteogenesis, and CAVD[a, b]

Many of the signaling pathways important for endocardial cushion formation also have later functions in valve lineage diversification, remodeling, and stratification. However, these functions have been difficult to elucidate due to limitations of available genetic tools and critical requirements for these same regulatory pathways in endocardial cushion formation. BMP signaling, as indicated by phosphorylation of the intermediate signaling molecules Smad1/5/8, is active throughout endocardial cushion mesenchymal cells, is associated with mesenchymal cell proliferation [55], and also is active later in valve cell lineage diversification [48]. *BMP Receptor II* mutations and conditional mutagenesis results in thickening of semilunar valve leaflets at late fetal stages [56, 57]. Loss of inhibitory Smad6 leads to increased BMP signaling, in addition to thickening of valve leaflets and CAVD in adult animals [58]. Studies in explanted avian valve progenitors have revealed antagonistic regulatory roles for BMP and fibroblast growth factor (FGF) signaling in promoting diversified ECM gene expression, conserved with mechanisms that control cartilage and tendon lineage development [11, 48, 59]. Wnt pathway activation is evident throughout the remodeling AV and semilunar valve primordia, as indicated in TopGal reporter mice [60]. Multiple Wnt ligands are expressed during valvulogenesis, but the function of Wnt signaling in heart valve remodeling has not yet been determined [60]. Thus, additional in vivo studies are necessary to determine the specific functions and intersecting regulatory mechanisms of these critical signaling pathways in valve leaflet development and also to determine specific contributions to valve degeneration and disease.

The later stages of heart valve development are characterized by leaflet elongation, ECM remodeling, and stratification, all of which are critical for mature valve structure and function [24]. Limited information is available on the regulation of these processes, but several regulatory pathways have been implicated in late valve remodeling and morphogenesis. Strikingly these same pathways have been implicated in adult CAVD (see below). RANKL, expressed by valve endothelial cells, promotes ECM remodeling and Cathepsin K (Ctsk) expression by NFATc1 in a mechanism partially conserved with osteoclast differentiation and function [11, 47, 61]. The signaling mechanisms that control stratification and ECM organization of the valve leaflets are relatively unknown. Notch signaling is localized on the ventricularis surface of the remodeling aortic valve in mice [62], and Wnt/β-catenin signaling is active throughout aortic valve primordia at late gestation and in a subpopulation of VICs after birth [60]. Likewise, Wnt signaling promotes expression of fibrosa genes *periostin* and *matrix gla-protein* (*mgp)* in cultured chicken embryo aortic VICs, but a role in valve stratification or lineage diversification has not yet been established in vivo [60]. Additional studies are necessary to demonstrate the specific functions and potential biomechanical stimulation of these pathways in an in vivo context. Since, both Notch and Wnt signaling pathways are required for initial stages of endocardial cushion formation, it has been difficult to establish their roles in the later stages of valvulogenesis in vivo using available conditional targeting approaches.

Bicuspid aortic valve is arguably the most common congenital heart malformation with an incidence of 1-2% in the US adult population [63]. BAV often does not often manifest in valve dysfunction in early life, but malformed aortic valves are predisposed to calcification. Strikingly, the majority of stenotic aortic valves that are replaced in adults are congenitally malformed [4]. However, the molecular and cellular mechanisms of BAV are not well defined. In humans, mutations in *NOTCH1* are associated with BAV, but the mechanisms by which valve leaflet number is regulated by Notch signaling have not yet been identified [64]. Likewise, Notch1 haploinsufficiency in mice leads to BAV at very low penetrance and there are likely to be additional factors necessary for congenital malformation of the aortic valve leaflets [65]. Loss of the zinc finger transcription factor GATA5 in mice [66] and mutations in human *GATA5* [67] are associated with BAV with incomplete penetrance. Likewise eNOS haploinsufficiency also leads to BAV, albeit with incomplete penetrance [68]. The mechanisms by which these genetic lesions lead to BAV in some individuals and not others are not known. However, based on the expression and function of Notch1, GATA5, and eNOS in endothelial cells, it is likely that these cells contribute to development of BAV in these models. The link between BAV and CAVD could be due to similar regulatory mechanisms in development and disease or could, alternatively, result from induction of calcification in a hemodynamically compromised congenitally malformed aortic valve (see other chapters for a more complete discussion of BAV and CAVD).

2.5. Extracellular matrix composition and stratification of the developing valves

The mature valve leaflets are composed of stratified ECM with layered compartments of fibrillar collagen, proteoglycan, and elastin (Figure 1) (reviewed in [10, 69]). During heart valve remodeling, there is little proliferation of VICs, but the cells are highly synthetic and produce multiple ECM proteins of the mature leaflets [24, 44]. The distinct layers of matrix are integral to heart valve function and confer specific biomechanical properties to the valve leaflets [69]. The regulatory mechanisms for ECM remodeling and stratification are not well defined but are relevant to heart valve disease mechanisms. Periostin is required for collagen remodeling, and loss of periostin in mice leads to adult valve malformations and cardiac dysfunction [70, 71]. Likewise, mutations in *Collagen 1a2* or elastin haploinsufficiency also result in aortic valve dysmorphogenesis and adult disease [72, 73]. Gene expression of *CtsK*, a matrix remodeling enzyme expressed during heart valve elongation, is regulated by the RANKL/NFATc1 regulatory pathway [47, 61]. Additional ECM remodeling enzymes, including matrix metalloproteinase (MMP)13, a collagenase, and Adam-TS5 and 9 proteoglycan proteases, also are expressed during late valve morphogenesis and have been implicated in ECM maturation and organization [39, 74, 75]. Several ECM molecules required for normal valve structure/function also are expressed during osteogenesis, and valve progenitors have gene expression profiles similar to bone progenitors [43]. *Osteopontin, osteonectin,* and *periostin* gene expression and collagen fiber deposition are increased during heart valve remodeling [24, 43, 60]. However, the regulatory mechanisms for expression of these genes in valve development are not well defined. These proteins also are induced and mislocalized in pediatric and adult heart valve disease [13, 24, 70], but the pathways leading to their dysregulation have not yet been fully characterized.

3. Molecular mechanisms of osteogenesis

3.1. Overview of skeletal development

Many osteogenic regulatory interactions identified in developing bone also are active in CAVD (Table 1). The regulatory hierarchies and ECM composition of the developing valves, most notably the collagen rich fibrosa layer, are similar to those observed in osteoblast precursor cells [43]. Both the bone substratum and valve ECM are composed primarily of fibrillar collagen. Thus, it is not surprising that there are extensive similarities in their composition and developmental regulation. Normally, heart valves do not progress to mineralization, but striking similarities have been identified between osteogenic pathways that regulate bone mineralization and CAVD mechanisms [7]. Thus the molecular understanding of normal development of bone has clear implications for pathogenic mechanisms of connective tissue mineralization, including CAVD.

The osteogenic precursors of the developing axial skeleton and long bones of the limbs are derived primarily from paraxial mesoderm of the developing somites and also lateral plate mesoderm, the main source of cardiac precursor cells [76, 77]. Additional progenitors of the craniofacial skeleton are derived from cranial neural crest [78]. Most axial skeletal elements develop by endochondral bone formation that occurs through a cartilage intermediate [76, 77]. Alternatively, the craniofacial bones of the skull form through membranous ossification in which condensed osteogenic progenitors differentiate directly into bone and do not go through a cartilage intermediate [76]. The osteochondroprogenitors present in the axial and appendicular skeletal elements develop into both bone and cartilage lineages [77, 79, 80]. Extensive research over the past several years has defined transcriptional regulatory mechanisms and signaling events that control the development of cartilage and bone (Figure 2) [79, 80].

Mature cartilage is composed predominantly of chondroitin sulfate proteoglycans that provides cushioning and flexibility to cartilaginous structures [77, 81]. In addition, the proteoglycan-rich ECM is angiostatic and mature cartilage is avascular [81]. Interestingly, the predominant proteoglycan composition and lack of vasculature also are features of the mature aortic valve leaflet spongiosa layer [82]. Likewise, the cartilage ECM inhibits mineralization, and a similar role has been hypothesized for the proteoglycan-rich matrix of the aortic valve [49]. During normal axial bone development, osteoblasts from the laterally placed periostium differentiate into trabecular bone, and secondary ossification centers at the ends of the bone displace the growth plate hypertrophic cartilage [79, 80]. During bone differentiation, hypertrophic cartilage cells must die for mineralization to occur in a process of endochondral ossification, which could be related to dystrophic mechanisms of CAVD [79, 80].

Bone cell lineage maturation goes through multiple stages defined by molecular regulatory mechanisms that also are active in valve development and disease processes [80]. Osteochondroprogenitor cells express several mesenchymal transcription factors, including Twist1, Msx2, and Sox9, that also are predominant in valve progenitor cells and diseased aortic valves [79]. Immature pre-osteoblasts express high levels of fibrillar type 1 collagen, in addition to periostin, osteonectin, and osteopontin, similar to normal differentiated VICs [43, 60]. Differentiated osteoblasts are not yet mineralized but express the transcription factor Runx2, in addition to osteocalcin and bone sialoprotein involved in bone mineralization and also in valve calcification, [7, 80]. Later stage osteoblasts and osteocytes express the transcription factor Osterix (Osx), which is regulated by Runx2 and is required for mature bone formation [83]. Bone mineralization occurs with the deposition of calcium phosphate and hydroxyapatite by osteocytes and is dependent on Runx2 and Osx function [80]. Bone homeostasis is maintained throughout life by the osteogenic activity of osteocytes and bone resorption activity of osteoclasts [80].

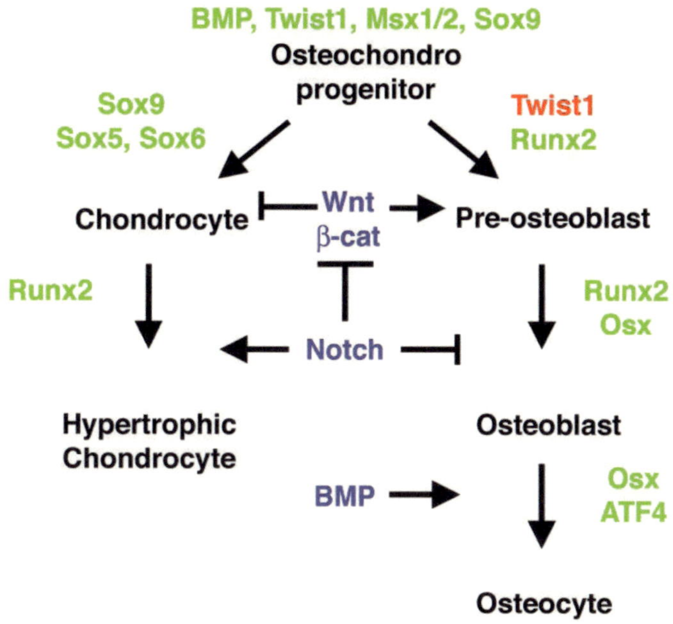

Figure 2. Hierarchies of signaling pathways and transcription factors regulate the differentiation of chondrogenic and osteogenic progenitor cells during skeletal development. Early osteochondrogenic progenitor cells express BMPs, Twist1, Msx1/2, and Sox9. Wnt/β-catenin signaling promotes pre-osteoblast differentiation while inhibiting chondrocyte differentiation. In contrast, Notch signaling promotes cartilage differentiation and inhibits osteoblast differentiation. BMP signaling is further required for osteocyte differentiation in the final stages of bone maturation. Sox5, 6, and 9 are transcription factors crucial for maintaining the chondrogenic lineage, whereas, Runx2, Osx, and ATF4 are transcription factors necessary for osteoblast and osteocyte differentiation and maturation. Many of these factors are also expressed during calcific aortic valve disease and have been implicated in pathologic calcification. Please see text for details and references. Activating factors are shown in green, inhibitory factors are shown in red, and signaling pathways are indicated in blue.

3.2. Transcriptional regulation of osteoblast lineage development and bone differentiation

Twist1 is expressed early in the osteochondroprogenitor lineage and inhibits terminal differentiation of cartilage and bone [84]. In preosteoblasts, Twist1 binds to Runx2 and inhibits its transcriptional activation of bone differentiation genes including *osteocalcin* [84]. Similarly, Twist1 can inhibit cartilage differentiation by binding to Sox9 and preventing activation of cartilage-specific gene expression [85]. Mutations in human *TWIST1* cause Saethre-Chotzen syndrome, characterized by premature bone differentiation evident in premature fusion of cranial sutures of the skull [86]. Msx2 also is involved in early mesenchymal stages of osteochondroprogenitor development and is down regulated during osteoblast differentiation [79]. Persistent Msx2 expression in osteoblasts prevents differentiation and mineralization, while antisense mRNA-mediated loss of Msx2 accelerates these processes [87]. Thus Msx2 is expressed in osteoblast progenitor cells but has an inhibitory role in osteogenic differentiation. Together Twist1 and Msx2 act to maintain undifferentiated osteochondroprogenitors during development.

Sox9 functions in the expansion of cartilage progenitors and promotes cartilage differentiation, while inhibiting bone differentiation [77, 80]. Sox9 is required for osteochondroprogenitor lineage specification but is not expressed in differentiated osteoblasts [88]. At early stages of cartilage lineage development, Sox9 promotes cell proliferation and later is required for cartilage lineage differentiation [88]. BMP signaling induces *Sox9* gene expression in cartilage progenitor cells [89], and Sox9 regulates expression of cartilage marker genes *Col2a1* and *aggrecan* [90, 91]. Sox9 transcriptional activity can be inhibited by binding to Twist1, thus inhibiting differentiation of early stage osteochondroprogenitor cells [85]. At later stages of cartilage maturation, Sox9 inhibits Runx2 transcriptional activity, thus promoting hypertrophic cartilage and inhibiting osteogenic differentiation [92]. Thus downregulation of Sox9 is required in osteoblasts for differentiation and mineralization of bone.

Runx2, originally called Cbfa1, has been defined as a master regulatory gene in bone formation [79, 93]. Gain and loss of function studies in mice demonstrate that Runx2 is both necessary and sufficient for osteoblast differentiation [93]. During bone development, Runx2 directly regulates *osteocalcin* gene expression [93]. Runx2 transcriptional function can be inhibited by interaction with Twist1 and also by Hey1, downstream of Notch signaling [84, 94]. Mice lacking Runx2 lack mineralized bone, and haploinsufficiency of Runx2 results in reduced bone formation in mice and humans [80]. Induction of a dominant negative form of Runx2 in differentiated osteoblasts after birth also leads to reduced bone mineralization, demonstrating a role for Runx2 in bone homeostasis and mineralization throughout life [95]. Runx2 has not been implicated in normal heart valve development, and its expression in developing valves has not been reported, consistent with the lack of calcification in normal valves. Likewise, in adult valves Runx2 is not normally expressed, but its expression is induced in CAVD in both humans and mice [13, 73]. The presence of Runx2 in diseased aortic valves and association with calcification is consistent with a role in mineralization, as has been established for bone cell lineages.

NFATc1 is a critical transcription factor in osteoclast differentiation and also has been implicated in osteoblast development [80, 96]. Osteoclasts, derived from a macrophage lineage, have bone resorptive activity and are necessary for bone homeostasis [96]. During osteoclast development, RANKL signaling induces activation of NFATc1, which promotes the transcription of bone matrix remodeling genes including *CtsK* and *mmp9* [97, 98]. RANKL activity in bone is antagonized by the receptor decoy osteoprotegerin (OPG) that promotes bone calcification [99, 100]. In osteoblasts, NFATc1 promotes cell proliferation and also enhances differentiation by cooperating with Osx to promote *Col1a1* gene expression [101, 102]. Thus, the balance of RANKL and OPG signaling acting on NFATc1 transcriptional function is a critical mediator of bone calcification and resorption [96]. A similar balance of OPG and RANKL signaling in CAVD has been proposed [103]. While NFATc1 is a critical regulator of heart valve remodeling during development and activates valvular *CtsK* expression [47, 61], its role in CAVD and adult valve homeostasis has not been determined.

Additional transcription factors involved in bone differentiation are not generally found in CAVD, although there are conflicting reports. Most notable is Osx, which is required for terminal differentiation of osteoblasts and mineralization of bone [83]. Osx, promotes expression of *collagen 1a1* and the matrix metalloproteinase *mmp13*, which also are upregulated in aortic valve disease [73, 101, 104, 105]. Studies based on antibody staining demonstrate Osx expression in Notch signaling-deficient calcified mouse valves [65] and human CAVD [106]. ATF4 is an additional transcription factor critical for bone differentiation, mineralization, and homeostasis that has not been found in developing or diseased valves [79]. Further studies are necessary to determine if *ATF4* or *Osx* gene expression is induced or if they contribute to valve mineralization in CAVD.

3.3. Signaling pathways involved in bone development

Multiple signaling pathways control the stages of bone cell lineage determination, differentiation and maturation [80, 107]. These include BMP, Wnt, and Notch pathways, also active in developing and diseased heart valves, as well as FGF, hedgehog, insulin-like growth factor (IGF), and retinoic acid (RA) pathways, not yet characterized in heart valve pathogenesis [80]. BMP, Wnt, and Notch pathways are required at multiple stages of osteogenesis and have distinct regulatory interactions that control transcription factor function and cell type-specific gene expression in cartilage and bone cell lineages (Figure 2). In addition, these pathways crosstalk with each other in synergistic and antagonistic regulatory interactions. Strikingly many of these same regulatory interactions occur in heart valve development and pathogenesis (Table 1) [8].

Bone morphogenetic proteins were originally identified based on their ability to induce ectopic bone formation [108]; however, in vivo functions in normal bone development are less clear [109]. In the developing limb buds, BMP signaling has a critical role in mesenchymal condensation, Sox9 activation, and cartilage lineage differentiation [89]. Thus BMP signaling is an important regulator of the earliest stages of skeletal development. Later in differentiating osteoblasts, BMP signaling through Smad1/5/8 phosphorylation (pSmad1/5/8) promotes osteogenic differentiation and calcification [110]. Runx2 directly binds to activated Smads1 and 5 to cooperatively activate osteoblast gene expression in response to BMP signaling [109]. Conditional loss of BMP2 and BMP4 in the osteoblast lineage in mice inhibits late stage differentiation into Osx1-positive osteocytes, and BMP signaling is required for bone homeostasis after birth [80, 109]. Surprisingly, earlier stages of bone lineage development are apparently unaffected with conditional loss of these ligands.

Wnt/β-catenin signaling is required for osteoblast differentiation as demonstrated by loss of osteoblast differentiation with conditional loss of β-catenin in osteochondroprogenitor cells in mice [80]. In addition, loss of β-catenin in pre-osteoblasts leads to ectopic cartilage formation, thus implicating Wnt signaling in osteogenic versus chondrogenic cell fate determination. At a molecular level, Wnt/β-catenin signaling promotes osteoblast lineage differentiation, while inhibiting chondrogenesis, by activating Runx2, while inhibiting Sox9 [77]. In bone lineages, BMP and Wnt signaling act synergistically to promote calcification, although neither pathway alone is sufficient to induce a full osteogenic response [111]. During the initial differentiation of bone progenitor cells, regulatory elements of *Runx2* and *Msx2* genes are bound by Smad1, downstream of BMP signaling, and also by Lef1, activated by Wnt signaling, for cooperative gene activation [112]. Postnatally, Wnt signaling through the Lrp5 receptor is required for bone accrual in mice and humans [80]. In developing bone, osteogenic differentiation and calcification are dependent on sequential activation of BMP, followed by Wnt/β-catenin, signaling [110]. It is possible that a similar regulatory relationship exists in CAVD, but this has not yet been demonstrated.

Notch activation inhibits osteogenesis through suppression of the Wnt/β-catenin pathway and Runx2 transcription factor activity [94, 113, 114]. Loss of Notch1 or Notch2 function promotes osteoblast differentiation and leads to increased bone mass in mice [115]. Notch pathway activation inhibits the progression of osteoblast differentiation through direct binding of the activated Notch1 intracellular domain (N1ICD) to β-catenin, thereby counteracting Wnt-mediated induction of osteogenesis [113, 114]. In addition, the Notch target gene *Hey1* encodes a transcriptional repressor that binds and inhibits Runx2 transcriptional function [115]. Precise levels of Notch signaling are required for cell proliferation and chondrogenic differentiation, with defects in these processes occurring with increased or decreased Notch signaling in mice [116]. In early cartilage precursors, Notch signaling is required for cell proliferation, but increased Notch signaling inhibits terminal differentiation of chondrocytes and endochondral ossification [116]. Loss of Notch signaling has been implicated in CAVD [64], but it is not known if this occurs through inhibition of Wnt/β-catenin signaling, as has been demonstrated for osteoblast differentiation and bone mineralization.

4. Molecular and cellular mechanisms of CAVD

4.1. Overview of CAVD progression

The mature aortic valves are comprised of three ECM layers critical for normal leaflet structure and function [24, 44, 117]. Collagen predominates in the fibrosa layer, which is oriented on the opposite side of blood flow, whereas elastin is enriched in the ventricularis layer on the flow side of the valve. Between the fibrosa and ventricularis layers, is the proteoglycan-rich spongiosa layer [24, 44, 117]. This trilaminar ECM arrangement is preserved among species, and lends both strength and elasticity to the aortic valves [24]. In CAVD, the aortic valve becomes thickened and displays extensive ECM remodeling and mineralization [118-121]. Abnormal thickening (aortic valve sclerosis) and calcification of the aortic valve lead to stiffening of the valve leaflets and can reduce the effective valve opening (aortic valve stenosis), which can impede blood flow and lead to clinical symptoms such as syncope and angina [119, 122, 123]. Histologically, human explanted diseased aortic valves have

http://dx.doi.org/10.5772/54356

extensive ECM remodeling and elastic fiber fragmentation with evidence of both macroscopic calcific nodule formation as well as microscopic mineral deposits [119].

Changes in the resident VICs are apparent in CAVD. Under normal conditions, aortic VICs are quiescent and non-proliferative [13, 24, 104, 124]. However, in disease, a subset of aortic VICs exhibits features of myofibroblast activation, which is characterized by expression of α-smooth muscle actin (αSMA), MMP13, non-muscle myosin heavy chain (SMemb), and markers of proliferation [13, 104, 119, 124, 125]. In vivo, the factors responsible for inducing myofibroblast activation are not well defined. However, in culture, TGFβ1 stimulation and mechanical strain are potent inducers of VIC myofibroblast activation [125, 126]. Activated VICs also exhibit characteristics of valve and bone precursor cells as they induce expression of the common mesenchymal markers Sox9, Twist1, and Msx2 [13]. Currently it is unknown where the mesenchymal-like cells come from and what role these proliferative cells play in the progression of CAVD pathogenesis.

Valve calcification, apparent as hydroxyapatite deposits on the surface of or within the leaflets, is a prominent feature of CAVD [119, 127, 128]. Histologically, valve calcific nodules are primarily acellular [13, 129]. Although traditionally thought to be a completely passive deposition of mineral, in some cases, valve calcification is coincident with endochondral bone-like and cartilaginous-like nodules [129, 130]. Aortic valve calcification is observed primarily in the regions of the valves exposed to the greatest physical strain, specifically at the hinge region of the valve and along the line of leaflet coaptation [120]. Furthermore, calcification is predominantly found in the fibrosa layer of the diseased valve, which is similar to early bone matrix as it is contains primarily fibrillar collagen [44]. Expression of other bone matrix molecules, such as osteocalcin and osteopontin, are induced during disease [5]. Furthermore, expression of osteogenic factors, such as Runx2, BMP2, and alkaline phosphatase, also is induced in VICs from calcified valves, suggesting that resident VICs may have the potential to undergo osteogenic transdifferentiation and actively contribute to valve calcification (reviewed in [131]).

Extrinsic factors have been implicated in valve calcification. For example, lipid deposition and immune cell infiltration are common histopathological features of CAVD, and it has been proposed that aortic valve calcification occurs by mechanisms similar to arterial calcification in atherosclerosis [119, 132-135]. In addition, altered external physical forces elicit changes in resident VICs, which play an active role in pathological valve calcification [126]. In contrast to VIC response to immune cell infiltration and altered physical forces, cell intrinsic mechanisms may also contribute to valve calcification, as stimulation with factors such as BMP2 or TGFβ1 in cell culture studies can induce VIC calcification in the absence of inflammatory stimulation or altered physical forces [126, 136-138]. Together, these studies suggest that not only is valve calcification an active cell-regulated process, but that many factors likely contribute to progression of calcification during disease. It is also likely that not all CAVD is created equal. Genetic predisposition, the presence of a malformed aortic valve, and other disease comorbidities, such as coronary artery disease, hypertension, and kidney disease, likely affect the pathology and underlying cause of CAVD [64, 139-142].

4.2. Activation of progenitor cell and osteogenesis-related molecular pathways in CAVD

4.2.1. Expression of valve and bone progenitor cell genes in CAVD

The mesenchymal markers Twist1, Msx2, and Sox9 are expressed in adult calcific aortic valves in mesenchymal-like activated VICs [12, 13, 106, 143, 144]. As discussed, these genes are expressed in both valve and bone mesenchymal progenitor cells. A recent study has compared gene expression in pediatric versus adult aortic valve disease and shown that the mesenchymal markers Twist1, Msx2, and Sox9 are increased in both [13]. The observation that both pediatric and adult diseased valves have increased expression of the mesenchymal markers suggests that this expression is related to VIC activation and proliferation, which is common to both, and not related to valve calcification, which is found only in advanced adult disease [13]. In both valve and bone progenitors, Twist1, Msx2, and Sox9 induce proliferation and promote a mesenchymal phenotype, thus reactivation in diseased valves is suggestive of a similar role in valve pathogenesis [38, 40-42, 84, 88, 145]. Although it is presumed that resident VICs re-activate these early mesenchymal markers, other possibilities exist. EMT as a mechanism for VIC activation has not been established in CAVD, however, recent studies report EMT-like events in adult valves. Increased cyclic strain and altered hemodynamics, both recognized features of CAVD, can induce EMT in isolated sheep valve endothelial cells [146, 147]. In addition, cultured valve endothelial cells stimulated with TGFβ adapt a mesenchymal-like phenotype and express markers of both endothelial and mesenchymal cells, suggesting that they can undergo EMT [148, 149]. Likewise, disruption of Notch signaling in adult mice induces aortic valve thickening with evidence of endocardial EMT, as indicated by endocardial cells with more pseudopodial projections, loose endocardial cell-cell junctions, and αSMA expression [150]. Additional sources of mesenchymal-like cells have been suggested. For example, circulating bone marrow-derived hematopoietic stem cells have been shown to integrate into the valve interstitium, adapt fibroblast-like characteristics, and surround regions of prominent valve calcification in human end stage CAVD [33, 130, 151]. It is uncertain what role reactivation of the mesenchymal markers Twist1, Msx2, and Sox9 have in potential valve repair mechanisms or in the progression of CAVD. It is possible that adult VICs maintain a certain "mesenchymal-plasticity" and are able to revert back to an early progenitor-like mesenchymal cell during disease. Alternatively, they may be indicators of newly derived VICs arising from EMT or circulating progenitor cell populations in response to disease conditions.

4.2.2. Osteogenic factors in CAVD

Molecular mechanisms of endochondral ossification and cartilaginous nodule formation are active in CAVD [7, 13]. Studies in human explanted diseased aortic valve tissues have demonstrated increased expression of the osteogenic factors BMP2, TGFβ1, Runx2, osteocalcin (OCN), osteopontin (OPN), osteoprotegerin (OPG), bone sialoprotein (BSP), alkaline phosphatase (ALP), and Osx in disease [5, 13, 106, 118, 137, 152]. At a molecular level, BMP2 signaling is a key inducer of VIC calcification, which is thought to act through p-SMAD1/5/8 and phospho-ERK1/2 signaling to stimulate increases in both Runx2 and OPN expression [138]. Induction of VIC calcification by BMP2 stimulation is highly reminiscent of BMP signaling in bone development, suggesting that some parallels exist between osteogenic bone formation and VIC calcification [9]. Histological studies of explanted human valves further support a role for BMP signaling in valve calcification. Comparison of pediatric diseased valves, which do not acquire calcification, and adult calcified valves demonstrates that increased BMP signaling, evident in p-SMAD1/5/8 activation, is exclusive to adult valves with calcification, indicating that BMP signaling may contribute to valve calcification in human disease [13]. Additionally, TGFβ1 is also a potent inducer of osteogenic-like differentiation of VICs in cell culture, as it stimulates VIC activation and calcification, increases ALP activity, and increases expression of ECM remodeling enzymes [126, 136, 137]. Negative regulators of valve calcification have been demonstrated through in vivo studies. One negative regulator of valve calcification is Notch signaling. Animals haploinsufficient for Notch signaling develop aortic valve calcification with increased BMP signaling and increased expression of Runx2 in the valve leaflets [65, 153]. Studies in isolated aortic VICs further demonstrate that Notch signaling plays an important role in suppressing valve calcification as treatment of VICs with Notch inhibitors induces BMP signaling and subsequent increases in osteogenic gene expression [65, 153]. Another negative regulator of valve calcification is Sox9, which potentially acts through induction of proteoglycan expression, similar to what has been observed in developing cartilage [40, 49]. Conditional heterozygous Sox9 mutant mice develop valve calcification along with increased valve thickness and expression of the osteogenic genes *Runx2*, *osteonectin*, *OPN*, and *OPG* [40, 49]. Based on these studies, it is apparent that many factors involved in endochondral bone formation are active in the process of aortic valve calcification.

CAVD has been linked to chronic kidney disease in human patients and animal models [140, 154-157]. A prominent pathological feature of kidney disease is the inability to regulate calcium and phosphate metabolism [158]. Increased blood phosphate levels (hyperphosphatemia) are highly associated with aortic valve sclerosis and valve calcification in humans [140]. Klotho-null mice are a model of accelerated aging that includes development of kidney failure and hyperphosphatemia, along with cardiovascular disease [159-162]. Klotho-null mice exhibit extensive valve annulus calcification with increased expression of osteogenic genes, but minimal CD68 positive macrophage infiltration [73]. Thus, valve calcification in the klotho-null animals parallels bone formation, where increases in crucial osteogenic genes, such as *Col10a1, Runx2, OPN*, and *BSP*, are observed [73]. These observations suggest that increased blood phosphate levels could be one stimulus for inducing advanced aortic valve calcification with osteogenic gene expression, but this has not been definitively demonstrated [73, 140].

Atherogenic lipid deposition and inflammation in the valves also has been linked to induction of osteogenic gene expression and disease [163-165]. Rabbit and mouse models of CAVD, induced with hypercholesterolemic or high fat diets, have increased lipid deposition and macrophage infiltration associated with induction of osteogenic markers such as ALP, OCN, OPN, Runx2, and Osx [165-167]. Although osteogenic gene expression is induced in these models, this type of valve calcification closely mimics vascular calcification observed in atherosclerosis, rather than endochondral bone formation, due to the presence of extensive immune cell infiltration [165, 166]. In support, human aortic VICs stimulated with pro-inflammatory mimetics not only induce the expression of inflammatory cytokines, but also induce the expression of osteogenic factors, such as BMP2 and Runx2, again suggesting that this process may be similar to what is occurring in atherosclerotic disease [164, 168]. Based on this evidence, multiple physiologic factors likely contribute to osteogenic gene induction in calcified diseased aortic valves.

4.2.3. Valvulogenic- and osteogenic-related signaling pathways in CAVD

As in both heart valve and endochondral bone development, BMP, TGFβ, Notch, and Wnt signaling have been implicated in the progression of CAVD (Figure 2; Table 1). Increased BMP ligand expression, particularly BMP2 and BMP4, has been demonstrated histologically in human explanted calcific aortic valves surrounding and throughout regions of valvular calcification [118, 129]. Furthermore, active BMP signaling, as indicated by pSMAD1/5/8 expression, is present in both human explanted diseased aortic valves and animal models of CAVD [13, 169, 170]. Comparison of pediatric diseased valves void of calcification to heavily calcified adult diseased valves demonstrates extensive ECM remodeling and evidence of VIC activation in both; however, increased pSMAD1/5/8 signaling is exclusive to calcified valves [13]. The observation that pSMAD1/5/8 expression is found only in adult calcified valves is suggestive of a critical role for BMP signaling as an initiating osteogenic factor in CAVD [13]. Furthermore, increased pSMAD1/5/8 expression reportedly localizes to the fibrosa layer of human calcific aortic valves, which is the primary sight of aortic valve calcification [169]. Cell culture studies support this and show that BMP2 stimulation promotes osteogenic-like aortic valve calcification in human aortic VICs by inducing the expression of the osteogenic factors Runx2, OPN, and ALP [138, 171]. Based on this evidence, active BMP signaling may be a potential therapeutic target to treat CAVD, however it has not yet been tested.

TGFβ signaling induces α SMA expression and myofibroblast differentiation of porcine aortic VICs, suggesting that TGFβ promotes VIC activation, potentially in response to physical strain [125, 172]. Furthermore, TGFβ signaling may also have a role in aortic valve calcification, as human explanted calcific aortic valves have increased levels of TGFβ1 expression and ovine aortic VICs in culture calcify in response to TGFβ1 induction [136, 137]. TGFβ signaling has also been linked to both Wnt/β-catenin and FGF signaling pathways in CAVD [173, 174]. Specifically, FGF signals have been shown to induce MAPK signaling, which inhibits aortic VIC αSMA expression and myofibroblast response to TGFβ [174]. In addition, TGFβ stimulation of aortic VICs induces nuclear localization and activation of β-catenin, which promotes VIC myofibroblast differentiation [173]. Although the role of TGFβ in CAVD is not well established in vivo, there is accumulating evidence for a role in VIC activation and calcification from studies in cell culture systems.

http://dx.doi.org/10.5772/54356

Whereas both BMP and TGFβ signaling have been found to induce VIC calcification, Notch signaling has been implicated as a negative regulator of valve calcification. Familial studies demonstrated that Notch1 haploinsufficiency is associated with CAVD and aortic stenosis (AS) [64]. During development, Notch1 is expressed in the endothelial cells lining the aortic valve cusps and is also observed at lower levels in the VICs, and this expression pattern is maintained into adulthood [64, 175]. Histological analysis of human explanted aortic valves demonstrates that activated Notch1 intracellular domain (NICD) expression is dramatically reduced in VICs directly adjacent to regions of aortic valve calcification [175]. This observation is consistent with a mechanism whereby Notch signaling inhibits valve calcification and downregulation of Notch expression promotes valve calcification [175]. The idea that Notch signaling functions as a negative regulator of calcification was originally defined in endochondral bone formation, where downstream effectors of Notch signaling, Hes1 and Hey1, repress Runx2 transcriptional function, leading to expansion of hypertrophic cartilage and impaired osteoblast differentiation [115]. Notch1 heterozygous or RBPJ heterozygous mice develop CAVD, as evidenced by increased aortic valve calcification, and also display significant increases in BMP/pSMAD1/5/8 signaling and Runx2 expression in the aortic valves [65, 153]. Likewise, deletion of RBPJ in adult mice results in increased aortic valve thickness with evidence of VIC proliferation and potentially, endothelial EMT [150]. Together these in vivo studies support the idea that Notch signaling represses BMP expression, thereby indirectly repressing other osteogenic factors [65, 153]. Cell culture studies indicate that Notch inhibition promotes calcification of VICs by repressing chondrogenic genes, including *Sox9*, and inducing expression of the osteogenic genes *OPN, osteonectin, Runx2, ALP*, and *BMP2* [65, 153, 175]. Specifically, Notch signaling in the aortic valves is thought to induce expression of Sox9, which is a negative regulator of calcification, and to repress the expression of both Runx2 and BMP2, which are known to stimulate osteogenic differentiation [64, 153, 175]. These studies suggest that, in the absence of a negative regulator of calcification, the resident VICs possess an intrinsic calcification mechanism, which becomes activated and subsequently induces valve calcification. Combined, the evidence suggests that Notch signaling is a negative regulator of VIC osteogenic differentiation, and that the absence or dysregulation of Notch signaling can induce valvular calcification.

Wnt/β-catenin signaling is important for osteoblast maturation during embryonic development and contributes to mineralized bone formation (reviewed in [80]). A number of studies have also shown activation of Wnt/β-catenin signaling in aortic valve calcification. Canonical Wnt signaling acts through the frizzled receptors and the Wnt co-receptors Lrp5 and Lrp6, resulting in β-catenin nuclear localization and TCF/LEF1 activation [176]. Human explanted calcific AoVs have increased expression of Lrp5, β-catenin, and Wnt3a ligand as compared to control valves [143]. Increased Wnt signaling in diseased aortic valves also has been observed in multiple animal models of CAVD. Pigs and rabbits maintained on an atherogenic diet develop aortic valve disease and display increased expression levels of β-catenin and Lrp5 receptor [173, 177]. Likewise, in a subset of endothelial nitric oxide synthase (eNOS) deficient mice that develop BAV, expression of Wnt3a ligand and Lrp5 receptor is increased when the animals are fed a high cholesterol diet [178]. Cell culture studies also support the idea that Wnt/β-catenin signaling is important for VIC myofibroblast activation, proliferation, and chondrogenic gene induction. Studies in porcine aortic VICs show that Wnt3a treatment induces significant VIC proliferation and myofibroblast activation [173, 179]. Furthermore, Wnt3a treatment of embryonic chicken aortic VICs results in increased expression of *periostin* and *mgp*, but does not induce the expression of osteogenic-related genes, suggesting that Wnt3a signaling is not sufficient for VIC osteogenic differentiation [60]. However in adult valves, Wnt signaling can promote the VIC calcification response, as loss of Wnt signaling through the Lrp5 receptor in ApoE knockout mice results in decreased aortic valve calcification [180]. Together these studies demonstrate that Wnt signaling likely contributes to VIC activation, proliferation, and calcification in CAVD.

4.3. Matrix remodeling in CAVD

Diseased aortic valves are characterized by changes in the ECM; in particular, disorganized collagen bundles and extensive elastic fiber fragmentation are observed [181, 182]. Insight into the role of elastin fiber disorganization in the pathogenesis of CAVD has been provided through studies of elastin haploinsufficient mice, which display elastin fiber fragmentation, abnormal ECM remodeling, and increased valve stiffness, suggesting that elastin homeostasis is important for maintaining valve function [72, 183]. Collagen synthesis and remodeling are dramatically increased in CAVD, however, overall collagen content in the valve is actually decreased, suggesting that there is extensive collagen proteolysis during disease [184-186]. In contrast to collagens, expression of proteoglycans, including decorin, biglycan, versican, and hyaluronan, is increased particularly in regions of the diseased valve adjacent to calcific nodules [187]. These changes in ECM composition during CAVD can be compared to matrix remodeling events that occur during valve development and also in bone formation. The decreased collagen content and increased proteoglycan matrix found in CAVD is similar to the primitive ECM characteristic of early valve development [188]. Furthermore, parallels can also be drawn between matrix remodeling in CAVD and bone development. Specifically, matrix remodeling in the immature bone is essential for providing a scaffold upon which the calcified matrix is deposited, and subsequent ECM degradation is essential for expansion of the calcified regions of newly forming bone [189]. The parallels between matrix remodeling in bone development and the disease process of CAVD suggest that valve matrix remodeling may contribute to valvular calcification.

Matrix degradation and remodeling in valvulogenesis, osteogenesis, and CAVD occurs concomitant with increased activity of MMPs and cathepsins, along with increased RANKL signaling. A number of studies have shown significant increases in expression of multiple MMPs, including MMP1, MMP3, MMP7, MMP9, and MMP12, with increased cathepsins B, K, and S in human calcific diseased aortic valves, suggesting that extensive ECM remodeling is a key feature of disease [124, 163, 181, 182, 184, 190]. In bone, RANKL signals through the RANK receptor, which can be inhibited via binding to the soluble receptor OPG, and promotes the expression of proteolytic enzymes, such as MMPs and cathepsin K, through activation of NFATc1 [191, 192]. A similar mechanism has been identified in heart valve remodeling [47, 61]. Comparison of sclerotic diseased aortic valves and advanced stenotic aortic valves determined that OPG levels are significantly higher in sclerotic valves without calcification, whereas RANKL expression is higher in stenotic calcified valves [103, 193]. This study concluded that OPG may be protective against valve calcification, whereas elevated RANKL expression may promote valve calcification by promoting upregulation of matrix remodeling enzymes [103, 193]. Furthermore, treatment of human aortic VICs with RANKL results in increased MMP1 and MMP2 activity with increased VIC proliferation, concomitant with increased calcification and osteogenic gene expression [103, 191]. In addition, NFATc1 expression is increased in human explanted aortic valve leaflets with CAVD [106]. Together, these studies are consistent with signaling events during bone development, namely RANKL activation of NFATc1, stimulating matrix remodeling enzymes, and promoting calcification [192].

A number of other signaling pathways are likely involved in ECM changes that occur during CAVD. In particular, TGFβ1 stimulation of cultured VICs stimulates myofibroblast differentiation, leading to increased levels of αSMA stress fibers in the VICs [125, 172]. It has been suggested that these myofibroblasts then exert a contractile force on the surrounding valve ECM and stimulate rearrangement of the matrix, particularly in fibronectin fibers [125]. Furthermore, TGFβ1 stimulation also induces increased type I collagen production and expression of the matrix remodeling enzymes MMP9 and MMP2 in cultured aortic VICs [136, 172]. These studies indicate that TGFβ1 signaling may be a key factor in ECM-related changes during CAVD pathogenesis. Moreover, Wnt signaling may work in concert with TGFβ1 to induce changes in ECM during CAVD [173]. TGFβ1 stimulation promotes nuclear localization and activation of β-catenin in cultured VICs, and, when combined, Wnt and TGFβ1 signaling dramatically increases myofibroblast activation [173]. In contrast to TGFβ1 and Wnt signaling, FGF signaling may work to inhibit ECM remodeling during valve disease. FGF signaling has been shown to block TGFβ1 induced myofibroblast differentiation and αSMA expression in porcine aortic VICs through activation of phospho-ERK1/2 signaling [174]. In addition, FGF signaling inhibits myofibroblast contraction of a collagen matrix, supporting the idea that FGF signaling blocks TGFβ1 stimulation of matrix-related changes [174]. Many parallels exist between signaling factors involved in ECM changes in development and disease. In particular, RANKL, TGFβ1, Wnt, and FGF signaling have demonstrated roles in ECM production and regulation in both heart valve and endochondral bone formation [8, 76]. The shared signaling pathways in these tissues, both in development and disease, suggest that developmental pathways may be reactivated in CAVD to induce matrix changes characteristic of the disease.

5. Therapeutic mechanisms in CAVD

Currently, aortic valve replacement surgery is the only effective treatment option for CAVD [122]. There have been numerous studies, which are summarized below, testing the effectiveness of different pharmacotherapies on preventing the progression of AS. Unfortunately, studies on statin therapies, inhibitors of the renin-angiotensin-aldosterone system, and osteoporosis treatments have not been proven to be effective at preventing the symptoms or the progression of CAVD/AS. Following the summary of these studies, additional treatment options, related to the expression of developmental and osteogenic-related genes in CAVD, are discussed.

5.1. Statins

Lipid deposition and the accumulation of apolipoproteins (Apo) in the aortic valve leaflets have long been associated with CAVD, and many studies have compared the progression of CAVD to atherosclerotic disease [119, 133, 134, 194]. Therefore, it has been hypothesized that cholesterol lowering therapy with statin drugs may be an effective treatment strategy to delay the progression of CAVD. A specialized mouse model called "Reversa" mice develop signs of CAVD when fed a high cholesterol diet, however, when serum cholesterol is lowered via a genetic deletion of the microsomal triglyceride transfer protein (Mttp), reduced levels of aortic valve calcification, as well as decreased expression of the osteogenic markers pSMAD1/5/8, Msx2, Osx, β-catenin, and Runx2, are observed [167, 170]. Thus reducing plasma cholesterol may reduce CAVD pathogenesis, particularly in terms of reducing osteogenic gene expression in the diseased valves. Similarly, statin treatment of human or porcine aortic VICs cultured concomitantly with osteogenic media results in decreased expression of the osteogenic genes ALP, OCN, Lrp5, and OPN, and reduced calcific nodule formation [171, 177, 195]. However, when statin treatment of aortic VICs is initiated after osteogenic transformation or calcific nodule formation, it is ineffective at reducing calcification and expression of osteogenic markers, indicating that statin therapy cannot reverse aortic valve calcification and osteogenic differentiation once it has occurred [195, 196]. Results from animal studies are equally contradictory. Rabbits fed a high cholesterol diet supplemented with atorvastatin have decreased aortic valve thickness, reduced VIC proliferation, and reduced expression of Lrp5, β -catenin, OPN, *Runx2*, and *ALP*, compared to those animals fed only a high cholesterol diet [165, 177]. Similarly, endothelial nitric oxide synthase (eNOS) deficient mice, displaying a BAV phenotype and fed a high cholesterol diet, have reduced *Lrp5* and *Wnt3a* expression as well as reduced aortic valve calcification when treated with statins, compared to animals fed only a high cholesterol diet [178]. In contrast, a long term study in rabbits fed a high cholesterol diet showed that atorvastatin therapy initiated after aortic valve disease is established is not effective at reducing the amount of aortic valve calcification present, although some improvements in other histological parameters were noted [197]. Based on both cell culture and animal studies, statin therapy may improve some measures of aortic valve calcification, specifically in terms of reducing osteogenic gene expression, however, firm conclusions as to potential efficacy as a CAVD treatment cannot be drawn.

Clinicial studies investigating the use of statin therapy in patients with CAVD are also widely contradictory. An early study investigating the use of statin therapy in patients with moderate to severe aortic stenosis (AS) reported that patients treated with statins had less hemodynamic progression of AS over a 2 year time period than patients who were not on statin therapy [198]. In contrast, three larger prospective clinical studies, SALTIRE (Scottish Aortic Stenosis and Lipid Lowering Trial, Impact on Regression), SEAS (Simvastatin and Ezetimibe in Aortic Stenosis), and ASTRONOMER (Aortic Stenosis Progression Observation: Measuring Effects of Rosuvastatin), found that statin therapy was not effective at treating the progression of AS [199-201]. In these trials, three different statin therapies were investigated in patients with mild to moderate AS and it was determined that statin therapy did not alter the progression of CAVD/AS nor prevent outcomes such as the necessity to undergo aortic valve replacement surgery [199-201]. In response to the negative outcomes of these large clinical trials, the use of statin therapy was next investigated in patients with the earliest form of CAVD/AS, aortic valve sclerosis, to determine if statin use could prevent, rather than reverse, AS [202]. In this report, statin therapy was significantly associated with a decreased development of AS and a decreased need for aortic valve replacement surgery, suggesting that statin therapy may be an effective treatment if started at the earliest stages of the disease, prior to any indication of valve calcification [202]. Based on these studies, it can be concluded that in humans, statin therapy is ineffective at preventing the progression of AS and reversing aortic valve calcification. However, statin therapy may be useful at preventing the onset of AS in patients with the earliest stages of aortic valve thickening.

5.2. Angiotensin converting enzyme inhibitors/Angiotensin receptor blockers

Another potential therapy to prevent the progression of CAVD/AS is the use of the anti-hypertensive angiotensin-converting enzyme inhibitors (ACEI) and angiotensin receptor blockers (ARB). Currently, ACEIs and ARBs are prescribed to treat hypertension, and function by acting on the renin-angiotensin-aldosterone system to ultimately inhibit the vasoconstrictor effects of angiotensin II [203]. Previous reports have identified the overlapping expression of angiotensin-converting enzyme (ACE) and angiotensin II in calcified human aortic valves surrounding regions of valvular calcification [133]. It has been hypothesized that ACE inhibition may prevent the progression of CAVD by reducing ACE activity in the diseased valve leaflet [204-206]. A study conducted in ApoE knockout mice with induced chronic renal failure concluded that animals treated with the ACEI enalapril had significantly reduced levels of pathologic aortic valve leaflet thickening and valve fibrosis than untreated animals [206]. Similarly, in a rabbit model of CAVD in which the animals were fed a high vitamin D diet, treatment with the ACEI ramipril significantly reduced the progression to AS, improved valve endothelial cell integrity, and reduced aortic valve calcification [205]. It is uncertain how ACE and angiotensin receptor (AR) inhibition would directly affect molecular changes in the valve leaflets. However, in a study of rabbits fed a high cholesterol diet, treatment with the ARB olmesartan decreased the number of α SMA positive myofibroblasts and reduced expression of the osteogenic markers *Runx2* and OPN, compared to untreated control animals [204]. These animal studies suggest that ACE and/or AR inhibition may reduce pathologic changes in aortic valve disease by limiting valve fibrosis, reducing myofibroblast activation, and decreasing osteogenic gene expression.

Clinical studies testing the therapeutic benefits of ACEIs and ARBs in CAVD progression have had mixed results. In human explanted aortic valve tissues, ARB therapy is associated with reduced aortic valve remodeling and calcification [207]. As in animal studies, this histological analysis suggests that AR inhibition may limit aortic valve calcification [207]. In a small pilot clinical study (Symptomatic Cardiac Obstruction – Pilot Study of Enalapril in

Aortic Stenosis), use of the ACEI Enalapril was associated with improved clinical symptoms in patients with severe symptomatic AS [208]. The majority of studies investigating the use of ACEIs or ARBs in CAVD/AS with positive outcomes have been retrospective. In three different retrospective studies, ACEI or ARB use in patients with mild to moderate AS was associated with decreased mortality, decreased number of adverse cardiovascular events, slower progression of AS, and less accumulation of valvular calcification [209-211]. Additionally, one prospective study followed a small random population of patients over a 4-year period and reported that the use of ACEIs or ARBs was significantly associated with reduced CAVD/AS disease progression [212]. Together, these studies provide evidence that ACEI and ARB may delay CAVD progression. Conversely, there have also been a number of studies that show no association between ACEI and ARB use and improved outcomes in CAVD progression. The JASS study (Japanese Aortic Stenosis Study) reported that ARB therapy in patients with moderate to severe AS had no beneficial outcomes in CAVD progression, although patients with mild asymptomatic AS had some indication of reduced progression to AS [213]. Furthermore, a large study in patients with very mild asymptomatic AS found that patients on ACEI or ARB therapy had no improvement in the progression of AS compared against a control group [202]. Similarly, a small 2-year study observed no difference in the hemodynamic progression of AS with ACEI use versus non-use [198]. Based on both animal and clinical studies, it is unclear whether ACEI or ARB therapy is an effective treatment option to prevent the progression of CAVD/AS, however there are indications that perhaps this therapy may limit valve calcification [204, 207]. A placebo controlled, blinded trial will be necessary to determine the effectiveness of these therapies in treating CAVD.

5.3. Aldosterone-receptor antagonists

Aldosterone is a component of the renin-angiotensin-aldosterone system that plays a key role in the kidney to regulate water and sodium reabsorption and effectively raise blood pressure [203]. Aldosterone-receptor antagonists (ARA) are commonly prescribed for their diuretic effects [203]. Recently, there have been two studies investigating the use of ARAs in the treatment of CAVD/AS. In an animal study, rabbits fed a high cholesterol diet develop aortic valve sclerosis, with thickening of the valve leaflets and microscopic calcific deposits, which was blocked by treatment with the ARA eplerenone [214]. In addition to reducing valve fibrosis and mineralization, evidence of macrophage infiltration was also reduced [214]. Conversely, in a small placebo-controlled human trial of patients with moderate to severe asymptomatic AS, there was no difference in the progression of AS in those patients receiving the ARA eplerenone versus placebo [215]. To our knowledge, no molecular evidence has been reported in studies on ARA therapy in CAVD and it is unknown whether ARA therapy affects myofibroblast activation or osteogenic gene induction. Additional clinical studies will be necessary to determine if ARA use can prevent AS progression if therapy is started in early disease stages.

5.4. Bisphosphonates

Bisphosphonates (BP) are a class of drugs that mimic inorganic pyrophosphate and prevent ectopic soft tissue calcification and inhibit bone resorption [216]. In adults, especially women, BPs are commonly prescribed to treat excessive bone resorption associated with osteoporosis [216]. Human aortic VICs, grown on collagen gels in the presence of a specialized thiol bisphosphonate, have decreased ALP activity and reduced cellular aggregation, a step that precedes calcific nodule formation, as compared to cells grown on collagen alone [217]. This study suggests that bisphosphonates may inhibit VIC calcification in vitro and could serve as a potential therapeutic strategy to prevent aortic valve calcification [217]. Due to the ability of BPs to prevent ectopic calcification in bone and the availability of patient populations currently using BPs, a number of studies have investigated the use of BPs in the inhibition of aortic valve calcification. Three small retrospective human studies compared measurements of AS progression over a 2-year period in patients with AS taking BPs versus those not taking BPs [218-220]. The results of these studies suggest a modest reduction in the progression of AS in those patients taking BPs [218-220]. The large MESA study (Multi-Ethnic Study of Atherosclerosis) followed women taking BPs, compared to those not taking BPs, and their development of CAVD/AS over time [221]. The results of this study were mixed and showed that, in older women, BP therapy was associated with a slight benefit in terms of aortic valve calcification, whereas, younger women taking BPs had significantly more progression of aortic valve calcification compared to women not taking BPs [221]. Most recently, a large retrospective study investigated the progression of AS in women with mild to moderate AS over a 5-year period and compared the outcomes in patients on BP therapy versus those not taking BPs [222]. The evidence from this study shows that there was no change in survival, or in the number of aortic valve replacement surgeries, in women taking BPs compared to those not taking BPs, suggesting that BP therapy does not suppress the progression of CAVD/AS [222]. Thus far, the outcomes of the human studies investigating the use of bisphosphonate therapy in CAVD demonstrate that this therapy is ineffective at preventing or delaying the progression of CAVD/AS. To definitively determine whether or not BP therapy is effective at suppressing the progression of CAVD/AS, placebo-controlled prospective studies will be necessary.

5.5. Nitric oxide bioavailability

Endothelial nitric oxide synthase (eNOS) produces nitric oxide (NO) from L-arginine, and eNOS expression has been identified in the endothelial cells lining the aortic valves [68]. eNOS deficiency has been linked to defective aortic valve development, as approximately 50% of eNOS deficient mice develop a bicuspid, rather than tricuspid, aortic valve [68]. eNOS deficient mice with a BAV phenotype fed a high cholesterol diet develop hemodynamic symptoms of AS and also display microscopic mineralization in the aortic valve leaflets, indicating that eNOS activity may be important for suppressing aortic valve calcification [178]. Nitric Oxide deficiency is also an indicator of endothelial cell dysfunction, and systemic endothelial cell dysfunction is prevalent in patients with aortic valve sclerosis/stenosis [223-225]. The uncoupling, or dysfunction, of eNOS results in decreased NO production and increased generation of reactive oxygen species (ROS) [223]. ROS activity is present in calcific lesions of human stenotic aortic valves, and it has been suggested that ROS activity may speed aortic valve calcification [144, 226]. In animal studies, rabbits fed a high cholesterol/high vitamin D diet develop aortic valve thickening, small deposits of valve calcification, and increased ROS activity in cells surrounding regions of valve calcification [226]. Furthermore, ROS activity was co-localized to clusters of cells expressing Runx2 and OPN, suggesting that ROS activity is associated with VICs displaying an osteogenic-like phenotype [226]. In VIC culture studies, TGFβ1 stimulation induces increased ROS activity, along with calcific nodule formation and ALP activity [227]. Increasing the availability of NO, via NO donors such as sodium nitroprusside, partially blocks both nodule formation and ALP activity, suggesting that NO levels are important for reducing ROS and inhibiting calcification in VICs [227]. There have been a number of small clinical studies investigating the levels of the NOS inhibitor, asymmetric dimethylarginine (ADMA), an indicator of endothelial cell dysfunction, in patients with moderate to severe AS [228-230]. In these studies, plasma levels of ADMA are significantly higher in patients with moderate to severe AS, compared to patients with mild AS or no disease, suggesting that NO production is disrupted in CAVD/AS [228-230]. Combined, these studies suggest that increased ROS production is associated with aortic valve calcification and the induction of osteogenic gene expression. Thus, increasing the bioavailability of NO may be a potential therapeutic avenue to block ROS activity, and thereby disease progression, in CAVD.

5.6. NSAIDs/COX2 inhibitors

Previous reports have demonstrated that immune cell infiltration is common in CAVD [119, 132, 135]. Non-steroidal anti-inflammatory drugs (NSAIDS) are commonly used to treat pain and inflammation, and act by inhibiting the enzymes COX1 and/or COX2 [231-233]. These enzymes function by converting arachidonic acid to prostaglandins (PGs) [233, 234]. There has been one study conducted in human aortic VICs, demonstrating that stimulation of VICs with pro-inflammatory mimetics induces the expression of COX2 and the release of prostaglandins [235]. This study suggests that COX2 inhibition may be one way to treat the immune response associated with CAVD [235]. Interestingly, COX2 and PG signaling are also involved in bone formation as well as cellular responses to physical stress and strain, processes that also likely contribute to CAVD (reviewed in [131]). In bone, PG signaling has an anabolic effect, and PG treatment of osteoblast cultures results in increased expression of OCN, BMP2, Runx2, OPN, ALP, and BSP [236-244]. In osteoblast cultures, BMP2 stimulation induces COX2 expression through upregulation of Runx2, which binds to and activates the COX2 promoter [245, 246]. Downstream, PG signaling induces the expression of p38 MAPK through the activation of protein kinase A [243, 247]. Furthermore, fluid shear stress and other physical forces induce COX2 expression in osteoblast-like cells, suggesting that increased COX2 and PG signaling is a cellular response to altered mechanical forces [248, 249]. The combined results of these studies suggest that COX2/PG signaling may be an effective therapeutic target to treat CAVD progression, as COX2/PG signaling plays a role in inflammation, osteogenesis, and cellular response to physical strain, all of which are thought to be pathological mechanisms involved in CAVD [131, 243, 244, 248-251]. It would be interesting

http://dx.doi.org/10.5772/54356

to determine whether COX2 inhibition/NSAID use could reduce CAVD progression. However, one caveat is that COX2 inhibitor therapy can be associated with some rare but significant adverse cardiovascular events such as myocardial infarction and stroke [252, 253]. Perhaps therapeutics designed toward downstream targets of PG signaling, such as p38 MAPK, could improve outcomes of CAVD patients without the cardiovascular side effects of selective coxibs [254].

5.7. Development of new therapeutic approaches based on valvulogenic and osteogenic molecular mechanisms.

As reviewed above, Notch, Wnt, and BMP signaling have been implicated in the progression of CAVD. Pharmacotherapies designed to act as Wnt and BMP inhibitors, or Notch agonists, could be a potential avenue for new therapeutics to treat the progression of CAVD. BMP signaling is thought to be a specific indicator of aortic valve calcification as active BMP signaling is observed in adult diseased valves with prominent calcification and is not found in pediatric diseased valves void of calcification [13]. Furthermore, BMP2 signaling stimulates VIC calcific nodule formation and induces osteogenic gene expression [138, 171]. It is possible that therapies designed to inhibit BMP signaling will block osteogenic-like calcification in diseased aortic valves. Likewise, inhibition of the Wnt/β-catenin signaling pathway may also serve to reduce aortic valve calcification during disease, which is supported by evidence from animal studies in ApoE knockout mice. When fed an atherogenic diet, ApoE knockout mice reportedly develop aortic valve calcification, however, when the Wnt co-receptor Lrp5 is genetically deleted in these mice, the amount of aortic valve calcification is significantly reduced [180]. Therefore, Wnt inhibition may be another potential therapeutic approach for treating CAVD. Lastly, strategies to maintain Notch signaling in the valves may be another potential way to inhibit calcification in CAVD. Notch inhibition of calcification and osteogenic gene expression has been demonstrated in aortic VICs in culture and reduced Notch signaling in vivo leads to CAVD in mice [65, 153, 175]. Furthermore, Notch1 haploinsufficiency in humans is associated with CAVD, indicating that maintaining Notch signaling is important for valve homeostasis [64]. Thus, therapeutic strategies designed to affect one or more of these pathways may serve to prevent valve calcification in CAVD. A potential limitation of this approach is that BMP, Wnt, and Notch signaling pathways are involved in many homeostatic and disease processes. For example, Wnt signaling is increased in many types of cancer, and all three pathways are involved in bone homeostasis. Therefore the development of therapeutics based on these molecular mechanisms must take into account potential effects on multiple organ systems. Nevertheless, targeted approaches based on these pathways could represent a new therapeutic avenue in the development of pharmacologic based approaches to CAVD.

6. Conclusions and future directions

There are numerous examples of shared molecular pathways between valvulogenesis, osteogenesis, and disease pathogenesis of CAVD. In valvulogenesis, signaling factors involved in early cushion formation, such as BMP, Notch, and Wnt/β-catenin pathways are active in osteogenesis and in CAVD [7-9, 14]. Furthermore, transcription factors expressed in the early valve mesenchyme, such as Twist1, Msx2, and Sox9, can also be found in the primitive condensed bone mesenchyme and in the mesenchymal-like cells identified in diseased aortic valve tissues [8, 13, 80, 255]. In addition to signaling and transcription factors, molecular pathways governing ECM production and remodeling, such as the RANKL – NFATc1 – CtsK pathway are shared amongst valve progenitor, developing bone, and diseased valve tissues [11, 47, 103, 106, 193]. This commonality suggests that the mesenchymal cells found within these tissues are governed by common molecular pathways and that these developmental pathways are reactivated during disease. Additional parallels can be drawn between calcification of the embryonic bone tissues and calcification observed in diseased aortic valves. For example, the endochondral bone factors Runx2, OCN, and BSP are reactivated during aortic valve disease, suggesting that osteogenic molecular pathways are activated during CAVD and may contribute to pathogenic calcification [5, 13, 76, 80, 106, 152]. Effective pharmacological therapies to treat CAVD remain elusive and identifying potential targets for new pharmacotherapies is a priority, as the only effective treatment for CAVD with AS is valve replacement surgery [256]. Studies testing the effectiveness of statin therapy, inhibitors of the renin-angiotensin-aldosterone, and bisphosphonates in slowing the progression of CAVD have been disappointing (see therapeutic section). New therapeutic strategies are needed and, perhaps, targeted inhibition of BMP and Wnt signaling or maintenance of Notch signaling may provide new avenues for potential CAVD treatments.

Author details

Elaine E. Wirrig and Katherine E. Yutzey*

*Address all correspondence to: Katherine.yutzey@cchmc.org

The Heart Institute, Cincinnati Children's Hospital Medical Center, Cincinnati, Ohio, USA

References

[1] Roger VL, Go AS, Lloyd-Jones DM, Adams RJ, Berry JD, Brown TM, et al. Heart disease and stroke statistics--2011 update: A report from the American Heart Association Circulation. 2011;123:e18-e209.

[2] Otto CM. Valvular aortic stenosis: disease severity and timing of intervention. J Am Coll Cardiol. 2006;47:2141-2151.

[3] Bonow RO, Carabello BA, Kanu C, de Leon AC, Jr., Faxon DP, Freed MD, et al. ACC/AHA 2006 guidelines for the management of patients with valvular heart disease: a report of the American College of Cardiology/American Heart Association

Task Force on Practice Guidelines (writing committee to revise the 1998 Guidelines for the Management of Patients With Valvular Heart Disease). Circulation. 2006;114:e84-231.

[4] Roberts WC, Ko JM. Frequency by decades of unicuspid, bicuspid and tricuspid aortic valves in adults having isolated aortic valve replacement for aortic stenosis, with or without associated aortic regurgitation. Circulation. 2005;111:920-925.

[5] Rajamannan NM, Subramaniam M, Rickard DJ, Stock SR, Donovan J, Springett M, et al. Human aortic valve calcification is associated with an osteoblast phenotype. Circulation. 2003;107:2181-2184.

[6] O'Brien KD. Pathogenesis of calcific aortic valve disease: a disease process comes of age (and a good deal more). Arterioscler Thromb Vasc Biol. 2006;26:1721-1728.

[7] Bostrom K, Rajamannan NM, Towler DA. The regulation of valvular and vascular sclerosis by osteogenic morphogens. Circ Res. 2011;109:564-577.

[8] Combs MD, Yutzey KE. Heart valve development: Regulatory networks in development and disease. Circ Res. 2009;105:408-421.

[9] Karsenty G, Kronenberg HM, Settembre C. Genetic control of bone formation. Annu Rev Cell Dev Biol. 2009;25:629-648.

[10] Hinton RB, Yutzey KE. Heart valve structure and function in development and disease. Annu Rev Physiol. 2011;73:29-46.

[11] Lincoln J, Lange AW, Yutzey KE. Hearts and bones: Shared regulatory mechanisms in heart valve, cartilage, tendon, and bone development. Dev Biol. 2006;294:292-302.

[12] Chakraborty S, Wirrig EE, Hinton RB, Merrill WH, Spicer DB, Yutzey KE. Twist1 promotes heart valve cell proliferation and extracellular matrix gene expression during development in vivo and is expressed in human diseased aortic valves. Dev Biol. 2010;347:167-179.

[13] Wirrig EE, Hinton RB, Yutzey KE. Differential expression of cartilage and bone-related proteins in pediatric and adult diseased aortic valves. J Mol Cell Cardiol. 2011;50:561-569.

[14] Miller JD, Weiss RM, Heistad DD. Calcific aortic valve stenosis: Methods, models, and mechanisms. Circ Res. 2011;108:1392-1412.

[15] Schroeder JA, Jackson LF, Lee DC, Camenisch TD. Form and function of developing heart valves: coordination by extracellular matrix growth and signaling. J Mol Med. 2003;81:392-403.

[16] Person AD, Klewer SE, Runyan RB. Cell biology of cardiac cushion development. Int Rev Cytol. 2005;243:287-335.

[17] Camenisch TD, Molin DG, Person A, Runyan RB, Gittenberger-de Groot AC, McDonald JA, et al. Temporal and distinct TGFbeta ligand requirements during mouse and avian endocardial cushion morphogenesis. Dev Biol. 2002;248:170-181.

[18] Ma L, Lu MF, Schwartz RJ, Martin JF. Bmp2 is essential for cardiac cushion epithelial-mesenchymal transition and myocardial patterning. Development. 2005;132:5601-5611.

[19] Rivera-Feliciano J, Tabin CJ. Bmp2 instructs cardiac progenitors to form the heart-valve-inducing field. Dev Biol. 2006;295:580-588.

[20] McCulley DJ, Kang JO, Martin JF, Black BL. BMP4 is required in the anterior heart field and its derivatives for endocardial cushion remodeling, outflow tract septation, and semilunar valve development. Dev Dyn. 2008;237:3200-3209.

[21] Snarr BS, Kern CB, Wessels A. Origin and fate of cardiac mesenchyme. Dev Dyn. 2008;237:2804-2819.

[22] Lin C-J, Lin C-Y, Chen C-H, Zhou B, Chang C-P. Partitioning the heart: mechanisms of cardiac septation and valve development. Development. 2012;139:3277-3299.

[23] Lincoln J, Alfieri CM, Yutzey KE. Development of heart valve leaflets and supporting apparatus in chicken and mouse embryos. Dev Dyn. 2004;230:239-250.

[24] Hinton RB, Lincoln J, Deutsch GH, Osinska H, Manning PB, Benson DW, et al. Extracellular matrix remodeling and organization in developing and diseased aortic valves. Circ Res. 2006;98:1431-1438.

[25] deLange FJ, Moorman AFM, Anderson RH, Manner J, Soufan AT, deGier-deVries C, et al. Lineage and morphogenetic analysis of the cardiac valves. Circ Res. 2004;95:645-654.

[26] Rochais F, Mesbah K, Kelly RG. Signaling pathways controlling second heart field development. Circ Res. 2009;104:933-942.

[27] Nakamura T, Colbert MC, Robbins J. Neural crest cells retain multipotential characteristics in the developing valves and label the cardiac conduction system. Circ Res. 2006;98:1547-1554.

[28] Jiang X, Rowitch DH, Soriano P, McMahon AP, Sucov HM. Fate of the mammalian cardiac neural crest. Development. 2000;127:1607-1616.

[29] Jain R, Engleka KA, Rentschler SL, Manderfield LJ, Li L, Yuan L, et al. Cardiac neural crest orchestrates remodeling and functional maturation of mouse semilunar valves. J Clin Invest. 2011;121:422-430.

[30] Zhang J, Chang JY, Huang Y, Lin X, Schwartz RJ, Martin JF, et al. The FGF-BMP signaling axis regulates outflow tract valve primordium formation by promoting cushion neural crest cell differentiation. Circ Res. 2010;107:1209-1219.

[31] Wessels A, van den Hoff MJ, Adamo RF, Phelps AL, Lockhart MM, Sauls K, et al. Epicardially derived fibroblasts preferentially contribute to the parietal leaflets of the atrioventricular valves in the murine heart. Dev Biol. 2012;366:111-124.

[32] Zhou B, Ma Q, Rajagopal S, Wu SM, Domian I, Rivera-Feliciano J, et al. Epicardial progenitors contribute to the cardiomyocyte lineage in the developing heart. Nature. 2008;454:109-113.

[33] Visconti RP, Ebihara Y, LaRue AC, Fleming PA, McQuinn TC, Masuya M, et al. An in vivo analysis of hematopoietic stem cell potential: hematopoietic origin of cardiac valve interstitial cells. Circ Res. 2006;98:690-696.

[34] Hajdu Z, Romeo SJ, Fleming PA, Markwald RR, Visconti RP, Drake CJ. Recruitment of bone marrow-derived valve interstitial cells is a normal homeostatic process. J Mol Cell Cardiol. 2011;51:955-965.

[35] Chakraborty S, Combs MD, Yutzey KE. Transcriptional regulation of heart valve progenitor cells. Pediatr Cardiol. 2010;31:414-421.

[36] Timmerman LA, Grego-Bessa J, Raya A, Bertran E, Perez-Pomares JM, Diez J, et al. Notch promotes epithelial-mesenchymal transition during cardiac development and oncogenic transformation. Genes Dev. 2004;18:99-115.

[37] Tao G, Levay AK, Gridley T, Lincoln J. Mmp15 is a direct target of Snai1 during endothelial to mesenchymal transformation and endocardial cushion development. Dev Biol. 2011;359:209-221.

[38] Shelton EL, Yutzey KE. Twist1 function in endocardial cell proliferation, migration, and differentiation during heart valve development. Dev Biol. 2008;317:282-295.

[39] Shelton EL, Yutzey KE. Tbx20 regulation of endocardial cushion cell proliferation and extracellular matrix gene expression. Dev Biol. 2007;302:376-388.

[40] Lincoln J, Kist R, Scherer G, Yutzey KE. Sox9 is required for precursor cell expansion and extracellular matrix gene expression. Dev Biol. 2007;302:376-388.

[41] Chen YH, Ishii M, Sukov HM, Maxson RE. Msx1 and Msx2 are required for endothelial-mesenchymal transformation of the atrioventricular cushions and patterning of the atrioventricular myocardium. BMC Dev Biol. 2008;8:75.

[42] Lee MP, Yutzey KE. Twist1 directly regulates genes that promote cell proliferation and migration in developing heart valves. PLoS One. 2011;6:e29758.

[43] Chakraborty S, Cheek J, Sakthivel B, Aronow BJ, Yutzey KE. Shared gene expression profiles in developing heart valves and osteoblasts. Physiol Genomics. 2008;35:75-85.

[44] Aikawa E, Whittaker P, Farber M, Mendelson K, Padera RF, Aikawa M, et al. Human semilunar cardiac valve remodeling by activated cells from fetus to adult. Circulation. 2006;113:1344-1352.

[45] de la Pompa JL, Timmerman LA, Takimoto H, Yoshida H, Elia AJ, Samper E, et al. Role of NF-ATc transcription factor in morphogenesis of cardiac valves and septum. Nature. 1998;392:182-186.

[46] Ranger AM, Grusby MJ, Gravallese EM, de la Brousse FC, Hoey T, Mickanin C, et al. The transcription factor NF-ATc is essential for cardiac valve formation. Nature. 1998;392:186-190.

[47] Combs MD, Yutzey KE. VEGF and RANKL regulation of NFATc1 in heart valve development. Circ Res. 2009;105:565-574.

[48] Lincoln J, Alfieri CM, Yutzey KE. BMP and FGF regulatory pathways control cell lineage diversification of heart valve precursor cells. Dev Biol. 2006;292:290-302.

[49] Peacock JD, Levay AK, Gillaspie DB, Tao G, Lincoln J. Reduced Sox9 function promotes heart valve calcification phenotypes in vivo. Circ Res. 2010;106:712-719.

[50] Levay AK, Peacock JD, Lu Y, Koch M, Hinton RB, Kadler KE, et al. Scleraxis is required for cell lineage differentiation and extracellular matrix remodeling during murine heart formation in vivo. Circ Res. 2008;103:948-956.

[51] Luna-Zurita L, Prados B, Grego-Bessa J, Luxan G, del Monte G, Benguria A, et al. Integration of a Notch-dependent mesenchymal gene program and BMP2-driven cell invasiveness regulates murine cardiac valve formation. J Clin Invest. 2010;120:3493-3507.

[52] Dor Y, Camenisch TD, Itin A, Fishman GI, McDonald JA, Carmeliet P, et al. A novel role for VEGF in endocardial cushion formation and its potential contribution to congenital heart defects. Development. 2001;128:1531-1538.

[53] Liebner S, Cattelino A, Gallini R, Rudini N, Iurlaro M, Piccolo S, et al. β-catenin is required for endothelial-mesenchymal transformation during heart cushion development in the mouse. J Cell Biol. 2004;166:359-367.

[54] Person AD, Garriock RJ, Krieg PA, Runyan RB, Klewer SE. Frzb modulates Wnt-9a-mediated β-catenin signaling during avian atrioventricular cardiac cushion development. Dev Biol. 2005;278:35-48.

[55] Jackson LF, Qiu TH, Sunnarborg SW, Chang A, Zhang C, Patterson C, et al. Defective valvulogenesis in HB-EGF and TACE-null mice is associated with aberrant BMP signaling. EMBO J. 2003;22:2704-2716.

[56] Delot EC, Bahamonde ME, Zhao M, Lyons KM. BMP signaling is required for septation of the outflow tract of the mammalian heart. Development. 2003;130:209-220.

[57] Beppu H, Malhotra RR, Beppu Y, Lepore JJ, Parmacek MS, Bloch KD. BMP type II receptor regulates positioning of the outflow tract and remodeling of the atrioventricular cushion during cardiogenesis. Dev Biol. 2009;331:167-175.

[58] Galvin KM, Donovan MJ, Lynch CA, Meyer RI, Paul RJ, Lorenz JN, et al. A role for smad6 in development and homeostasis of the cardiovascular system. Nat Genet. 2000;24:171-174.

[59] Zhao B, Etter L, Hinton RB, Benson DW. BMP and FGF regulatory pathways in semilunar valve precursor cells. Dev Dyn. 2007;236:971-980.

[60] Alfieri CM, Cheek J, Chakraborty S, Yutzey KE. Wnt signaling in heart valve development and osteogenic gene induction. Dev Biol. 2010;338:127-135.

[61] Lange AW, Yutzey KE. NFATc1 expression in the developing heart valves is responsive to the RANKL pathway and is required for endocardial expression of cathepsin K. Dev Biol. 2006;292:407-417.

[62] del Monte G, Grego-Bessa J, Gozalez-Rajal A, Bolos V, delaPompa JL. Monitoring Notch1 activity in development: evidence for a feedback regulatory loop. Dev Dyn. 2007;236:2594-2614.

[63] Cripe L, Andelfinger G, Martin LJ, Shooner K, Benson DW. Bicuspid aortic valve is heritable. J Am Coll Cardiol. 2004;44:138-143.

[64] Garg V, Muth AN, Ransom JF, Schluterman MK, Barnes R, King IN, et al. Mutations in NOTCH1 cause aortic valve disease. Nature. 2005;437:270-274.

[65] Nus M, MacGrogan D, Martinez-Poveda B, Benito Y, Casanova JC, Fernandez-Aviles F, et al. Diet-induced aortic valve disease in mice haploinsufficient for the Notch pathway effector RBPJK/CSL. Arterioscler Thromb Vasc Biol. 2011;31:1580-1588.

[66] Laforest B, Andelfinger G, Nemer M. Loss of Gata5 in mice leads to bicuspid aortic valve. J Clin Invest. 2011;121:2876-2887.

[67] Padang R, Bagnall RD, Richmond DR, Bannon PG, Semsarian C. Rare non-synonymous variations in the transcriptional activation domains of GATA5 in bicupid aortic valve disease. J Mol Cell Cardiol. 2012;53:277-291.

[68] Lee TC, Zhao YD, Courtman DW, Stewart DJ. Abnormal aortic valve development in mice lacking endothelial nitric oxide synthase. Circulation. 2000;101:2345-2348.

[69] Schoen FJ. Evolving concepts of cardiac valve dynamics. Circulation. 2008;118:1864-1880.

[70] Snider P, Hinton RB, Moreno-Rodriguez R, Wang J, Rogers R, Lindsley A, et al. Periostin is required for maturation and extracellular matrix stabilization of noncardiomyocyte lineages of the heart. Circ Res. 2008;102:752-760.

[71] Norris RA, Moreno-Rodriguez RA, Sugi Y, Hoffman S, Amos J, Hart MM, et al. Periostin regulates atrioventricular valve maturation. Dev Biol. 2008;316:200-213.

[72] Hinton RB, Adelman-Brown J, Witt S, Krishnamurthy VK, Osinska H, Sakthivel B, et al. Elastin haploinsufficiency results in progressive aortic valve malformation and latent valve disease in a mouse model. Circ Res. 2010;107:549-557.

[73] Cheek JD, Wirrig EE, Alfieri CM, James JF, Yutzey KE. Differential activation of valvulogenic, chondrogenic, and osteogenic pathways in mouse models of myxomatous and calcific aortic valve disease. J Mol Cell Cardiol. 2012;52:689-700.

[74] Kern CB, Wessels A, McGarity J, Dixon LJ, Alston E, Argraves WS, et al. Reduced versican cleavage due to Adamts9 haploinsufficiency is associated with cardiac and aortic anomalies. Matrix Biol. 2010;29:304-316.

[75] Dupuis LE, McCulloch DR, McGarity JD, Bahan A, Wessels A, Weber D, et al. Altered versican cleavage in ADAMTS5 deficient mice; a novel etiology of myxomatous valve disease. Dev Biol. 2011;357:152-164.

[76] Karsenty G, Wagner EF. Reaching a genetic and molecular understanding of skeletal development. Dev Cell. 2002;2:389-406.

[77] Lefebvre V, Bhattaram P. Vertebrate skeletogenesis. Curr Top Dev Biol. 2010;90:291-317.

[78] Chai Y, Jiang X, Ito Y, Bringas P, Jr., Han J, Rowitch DH, et al. Fate of the mammalian cranial neural crest during tooth and mandibular morphogenesis. Development. 2000;127:1671-1679.

[79] Karsenty G. Transcriptional control of skeletogenesis. Annu Rev Genomics Hum Genet. 2008;9:183-196.

[80] Long F. Building strong bones: molecular regulation of the osteoblast lineage. Nat Rev Mol Cell Biol. 2012;13:27-38.

[81] Goldring MB, Tsuchimochi K, Ijiri K. The control of chondrogenesis. J Cell Biochem. 2006;97:33-44.

[82] Yoshioka M, Yuasa S, Matsumura K, Kimura K, Shiomi T, Kimura N, et al. Chondromodulin-I maintains cardiac valvular function by preventing angiogenesis. Nat Med. 2006;12:1151-1159.

[83] Nakashima K, Zhou X, Kunkel G, Zhang Z, Deng JM, Behringer RR, et al. The novel zinc finger-containing transcription factor osterix is required for osteoblast differentiation and bone formation. Cell. 2002;108:17-29.

[84] Bialek P, Kern B, Yang X, Schrock M, Sosoc D, Hong N, et al. A Twist code determines the onset of osteoblast differentiation. Dev Cell. 2004;6:423-435.

[85] Gu S, Boyer TG, Naski M. Basic helix-loop-helix transcription factor Twist1 inhibits transactivator function of master chondrogenic regulator Sox9. J Biol Chem. 2012;287:21082-21092.

[86] Yousfi M, Lasmoles F, Lomri A, Delannoy P, Marie PJ. Increased bone formation and decreased osteocalcin expression induced by reduced Twist dosage in Saethre-Chotzen syndrome. J Clin Invest. 2001;107:1153-1161.

[87] Dodig M, Tadic T, Kronenberg MS, Dacic S, Liu YH, Maxson RE, et al. Ectopic Msx2 overexpression inhibits and Msx2 antisense stimulates calvarial osteoblast differentiation. Dev Biol. 1999;209:298-307.

[88] Akiyama H, Chaboissier M-C, Martin JF, Schedl A, de Crombrugghe B. The transcription factor Sox9 has essential roles in successive steps of the chondrocyte differentiation pathway and is required for expression of Sox5 and Sox6. Genes Dev. 2002;16:2813-2828.

[89] Chimal-Monroy J, Rodriguez-Leon J, Montero JA, Ganan Y, Macias D, Merino R, et al. Analysis of the molecular cascade responsible for mesodermal limb chondrogenesis: Sox genes and BMP signaling. Dev Biol. 2003;257:292-301.

[90] Lefebvre V, Huang W, Harley VR, Goodfellow PN, de Crombrugghe B. SOX9 is a potent activator of the chondrocyte-specific enhancer of the pro alpha1(II) collagen gene. Mol Cell Biol. 1997;17:2336-2346.

[91] Sekiya I, Tsuji K, Koopman P, Watanabe T, Yamada Y, Shinomiya K, et al. SOX9 enhances aggrecan gene promoter/enhancer activity and is up-regulated by retinoic acids in a cartilage-derived cell line, TC6. J Biol Chem. 2000;275:10738-10744.

[92] Dy P, Wang W, Bhattaram P, Wang Q, Wang L, Ballock RT, et al. Sox9 directs hypertrophic maturation and blocks osteoblast differentiation of growth plate chondrocytes. Dev Cell. 2012;22:597-609.

[93] Ducy P, Zhang R, Geoffroy V, Ridall AL, Karsenty G. Osf/Cbfa1: a transcriptional activator of osteoblast differentiation. Cell. 1997;89:747-754.

[94] Zamurovic N, Cappellen D, Rohner D, Susa M. Coordinated activation of Notch, Wnt, and transforming growth factor-beta signaling pathways in bone morphogenetic 2-induced osteogenesis. J Biol Chem. 2004;279:37704-37715.

[95] Ducy P, Starbuck M, Priemel M, Shen J, Pinero G, Geoffroy V, et al. A Cbfa1-dependent genetic pathway controls bone formation beyond embryonic development. Genes Dev. 1999;13:1025-1036.

[96] Boyle WJ, Simonet WS, Lacey DL. Osteoclast differentiation and activation. Nature. 2003;423:337-342.

[97] Takayanagi H, Kim S, Koga T, Nishina H, Isshiki M, Yoshida H, et al. Induction and activation of the transcription factor NFATc1 (NFAT2) integrate RANKL signaling and terminal differentiation of osteoclasts. Dev Cell. 2002;8:889-901.

[98] Ishida N, Hayashi K, Hoshijima M, Ogawa T, Koga S, Miyatake Y, et al. Large scale gene expression analysis of osteoclastogenesis in vitro and elucidation of NFAT2 as a key regulator. J Biol Chem. 2002;277:41147-41156.

[99] Simonet WS, Lacey DL, Dunstan CR, Kelley M, Chang MS, Luthy R, et al. Osteoprotegerin: a novel secreted protein involved in the regulation of bone density. Cell. 1997;89:309-319.

[100] Yasuda H, Shima N, Nakagawa N, Mochizuki SA, Yano K, Fujise N, et al. Identity of osteoclastogenesis inhibitor factor (OCIF) and osteoprotegerin (OPG): a mechanism by which OPG/OCIF inhibits osteoclastogenesis in vitro. Endocrinology. 1998;139:1329-1337.

[101] Koga T, Matsui Y, Asagiri M, Kodama T, de Crombrugge B, Nakashima K, et al. NFAT and Osterix cooperatively regulate bone formation. Nat Med. 2005;11:880-885.

[102] Winslow MM, Pan M, Starbuck M, Gallo EM, Deng L, Karsenty G, et al. Calcineurin/ NFAT signaling in osteoblasts regulates bone mass. Dev Cell. 2006;10:771-782.

[103] Kaden JJ, Bickelhaupt S, Grobholz R, Haase KK, Sarikoc A, Kilic R, et al. Receptor activator of nuclear factor kB ligand and osteoprotegerin regulate aortic valve calcification. J Mol Cell Cardiol. 2004;36:57-66.

[104] Rabkin-Aikawa E, Farber M, Aikawa M, Schoen FJ. Dynamic and reversible changes in interstitial cell phenotype during remodeling of cardiac valves. J Heart Valve Disease. 2004;13:841-847.

[105] Nishimura R, Wakabayashi M, Hata K, Matsubara T, Honma S, Wakisaka S, et al. Osterix regulates calcification and degradation of chondrogenic matrices through matrix metalloproteinase (MMP13) expression in association with transcription factor Runx2 during endochondral ossification. J Biol Chem. 2012;287:33179-33190.

[106] Alexopoulos A, Bravou V, Peroukides S, Kaklamanis L, Varakis J, Alexopoulos D, et al. Bone regulatory factors NFATc1 and Osterix in human calcific aortic valves. Int J Cardiol. 2010;139:142-149.

[107] Kobayashi T, Kronenberg H. Trascriptional regulation in development of bone. Endocrinology. 2005;146:1012-1017.

[108] Wozney JM, Rosen V, A.J. C, Mitsock LM, Whitters MJ, Kriz RW, et al. Novel regulators of bone formation: molecular clones and activities. Science. 1988;242:1528-1534.

[109] Nishimura R, Hata K, Matsubara T, Wakabayashi M, Yoneda T. Regulation of bone and cartilage development by network between BMP signaling and transcription factors. J Biochem. 2012;151:247-254.

[110] Lin GL, Hakenson KD. Integration of BMP, Wnt, and Notch signaling pathways in osteoblast differentiation. J Cell Biochem. 2011;112:3491-3501.

[111] Rawadi G, Vayssiere B, Dunn F, Baron R, Roman-Roman S. BMP-2 controls alkaline phosphatase expression and osteoblast mineralization by a Wnt auotcrine loop. J Bone Min Res. 2003;18:1842-1853.

[112] Rodriguez-Carballo E, Ulsamer A, Susperregui AR, Manzanares-Cespedes C, Sanchez-Garcia E, Bartrons R, et al. Conserved regulatory motifs in osteogenic gene promoters integrate cooperative effects of canonical Wnt and BMP pathways. J Bone Miner Res. 2011;26:718-729.

[113] Sciaudone M, Gazzerro E, Priest L, Delanty AM, Canalis E. Notch1 impairs osteoblastic cell differentiation. Endocrinology. 2003;144:5631-5639.

[114] Deregowski V, Gazzerro E, Priest L, Rydziel S, Canalis E. Notch 1 overexpression inhibits osteoblastogenesis by suppressing Wnt/β-catenin but not bone morphogenetic protein signaling. J Biol Chem. 2006;218:6203-6210.

[115] Hilton MJ, Tu X, Wu X, Bai S, Zhao H, Kobayashi T, et al. Notch signaling maintains bone marrow mesenchyme progenitors by suppressing osteoblast differentiation. Nat Med. 2008;14:306-314.

[116] Mead TJ, Yutzey KE. Notch pathway regulation of chondrocyte differentiation and proliferation during appendicular and axial skeleton development. Proc Natl Acad Sci USA. 2009;106:14420-14425.

[117] Gross L, Kugel MA. Topographic Anatomy and Histology of the Valves in the Human Heart. Am J Pathol. 1931;7:445-474.

[118] Kaden JJ, Bickelhaupt S, Grobholz R, Vahl CF, Hagl S, Brueckmann M, et al. Expression of bone sialoprotein and bone morphogenetic protein-2 in calcific aortic stenosis. J Heart Valve Dis. 2004;13:560-566.

[119] Otto CM, Kuusisto J, Reichenbach DD, Gown AM, O'Brien KD. Characterization of the early lesion of 'degenerative' valvular aortic stenosis. Histological and immunohistochemical studies. Circulation. 1994;90:844-853.

[120] Thubrikar MJ, Jaffar A, Nolan SP. Patterns of calcific deposits in operatively excised stenotic or purely regurgitant aortic valves and their relation to mechanical stress. Am J Cardiol. 1986;58:304-308.

[121] Turri M, Thiene G, Bortolotti U, Milano A, Mazzucco A, Gallucci V. Surgical pathology of aortic valve disease. A study based on 602 specimens. Eur J Cardiothorac Surg. 1990;4:556-560.

[122] Bonow RO, Carabello BA, Chatterjee K, de Leon AC, Jr., Faxon DP, Freed MD, et al. 2008 Focused update incorporated into the ACC/AHA 2006 guidelines for the management of patients with valvular heart disease: a report of the American College of Cardiology/American Heart Association Task Force on Practice Guidelines (Writing Committee to Revise the 1998 Guidelines for the Management of Patients With Valvular Heart Disease). Circulation. 2008;118:e523-661.

[123] Cosmi JE, Kort S, Tunick PA, Rosenzweig BP, Freedberg RS, Katz ES, et al. The risk of the development of aortic stenosis in patients with "benign" aortic valve thickening. Arch Intern Med. 2002;162:2345-2347.

[124] Rabkin E, Aikawa M, Stone JR, Fukumoto Y, Libby P, Schoen FJ. Activated interstitial myofibroblasts express catabolic enzymes and mediate matrix remodeling in myxomatous heart valves. Circulation. 2001;104:2525-2532.

[125] Walker GA, Masters KS, Shah DN, Anseth KS, Leinwand LA. Valvular myofibroblast activation by transforming growth factor β. Circ Res. 2004;95:253-260.

[126] Fisher CI, Chen J, Merryman WD. Calcific nodule morphogenesis by heart valve interstitial cells is strain dependent. Biomech Model Mechanobiol. 2012; In Press.

[127] Ortlepp JR, Schmitz F, Mevissen V, Weiss S, Huster J, Dronskowski R, et al. The amount of calcium-deficient hexagonal hydroxyapatite in aortic valves is influenced by gender and associated with genetic polymorphisms in patients with severe calcific aortic stenosis. Eur Heart J. 2004;25:514-522.

[128] Weska RF, Aimoli CG, Nogueira GM, Leirner AA, Maizato MJ, Higa OZ, et al. Natural and prosthetic heart valve calcification: morphology and chemical composition characterization. Artif Organs. 2010;34:311-318.

[129] Mohler ER, Gannon F, Reynolds C, Zimmerman R, Keane MG, Kaplan FS. Bone formation and inflammation in cardiac valves. Circulation. 2001;103:1522-1528.

[130] Egan KP, Kim JH, Mohler ER, 3rd, Pignolo RJ. Role for circulating osteogenic precursor cells in aortic valvular disease. Arterioscler Thromb Vasc Biol. 2011;31:2965-2971.

[131] Li C, Xu S, Gotlieb AI. The progression of calcific aortic valve disease through injury, cell dysfunction, and disruptive biologic and physical force feedback loops. Cardiovasc Pathol. 2012; In Press.

[132] Mazzone A, Epistolato MC, De Caterina R, Storti S, Vittorini S, Sbrana S, et al. Neoangiogenesis, T-lymphocyte infiltration, and heat shock protein-60 are biological hallmarks of an immunomediated inflammatory process in end-stage calcified aortic valve stenosis. J Am Coll Cardiol. 2004;43:1670-1676.

[133] O'Brien KD, Shavelle DM, Caulfield MT, McDonald TO, Olin-Lewis K, Otto CM, et al. Association of angiotensin-converting enzyme with low-density lipoprotein in aortic valvular lesions and in human plasma. Circulation. 2002;106:2224-2230.

[134] Olsson M, Thyberg J, Nilsson J. Presence of oxidized low density lipoprotein in nonrheumatic stenotic aortic valves. Arterioscler Thromb Vasc Biol. 1999;19:1218-1222.

[135] Steiner I, Krbal L, Rozkos T, Harrer J, Laco J. Calcific aortic valve stenosis: Immunohistochemical analysis of inflammatory infiltrate. Pathol Res Pract. 2012;208:231-234.

[136] Clark-Greuel JN, Connolly JM, Sorichillo E, Narula NR, Rapoport HS, Mohler ER, et al. Transforming growth factor-β1 mechanisms in aortic valve calcification: increased alkaline phosphatase and related events. Ann Thorac Surg. 2007;83:946-953.

[137] ian B, Narula N, Li QY, Mohler ER, 3rd, Levy RJ. Progression of aortic valve stenosis: TGF-beta1 is present in calcified aortic valve cusps and promotes aortic valve interstitial cell calcification via apoptosis. Ann Thorac Surg. 2003;75:457-465.

[138] Yang X, Meng X, Su X, Mauchley DC, Ao L, Cleveland JC, et al. Bone morphogenetic protein 2 induces Runx2 and osteopontin expression in human aortic valve intersti-

http://dx.doi.org/10.5772/54356

tial cells: Role of Smad1 and extracellular signal-regulated kinase 1/2. J Thorac Cardiovasc Surg. 2009;138:1008-1015.

[139] Beppu S, Suzuki S, Matsuda H, Ohmori F, Nagata S, Miyatake K. Rapidity of progression of aortic stenosis in patients with congenital bicuspid aortic valves. Am J Cardiol. 1993;71:322-327.

[140] Linefsky JP, O'Brien KD, Katz R, de Boer IH, Barasch E, Jenny NS, et al. Association of serum phosphate levels with aortic valve sclerosis and annular calcification: the cardiovascular health study. J Am Coll Cardiol. 2011;58:291-297.

[141] Rosenhek R, Klaar U, Schemper M, Scholten C, Heger M, Gabriel H, et al. Mild and moderate aortic stenosis. Natural history and risk stratification by echocardiography. Eur Heart J. 2004;25:199-205.

[142] Varadarajan P, Kapoor N, Bansal RC, Pai RG. Clinical profile and natural history of 453 nonsurgically managed patients with severe aortic stenosis. Ann Thorac Surg. 2006;82:2111-2115.

[143] Caira FC, Stock SR, Gleason TG, McGee EC, Huang J, Bonow RO, et al. Human degenerative valve disease is associated with up-regulation of low-density lipoprotein-related protein 5 receptor-mediated bone formation J Am Coll Cardiol. 2006;47:1707-1712.

[144] Miller JD, Chu Y, Brooks RM, Richenbacher WE, Pena-Silva R, Heistad DD. Dysregulation of antioxidant mechanisms contributes to increased oxidative stress in calcific aortic valvular stenosis in humans. J Am Coll Cardiol. 2008;52:843-850.

[145] Satokata I, Ma L, Ohshima H, Bei M, Woo I, Nishizawa K, et al. Msx2 deficiency in mice causes pleiotropic defects in bone growth and ectodermal organ formation. Nat Genet. 2000;24:391-395.

[146] Balachandran K, Alford PW, Wylie-Sears J, Goss JA, Bischoff J, Aikawa E, et al. Cyclic strain induces dual-mode endothelial-mesenchymal transformation of the cardiac valve. Proc Natl Acad Sci USA. 2011;108:19943-19948.

[147] Dal-Bianco JP, Aikawa E, Bischoff J, Guerrero JL, Handschumacher MD, Sullivan S, et al. Active adaptation of the tethered mitral valve: Insights into a compensatory mechanism for functional mitral regurgitation. Circulation. 2009;120:334-342.

[148] Paranya G, Vineberg S, Dvorin E, Kaushal S, Roth SJ, Rabkin E, et al. Aortic valve endothelial cells undergo transforming growth factor-beta-mediated and non-transforming growth factor-beta-mediated transdifferentiation in vitro. Am J Pathol. 2001;159:1335-1343.

[149] Paruchuri S, Yang JH, Aikawa E, Melero-Martin JM, Khan ZA, Loukogeorgakis S, et al. Human pulmonary valve progenitor cells exhibit endothelial/mesenchymal plasticity in response to vascular endothelial growth factor-A and transforming growth factor-beta2. Circ Res. 2006;99:861-869.

[150] Li Z, Feng L, Wang CM, Zheng QJ, Zhao BJ, Yi W, et al. Deletion of RBP-J in adult mice leads to the onset of aortic valve degenerative diseases. Mol Biol Rep. 2012;39:3837-3845.

[151] Hajdu Z, Romeo SJ, Fleming PA, Markwald RR, Visconti RP, Drake CJ. Recruitment of bone marrow-derived valve interstitial cells is a normal homeostatic process. J Mol Cell Cardiol. 2011;51:955-965.

[152] Pohjolainen V, Taskinen P, Soini Y, Rysa J, Ilves M, Juvonen T, et al. Noncollagenous bone matrix proteins as a part of calcific aortic valve disease regulation. Hum Pathol. 2008;39:1695-1701.

[153] Nigam V, Srivastava D. Notch1 represses osteogenic pathways in aortic valve cells. J Mol Cell Cardiol. 2009;47:828-834.

[154] Aikawa E, Aikawa M, Libby P, Figueiredo J-L, Rusanescu G, Iwamoto Y, et al. Arterial and aortic valve calcification abolished by elastolytic cathepsin S deficiency in chronic renal disease. Circulation. 2009;119:1785-1794.

[155] Hjortnaes J, Butcher J, Figueiredo J-L, Riccio M, Kohler RH, Kozloff KM, et al. Arterial and aortic valve calcification inversely correlates with osteoporotic bone remodeling: a role for inflammation. Eur Heart J. 2010;31:1975-1984.

[156] Ix JH, Shlipak MG, Katz R, Budoff MJ, Shavelle DM, Probstfield JL, et al. Kidney function and aortic valve and mitral annular calcification in the Multi-Ethnic Study of Atherosclerosis (MESA). Am J Kidney Dis. 2007;50:412-420.

[157] Shuvy M, Abedat S, Beeri R, Danenberg HD, Planer D, Ben-Dov IZ, et al. Uraemic hyperparathyroidism causes a reversible inflammatory process of aortic valve calcification in rats. Cardiovasc Res. 2008;79:492-499.

[158] Shanahan CM, Crouthamel MH, Kapustin A, Giachelli C. Arterial calcification in chronic kidney disease: key roles for calcium and phosphate. Circ Res. 2011;109:697-711.

[159] Hu MC, Kuro-o M, Moe OW. Klotho and kidney disease. J Nephrol. 2010;23 Suppl 16:S136-144.

[160] Kuro-o M, Matsumura Y, Aizawa H, Kawaguchi H, Suga T, Utsugi T, et al. Mutation of the mouse klotho gene leads to a syndrome resembling ageing. Nature. 1997;390:45-51.

[161] Segawa H, Yamanaka S, Ohno Y, Onitsuka A, Shiozawa K, Aranami F, et al. Correlation between hyperphosphatemia and type II Na-Pi cotransporter activity in klotho mice. Am J Physiol Renal Physiol. 2007;292:F769-779.

[162] Takeshita K, Fujimori T, Kurotaki Y, Honjo T, Tsujikawa H, Yasui K, et al. Sinoatrial node dysfunction and early unexpected death of mice with a defect of klotho gene expression. Circulation. 2004;109:1776-1782.

[163] Aikawa E, Nahrendorf M, Sosnovik D, Lok VM, Jaffer FA, Aikawa M, et al. Multimodality molecular imaging identifies proteolytic and osteogenic activities in early aortic valve disease. Circulation. 2007;115:377-386.

[164] Meng X, Ao L, Song Y, Babu A, Yang X, Wang M, et al. Expression of functional Toll-like receptors 2 and 4 in human aortic valve interstitial cells: potential roles in aortic valve inflammation and stenosis. Am J Physiol Cell Physiol. 2008;294:C29-35.

[165] Rajamannan NM, Subramaniam M, Springett M, Sebo TC, Niekrasz M, McConnell JP, et al. Atorvastatin inhibits hypercholesterolemia-induced cellular proliferation and bone matrix production in the rabbit aortic valve. Circulation. 2002;105:2660-2665.

[166] Aikawa E, Nahrendorf M, Figueiredo JL, Swirski FK, Shtatland T, Kohler RH, et al. Osteogenesis associates with inflammation in early-stage atherosclerosis evaluated by molecular imaging in vivo. Circulation. 2007;116:2841-2850.

[167] Miller JD, Weiss RM, Serrano KM, Brooks RM, Berry CJ, Zimmerman K, et al. Lowering plasma cholesterol levels halts progression of aortic valve disease in mice. Circulation. 2009;119:2693-2701.

[168] Babu AN, Meng X, Zou N, Yang X, Wang M, Song Y, et al. Lipopolysaccharide stimulation of human aortic valve interstitial cells activates inflammation and osteogenesis. Ann Thorac Surg. 2008;86:71-76.

[169] Ankeny RF, Thourani VH, Weiss D, Vega JD, Taylor WR, Nerem RM, et al. Preferential activation of SMAD1/5/8 on the fibrosa endothelium in calcificed human aortic valves - Association with low BMP antagonists and SMAD6. PLoS One. 2011;6:e20969.

[170] Miller JD, Weiss RM, Serrano KM, Casteneda LE, Brooks RM, Zimmerman K, et al. Evidence for active regulation of pro-osteogenic signaling in advanced aortic valve disease. Arterioscler Thromb Vasc Biol. 2010;30:2482-2486.

[171] Osman L, Yacoub MH, Latif N, Amrani M, Chester AH. Role of human valve interstitial cells in valve calcification and their response to atorvastatin. Circulation. 2006;114:I-547-I-552.

[172] Merryman WD, Lukoff HD, Long RA, Engelmayr GC, Jr., Hopkins RA, Sacks MS. Synergistic effects of cyclic tension and transforming growth factor-beta1 on the aortic valve myofibroblast. Cardiovasc Pathol. 2007;16:268-276.

[173] Chen JH, Chen WLK, Sider KL, Yip CYY, Simmons CA. beta-catenin mediated mechanically regulated, transforming growth factor-beta1-induced myofibroblast differentiation of aortic valve interstitial cells. Arterioscler Thromb Vasc Biol. 2011;31:590-597.

[174] Cushing MC, Mariner PD, Liao JT, Sims EA, Anseth KS. Fibroblast growth factor represses Smad-mediated myofibroblast activation in aortic valvular interstitial cells. FASEB J. 2008;22:1769-1777.

[175] Acharya A, Hans CP, Keonig SN, Nichols HA, Galindo CL, Garner HR, et al. Inhibitory role for Notch1 in calcific aortic valve disease. PLoS One. 2011;6:e27743.

[176] Tamai K, Zeng X, Liu C, Zhang X, Harada Y, Chang Z, et al. A mechanism for Wnt coreceptor activation. Mol Cell. 2004;13:149-156.

[177] Rajamannan NM, Subramaniam M, Caira F, Stock SR, Spelsberg TC. Atorvastatin inhibits hypercholesterolemia-induced calcification in the aortic valves via the Lrp5 receptor pathway. Circulation. 2005;112:I229-I234.

[178] Rajamannan NM. Oxidative-mechanical stress signals stem cell niche mediated Lrp5 osteogenesis in eNOS(-/-) null mice. J Cell Biochem. 2012;113:1623-1634.

[179] Xu S, Gotlieb AI. Wnt3a/beta-catenin increases proliferation in heart valve interstitial cells. Cardiovasc Pathol. 2012; In Press.

[180] Rajamannan NM. The role of Lrp5/6 in cardiac valve disease: experimental hypercholesterolemia in the ApoE-/- /Lrp5-/- mice. J Cell Biochem. 2011;112:2987-2991.

[181] Fondard O, Detaint D, Iung B, Choqueux C, Adle-Biassette H, Jarraya M, et al. Extracellular matrix remodelling in human aortic valve disease: the role of matrix metalloproteinases and their tissue inhibitors. Eur Heart J. 2005;26:1333-1341.

[182] Perrotta I, Russo E, Camastra C, Filice G, Di Mizio G, Colosimo F, et al. New evidence for a critical role of elastin in calcification of native heart valves: immunohistochemical and ultrastructural study with literature review. Histopathology. 2011;59:504-513.

[183] Krishnamurthy VK, Opoka AM, Kern CB, Guilak F, Narmoneva DA, Hinton RB. Maladaptive matrix remodeling and regional biomechanical dysfunction in a mouse model of aortic valve disease. Matrix Biol. 2012;31:197-205.

[184] Bosse Y, Miqdad A, Fournier D, Pepin A, Pibarot P, Mathieu P. Refining molecular pathways leading to calcific aortic valve stenosis by studying gene expression profile of normal and calcified stenotic human aortic valves. Circ Cardiovasc Genet. 2009;2:489-498.

[185] Eriksen HA, Satta J, Risteli J, Veijola M, Vare P, Soini Y. Type I and type III collagen synthesis and composition in the valve matrix in aortic valve stenosis. Atherosclerosis. 2006;189:91-98.

[186] Matsumoto KI, Satoh K, Maniwa T, Araki A, Maruyama R, Oda T. Noticeable Decreased Expression of Tenascin-X in Calcific Aortic Valves. Connect Tissue Res. 2012; In Press.

[187] Stephens EH, Shangkuan J, Kuo JJ, Carroll JL, Kearney DL, Carberry KE, et al. Extracellular matrix remodeling and cell phenotypic changes in dysplastic and hemodynamically altered semilunar human cardiac valves. Cardiovasc Pathol. 2011;20:e157-167.

[188] Lockhart M, Wirrig E, Phelps A, Wessels A. Extracellular matrix and heart development. Birth Defects Res A Clin Mol Teratol. 2011;91:535-550.

[189] Mackie EJ, Tatarczuch L, Mirams M. The skeleton: a multi-functional complex organ: the growth plate chondrocyte and endochondral ossification. J Endocrinol. 2011;211:109-121.

[190] Balachandran K, Sucosky P, Jo H, Yoganathan AP. Elevated cyclic stretch alters matrix remodeling in aortic valve cusps: implications for degenerative aortic valve disease. Am J Physiol Heart Circ Physiol. 2009;296:H756-764.

[191] Kaden JJ, Dempfle CE, Kilic R, Sarikoc A, Hagl S, Lang S, et al. Influence of receptor activator of nuclear factor kappa B on human aortic valve myofibroblasts. Exp Mol Pathol. 2005;78:36-40.

[192] Takayanagi H. Mechanistic insight into osteoclast differentiation in osteoimmunology. J Mol Med (Berl). 2005;83:170-179.

[193] Steinmetz M, Skowasch D, Wernert N, Welsch U, Preusse CJ, Welz A, et al. Differential profile of the OPG/RANKL/RANK-system in degenerative aortic native and bioprosthetic valves. J Heart Valve Dis. 2008;17:187-193.

[194] O'Brien KD, Reichenbach DD, Marcovina SM, Kuusisto J, Alpers CE, Otto CM. Apolipoproteins B, (a), and E accumulate in the morphologically early lesion of 'degenerative' valvular aortic stenosis. Arterioscler Thromb Vasc Biol. 1996;16:523-532.

[195] Benton JA, Kern HB, Leinwand LA, Mariner PD, Anseth KS. Statins block calcific nodule formation of valvular interstitial cells by inhibiting alpha-smooth muscle actin expression. Arterioscler Thromb Vasc Biol. 2009;29:1950-1957.

[196] Monzack EL, Masters KS. A time-course investigation of the statin paradox among valvular interstitial cell phenotypes. Am J Physiol Heart Circ Physiol. 2012; 303:H903-9.

[197] Hamilton AM, Boughner DR, Drangova M, Rogers KA. Statin treatment of hypercholesterolemic-induced aortic valve sclerosis. Cardiovasc Pathol. 2011;20:84-92.

[198] Rosenhek R, Rader F, Loho N, Gabriel H, Heger M, Klaar U, et al. Statins but not angiotensin-converting enzyme inhibitors delay progression of aortic stenosis. Circulation. 2004;110:1291-1295

[199] Chan KL, Teo K, Dumesnil JG, Ni A, Tam J. Effect of Lipid lowering with rosuvastatin on progression of aortic stenosis: results of the aortic stenosis progression observation: measuring effects of rosuvastatin (ASTRONOMER) trial. Circulation. 2010;121:306-314.

[200] Cowell SJ, Newby DE, Prescott RJ, Bloomfield P, Reid J, Northridge DB, et al. A randomized trial of intensive lipid-lowering therapy in calcific aortic stenosis. N Engl J Med. 2005;352:2389-2397.

[201] Rossebo AB, Pedersen TR, Boman K, Brudi P, Chambers JB, Egstrup K, et al. Intensive lipid lowering with simvastatin and ezetimibe in aortic stenosis. N Engl J Med. 2008;359:1343-1356.

[202] Ardehali R, Leeper NJ, Wilson AM, Heidenreich PA. The effect of angiotensin-converting enzyme inhibitors and statins on the progression of aortic sclerosis and mortality. J Heart Valve Dis. 2012;21:337-343.

[203] Powers B, Greene L, Balfe LM. Updates on the treatment of essential hypertension: a summary of AHRQ's comparative effectiveness review of angiotensin-converting enzyme inhibitors, angiotensin II receptor blockers, and direct renin inhibitors. J Manag Care Pharm. 2011;17(8 Suppl):S1-14.

[204] Arishiro K, Hoshiga M, Negoro N, Jin D, Takai S, Miyazaki M, et al. Angiotensin receptor-1 blocker inhibits atherosclerotic changes and endothelial disruption of the aortic valve in hypercholesterolemic rabbits. J Am Coll Cardiol. 2007;49:1482-1489.

[205] Ngo DT, Stafford I, Sverdlov AL, Qi W, Wuttke RD, Zhang Y, et al. Ramipril retards development of aortic valve stenosis in a rabbit model: mechanistic considerations. Br J Pharmacol. 2011;162:722-732.

[206] Simolin MA, Pedersen TX, Bro S, Mayranpaa MI, Helske S, Nielsen LB, et al. ACE inhibition attenuates uremia-induced aortic valve thickening in a novel mouse model. BMC Cardiovasc Disord. 2009;9:10.

[207] Cote N, Couture C, Pibarot P, Despres JP, Mathieu P. Angiotensin receptor blockers are associated with a lower remodelling score of stenotic aortic valves. Eur J Clin Invest. 2011;41:1172-1179.

[208] Chockalingam A, Venkatesan S, Subramaniam T, Jagannathan V, Elangovan S, Alagesan R, et al. Safety and efficacy of angiotensin-converting enzyme inhibitors in symptomatic severe aortic stenosis: Symptomatic Cardiac Obstruction-Pilot Study of Enalapril in Aortic Stenosis (SCOPE-AS). Am Heart J. 2004;147:E19.

[209] Nadir MA, Wei L, Elder DH, Libianto R, Lim TK, Pauriah M, et al. Impact of renin-angiotensin system blockade therapy on outcome in aortic stenosis. J Am Coll Cardiol. 2011;58:570-576.

[210] O'Brien KD, Probstfield JL, Caulfield MT, Nasir K, Takasu J, Shavelle DM, et al. Angiotensin-converting enzyme inhibitors and change in aortic valve calcium. Arch Intern Med. 2005;165:858-862.

[211] Wakabayashi K, Tsujino T, Naito Y, Ezumi A, Lee-Kawabata M, Nakao S, et al. Administration of angiotensin-converting enzyme inhibitors is associated with slow progression of mild aortic stenosis in Japanese patients. Heart Vessels. 2011;26:252-257.

[212] Sverdlov AL, Ngo DT, Chan WP, Chirkov YY, Gersh BJ, McNeil JJ, et al. Determinants of aortic sclerosis progression: implications regarding impairment of nitric oxide signaling and potential therapeutics. Eur Heart J. 2012; 33:2419-2425.

[213] Yamamoto K, Yamamoto H, Yoshida K, Kisanuki A, Hirano Y, Ohte N, et al. Prognostic factors for progression of early- and late-stage calcific aortic valve disease in Japanese: the Japanese Aortic Stenosis Study (JASS) Retrospective Analysis. Hypertens Res. 2010;33:269-274.

[214] Gkizas S, Koumoundourou D, Sirinian X, Rokidi S, Mavrilas D, Koutsoukos P, et al. Aldosterone receptor blockade inhibits degenerative processes in the early stage of calcific aortic stenosis. Eur J Pharmacol. 2010;642:107-112.

[215] Stewart RA, Kerr AJ, Cowan BR, Young AA, Occleshaw C, Richards AM, et al. A randomized trial of the aldosterone-receptor antagonist eplerenone in asymptomatic moderate-severe aortic stenosis. Am Heart J. 2008;156:348-355.

[216] Russell RG. Bisphosphonates: mode of action and pharmacology. Pediatrics. 2007;119 Suppl 2:S150-162.

[217] Rapoport HS, Connolly JM, Fulmer J, Dai N, Murti BH, Gorman RC, et al. Mechanisms of the in vivo inhibition of calcification of bioprosthetic porcine aortic valve cusps and aortic wall with triglycidylamine/mercapto bisphosphonate. Biomaterials. 2007;28:690-699.

[218] Innasimuthu AL, Katz WE. Effect of bisphosphonates on the progression of degenerative aortic stenosis. Echocardiography. 2011;28:1-7.

[219] Skolnick AH, Osranek M, Formica P, Kronzon I. Osteoporosis treatment and progression of aortic stenosis. Am J Cardiol. 2009;104:122-124.

[220] Sterbakova G, Vyskocil V, Linhartova K. Bisphosphonates in calcific aortic stenosis: association with slower progression in mild disease--a pilot retrospective study. Cardiology. 2010;117:184-189.

[221] Elmariah S, Delaney JA, O'Brien KD, Budoff MJ, Vogel-Claussen J, Fuster V, et al. Bisphosphonate Use and Prevalence of Valvular and Vascular Calcification in Women MESA (The Multi-Ethnic Study of Atherosclerosis). J Am Coll Cardiol. 2010;56:1752-1759.

[222] Aksoy O, Cam A, Goel SS, Houghtaling PL, Williams S, Ruiz-Rodriguez E, et al. Do bisphosphonates slow the progression of aortic stenosis? J Am Coll Cardiol. 2012;59:1452-1459.

[223] Kietadisorn R, Juni RP, Moens AL. Tackling endothelial dysfunction by modulating NOS uncoupling: new insights into its pathogenesis and therapeutic possibilities. Am J Physiol Endocrinol Metab. 2012;302:E481-495.

[224] Matsumoto Y, Adams V, Walther C, Kleinecke C, Brugger P, Linke A, et al. Reduced number and function of endothelial progenitor cells in patients with aortic valve stenosis: a novel concept for valvular endothelial cell repair. Eur Heart J. 2009;30:346-355.

[225] Poggianti E, Venneri L, Chubuchny V, Jambrik Z, Baroncini LA, Picano E. Aortic valve sclerosis is associated with systemic endothelial dysfunction. J Am Coll Cardiol. 2003;41:136-141.

[226] Liberman M, Bassi E, Martinatti MK, Lario FC, Wosniak J, Jr., Pomerantzeff PM, et al. Oxidant generation predominates around calcifying foci and enhances progression of aortic valve calcification. Arterioscler Thromb Vasc Biol. 2008;28:463-470.

[227] Kennedy JA, Hua X, Mishra K, Murphy GA, Rosenkranz AC, Horowitz JD. Inhibition of calcifying nodule formation in cultured porcine aortic valve cells by nitric oxide donors. Eur J Pharmacol. 2009;602:28-35.

[228] Cagirci G, Cay S, Canga A, Karakurt O, Yazihan N, Kilic H, et al. Association between plasma asymmetrical dimethylarginine activity and severity of aortic valve stenosis. J Cardiovasc Med. 2011;12:96-101.

[229] Ngo DT, Heresztyn T, Mishra K, Marwick TH, Horowitz JD. Aortic stenosis is associated with elevated plasma levels of asymmetric dimethylarginine (ADMA). Nitric Oxide. 2007;16:197-201.

[230] Schumm J, Luetzkendorf S, Rademacher W, Franz M, Schmidt-Winter C, Kiehntopf M, et al. In patients with aortic stenosis increased flow-mediated dilation is independently associated with higher peak jet velocity and lower asymmetric dimethylarginine levels. Am Heart J. 2011;161:893-899.

[231] Boursinos LA, Karachalios T, Poultsides L, Malizos KN. Do steroids, conventional non-steroidal anti-inflammatory drugs and selective Cox-2 inhibitors adversely affect fracture healing? J Musculoskelet Neuronal Interact. 2009;9:44-52.

[232] Grosser T. Variability in the response to cyclooxygenase inhibitors: toward the individualization of nonsteroidal anti-inflammatory drug therapy. J Investig Med. 2009;57:709-716.

[233] Smith WL, DeWitt DL, Garavito RM. Cyclooxygenases: structural, cellular, and molecular biology. Annu Rev Biochem. 2000;69:145-182.

[234] Narumiya S, Sugimoto Y, Ushikubi F. Prostanoid receptors: structures, properties, and functions. Physiol Rev. 1999;79:1193-1226.

[235] Lopez J, Fernandez-Pisonero I, Duenas AI, Maeso P, Roman JA, Crespo MS, et al. Viral and bacterial patterns induce TLR-mediated sustained inflammation and calcification in aortic valve interstitial cells. Int J Cardiol. 2012;158:18-25.

[236] Alander CB, Raisz LG. Effects of selective prostaglandins E2 receptor agonists on cultured calvarial murine osteoblastic cells. Prostaglandins Other Lipid Mediat. 2006;81:178-183.

[237] Choudhary S, Alander C, Zhan P, Gao Q, Pilbeam C, Raisz L. Effect of deletion of the prostaglandin EP2 receptor on the anabolic response to prostaglandin E2 and a selective EP2 receptor agonist. Prostaglandins Other Lipid Mediat. 2008;86:35-40.

[238] Chyun YS, Raisz LG. Stimulation of bone formation by prostaglandin E2. Prostaglandins. 1984;27:97-103.

[239] Gao Q, Xu M, Alander CB, Choudhary S, Pilbeam CC, Raisz LG. Effects of prostaglandin E2 on bone in mice in vivo. Prostaglandins Other Lipid Mediat. 2009;89:20-25.

[240] Jee WS, Ueno K, Kimmel DB, Woodbury DM, Price P, Woodbury LA. The role of bone cells in increasing metaphyseal hard tissue in rapidly growing rats treated with prostaglandin E2. Bone. 1987;8:171-178.

[241] Kaneki H, Takasugi I, Fujieda M, Kiriu M, Mizuochi S, Ide H. Prostaglandin E2 stimulates the formation of mineralized bone nodules by a cAMP-independent mechanism in the culture of adult rat calvarial osteoblasts. J Cell Biochem. 1999;73:36-48.

[242] Li M, Healy DR, Li Y, Simmons HA, Crawford DT, Ke HZ, et al. Osteopenia and impaired fracture healing in aged EP4 receptor knockout mice. Bone. 2005;37:46-54.

[243] Minamizaki T, Yoshiko Y, Kozai K, Aubin JE, Maeda N. EP2 and EP4 receptors differentially mediate MAPK pathways underlying anabolic actions of prostaglandin E2 on bone formation in rat calvaria cell cultures. Bone. 2009;44:1177-1185.

[244] Zhang X, Schwarz EM, Young DA, Puzas JE, Rosier RN, O'Keefe RJ. Cyclooxygenase-2 regulates mesenchymal cell differentiation into the osteoblast lineage and is critically involved in bone repair. J Clin Invest. 2002;109:1405-1415.

[245] Chikazu D, Li X, Kawaguchi H, Sakuma Y, Voznesensky OS, Adams DJ, et al. Bone morphogenetic protein 2 induces cyclo-oxygenase 2 in osteoblasts via a Cbfal binding site: role in effects of bone morphogenetic protein 2 in vitro and in vivo. J Bone Miner Res. 2002;17:1430-1440.

[246] Susperregui AR, Gamell C, Rodriguez-Carballo E, Ortuno MJ, Bartrons R, Rosa JL, et al. Noncanonical BMP signaling regulates cyclooxygenase-2 transcription. Mol Endocrinol. 2011;25:1006-1017.

[247] Kakita A, Suzuki A, Ono Y, Miura Y, Itoh M, Oiso Y. Possible involvement of p38 MAP kinase in prostaglandin E1-induced ALP activity in osteoblast-like cells. Prostaglandins Leukot Essent Fatty Acids. 2004;70:469-474.

[248] Celil Aydemir AB, Minematsu H, Gardner TR, Kim KO, Ahn JM, Lee FY. Nuclear factor of activated T cells mediates fluid shear stress- and tensile strain-induced Cox2 in human and murine bone cells. Bone. 2010;46:167-175.

[249] Mehrotra M, Saegusa M, Voznesensky O, Pilbeam C. Role of Cbfa1/Runx2 in the fluid shear stress induction of COX-2 in osteoblasts. Biochem Biophys Res Commun. 2006;341:1225-1230.

[250] Boniface K, Bak-Jensen KS, Li Y, Blumenschein WM, McGeachy MJ, McClanahan TK, et al. Prostaglandin E2 regulates Th17 cell differentiation and function through cyclic AMP and EP2/EP4 receptor signaling. J Exp Med. 2009;206:535-548.

[251] Yao C, Sakata D, Esaki Y, Li Y, Matsuoka T, Kuroiwa K, et al. Prostaglandin E2-EP4 signaling promotes immune inflammation through Th1 cell differentiation and Th17 cell expansion. Nat Med. 2009;15:633-640.

[252] Garcia Rodriguez LA, Gonzalez-Perez A, Bueno H, Hwa J. NSAID use selectively increases the risk of non-fatal myocardial infarction: a systematic review of randomised trials and observational studies. PLoS One. 2011;6:e16780.

[253] Salvo F, Fourrier-Reglat A, Bazin F, Robinson P, Riera-Guardia N, Haag M, et al. Cardiovascular and gastrointestinal safety of NSAIDs: a systematic review of meta-analyses of randomized clinical trials. Clin Pharmacol Ther. 2011;89:855-866.

[254] Willette RN, Eybye ME, Olzinski AR, Behm DJ, Aiyar N, Maniscalco K, et al. Differential effects of p38 mitogen-activated protein kinase and cyclooxygenase 2 inhibitors in a model of cardiovascular disease. J Pharmacol Exp Ther. 2009;330:964-970.

[255] Wirrig EE, Yutzey KE. Transcriptional regulation of heart valve development and disease. Cardiovasc Pathol. 2011;20:162-167.

[256] Rajamannan NM, Evans FJ, Aikawa E, Grande-Allen KJ, Demer LL, Heistad DD, et al. Calcific aortic valve disease: not simply a degenerative process: A review and agenda for research from the National Heart and Lung and Blood Institute Aortic Stenosis Working Group. Executive summary: Calcific aortic valve disease-2011 update. Circulation. 2011;124:1783-1791.

Chapter 4

Notch Signaling in Congenital and Acquired Aortic Valve Disease

Erik Fung and Masanori Aikawa

Additional information is available at the end of the chapter

http://dx.doi.org/10.5772/56533

1. Introduction

Calcific aortic valve disease represents the predominant pathology of tricuspid (trileaflet) and bicuspid aortic valves in developed countries (Ladich et al., 2011). Accounting for approximately half of anatomically isolated aortic stenosis and 25 percent of patients with aortic regurgitation (Roberts, 1970), calcific bicuspid aortic valves requiring surgical intervention present at least two decades earlier than the tricuspid counterpart (Ward, 2000). Mechanisms important in cardiac and organ development — notably, the Notch pathway — have emerged as central players recapitulated and reused during the pathogenesis of calcific aortic valve disease, and support also a common etiology for bicuspid aortic valve and aortic valve calcification (Garg et al., 2005) (Table 1). Active engagement of inflammatory, remodeling, neovascularization and osteogenic (Aikawa et al., 2007a; Aikawa et al., 2007b; Miller et al., 2010; Rajamannan et al., 2003) pathways has conceptually replaced 'degeneration' in calcific aortic valve disease pathogenesis and progression (Dweck et al., 2012). Moreover, these pathways invoke similar mechanisms during cardiac morphogenesis. Dysregulated Notch activity has also been reported in vascular inflammation, macrophage activation (Fung et al., 2007), cardiometabolic disorder, and vascular and aortic valve calcification (Fukuda et al., 2012). Preclinical studies suggest that specific blockade of Notch ligand–receptor signaling potently suppresses vascular calcification and calcific aortic valve disease (Fukuda et al., 2012). In this chapter, we review the mechanisms of Notch signaling, aortic valve dysmorphology pertinent to accelerated valve calcification, and discuss the pathways involving Notch that lead to aortic valve calcification and disease.

	Role in cardiac and aortic valve development	*Role in aortic valve calcification*
NOTCH1	cardiac morphogenesis	inhibits calcification
Hey1/2	downstream effector of Notch inhibits action of BMP2	inhibits calcification, decreases ostepontin
BMP2	coordination of cardiac patterning and EMT required for valve formation	promotes calcification
Sox9	increased by Hey2 and mediates chondrogenesis	suppresses osteogenesis
Runx2	repressed by NOTCH1 and Hey1/2	promotes calcification
JAG1	boundary definition in myocardium; vasculogenesis	inhibits calcification
DLL4	formation of heart fields and boundary definition in endocardium; vasculogenesis	neovascularization (angioneogenesis) & hemorrhage leading to calcific aortic valve disease

Table 1. Major components of the Notch1-Hey-BMP2 axis and their actions in cardiac and aortic valve development, and in aortic valve calcification. BMP, bone morphogenetic protein. DLL4, Delta-like 4. JAG1, Jagged1.

2. Notch signaling

The human Notch receptor family comprises four members, Notch1 through Notch4, expressed as transmembrane molecules on the cell surface of neighboring cells that enable canonical signaling in a contact-dependent manner (Bray, 2006; Kopan and Ilagan, 2009). Canonical Notch signaling describes the 'classic' interaction between membrane-bound receptors and ligands expressed on the surface of neighboring (signaling and receiving) cells, whereas non-canonical signaling encompasses a diverse group of structurally unrelated ligands that contribute to the pleiotropic effect of Notch signaling (Kopan and Ilagan, 2009). In mammals, five members of the Delta-Serrate-LAG-2 (DSL) family have the capacity to activate or modify canonical Notch signaling — Delta-like 1 (Dll1), Dll3, Dll4, Jagged1, and Jagged2. Interaction between Notch receptor and ligand is tightly controlled, and the signaling outcome is determined by the receptor:ligand ratio (Artavanis-Tsakonas and Muskavitch, 2010; Gibert and Simpson, 2003; Heitzler and Simpson, 1991; Wilkinson et al., 1994) that critically determines asymmetry in cell fate and development of neighboring cells. This interaction between receptor and ligand can be modified posttranslationally through Notch glycosylation by lunatic, manic and radical glycosyltransferases (Bray, 2006). The receptor:ligand ratio is dependent on the differential expression of competing ligands on neighboring cells in *trans*, as opposed to *cis* interaction through which receptor and ligand expressed on the same cell can also modulate Notch signaling. The complexity of receptor–ligand interaction is further increased by the requirement of heterodimerization of the receptor (Kopan and Ilagan, 2009). Canonical interaction between Notch receptor and ligand leads to two sequential cleavage events at site 2 (S2) and S3. S2 is a 'permissive' extracellular juxtamembrane cleavage by a disintegrin and metalloprotease 17 (ADAM17, known also as tumor necrosis factor-α converting enzyme/TACE) and/or ADAM10 (Artavanis-Tsakonas and Muskavitch, 2010;

Bray, 2006), whereas S3 is executed by γ-secretase, a protease with many substrates (McCarthy et al., 2009; Wakabayashi and De Strooper, 2008). S1 cleavage is carried out by a furin-like convertase occurring posttranslationally in the trans-Golgi apparatus before translocation of the nascent Notch receptor to the cell surface (Bray, 2006; Kopan and Ilagan, 2009). Following S3 cleavage, the Notch intracellular domain is liberated and enters the nucleus to form a transcription activational complex with the transcriptional factor RBP-Jκ, and the transcriptional coactivator Mastermind to promote target gene transcription (Bray, 2006; Kopan and Ilagan, 2009). Targets indicative of Notch activity include the basic-helix-loop-helix genes of the hairy and enhancer of split (HES) and the hairy-related (HRT or Hey) family (Bray, 2006; Kopan and Ilagan, 2009).

Functionality of Notch signaling components is highly context-dependent and conventionally requires cell-to-cell contact to specify cell fate, differentiation, growth, proliferation, survival and apoptosis (Bray, 2006; Fiuza and Arias, 2007; Guruharsha et al., 2012). Interaction between Notch receptor and ligand on adjacent cells results in asymmetric signal transduction, leading to potentially divergent cell fate decision, phenotypic development and growth (Bray, 2006; Kopan and Ilagan, 2009).

3. Congenital aortic valve disease

3.1. Notch dysfunction in aortic valve anomalies and other congenital heart diseases

Congenital aortic valve anomalies frequently associate with other abnormalities in neighboring structures, including the aortic root (e.g. dilatation, aneurysm), aorta (e.g. coarctation of aorta), ventricular outflow tract (e.g. septal defect, transposition of great vessels), and/or coronary arteries (e.g. coronary anomalies) (Perloff, 2003; Ward, 2000). The association of anomalies is due in part to the complexity and critical function of the endocardial cushion, and its formation during cardiac valve and septum development (Camenisch et al., 2010).

The tight regulation of Notch signaling during murine cardiac morphogenesis, particularly of the cardiac outflow tract and semilunar (aortic and pulmonary) valves, have been recently reviewed in detail by de la Pompa and Epstein (de la Pompa and Epstein, 2012). The evolutionarily conserved nature of Notch across mammalian species is generally recognized to be applicable to human. The highly coordinated action of Notch in progenitor cell proliferation and differentiation is instrumental during development. Earliest signs of cardiac morphogenesis occur with formation of the cardiac crescent by midline fusion of first and second heart fields that feature expression of Notch1, Dll4 and Jagged1 in the primitive endocardium (de la Pompa and Epstein, 2012; del Monte et al., 2007; Duarte et al., 2004). Continuing cell proliferation and development leads to the generation of the heart tube, consisting of an outer myocardial layer, middle cardiac jelly of extracellular matrix, and an inner endocardial endothelium (Camenisch et al., 2010; de la Pompa and Epstein, 2012). Demarcation of boundary and tissue layers is marked by expression of Jagged1 limited to the myocardial layer, and Dll4, Notch1, Notch2 and Notch4 in the endocardium. The heart tube gradually undergoes a complex morphologic change with a rightward bend, converting the anterior-posterior polarity of the heart tube into a right-left (R-) loop. As the looped heart further develops, the valve territories of the atrioventricular canal (AVC) and outflow tract (OFT) are demarcated. The AVC and OFT cushions become the sites for formation of the mitral and aortic valves, respectively, in the left ventricle and the tricuspid and pulmonary valves in the right ventricule (Person et al., 2005). Contribution of endocardium-derived mesenchyme to the development of AVC and OFT valve primordia diverge as the neural crest contribute additionally to the development of the OFT valve primordium (de la Pompa and Epstein, 2012; Zhang et al., 2010). At this stage of development, Jagged1 expression is present in the endocardium and chamber myocardium, whereas expression of Dll4 and Notch1 localizes to the valve and atrial endocardium. Here, Notch coordinates cardiac patterning through regulation of the Notch-Hey-Bmp2 axis (MacGrogan et al., 2011). Bmp2, or bone morphogenetic protein 2, is responsible for AVC specification together with Tbx2/3, members of the T-box transcription factor family with crucial roles in cardiac development (de la Pompa and Epstein, 2012; Ma et al., 2005). Tbx2 is repressible by Tbx20, which has regulatory function in ion channel expression (Shen et al., 2011). Importantly, *TBX20* nonsense and missense germline mutations result in complex septal, chamber and valvular anomalies in human (Kirk et al., 2007). Tbx transcription factors carry strong activation and repression domains and, especially Tbx20, interact with other important cardiac developmental factors including Nkx2.5, Gata4, Gata5 and Tbx5 (Brown et al., 2005; Combs and Yutzey, 2009; Kirk et al., 2007; Plageman and Yutzey, 2005; Stennard et al., 2003). Targeted disruption of *Gata5* has been demonstrated to associate with the development of bicuspid aortic valve in the mouse (Laforest et al., 2011), and one study on patients with bicuspid aortic valve found that approximately 4% had rare non-synonymous mutations within the *GATA5* transcriptional activation domains (Padang et al., 2012). A functional connection between *gata5* and *notch1* was reported in a zebrafish study of endoderm formation (Kikuchi et al., 2004), and those findings may potentially be generalized to human, given the evolutionarily conserved nature of the Notch pathway (Artavanis-Tsakonas and Muskavitch, 2010).

Cardiac valve formation begins with myocardial cells signaling to endocardial cells in the AVC and OFT cushions to undergo epithelial-mesenchymal transformation (transition) (EMT) (de la Pompa and Epstein, 2012). Coordinated by Notch and RBP-Jκ (del Monte et al., 2007; Timmerman et al., 2004), Bmp2 instructs cushion endocardial cells to invade the extracellular matrix and become the cushion mesenchyme (Hinton and Yutzey, 2011), and acting via Snail1/2, the Notch–Hey–Bmp2/4 axis promotes EMT and subsequent completion of valve tissue development (MacGrogan et al., 2011) (Figure 1). Interference with Notch signaling results in abnormal development of the aortic valve and cardiac outflow tract as demonstrated in animal studies (de la Pompa and Epstein, 2012; Garg et al., 2005; Mohamed et al., 2006; van den Akker et al., 2012). As discussed below, BMP2 also mediates aortic valve calcification.

Bicuspid aortic valve represents one of the most common anomalies of the heart or vessels (Roberts, 1970; Roberts et al., 2012; Ward, 2000), and its association with other anomalies is well recognized. For instance, ~10% of relatives of patients with hypoplastic left heart syndrome have bicuspid aortic valve (Loffredo et al., 2004), and aortic abnormalities such as coarctation of aorta and interrupted aortic arch are present in 20–85% (Presbitero et al., 1987;

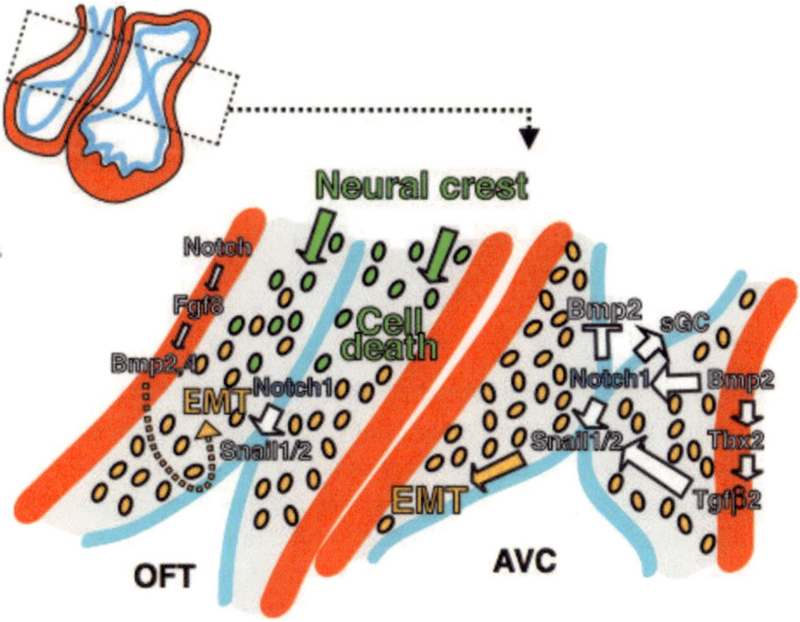

Figure 1. Diagram of a looped heart expanded to show the outflow tract (OFT) and the atrioventricular canal (AVC) endocardial cushions where epithelial-mesenchymal transition (EMT) occurs and precedes the development of semilunar and atrioventricular valves, respectively. Factors important during cardiac EMT and valve morphogenesis are shown. Myocardium, red; endocardium, blue; extracellular matrix, gray. Bmp, bone morphogenetic protein. Fgf, fibroblast growth factor. sGC, soluble guanylyl cyclase. Tbx, T-box transcription factor. Tgf, transforming growth factor. Adapted with permission from Elsevier.

Stewart et al., 1993) and ~27% (Roberts et al., 2012) of cases, respectively. Individuals with bicuspid aortic valve consistently have dilatation of the ascending aorta (Hahn et al., 1992). As a common variation noted by several investigators (Higgins and Wexler, 1975; Hutchins et al., 1978), a higher incidence of left coronary arterial system dominance (defined by the presence of the posterior descending artery arising from the left circumflex artery, as opposed to the right coronary artery) is observed in patients with bicuspid aortic valve. The phenotypic heterogeneity and overlap suggest common developmental mechanisms and gene networks that closely interact; the extent of the interactions may vary depending on the penetrance of the mutation(s), effect size of the variants, and the interaction between genes and signaling pathway.

In a study of two unrelated families, one of which included five generations, Garg and colleagues observed mutations in *NOTCH1* that segregated with aortic valve disease, particularly with bicuspid aortic valve and aortic valve calcification; but also, to a lesser extent, with tetralogy of Fallot, ventricular septal defect, mitral atresia, double-outlet right ventricle, or hypoplastic left ventricle (Garg et al., 2005). *NOTCH1* is located on chromosome 9q34.3 and encodes the 2,556-amino acid transmembrane Notch1 receptor. Affected members of one of the families analyzed had autosomal dominant inheritance of a point mutation (R1108X) resulting from a C-to-T transition of nucleotide 3322. Another unrelated family analyzed had a single base pair deletion leading to a frameshift mutation (H1505del) at position 4515. These mutations produced truncated transcripts that are believed to undergo nonsense-mediated decay, supporting haploinsufficiency of *NOTCH1* in the pathogenesis of congenital heart disease (Garg et al., 2005). Of note, despite the high propensity to development of bicuspid aortic valve and other cardiac anomalies in individuals with the *NOTCH1* mutation (R1108X) (Garg et al., 2005), aortic valve calcification was present even in a minority of family members with the mutation who did not have bicuspid or dysmorphic aortic valves, suggesting that the penetrance of the *NOTCH1* mutation is variable (or the effects compensated for by another Notch receptor or other mechanisms), and that maldistribution of mechanical stress alone can not explain accelerated valve calcification in these individuals.

Mutations or abnormal copy number variants in the gene (*JAG1*) encoding Jagged1, a Notch ligand, on chromosome 20p12 can cause a range of cardiovascular anomalies (McElhinney et al., 2002; Oda et al., 1997). However, the distribution and manifestations of cardiovascular anomalies, including the frequency of bicuspid aortic valve and calcific aortic valve disease, differ considerably between the *JAG1* and *NOTCH1* mutations (Garg et al., 2005; McElhinney et al., 2002). Although *JAG1* mutation is well recognized as a primary cause of Alagille syndome, familial as well as 'sporadic' tetralogy of Fallot, among other anomalies, has been reported (Eldadah et al., 2001; Greenway et al., 2009). Tetralogy of Fallot is a syndrome that comprises ventricular septal defect, pulmonary stenosis, right ventricular hypertrophy and an overriding aorta, in association with aortic regurgitation in ~6% of patients (Abraham et al., 1979). Mutations in *JAG1* have been identified in 60–75% of individuals with Alagille syndrome (Colliton et al., 2001; Li et al., 1997; Oda et al., 1997; Spinner et al., 2001), a condition characterized by cholestatic jaundice due to biliary tree anomalies, skeletal deformities, systemic vascular malformations and aneurysms (Kamath et al., 2004), and a high frequency of right-sided cardiovascular anomalies (62% of 200 patients) (McElhinney et al., 2002). In patients with left-sided anomalies (22 of 200 individuals (McElhinney et al., 2002)), a comparison of those with ($n = 17$) and without ($n = 5$) *JAG1* mutation did not reveal an obvious trend favoring the distribution nor preponderance of valvular aortic stenosis, supravalvular aortic stenosis, aortic coarctation, or bicuspid aortic stenosis without stenosis (McElhinney et al., 2002). Those findings suggest that aortic valve disease, such as bicuspid aortic valve and at least moderate-severe aortic stenosis, is relatively uncommon (<5%) in patients with Alagille syndrome (McElhinney et al., 2002), and implies that *JAG1* mutation *per se* does not predispose to aortic valve calcification in human, as evidenced by the paucity of left-sided abnormalities. Interestingly, although previous mouse studies have reported high lethality associated with endothelial-specific deletion of *Jag1* (Benedito et al., 2009; High et al., 2008), one recent study demonstrated a high frequency of cardiac, great vessel, coronary, and valve defects resembling features of tetralogy of Fallot in human; and in animals, chondrogenic nodules and calcification were observed in the aortic valve (5 of 10 transgenic animals versus 0 of 10 controls) (Hofmann et al., 2012). The authors of the study postulated that murine *Jag1* was essential to morphogenesis of the interventricular septum and cardiac valves, and particularly, in valve remodeling postnatally through modulation of extracellular matrix (Hofmann et al., 2012).

The complexity of gene-phenotype effects in human is highlighted by variable penetrance of *JAG1* mutation (e.g. G274D missense mutation) and phenotypic expression, as demonstrated by differences in the degree of glycosylation, protein trafficking and cell-surface protein expression given the same mutation (Lu et al., 2003). This heterogeneity is reminiscent of the variable effects of *NOTCH1* in the pathogenesis of bicuspid aortic valve and other cardiovascular anomalies (Garg et al., 2005), and epigenetic factors such as intracardiac fluid forces may be important contributors that couple with transcription factors to affect cardiogenesis and valve development (Hove et al., 2003; Lee et al., 2006; Vermot et al., 2009).

3.2. Aortic valve dysmorphology, bicuspid aortic valve and calcification

Anomalies of the aortic valve can be classified based on size, shape, the number of valve leaflets, cuspal inequality, nature of commissures (e.g. unicomissural, acquired fusion), and location of a false raphé if present (Perloff, 2003; Ward, 2000). Unicuspid, quadricuspid and six-cuspid aortic valves occur rarely (Perloff, 2003), and associated mutations have not been reported, unlike bicuspid aortic valves resulting from impaired Notch1 signaling (Garg et al., 2005). Unicuspid and bicuspid aortic valves often prematurely develop valve calcification at least two decades earlier than their normal trileaflet counterpart (Pachulski and Chan, 1993). Although maldistribution of mechanical stress contributes to the fibrocalcific process, additional factors apart from biomechanical forces including inflammatory and profibrotic processes direct the differentiation of valve fibroblasts into myofibroblasts and osteoblasts that promote osteogenesis (Dweck et al., 2012; Rajamannan et al., 2003).

Maldistribution of shear stress on valve cusps is thought to promote calcification of the aortic valve seen in unicuspid, bicuspid, and tricuspid aortic valve with cuspal inequality (Perloff, 2003). Bicuspid aortic valve is found in 1–2% of the general population in the United States, with a slight male predominance reported in some studies (Roberts et al., 2012; Ward, 2000). Maldistribution of diastolic force among valve cusps and sinus attachment is thought also to promote ascending aortic dilatation or aneurysm (Burks et al., 1998; Perloff, 2003; Roberts, 1970). However, it remains unclear whether these aortic manifestations are genetically determined or represent a byproduct of mechanical stress, given that aortic dilatation is indistinct among regurgitant, stenotic and functionally normal bicuspid aortic valves (Hahn et al., 1992). Emerging evidence supports increased proteolytic activity in the aortic valve and adjacent areas including the aorta that may enhance the remodeling processes (Aikawa et al., 2007b).

Valvular calcification in the early stages causes aortic sclerosis, which predicts increased risks for cardiovascular morbidity and mortality (Otto et al., 1999). As the process progresses, the aortic valve orifice narrows while the valve anatomy and function become gradually distorted to produce valvular aortic stenosis with or without regurgitation, myocardial hypertrophic response, myocardial fibrosis, heart failure, and hemodynamic instability (Dweck et al., 2012). In recent years, the concept of degeneration in the pathogenesis of calcific aortic valve disease has been superseded by that of phenotypic modulation recapitulating embryonic development, angiogenesis, acquired and innate immune activation, wound healing and bone formation (Hakuno et al., 2009).

4. Acquired aortic valve disease

4.1. Aortic valve calcification and systemic inflammation

Aortic valve sclerosis has been estimated to affect at least 20% of adults over 65 years of age in the general population (Lindroos et al., 1993; Stewart et al., 1997). Calcific aortic valve disease represents a continuum of maladapted calcification in the aortic valve arising from active inflammatory and oxidative processes (Kaden et al., 2004; New and Aikawa, 2011; Towler, 2008), as well as a shift in the valve interstitial phenotype from chondrogenic to osteogenic. Early calcification of the aortic valve leads to increased valve leaflet thickness and stiffness in a condition termed aortic valve sclerosis (Otto et al., 1999). Continuation of the inflammatory process propagates angioneogenesis and biomineralization, leading to formation of calcium nodules that distort valve geometry and function, culminating in outflow-limiting aortic stenosis with or without regurgitation (Dweck et al., 2012; Rajamannan et al., 2011). Conditions that promote systemic inflammation, such as atherosclerosis, dyslipidemia and diabetes mellitus, have been shown to exacerbate the development of calcific aortic valve disease (Rajamannan et al., 2011). While statins may stabilize atheromatous plaques, reduce vascular calcification and clinical adverse outcomes, they have unfortunately not been shown to benefit calcific aortic valve disease in disease progression or patient outcomes (Chan et al., 2010; Cowell et al., 2005; Rossebo et al., 2008).

Studies exploring Notch signaling beyond congenital disorders and developmental biology identified Dll4 in macrophage-mediated inflammation (Fung et al., 2007). Recently, Fukuda and colleagues demonstrated that blockade of Dll4-Notch signaling using anti-Dll4 monoclonal antibody decreased BMP2, a central regulator of osteogenesis and bone mineralization (Fukuda et al., 2012), in line with other studies showing reduced aortic valve calcification with BMP2 knockdown by siRNA (Nigam and Srivastava, 2009), and the proinflammatory cytokine, TNF-α, accelerated BMP2-mediated calcification of human aortic valve interstitial cells from patients with calcific aortic valve stenosis (Yu et al., 2011). BMP2 mediates aortic valve calcification via Runx2 (Osf2/Cbfa1), a transcriptional activator of osteoblast development or gene expression (Ducy et al., 1997; Kaden et al., 2004; Mohler et al., 2001), and is suppressible by activation of Notch1 via Hey (HRT) (Acharya et al., 2011; Nigam and Srivastava, 2009). Moreover, the marked attenuation of aortic valvular calcification and stenosis through the blockade of angiogenesis-promoting Dll4 in a mouse model of hypercholesterolemia (Figure 2) also supports the current theory that angioneogenesis is a crucial stage in the natural history of calcific aortic valve disease (Dweck et al., 2012), recapitulating cardiogenesis and valve development (de la Pompa and Epstein, 2012; van den Akker et al., 2012). Thus, Dll4 critically bridges inflammation and angioneogenesis to osteogenesis in calcific aortic valve disease (Fukuda et al., 2012). These effects are probably independent of Notch 1 (Nus et al., 2011), since activation of the receptor presumably leads to inhibition of valve calcification (Acharya et al., 2011), whereas evidence on the benefits of Dll4 blockade (i.e. interruption of Dll4–Notch signaling) suggests that a Notch receptor other than Notch1, when activated, potentiates the development and progression of valve calcification. A shift in the Notch receptor:ligand ratio and/or the DLL:Jagged (Notch ligands) ratio may plausibly alter the cell-to-cell signalling strength and modality *in cis* and/or *in trans*, thus, modifying the final functional outcome. Much work remains to be done to fully delineate the mechanisms through which anti-Dll4 antibody exert inhibitory effects on inflammation and calcification.

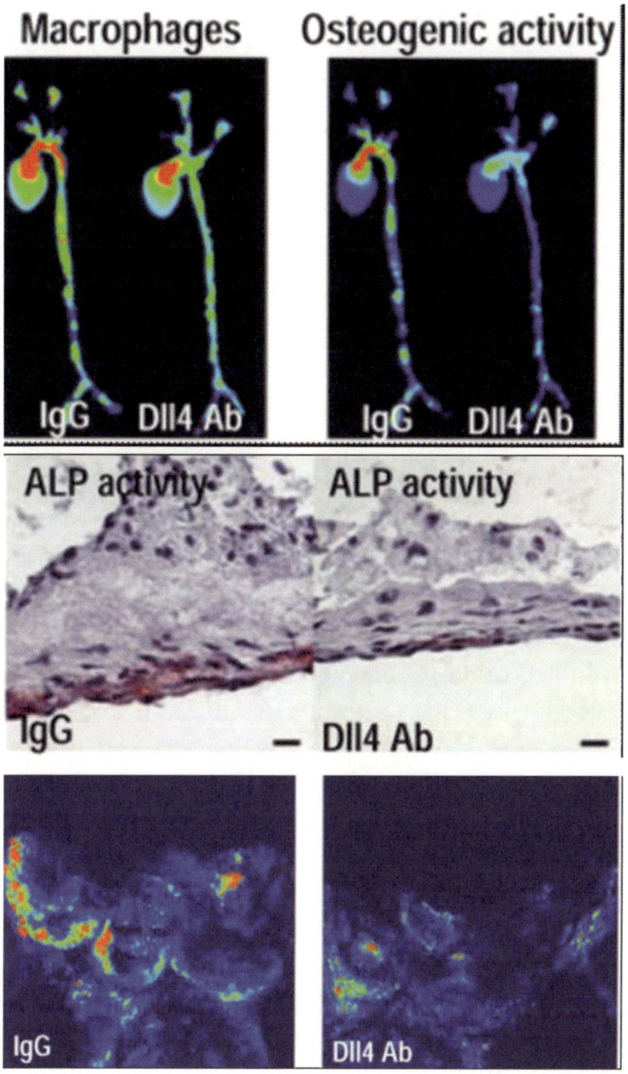

Figure 2. *Ex vivo* mapping using fluorescence reflectance imaging to grossly visualize the biomineralization of the hearts and vessels of atherosclerosis-prone (low-density lipoprotein receptor-deficient, *Ldlr*$^{-/-}$) animals fed a hypercholesterolemic diet, and independently treated with IgG isotype control or anti-Dll4 monoclonal antibody (Dll4 Ab). 750-nm CLIO750 nanoparticles were used to image macrophages, and 680-nm VisEn OsteoSense680 was used for the detection of osteogenic activity (top and bottom rows). Decreased osteogenic activity in the anti-Dll4 monoclonal antibody treated specimen is visualized using alkaline phosphatase (ALP) staining (middle row). Adapted from Fukuda and colleagues (Fukuda et al., 2012).

5. Clinical implications

Calcific aortic valve disease in individuals with severe aortic stenosis can progress quickly after presentation with symptoms, usually portending limited short-term survival (Turina et al., 1987). Clinical trials on medical therapy including statins have found little benefit and utility in forestalling disease progression, with no demonstrated impact on survival. Since the evidence suggests that inflammatory cells, particularly macrophages, play a crucial role in calcification, anti-inflammatory therapies may prevent development of arterial and valvular calcification. We and others have demonstrated that lipid lowering reduces inflammation (Aikawa et al., 1998; Aikawa et al., 2001; Chu et al., 2012; Libby and Aikawa, 2002; Libby et al., 2011). However, clinical trials (e.g. SALTIRE, SEAS, etc.) have failed to demonstrate that lipid lowering attenuates development of aortic stenosis. Preclinical findings suggest that macrophage accumulation precedes calcific changes in arteries and valves while lesions with advanced calcification are often unassociated with macrophages (Aikawa et al., 2007a; Aikawa et al., 2007b). This may suggest that anti-inflammatory therapies need to be initiated early (Aikawa and Otto, 2012), and thus clinical trials involving patients who had been diagnosed with aortic stenosis due to advanced calcification did not show substantial benefits of lipid lowering therapy. To establish more effective therapies, it is crucial to better understand the complex mechanisms for aortic valve calcification. To identify individuals with subclinical aortic valve calcification and those with high probability or propensity of developing severe aortic valvular stenosis, methods for early detection of calcific changes (e.g., molecular imaging, biomarkers) need to be developed. National Institutes of Health of the United States of America has formed the Working Group of Calcific Aortic Valve Disease to facilitate basic research on this devastating global health threat and initiated federal funding (Rajamannan et al., 2011).

Author details

Erik Fung[1,2] and Masanori Aikawa[3]

1 Section of Cardiology, Heart & Vascular Center, Dartmouth-Hitchcock Medical Center, Lebanon, New Hampshire, USA

2 Geisel School of Medicine at Dartmouth, Dartmouth College, Hanover, New Hampshire, USA

3 Center for Excellence in Vascular Biology, Cardiovascular Division, Brigham and Women's Hospital and Harvard Medical School, Boston, Massachusetts, USA

References

[1] Abraham, K.A., Cherian, G., Rao, V.D., Sukumar, I.P., Krishnaswami, S., and John, S. (1979). Tetralogy of Fallot in adults. A report on 147 patients. Am J Med 66, 811-816.

[2] Acharya, A., Hans, C.P., Koenig, S.N., Nichols, H.A., Galindo, C.L., Garner, H.R., Merrill, W.H., Hinton, R.B., and Garg, V. (2011). Inhibitory role of Notch1 in calcific aortic valve disease. PLoS One 6, e27743.

[3] Aikawa, E., Nahrendorf, M., Figueiredo, J.L., Swirski, F.K., Shtatland, T., Kohler, R.H., Jaffer, F.A., Aikawa, M., and Weissleder, R. (2007a). Osteogenesis associates with inflammation in early-stage atherosclerosis evaluated by molecular imaging in vivo. Circulation 116, 2841-2850.

[4] Aikawa, E., Nahrendorf, M., Sosnovik, D., Lok, V.M., Jaffer, F.A., Aikawa, M., and Weissleder, R. (2007b). Multimodality molecular imaging identifies proteolytic and osteogenic activities in early aortic valve disease. Circulation 115, 377-386.

[5] Aikawa, E., and Otto, C.M. (2012). Look more closely at the valve: imaging calcific aortic valve disease. Circulation 125, 9-11.

[6] Aikawa, M., Rabkin, E., Okada, Y., Voglic, S.J., Clinton, S.K., Brinckerhoff, C.E., Sukhova, G.K., and Libby, P. (1998). Lipid lowering by diet reduces matrix metalloproteinase activity and increases collagen content of rabbit atheroma: a potential mechanism of lesion stabilization. Circulation 97, 2433-2444.

[7] Aikawa, M., Rabkin, E., Sugiyama, S., Voglic, S.J., Fukumoto, Y., Furukawa, Y., Shiomi, M., Schoen, F.J., and Libby, P. (2001). An HMG-CoA reductase inhibitor, cerivastatin, suppresses growth of macrophages expressing matrix metalloproteinases and tissue factor in vivo and in vitro. Circulation 103, 276-283.

[8] Artavanis-Tsakonas, S., and Muskavitch, M.A. (2010). Notch: the past, the present, and the future. Curr Top Dev Biol 92, 1-29.

[9] Benedito, R., Roca, C., Sorensen, I., Adams, S., Gossler, A., Fruttiger, M., and Adams, R.H. (2009). The notch ligands Dll4 and Jagged1 have opposing effects on angiogenesis. Cell 137, 1124-1135.

[10] Bray, S.J. (2006). Notch signalling: a simple pathway becomes complex. Nat Rev Mol Cell Biol 7, 678-689.

[11] Brown, D.D., Martz, S.N., Binder, O., Goetz, S.C., Price, B.M., Smith, J.C., and Conlon, F.L. (2005). Tbx5 and Tbx20 act synergistically to control vertebrate heart morphogenesis. Development 132, 553-563.

[12] Burks, J.M., Illes, R.W., Keating, E.C., and Lubbe, W.J. (1998). Ascending aortic aneurysm and dissection in young adults with bicuspid aortic valve: implications for echocardiographic surveillance. Clin Cardiol 21, 439-443.

[13] Camenisch, T.D., Runyan, R.B., and Markwald, R.R., eds.Molecular regulation of cushion morphogenesis, In: Heart Development and Regeneration, 363-413, 1st edn (London, UK, Academic Press).

[14] Chan, K.L., Teo, K., Dumesnil, J.G., Ni, A., and Tam, J. (2010). Effect of Lipid lowering with rosuvastatin on progression of aortic stenosis: results of the aortic stenosis progression observation: measuring effects of rosuvastatin (ASTRONOMER) trial. Circulation 121, 306-314.

[15] Chu, A.Y., Guilianini, F., Barratt, B.J., Nyberg, F., Chasman, D.I., and Ridker, P.M. (2012). Pharmacogenetic determinants of statin-induced reductions in C-reactive protein. Circ Cardiovasc Genet 5, 58-65.

[16] Colliton, R.P., Bason, L., Lu, F.M., Piccoli, D.A., Krantz, I.D., and Spinner, N.B. (2001). Mutation analysis of Jagged1 (JAG1) in Alagille syndrome patients. Hum Mutat 17, 151-152.

[17] Combs, M.D., and Yutzey, K.E. (2009). Heart valve development: regulatory networks in development and disease. Circ Res 105, 408-421.

[18] Cowell, S.J., Newby, D.E., Prescott, R.J., Bloomfield, P., Reid, J., Northridge, D.B., and Boon, N.A. (2005). A randomized trial of intensive lipid-lowering therapy in calcific aortic stenosis. N Engl J Med 352, 2389-2397.

[19] de la Pompa, J.L., and Epstein, J.A. (2012). Coordinating tissue interactions: Notch signaling in cardiac development and disease. Dev Cell 22, 244-254.

[20] Del Monte, G., Grego-Bessa, J., Gonzalez-Rajal, A., Bolos, V., and De La Pompa, J.L. (2007). Monitoring Notch1 activity in development: evidence for a feedback regulatory loop. Dev Dyn 236, 2594-2614.

[21] Duarte, A., Hirashima, M., Benedito, R., Trindade, A., Diniz, P., Bekman, E., Costa, L., Henrique, D., and Rossant, J. (2004). Dosage-sensitive requirement for mouse Dll4 in artery development. Genes Dev 18, 2474-2478.

[22] Ducy, P., Zhang, R., Geoffroy, V., Ridall, A.L., and Karsenty, G. (1997). Osf2/Cbfa1: a transcriptional activator of osteoblast differentiation. Cell 89, 747-754.

[23] Dweck, M.R., Boon, N.A., and Newby, D.E. (2012). Calcific aortic stenosis: a disease of the valve and the myocardium. J Am Coll Cardiol 60, 1854-1863.

[24] Eldadah, Z.A., Hamosh, A., Biery, N.J., Montgomery, R.A., Duke, M., Elkins, R., and Dietz, H.C. (2001). Familial Tetralogy of Fallot caused by mutation in the jagged1 gene. Hum Mol Genet 10, 163-169.

[25] Fiuza, U.M., and Arias, A.M. (2007). Cell and molecular biology of Notch. J Endocrinol 194, 459-474.

[26] Fukuda, D., Aikawa, E., Swirski, F.K., Novobrantseva, T.I., Kotelianski, V., Gorgun, C.Z., Chudnovskiy, A., Yamazaki, H., Croce, K., Weissleder, R., et al. (2012). Notch

ligand Delta-like 4 blockade attenuates atherosclerosis and metabolic disorders. Proc Natl Acad Sci U S A 109, E1868-1877.

[27] Fung, E., Tang, S.M., Canner, J.P., Morishige, K., Arboleda-Velasquez, J.F., Cardoso, A.A., Carlesso, N., Aster, J.C., and Aikawa, M. (2007). Delta-like 4 induces notch signaling in macrophages: implications for inflammation. Circulation 115, 2948-2956.

[28] Garg, V., Muth, A.N., Ransom, J.F., Schluterman, M.K., Barnes, R., King, I.N., Grossfeld, P.D., and Srivastava, D. (2005). Mutations in NOTCH1 cause aortic valve disease. Nature 437, 270-274.

[29] Gibert, J.M., and Simpson, P. (2003). Evolution of cis-regulation of the proneural genes. Int J Dev Biol 47, 643-651.

[30] Greenway, S.C., Pereira, A.C., Lin, J.C., DePalma, S.R., Israel, S.J., Mesquita, S.M., Ergul, E., Conta, J.H., Korn, J.M., McCarroll, S.A., et al. (2009). De novo copy number variants identify new genes and loci in isolated sporadic tetralogy of Fallot. Nat Genet 41, 931-935.

[31] Guruharsha, K.G., Kankel, M.W., and Artavanis-Tsakonas, S. (2012). The Notch signalling system: recent insights into the complexity of a conserved pathway. Nat Rev Genet 13, 654-666.

[32] Hahn, R.T., Roman, M.J., Mogtader, A.H., and Devereux, R.B. (1992). Association of aortic dilation with regurgitant, stenotic and functionally normal bicuspid aortic valves. J Am Coll Cardiol 19, 283-288.

[33] Hakuno, D., Kimura, N., Yoshioka, M., and Fukuda, K. (2009). Molecular mechanisms underlying the onset of degenerative aortic valve disease. J Mol Med (Berl) 87, 17-24.

[34] Heitzler, P., and Simpson, P. (1991). The choice of cell fate in the epidermis of Drosophila. Cell 64, 1083-1092.

[35] Higgins, C.B., and Wexler, L. (1975). Reversal of dominance of the coronary arterial system in isolated aortic stenosis and bicuspid aortic valve. Circulation 52, 292-296.

[36] High, F.A., Lu, M.M., Pear, W.S., Loomes, K.M., Kaestner, K.H., and Epstein, J.A. (2008). Endothelial expression of the Notch ligand Jagged1 is required for vascular smooth muscle development. Proc Natl Acad Sci U S A 105, 1955 1959.

[37] Hinton, R.B., and Yutzey, K.E. (2011). Heart valve structure and function in development and disease. Annu Rev Physiol 73, 29-46.

[38] Hofmann, J.J., Briot, A., Enciso, J., Zovein, A.C., Ren, S., Zhang, Z.W., Radtke, F., Simons, M., Wang, Y., and Iruela-Arispe, M.L. (2012). Endothelial deletion of murine Jag1 leads to valve calcification and congenital heart defects associated with Alagille syndrome. Development 139, 4449-4460.

[39] Hove, J.R., Koster, R.W., Forouhar, A.S., Acevedo-Bolton, G., Fraser, S.E., and Gharib, M. (2003). Intracardiac fluid forces are an essential epigenetic factor for embryonic cardiogenesis. Nature 421, 172-177.

[40] Hutchins, G.M., Nazarian, I.H., and Bulkley, B.H. (1978). Association of left dominant coronary arterial system with congenital bicuspid aortic valve. Am J Cardiol 42, 57-59.

[41] Kaden, J.J., Bickelhaupt, S., Grobholz, R., Vahl, C.F., Hagl, S., Brueckmann, M., Haase, K.K., Dempfle, C.E., and Borggrefe, M. (2004). Expression of bone sialoprotein and bone morphogenetic protein-2 in calcific aortic stenosis. J Heart Valve Dis 13, 560-566.

[42] Kamath, B.M., Spinner, N.B., Emerick, K.M., Chudley, A.E., Booth, C., Piccoli, D.A., and Krantz, I.D. (2004). Vascular anomalies in Alagille syndrome: a significant cause of morbidity and mortality. Circulation 109, 1354-1358.

[43] Kikuchi, Y., Verkade, H., Reiter, J.F., Kim, C.H., Chitnis, A.B., Kuroiwa, A., and Stainier, D.Y. (2004). Notch signaling can regulate endoderm formation in zebrafish. Dev Dyn 229, 756-762.

[44] Kirk, E.P., Sunde, M., Costa, M.W., Rankin, S.A., Wolstein, O., Castro, M.L., Butler, T.L., Hyun, C., Guo, G., Otway, R., et al. (2007). Mutations in cardiac T-box factor gene TBX20 are associated with diverse cardiac pathologies, including defects of septation and valvulogenesis and cardiomyopathy. Am J Hum Genet 81, 280-291.

[45] Kopan, R., and Ilagan, M.X. (2009). The canonical Notch signaling pathway: unfolding the activation mechanism. Cell 137, 216-233.

[46] Ladich, E., Nakano, M., Carter-Monroe, N., and Virmani, R. (2011). Pathology of calcific aortic stenosis. Future Cardiol 7, 629-642.

[47] Laforest, B., Andelfinger, G., and Nemer, M. (2011). Loss of Gata5 in mice leads to bicuspid aortic valve. J Clin Invest 121, 2876-2887.

[48] Lee, J.S., Yu, Q., Shin, J.T., Sebzda, E., Bertozzi, C., Chen, M., Mericko, P., Stadtfeld, M., Zhou, D., Cheng, L., et al. (2006). Klf2 is an essential regulator of vascular hemodynamic forces in vivo. Dev Cell 11, 845-857.

[49] Li, L., Krantz, I.D., Deng, Y., Genin, A., Banta, A.B., Collins, C.C., Qi, M., Trask, B.J., Kuo, W.L., Cochran, J., et al. (1997). Alagille syndrome is caused by mutations in human Jagged1, which encodes a ligand for Notch1. Nat Genet 16, 243-251.

[50] Libby, P., and Aikawa, M. (2002). Stabilization of atherosclerotic plaques: new mechanisms and clinical targets. Nat Med 8, 1257-1262.

[51] Libby, P., Ridker, P.M., and Hansson, G.K. (2011). Progress and challenges in translating the biology of atherosclerosis. Nature 473, 317-325.

[52] Lindroos, M., Kupari, M., Heikkila, J., and Tilvis, R. (1993). Prevalence of aortic valve abnormalities in the elderly: an echocardiographic study of a random population sample. J Am Coll Cardiol 21, 1220-1225.

[53] Loffredo, C.A., Chokkalingam, A., Sill, A.M., Boughman, J.A., Clark, E.B., Scheel, J., and Brenner, J.I. (2004). Prevalence of congenital cardiovascular malformations among relatives of infants with hypoplastic left heart, coarctation of the aorta, and d-transposition of the great arteries. Am J Med Genet A 124A, 225-230.

[54] Lu, F., Morrissette, J.J., and Spinner, N.B. (2003). Conditional JAG1 mutation shows the developing heart is more sensitive than developing liver to JAG1 dosage. Am J Hum Genet 72, 1065-1070.

[55] Ma, L., Lu, M.F., Schwartz, R.J., and Martin, J.F. (2005). Bmp2 is essential for cardiac cushion epithelial-mesenchymal transition and myocardial patterning. Development 132, 5601-5611.

[56] MacGrogan, D., Luna-Zurita, L., and de la Pompa, J.L. (2011). Notch signaling in cardiac valve development and disease. Birth Defects Res A Clin Mol Teratol 91, 449-459.

[57] McCarthy, J.V., Twomey, C., and Wujek, P. (2009). Presenilin-dependent regulated intramembrane proteolysis and gamma-secretase activity. Cell Mol Life Sci 66, 1534-1555.

[58] McElhinney, D.B., Krantz, I.D., Bason, L., Piccoli, D.A., Emerick, K.M., Spinner, N.B., and Goldmuntz, E. (2002). Analysis of cardiovascular phenotype and genotype-phenotype correlation in individuals with a JAG1 mutation and/or Alagille syndrome. Circulation 106, 2567-2574.

[59] Miller, J.D., Weiss, R.M., Serrano, K.M., Castaneda, L.E., Brooks, R.M., Zimmerman, K., and Heistad, D.D. (2010). Evidence for active regulation of pro-osteogenic signaling in advanced aortic valve disease. Arterioscler Thromb Vasc Biol 30, 2482-2486.

[60] Mohamed, S.A., Aherrahrou, Z., Liptau, H., Erasmi, A.W., Hagemann, C., Wrobel, S., Borzym, K., Schunkert, H., Sievers, H.H., and Erdmann, J. (2006). Novel missense mutations (p.T596M and p.P1797H) in NOTCH1 in patients with bicuspid aortic valve. Biochem Biophys Res Commun 345, 1460-1465.

[61] Mohler, E.R., 3rd, Gannon, F., Reynolds, C., Zimmerman, R., Keane, M.G., and Kaplan, F.S. (2001). Bone formation and inflammation in cardiac valves. Circulation 103, 1522-1528.

[62] New, S.E., and Aikawa, E. (2011). Molecular imaging insights into early inflammatory stages of arterial and aortic valve calcification. Circ Res 108, 1381-1391.

[63] Nigam, V., and Srivastava, D. (2009). Notch1 represses osteogenic pathways in aortic valve cells. J Mol Cell Cardiol 47, 828-834.

[64] Nus, M, MacGrogan, D, Martínez-Poveda, B, Benito, Y, Casanova, J. C, Fernández-Avilés, F, Bermejo, J, de la Pompa J. L. (2011). Diet-induced aortic valve disease in mice haploinsufficient for the Notch pathway effector RBPJK/CSL. Arterioscler Thromb Vasc Biol, 31, 1580-1588.

[65] Oda, T., Elkahloun, A.G., Pike, B.L., Okajima, K., Krantz, I.D., Genin, A., Piccoli, D.A., Meltzer, P.S., Spinner, N.B., Collins, F.S., et al. (1997). Mutations in the human Jagged1 gene are responsible for Alagille syndrome. Nat Genet 16, 235-242.

[66] Otto, C.M., Lind, B.K., Kitzman, D.W., Gersh, B.J., and Siscovick, D.S. (1999). Association of aortic-valve sclerosis with cardiovascular mortality and morbidity in the elderly. N Engl J Med 341, 142-147.

[67] Pachulski, R.T., and Chan, K.L. (1993). Progression of aortic valve dysfunction in 51 adult patients with congenital bicuspid aortic valve: assessment and follow up by Doppler echocardiography. Br Heart J 69, 237-240.

[68] Padang, R., Bagnall, R.D., Richmond, D.R., Bannon, P.G., and Semsarian, C. (2012). Rare non-synonymous variations in the transcriptional activation domains of GATA5 in bicuspid aortic valve disease. J Mol Cell Cardiol 53, 277-281.

[69] Perloff, J.K. (2003). Congenital aortic stenosis, In: The Clinical Recognition of Congenital Heart Disease, 81-112, 3rd edn (Philadelphia, PA, Saunders).

[70] Person, A.D., Klewer, S.E., and Runyan, R.B. (2005). Cell biology of cardiac cushion development. Int Rev Cytol 243, 287-335.

[71] Plageman, T.F., Jr., and Yutzey, K.E. (2005). T-box genes and heart development: putting the "T" in heart. Dev Dyn 232, 11-20.

[72] Presbitero, P., Demarie, D., Villani, M., Perinetto, E.A., Riva, G., Orzan, F., Bobbio, M., Morea, M., and Brusca, A. (1987). Long term results (15-30 years) of surgical repair of aortic coarctation. Br Heart J 57, 462-467.

[73] Rajamannan, N.M., Evans, F.J., Aikawa, E., Grande-Allen, K.J., Demer, L.L., Heistad, D.D., Simmons, C.A., Masters, K.S., Mathieu, P., O'Brien, K.D., et al. (2011). Calcific aortic valve disease: not simply a degenerative process: A review and agenda for research from the National Heart and Lung and Blood Institute Aortic Stenosis Working Group. Executive summary: Calcific aortic valve disease-2011 update. Circulation 124, 1783-1791.

[74] Rajamannan, N.M., Subramaniam, M., Rickard, D., Stock, S.R., Donovan, J., Springett, M., Orszulak, T., Fullerton, D.A., Tajik, A.J., Bonow, R.O., et al. (2003). Human aortic valve calcification is associated with an osteoblast phenotype. Circulation 107, 2181-2184.

[75] Roberts, W.C. (1970). The structure of the aortic valve in clinically isolated aortic stenosis: an autopsy study of 162 patients over 15 years of age. Circulation 42, 91-97.

[76] Roberts, W.C., Vowels, T.J., and Ko, J.M. (2012). Natural history of adults with congenitally malformed aortic valves (unicuspid or bicuspid). Medicine (Baltimore) 91, 287-308.

[77] Rossebo, A.B., Pedersen, T.R., Boman, K., Brudi, P., Chambers, J.B., Egstrup, K., Gerdts, E., Gohlke-Barwolf, C., Holme, I., Kesaniemi, Y.A., et al. (2008). Intensive lipid lowering with simvastatin and ezetimibe in aortic stenosis. N Engl J Med 359, 1343-1356.

[78] Shen, T., Aneas, I., Sakabe, N., Dirschinger, R.J., Wang, G., Smemo, S., Westlund, J.M., Cheng, H., Dalton, N., Gu, Y., et al. (2011). Tbx20 regulates a genetic program essential to adult mouse cardiomyocyte function. J Clin Invest 121, 4640-4654.

[79] Spinner, N.B., Colliton, R.P., Crosnier, C., Krantz, I.D., Hadchouel, M., and Meunier-Rotival, M. (2001). Jagged1 mutations in alagille syndrome. Hum Mutat 17, 18-33.

[80] Stennard, F.A., Costa, M.W., Elliott, D.A., Rankin, S., Haast, S.J., Lai, D., McDonald, L.P., Niederreither, K., Dolle, P., Bruneau, B.G., et al. (2003). Cardiac T-box factor Tbx20 directly interacts with Nkx2-5, GATA4, and GATA5 in regulation of gene expression in the developing heart. Dev Biol 262, 206-224.

[81] Stewart, A.B., Ahmed, R., Travill, C.M., and Newman, C.G. (1993). Coarctation of the aorta life and health 20-44 years after surgical repair. Br Heart J 69, 65-70.

[82] Stewart, B.F., Siscovick, D., Lind, B.K., Gardin, J.M., Gottdiener, J.S., Smith, V.E., Kitzman, D.W., and Otto, C.M. (1997). Clinical factors associated with calcific aortic valve disease. Cardiovascular Health Study. J Am Coll Cardiol 29, 630-634.

[83] Timmerman, L.A., Grego-Bessa, J., Raya, A., Bertran, E., Perez-Pomares, J.M., Diez, J., Aranda, S., Palomo, S., McCormick, F., Izpisua-Belmonte, J.C., et al. (2004). Notch promotes epithelial-mesenchymal transition during cardiac development and oncogenic transformation. Genes Dev 18, 99-115.

[84] Towler, D.A. (2008). Oxidation, inflammation, and aortic valve calcification peroxide paves an osteogenic path. J Am Coll Cardiol 52, 851-854.

[85] Turina, J., Hess, O., Sepulcri, F., and Krayenbuehl, H.P. (1987). Spontaneous course of aortic valve disease. Eur Heart J 8, 471-483.

[86] van den Akker, N.M., Caolo, V., and Molin, D.G. (2012). Cellular decisions in cardiac outflow tract and coronary development: an act by VEGF and NOTCH. Differentiation 84, 62-78.

[87] Vermot, J., Forouhar, A.S., Liebling, M., Wu, D., Plummer, D., Gharib, M., and Fraser, S.E. (2009). Reversing blood flows act through klf2a to ensure normal valvulogenesis in the developing heart. PLoS Biol 7, e1000246.

[88] Wakabayashi, T., and De Strooper, B. (2008). Presenilins: members of the gamma-secretase quartets, but part-time soloists too. Physiology (Bethesda) 23, 194-204.

[89] Ward, C. (2000). Clinical significance of the bicuspid aortic valve. Heart 83, 81-85.

[90] Wilkinson, H.A., Fitzgerald, K., and Greenwald, I. (1994). Reciprocal changes in expression of the receptor lin-12 and its ligand lag-2 prior to commitment in a C. elegans cell fate decision. Cell 79, 1187-1198.

[91] Yu, Z., Seya, K., Daitoku, K., Motomura, S., Fukuda, I., and Furukawa, K. (2011). Tumor necrosis factor-alpha accelerates the calcification of human aortic valve interstitial cells obtained from patients with calcific aortic valve stenosis via the BMP2-Dlx5 pathway. J Pharmacol Exp Ther 337, 16-23.

[92] Zhang, J., Chang, J.Y., Huang, Y., Lin, X., Luo, Y., Schwartz, R.J., Martin, J.F., and Wang, F. (2010). The FGF-BMP signaling axis regulates outflow tract valve primordium formation by promoting cushion neural crest cell differentiation. Circ Res 107, 1209-1219.

Chapter 5

Role of MicroRNAs in Cardiovascular Calcification

Claudia Goettsch and Elena Aikawa

Additional information is available at the end of the chapter

http://dx.doi.org/10.5772/55326

1. Introduction

With a growing older population, cardiovascular diseases are becoming an increasing economic and social burden in Western societies. Cardiovascular calcification is a major characteristic of chronic inflammatory disorders — such as chronic renal disease (CRD), type 2 diabetes (T2D), atherosclerosis and calcific aortic valve disease (CAVD) — that associate with significant morbidity and mortality. Cardiovascular calcification also associates with osteoporosis in humans and animal models [1, 2] — the so-called "calcification paradox" [3]. The concept that similar pathways control both bone remodeling and vascular calcification is currently widely accepted, but the precise mechanisms of calcification remain largely unknown. Osteogenic transition of vascular smooth muscle cells (SMCs), valvular interstitial cells (VIC) or stem cells is induced by bone morphogenetic proteins, inflammation, oxidative stress, or high phosphate levels, and leads to a unique molecular pattern marked by osteogenic transcription factors [4]. Loss of mineralization inhibitors, such as matrix γ-carboxyglutamic acid Gla protein (MGP) and fetuin-A also contribute to cardiovascular calcification. The physiological balance between induction and inhibition of calcification becomes dysregulated in CRD, T2D, atherosclerosis, and CAVD. Consequently, calcification may occur at several sites in the cardiovascular system, including the intima and media of vessels and cardiac valves [3].

The central role of miRNAs as fine-tune regulators in the cardiovascular system and bone biology has gained acceptance and has raised the possibility for novel therapeutic targets. Circulating miRNAs have been proposed as biomarkers for a wide range of cardiovascular diseases, but knowledge of miRNA biology in cardiovascular calcification is very limited.

2. Micro-RNA biology: Biosynthesis and function

Micro-RNAs (miRNAs) are a large class of evolutionarily conserved, small, endogenous, non-coding RNAs serving as essential post-transcriptional modulators of gene expression [5]. miRNAs regulate biological processes by binding to mRNA 3'-untranslated region (UTR) sequences to attenuate protein synthesis or messenger RNA (mRNA) stability [6]. Acting as genetic switches or fine-tuners, miRNAs are key regulators of diverse biological and pathological processes, including development, organogenesis, apoptosis, and cell proliferation and differentiation. miRNA dysregulation often results in impaired cellular function and disease progression. It has been estimated that the whole human genome encodes for about 1000 miRNAs which may be located within introns of coding or non-coding genes, within host exons or within intergenic regions [7].

miRNA biogenesis is shown in Figure 1. The transcription process is mediated by the RNA-polymerase II that produces long precursor RNAs known as "primary miRNA" (pri-miRNA) with a typical hairpin morphology [8]. A nuclear endonuclease, called DROSHA, then crops the distal stem portion of pri-RNA obtaining shorter chains (pre-miRNA) [9]. Pre-miRNA is transported to the cytoplasm by the nuclear receptor Exportin-5 [10] and processed by DICER, an RNase III, to short double-stranded RNA sequence containing the miRNA and the 'star strand' (miRNA*). miRNA* is degraded after stripping the miRNA strand to obtain mature miRNA [11]. Mature miRNA interact with proteins like Argonaute endonuclease (Arg 2), in order to form the RNA-induced silencing complex (RICS), which directs mature miRNA towards the targeted mRNA and bind on their 3' untranslated region (UTR) [6].

A single miRNA may modulate hundreds of miRNAs, and one mRNA has multiple predicted binding sites for miRNAs in their 3'UTR. Furthermore, after cleavage of a target mRNA, miRNAs are not Destroyed; so they may recognise and modulate other mRNAs [5, 12].

3. miRNAs and cardiovascular disease

Cardiovascular calcification is an independent risk factor for cardiovascular morbidity and mortality. Several risk factors can accelerate atherosclerosis and cardiovascular calcification, including age, hypercholesterolemia, metabolic syndrome, CRD, and T2D. Cardiovascular calcification can be distinguished by location — as intimal (atherosclerotic) , medial (CRD, T2D), or valvular [3]. Atherosclerotic calcification occurs as a part of atherogenic progress in the vessel intima. Small hydroxyapatite mineral crystals (microcalcification) can be visualized in early lesions [13]. Medial calcification occurs primarily in association with CRD and T2D, independently of hypercholesterolemia. Aortic valve calcification leads to impaired movement of aortic valve leaflets, and causes valve dysfunction [2]. All three processes shared risk factors and etiological factors, including inflammation and oxidative stress.

The identification of circulating miRNA as a novel biomarker in various diseases is a growing area of research investigation. Many pioneering studies describe specific miRNA patterns in

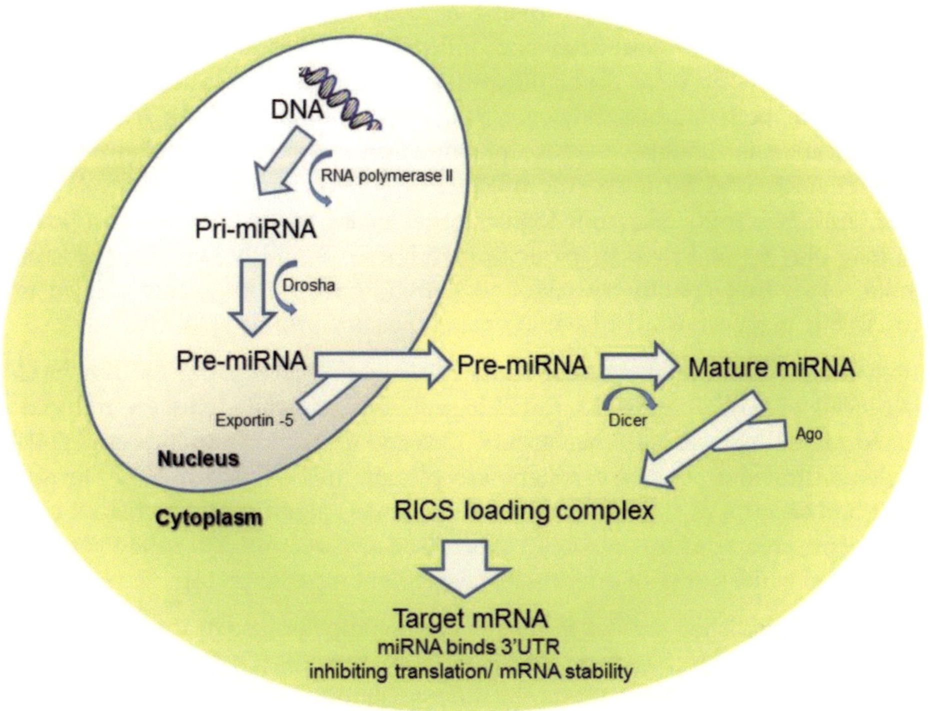

Figure 1. Schematic overview of miRNA biogenesis.

cardiovascular diseases. The first study reporting circulating miRNAs in patients with atherosclerosis was published in 2010, demonstrating a reduction of circulating vascular- and inflammation-associated miRNAs (miR-126, miR-17, miR-92a, miR-155) in patients with coronary artery disease (CAD) [14]. In addition, tissue levels of miRNAs were investigated.

Here we summarize and discuss the current knowledge on circulating and tissue miRNAs in diseases associated with cardiovascular calcification (Tables 1 and 2).

3.1. miRNAs in coronary artery disease

Studies about miRNA expression in calcified vessels are rare. Li *et al.* analyzed the expression of miRNAs in patients with peripheral artery disease (arteriosclerosis obliterans), characterized by fibrosis of the tunica intima and calcification of the tunica media [15]. miR-21, miR-130a, miR-27b, let-7f, and miR-210 were significantly increased, while miR-221 and miR-222 were decreased in the sclerotic intima, compared to normal vessels [15]. Higher levels of miR-21 and miR-210 were confirmed in a study that compared atherosclerotic with non-atherosclerotic left internal thoracic arteries [16]. In addition, the expression of miR-34a, miR-146a, miR146b-5p, and miR-210 increased more than 4-fold in atherosclerotic arteries. Several predicted targets were downregulated [16]. Another study found a different miRNA pattern using plaque material from the carotid artery, compared with the arteria mammaria interna as control tissue [17]. The healthy vessel expressed higher levels of miR-520b and miR-105, whereas miR-10b, miR-218, miR-30e, miR-26b, and miR-125a were predominantly expressed in atherosclerotic plaque [17]. The investigators in both studies, however, did not examine miRNAs in calcified lesions. Microcalcification is thought to cause plaque rupture [18, 19]. Destabilized human plaques are characterized by a specific miRNA expression profile (high levels of miR-100, miR-127, miR-145, miR-133a, miR-133b). Target genes of these miRNAs (Nox1, MMP9, CD40) may play a role in vascular calcification [7]. Thus, miRNAs could participate in the formation of hydroxyapatite crystals, and thereby have an important role in regulating atherosclerotic plaque toward unstable phenotypes and rupture [20].

Fichtlscherer *et al.* authored the first study investigating circulating miRNA in CAD [14]. Plasma levels of miR-17, miR-92a, miR-126, miR-145, and miR-155 were reduced in CAD compared to healthy controls, whereas miR-133a and miR-208a were increased [14]. Another study demonstrated a positive correlation of plasma miR-122 and miR-370 levels with the presence and severity of CAD [21]. Both miRNAs were significantly increased in hyperlipidemia patients, compared to controls [21]. Increased levels of miR-27b, miR-130a, and miR-210 were observed in the serum of arteriosclerosis obliterans patients [15].

Comparison of published studies is challenging mainly because of the different sources of circulating miRNAs, which include serum, whole blood, PBMCs, EPCs, and platelets (Table 1). The miRNA profiles obtained from the different studies, therefore, are often not the same. In this context, a recent report suggested the necessity of careful selection for reference miRNAs by showing that hemolysis may significantly affect the levels of plasma miRNAs previously used as controls [22].

Polymorphisms in the 3'UTR may alter miRNA binding, leading to post-transcriptional dysregulation of the target gene and aberrant protein level. Functional single-nucleotide polymorphisms (SNPs) of miRNA-binding sites associate with the risk of cardiovascular disease. Wu *et al.* discovered a SNP in the miR-149 binding site of the 5,10-methylenetetrahydrofolate reductase (MTHFR) gene that associated with increased risk for CAD [23]. Furthermore, a larger study in a Chinese population of 956 CAD patients and 620 controls revealed that a SNP in the binding sites for miR-196a2 and miR-499 associated with the occurrence and prognosis of CAD [24].

3.2. miRNAs in diabetes and chronic renal disease (CRD)

T2D is a major risk factor for cardiovascular disease. Zampetaki *et al.* identified a plasma miRNA signature for T2D that includes reduced levels of miR-223, miR-15, miR-20b, miR-21, miR-24, miR-29b, miR-126, miR-150, miR-191, miR-197, miR-320, and miR-486, and elevated levels of miR-28-3p [33]. Reduced miR-126 levels antedated diabetes manifestation, and might explain the impaired peripheral angiogenic signaling in patients with T2D. Reduction of circulating miR-21 and miR-126 was confirmed by Meng *et al.*, who also found a decrease of miR-27a,b and miR-130a in T2D patients [35]. Another study demonstrated mostly elevated miRNA levels (miR-9, miR-29a, miR-30d, miR-34a, miR-124a, miR-146a, and miR-375) in serum from T2D patients, compared with pre-diabetic and/or normal glucose tolerance

miRNA	Disease	Source	Finding	Reference number
miR-17, -21, -20a, -22a, -27a, -92a, -126, -145, -155, -221, -130a, -208b, let-7d miR-133a, -208a	CAD	Serum	Decreased Increased	[14]
miR-146a/b	CAD	PBMC	Increased	[25]
miR-34a	CAD	EPC	Increased	[26]
miR-221, -222	CAD	EPC	Increased	[27]
miR-135a, -147	CAD	PBMC	Decreased	[28]
miR-140, -182	CAD	Whole blood	Decreased	[29]
miR-122, -370	CAD	Plasma	Increased	[21]
miR-181a	CAD	Monocytes	Decreased	[30]
Let-7i	CAD	Monocytes	Decreased	[31]
miR-340, -624	CAD	Platelets	Increased	[32]
miR-20b, -21, -24, -29b, -15a, -126, -150, -191, -197, -223, -320, -486 miR-28-3p	T2D	Plasma	Decreased Increased	[33]
miR-146a	T2D	PBMC	Decreased	[34]
miR-21, -27a, b, -126, -130a	T2D	EPC	Decreased	[35]
miR-9, -29a, -30d, -34a, -124a, -146a, -375	T2D	Serum	Increased	[36]
miR-16, -21, -155, -210, -638	CRD	Plasma	Decreased	[37]
miR-188-5p, -135*, -323-3p, -509-3p, -520-3p, -572, -573, 629*, -632 miR-24, -106a, -191, -218, -222, -223, -342-3p, -412, let-7p	HC	HDL	Decreased Increased	[38]
miR-21, -27b, -130a, -210	AO	Serum	Increased	[15]

CRD, chronic renal disease; T2D, type 2 diabetes; CAD, coronary artery disease; AS, aortic stenosis; HC, familial hypercholesterolemia; AO, arteriosclerosis obliterans; PBMC, peripheral blood mononuclear cell; EPC, endothelial progenitor cell; HDL, high-density lipoprotein.

Table 1. Circulating miRNA in diseases associated with vascular calcification.

conditions [36]. In contrast, reduced miR-146a levels in PMBCs from Asian Indian T2D patients associated with insulin resistance, poor glycemic control, and several proinflammatory cytokine genes [34]. miR-146a participates in the transcriptional circuitry regulating fibronectin in T2D animals.[39].

The high incidence of cardiovascular complications in patients with CRD is partly explained by more aggressive development of atherosclerotic lesions and accelerated calcification [40]. To our knowledge, only one study reports circulating miRNA in patients with CRD. Neal *et al.* found that plasma levels of total and specific miRNAs (miR-16, miR-21, miR-155, miR-210, and miR-638) are reduced in CRD patients, compared to patients with normal renal function [37]. A strong correlation exists between detected circulating miRNAs and estimated glomerular filtration rate [37]. Interestingly, miR-638 was the only miRNA that showed a differential urine excretion in CRD patients [37]. Transforming growth factor beta (TGF-β), a pro-fibrotic key mediator of CRD, reduces levels of miR-192 [41] and miR-29a [42] and increases miR-377 levels [43] *in vitro* and *in vivo*, thereby promoting the expression of extracellular matrix components.

3.3. miRNAs and aortic valve disease

Aortic stenosis (AS) is typically caused by calcific aortic valve disease. To our knowledge, no study to date describes a specific miRNA signature in the circulation of patients with AS. Nigam *et al.* identified a miRNA pattern specific to AS using tissue from whole bicuspid valves and linking them to calcification-related genes, such as Smad1/3, Runx2, and BMP2 [44]. miR-26a, miR-30b, and miR-195 were decreased in the aortic valves of patients requiring replacement due to AS, compared to those requiring replacement due to aortic insufficiency [44]. Another group compared bicuspid with tricuspid aortic valve leaflets by miRNA microarray, and found a number of modulated miRNAs [45]. Particularly, miR-141 had the most dramatic change, showing a 14.5-fold decrease in the bicuspid versus tricuspid valve tissue, while the levels of calcification were comparable between the two groups.

3.4. Similar miRNA profiles may represent common miRNAs in diseases associated with cardiovascular calcification

Our detailed investigation using currently published literature revealed common circulating miRNAs in diseases associated with vascular calcification. Seven miRNAs (miR-21, miR-27, miR-34a, miR-126, miR-146a, miR-155, and miR210) were useful biomarkers in atherosclerosis, T2D, and/or CRD, and only miR-21 was common among all three diseases [14, 33, 37] (Table 3).

Atherosclerotic arteries [16] and sclerotic intima from lower-extremity vessels [15] expressed higher miR-21 levels than did healthy vessels. Circulating levels of miR-21 in atherosclerosis, T2D, and/or CRD were reduced [14, 33, 37]. The reason for this discrepancy is unknown, and requires further investigation.

miR-146a is an inflammation-related miRNA, implicated in atherosclerosis and osteoclastogenesis [46]. Circulating miR-146a is increased in CAD patients [25] and T2D [36]. In addition, miR-146a was more highly expressed in atherosclerotic arteries in an animal model [16], and associated with CRD *in vivo* [47]. miR-155, another inflammation-associated miRNA, is decreased in CAD [14] and CRD [37]. Deficiency of miR155 enhanced atherosclerotic plaque development and decreased plaque stability [48], suggesting that it acts as an anti-inflammatory and atheroprotective miRNA. miR-155 is also highly expressed in endothelial cells (ECs) and SMCs, where it targets angiotensin-II receptor [49]. The renin–angiotensin system participates in cardiovascular calcification [50, 51]. Angiotensin-receptor blockade can inhibit

miRNA	Disease	Tissue type	Finding	Reference number
miR-21, -34a, -146a, -146b-5p, -210	CAD	Atherosclerotic arteries	Increased	[16]
miR-105, -520b	CAD	Atherosclerotic carotid artery	Decreased	[17]
miR-10b, -26b, -30e, -125a, -218,			Increased	
miR-100, -127, -133a,b -145	CAD	Destabilized plaque	Increased	[20]
miR-221, -222	AO	Sclerotic intima from lower extremities vessels	Decreased	[15]
miR-21, -27b, -210, -130a, let-7f			Increased	
miR-22, -27a, -141, -124, -125b, -185, -187, -194, -211, -330, -370, -449, -486, -551, -564, -575, -585, -622, -637, -648, -1202, -1282, -1469, -1908, -1972	AS	Bicuspid aortic valve	Decreased	[45]
miR-30e, -32, -145, -151, -152, -190, -373, -768			Increased	
miR-26a, -30b, -195	AS	Whole bicuspid valves	Decreased	[44]

CAD, coronary artery disease; AS, aortic stenosis; AO, arteriosclerosis obliterans.

Table 2. miRNAs expressed in human calcified tissue.

CAD	T2D	CRD
miR-21 ↓	miR-21 ↓	miR-21 ↓
miR-27 ↓	miR-27 ↓	
miR-34a ↑	miR-34a ↑	
miR-126 ↓	miR-126 ↓	
miR-155 ↓		miR-155 ↓

CRD, chronic renal disease; T2D, type 2 diabetes; CAD, coronary artery disease

Table 3. Common circulating miRNA in diseases associated with vascular calcification.

arterial calcification by disrupting vascular osteogenesis *in vivo* [52]. In addition, an observational study showed reduced progression of AV disease in patients taking angiotensin-converting enzyme inhibitors [53]. Furthermore, miR-155 represses osteoblastogenesis by targeting Smad proteins [54]. Thus, high expression of miR-155 may prevent cardiovascular calcification by inhibiting the BMP signalling pathway or the renin–angiotensin system, making it a promising anti-calcification therapeutic target.

In summary, a set of circulating miRNAs (consisting of miR-21, miR-27, miR-34a, miR-126, miR-146a, miR-155, and miR-210) is dysregulated in various pro-inflammatory diseases and may represent a miRNA signature for cardiovascular calcification. Of note, systemic and local inflammation paradoxically affects cardiovascular calcification and bone loss, which supports the concept of inflammation-dependent cardiovascular calcification previously proposed by our group and others [13, 40, 55-57].

4. miRNA and osteogenesis in the vascular wall

Cardiovascular calcification is an active, cell-regulated process. Various studies provide evidence of phenotypic transition or transition/dedifferentiation of mature SMCs or VICs into an osteogenic phenotype — a key feature in cardiovascular calcification. In medial calcification, SMCs undergo dedifferentiation from a contractile to a pro-atherogenic synthestic phenotype, lose the expression of their marker genes, acquire osteogenic markers, and deposit a mineralized bone-like matrix. In valvular calcification, VICs can undergo the transition to osteoblast-like bone-forming cells [58]. Recently, a novel concept emerged of circulating cells harboring osteogenic potential that can home to atherosclerotic lesions and contribute to intimal calcification [59, 60]. Comparing the sources of cells that contribute to atherosclerotic intimal calcification revealed that SMCs are the major contributors that reprogram its lineage towards osteochondrogenesis/blastogenesis; circulating bone marrow-derived cells, however, also contribute to early osteochondrogenic differentiation in atherosclerotic vessels [61]. The master transcription factors, including Runx2/Cbfa1, Msx2, and Osterix, designate cells for osteoblast lineages through the induction of downstream genes such as alkaline phosphatase, osteopontin, and osteocalcin. Here we summarize miRNAs involved in SMC differentiation, as well as in osteogenesis, with targets involved in cardiovascular calcification.

The SMC phenotype is dependent on the miR-143/145 cluster [62-64]. Circulating miR-145 levels are reduced in CAD patients [14]. miR-145 is one of the most recognized arterial miRNAs [65]. Inhibition of miR-143/145 promotes a phenotypic switch to the synthetic, pro-atherogenic SMC state [62], including the inhibition of SMC marker-like alpha-smooth muscle actin and smooth muscle myosin heavy chain [66] — both diminished in osteogenic SMCs [67]. miR-145 modulates SMC differentiation by targeting Krüppel-like factor 4 (KLF4) [63]. KLF4 mediates high phosphate-induced conversion of SMCs into osteogenic cells [68]. Conversely, miR-145-deficient mice [69] and overexpression of miR-145 [66] both reduce neointima formation in vascular injury.

Similar to miR-145, miR-133 has a potent inhibitory role on the vascular SMC phenotypic switch [70]. Runx2, a cell-fate determining osteoblastic transcription factor, is a target of miR-133 [71]. Runx2 acts as a critical regulator of osteogenic lineage and a modulator of bone-related genes [72]. Runx2 is essential and sufficient for regulating osteogenesis in SMC and VIC [73, 74, 75, 76]. Discovered in the bone biology field, a program of miRNAs controls Runx2 expression to prevent skeletal disorders [77]. Three of these miRNAs (miR-133a, miR-135a, and miR-218) are altered in cardiovascular diseases associated with vascular calcification [14, 17, 20, 28]. Klotho mutant mice, which display vascular calcification due to hyperphosphatemia and through a Runx2-dependent mechanism [78], show overexpression of miR-135a (together with miR-762, miR-714, and miR-712) in the aortic media, which causes SMC calcification by disruption of Ca^{2+} transporters and increasing intracellular Ca^{2+} concentrations [79]. More recently, miR-204, another candidate of the Runx2-cluster, was found to contribute to SMC calcification *in vitro* and *in vivo* [80]. Downstream targets of Runx2 are bone-specific genes like osteopontin, osterix and osteocalcin, all present in the cardiovascular osteogenic cell phenotype [2, 81]. We recently demonstrated that miR-125b, which inhibits osteoblast differentiation [82] regulates the transition of SMCs into osteoblast-like cells partially by targeting the transcription factor osterix, providing the first miR-dependent mechanism in the progression of vascular calcification [83]. Additionally, miRNA-processing enzymes — essential for SMC function [84] — were reduced in calcified SMCs [83].

Another potent regulator of vascular and valvular calcification is the BMP signaling pathway (reviewed in detail elsewhere [85]). BMP2 and BMP4 are potent osteogenic differentiation factors detected in calcified valve and atherosclerotic lesions [86-88]. BMPs elicit their effects through activation of receptor complex composed of type I and type II receptors and activate receptor-type–dependent and ligand-dependent Smad transcription factors, which modulate the expression of Runx2 [85]. MiR-26a, miR-135, and miR-155 were previously reported as Smad-regulating miRNAs related to osteoblastogenesis; they functionally repress osteoblast differentiation by targeting Smad1 and Smad5, respectively [54]. miR-155 is one of the circulating miRNAs that is decreased in CAD [14] and CRD [37] (discussed earlier). miR-26a was repressed in aortic valve leaflets of patients with aortic stenosis, and human aortic valvular interstitial cells showed decreased mRNA levels of BMP2 and Smad1 when treated with miR-26a mimic [44]. The same group found lower expression of miR-30b, which targets Smad1 and Smad3. Another group reported deceased miR-141 levels together with increased BMP2 levels in bicuspid versus tricuspid aortic valve leaflets, and showed *in vitro* that miR-141 represses the VIC response to calcification, in part through BMP2-dependent calcification [45]. Itoh *et al.* identified miR-141 as a pre-osteoblast differentiation-related miRNA, which modulated the BMP2-induced pre-osteoblast differentiation by direct translational repression of Dlx5, a transcription factor for osterix [89].

Activation of canonical wingless-type (WNT) signaling is crucial for osteoblast function [90] and for the programming of valvular and vascular cells during cardiovascular calcification [85]. Activation of the Wnt/β-catenin signaling pathway occurs in human calcified aortic valve stenosis [91], in LDL receptor (LDLR)-deficient mice [92, 93], and in osteogenic SMCs *in vitro* [94]. Dickkopf (Dkk)1 is an extracellular antagonist of the canonical Wnt signaling that plays a crucial role in bone remodeling by binding to and inactivating signaling from LDLR-related protein 5/6 [95, 96]. Dkk-1 may also play a role in vascular calcification. In CRD patients, Dkk1 serum levels correlated negatively with arterial stiffness [97]. Dkk-1 prevents warfarin-induced activation of β-catenin, and osteogenic transdifferentiation of SMCs [98] and TNF α-induced induction of alkaline phosphatase activity [92]. Remarkably, two miRNAs targeting bone Dkk-1 (miR-335-5p, miR-29a) increase with age [99, 100] — a risk for cardiovascular calcification. miR-335-5p directly targets and represses Wnt inhibitor Dkk-1, thereby enhancing Wnt signaling and promoting osteoblast differentiation [101]. To date, no publications exist regarding the role of miR-335-5p in the cardiovascular system. Yet, the age-dependent increase of miR-335 in rat renal tissue inhibited the expression and function of the enzymes implicated in oxidative stress defense [99]. Likewise, miR-29a potentiates osteoblastogenesis by modulating Wnt signaling. Canonical Wnt signaling induces miR-29a expression, which negatively targets regulators of Wnt signaling, including Dkk-1, sFRP2, Kremen, and osteonectin [102, 103]. miR-29 increased age-dependently in mouse aortic tissue and associated with reduced extracellular matrix components, such as collagen and elastin [100]. Elastolysis accelerates arterial and aortic valve calcification [40]. Furthermore, MMP-2, another target of miR-29 [104], was shown to promote arterial calcification in CRD [105] and valvular calcification [106].

The contribution of osteoclasts to cardiovascular calcification is still controversial [59]. The observation of osteoclast-like cells in calcified atherosclerotic lesions suggested this bone-related cell is active in the vessel wall. The evidence was strengthened recently by Sun et al., who demonstrated the functional role of SMC-derived Runx2 promoting infiltration of macrophages into the calcified lesion to form osteoclast-like cells — suggesting that the development of vascular calcification is coupled with the formation of osteoclast-like cells, paralleling the bone remodeling process [74]. The receptor activator of the nuclear factor-kappa B (NF-kappa B) ligand (RANKL)/osteoprotegerin (OPG) system controls proper osteoclastogenesis, and actes as a biomarker for CAD [107, 108]. *In silico* analysis revealed RANKL as a target of miR-126 [109], which is decreased in the plasma of CAD [14] and T2D [33] patients. miR-146a, highly expressed in atherosclerotic arteries [16], inhibits osteoclastogenesis [46]. The number of tartrate-resistant acid phosphatase-positive multinucleated cells was significantly reduced by miR-146a in a dose-dependent manner [46]. Furthermore, miR-155, which is decreased in plasma of CRD [37] and CAD [14] patients, was shown to inhibit osteoclast function [110].

Taken together, osteogenic processes in both bone and the cardiovascular system are tightly controlled by miRNAs (Figure 2). Further studies are needed to elucidate whether interplay of miRNAs could explain the bone-vascular axis "calcification paradox," or whether they act independently in the calcifying vessel and bone.

5. Circulating miRNAs as biomarkers and extracellular communicators

miRNAs are present in blood (plasma, platelets, erythrocytes, nucleated blood cells) with high stability. miRNAs can circulate in extracellular vesicles [111], in a protein complex (Ago2), or in a lipoprotein complex (HDL) [38], which prevents their degradation. Depending on the size and type, extracellular vesicles are broadly classified as ectosomes (also called shedding microvesicles), exosomes, matrix vesicles (MVs), and apoptotic bodies. Ectosomes are large extracellular vesicles 50-1000 nm in diameter; exosomes are small membranous vesicles of endocytic origin, 40-100 nm in diameter; MVs are 30-300 nm in diameter, are produced by

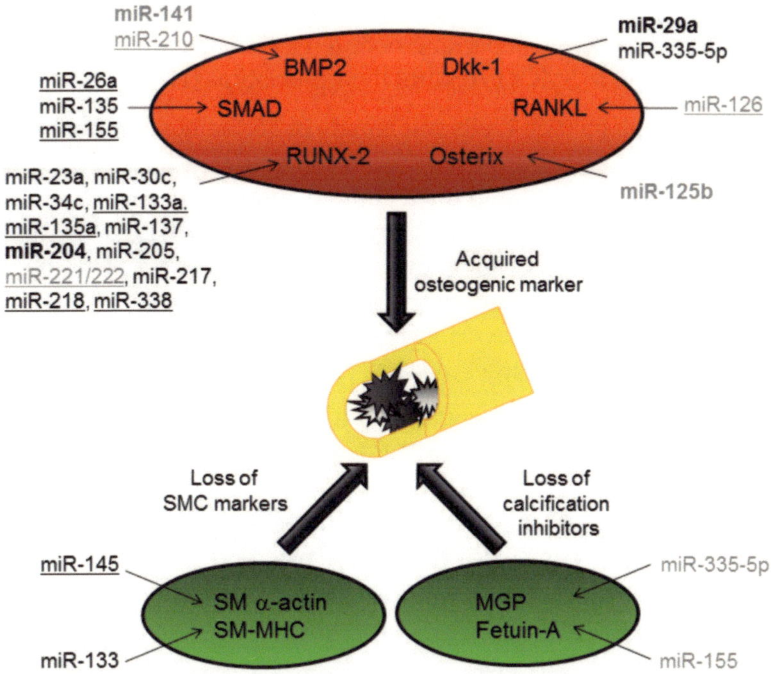

Figure 2. Potential and established miRNAs contributing to osteogenic regulation of vascular calcification. Bold, established miRNAs in vascular calcification; underlined, dysregulated in cardiovascular disease (circulating or tissue); gray, predicted miRNA binding sites.

blebbing of the plasma membrane, and can calcify; and apoptotic bodies, 50-5000 nm in diameter, are released from fragmented apoptotic cells.

The majority of miRNAs are independent of vesicles [111] and co-purify with the Ago2 complex [112, 113]. But in CAD patients, most plasma miRNAs associate with extracellular vesicles, and only a small amount are found in extracellular vesicle-free plasma [114]. A cell-type-specific miRNA release and different export systems are implicated, as the miRNA release pattern within vesicles is different from that associated with Ago2 complexes [112]. Thus, cells can select miRNA and pre-miRNA for controlled cellular release [115, 116]. miRNA profiles of extracellular vesicles are different from their maternal cell profiles, indicating an active mechanism of selective miRNA packing from cells into vesicles [114]. We have limited knowledge about miRNA secretion. Blockade of sphingomyelinase inhibits exosome generation and miRNA secretion, and intercellular miRNA transfer implicates a ceramide-dependent mechanism [117, 118]. Ago2–miRNA complexes may be passively produced by dead cells, released by live cells, or actively transported though cell-membrane–associated channels or receptors [119].

Extracellular vesicles use miRNA to mediate intercellular communication over long distances or on a local tissue level [120]. Endothelial apoptotic bodies can convey miR-126 to atherosclerotic lesions, which demonstrate uniquely paracrine-signaling function for miRNA during atherosclerosis [33, 121]. miRNA-containing vesicles can regulate intercellular communication between ECs and SMCs by selective packing of miR-143/145 in endothelial-derived vesicles, which are then transported to SMCs to control their phenotype [118].

How miRNAs are taken up by target cells and remain biologically active is still unknown. We know little about the mechanisms of vesicle-mediated cargo transfer. In physiological conditions, extracellular vesicles may bind to the membrane proteins of the surface of target cells through receptor–ligand interaction, resulting in intracellular stimulation of genetic pathways. They can also fuse with cell–target membranes and release genetic content in a nonselective manner. Furthermore, vesicles can bind to surface receptors on target cells with endocytotic internalization by recipient cells, followed by fusion with the membranes, leading to a release of their content into the cytosol of target cells [122].

A key event in the initiation and promotion of VIC and SMC calcification is the release of extracellular vesicles [81, 123]. Treatment of SMCs with elevated calcium levels promotes the production of calcifying vesicles (MVs), and the loss of fetuin-A, an inhibitor of mineral nucleation [124]. These vesicles act as early nucleation sites for calcification. The phosphatidylserine-membrane complex from SMC-derived and macrophage-derived MVs redistributes and nucleates hydroxyapatite [125-127]. In addition, hydroxyapatite nanocrystals shed from vesicles may further promote mineralization via direct effects on SMC phenotype [128].

Insight into the underlying mechanism of selective packing of miRNAs into extracellular vesicles and selective uptake into the target cell will help increase understanding of the role of miRNA-containing vesicles in physiological intercellular communication, which may prevent calcification in the cardiovascular system.

6. miRNAs in the "calcification paradox"

Osteoporosis frequently associates with cardiovascular calcification, and the severity of aortic calcification associates positively with bone loss [2, 129, 130]. The "calcification paradox" could be explained by the shared molecular pathways in bone remodeling and cardiovascular calcification [3]. How these two processes associate with each other and whether osteoporosis leads to cardiovascular calcification - or whether both disorders just share common risk factors - is unclear. In this section, we link cardiovascular calcification and bone loss and show commonalities in the systems' miRNA pathways/patterns.

Studies of miRNA in patients with bone disease are lacking. A recent clinical study first reported miRNA as a potential biomarker for postmenopausal osteoporosis. Wang *et al.* demonstrated an association of miR-133a levels in circulating monocytes - osteoclast precursors - with postmenopausal osteoporosis [131]. Women with low bone mineral density showed higher circulating miR-133a levels [131], but the number of patients per group was small (n=10). Circulating miR-133a levels were also higher in patients with CAD [14]. Unfortunately, the study investigating bone mineral density in patients with osteoporosis did not mention characteristics of the cardiovascular patient population. miR-133a belongs to the Runx2-targeting miRNA cluster [77].

http://dx.doi.org/10.5772/55326

Additionally, miR-2861 contributes to osteoporosis in mice and humans by targeting histone deacethylase 5, and thereby increasing Runx2 [132]. No studies of miR-2861 in the cardiovascular system have been reported. Patients with rheumatoid arthritis also suffer from vascular calcification in different vessel beds, in addition to osteoporosis; the pathogenesis includes pro-inflammatory cytokines and site-specific inflammation (reviewed in detail elsewhere [133]). miR-146a, a negative regulator of inflammation and osteoclastogenesis, also associates with rheumatoid arthritis [134]. Similar to patients with CAD, in patients with rheumatoid arthritis, miR-146a is up-regulated in PBMCs [25].

7. Conclusion and perspectives

In vitro and *in vivo* studies have established miRNAs as biomarkers focusing on different aspects and providing circulating miRNA signatures for different diseases. But these circulating miRNAs may not have biological functions within the cell while circulating — instead, they act as intercellular communicators, and this communication may be disturbed by calcified vesicles. More studies are needed to fully exploit this potentially novel mechanism of cardiovascular calcification.

Moreover, miRNA biology is very complex. Multiple miRNAs can target the same gene (e.g., Runx2–miRNA cluster), and one miRNA may have several targets. Only a small amount of these fine-tuned targets may alter biological responses and phenotypes. Understanding the role of miRNA in vascular calcification may be helpful in considering the paradoxical clinical observations of the concurrence of cardiovascular calcification and osteoporosis. Despite its global clinical burden, no medical therapies are available to treat cardiovascular calcification. Targeting of miRNA represents a novel therapeutic opportunity for treating calcification disorders. As vascular calcification and bone remodeling share common mechanisms, we have to understand in greater detail the functions of miRNAs and their association with the molecular pathogenesis of osteoporosis and vascular/valvular calcification.

Author details

Claudia Goettsch[1] and Elena Aikawa[1,2]

*Address all correspondence to: eaikawa@partners.org

1 Center for Interdisciplinary Cardiovascular Sciences, Cardiovascular Medicine, Brigham and Women's Hospital, Harvard Medical School, Boston, MA, USA

2 Center for Excellence in Vascular Biology, Cardiovascular Medicine, Brigham and Women's Hospital, Harvard Medical School, Boston, MA, USA

References

[1] Hjortnaes J, Bouten CV, Van Herwerden LA, Grundeman PF, Kluin J. Translating autologous heart valve tissue engineering from bench to bed. Tissue engineering Part B, Reviews 2009;15(3):307-17.

[2] Rajamannan NM, Evans FJ, Aikawa E, Grande-Allen KJ, Demer LL, Heistad DD, et al. Calcific aortic valve disease: not simply a degenerative process: A review and agenda for research from the National Heart and Lung and Blood Institute Aortic Stenosis Working Group. Executive summary: Calcific aortic valve disease-2011 update. Circulation 2011;124(16):1783-91.

[3] Sage AP, Tintut Y, Demer LL. Regulatory mechanisms in vascular calcification. Nature reviews Cardiology 2010;7(9):528-36.

[4] Johnson RC, Leopold JA, Loscalzo J. Vascular calcification: pathobiological mechanisms and clinical implications. Circulation research 2006;99(10):1044-59.

[5] Ambros V. The functions of animal microRNAs. Nature 2004;431(7006):350-5.

[6] Bartel DP. MicroRNAs: target recognition and regulatory functions. Cell 2009;136(2): 215-33.

[7] Santovito D, Mezzetti A, Cipollone F. MicroRNAs and atherosclerosis: New actors for an old movie. Nutrition, metabolism, and cardiovascular diseases : NMCD 2012.

[8] Lee Y, Kim M, Han J, Yeom KH, Lee S, Baek SH, et al. MicroRNA genes are transcribed by RNA polymerase II. The EMBO journal 2004;23(20):4051-60.

[9] Lee Y, Ahn C, Han J, Choi H, Kim J, Yim J, et al. The nuclear RNase III Drosha initiates microRNA processing. Nature 2003;425(6956):415-9.

[10] Yi R, Qin Y, Macara IG, Cullen BR. Exportin-5 mediates the nuclear export of premicroRNAs and short hairpin RNAs. Genes & development 2003;17(24):3011-6.

[11] Chendrimada TP, Gregory RI, Kumaraswamy E, Norman J, Cooch N, Nishikura K, et al. TRBP recruits the Dicer complex to Ago2 for microRNA processing and gene silencing. Nature 2005;436(7051):740-4.

[12] Hutvagner G, Zamore PD. A microRNA in a multiple-turnover RNAi enzyme complex. Science 2002;297(5589):2056-60.

[13] Aikawa E, Nahrendorf M, Figueiredo JL, Swirski FK, Shtatland T, Kohler RH, et al. Osteogenesis associates with inflammation in early-stage atherosclerosis evaluated by molecular imaging in vivo. Circulation 2007;116(24):2841-50.

[14] Fichtlscherer S, De Rosa S, Fox H, Schwietz T, Fischer A, Liebetrau C, et al. Circulating microRNAs in patients with coronary artery disease. Circulation research 2010;107(5):677-84.

[15] Li T, Cao H, Zhuang J, Wan J, Guan M, Yu B, et al. Identification of miR-130a, miR-27b and miR-210 as serum biomarkers for atherosclerosis obliterans. Clinica chimica acta; international journal of clinical chemistry 2011;412(1-2):66-70.

[16] Raitoharju E, Lyytikainen LP, Levula M, Oksala N, Mennander A, Tarkka M, et al. miR-21, miR-210, miR-34a, and miR-146a/b are up-regulated in human atherosclerotic plaques in the Tampere Vascular Study. Atherosclerosis 2011;219(1):211-7.

[17] Bidzhekov K, Gan L, Denecke B, Rostalsky A, Hristov M, Koeppel TA, et al. microRNA expression signatures and parallels between monocyte subsets and atherosclerotic plaque in humans. Thrombosis and haemostasis 2012;107(4):619-25.

[18] Vengrenyuk Y, Carlier S, Xanthos S, Cardoso L, Ganatos P, Virmani R, et al. A hypothesis for vulnerable plaque rupture due to stress-induced debonding around cellular microcalcifications in thin fibrous caps. Proceedings of the National Academy of Sciences of the United States of America 2006;103(40):14678-83.

[19] Hoshino T, Chow LA, Hsu JJ, Perlowski AA, Abedin M, Tobis J, et al. Mechanical stress analysis of a rigid inclusion in distensible material: a model of atherosclerotic calcification and plaque vulnerability. American journal of physiology Heart and circulatory physiology 2009;297(2):H802-10.

[20] Cipollone F, Felicioni L, Sarzani R, Ucchino S, Spigonardo F, Mandolini C, et al. A unique microRNA signature associated with plaque instability in humans. Stroke; a journal of cerebral circulation 2011;42(9):2556-63.

[21] Gao W, He HW, Wang ZM, Zhao H, Lian XQ, Wang YS, et al. Plasma levels of lipometabolism-related miR-122 and miR-370 are increased in patients with hyperlipidemia and associated with coronary artery disease. Lipids in health and disease 2012;11(1):55.

[22] Kirschner MB, Kao SC, Edelman JJ, Armstrong NJ, Vallely MP, van Zandwijk N, et al. Haemolysis during sample preparation alters microRNA content of plasma. PloS one 2011;6(9):e24145.

[23] Wu C, Gong Y, Sun A, Zhang Y, Zhang C, Zhang W, et al. The human MTHFR rs4846049 polymorphism increases coronary heart disease risk through modifying miRNA binding. Nutrition, metabolism, and cardiovascular diseases : NMCD 2012.

[24] Zhi H, Wang L, Ma G, Ye X, Yu X, Zhu Y, et al. Polymorphisms of miRNAs genes are associated with the risk and prognosis of coronary artery disease. Clinical research in cardiology : official journal of the German Cardiac Society 2012;101(4):289-96.

[25] Takahashi Y, Satoh M, Minami Y, Tabuchi T, Itoh T, Nakamura M. Expression of miR-146a/b is associated with the Toll-like receptor 4 signal in coronary artery disease: effect of renin-angiotensin system blockade and statins on miRNA-146a/b and Toll-like receptor 4 levels. Clin Sci (Lond) 2010;119(9):395-405.

[26] Tabuchi T, Satoh M, Itoh T, Nakamura M. MicroRNA-34a regulates the longevity-associated protein SIRT1 in coronary artery disease: effect of statins on SIRT1 and microRNA-34a expression. Clin Sci (Lond) 2012;123(3):161-71.

[27] Minami Y, Satoh M, Maesawa C, Takahashi Y, Tabuchi T, Itoh T, et al. Effect of atorvastatin on microRNA 221 / 222 expression in endothelial progenitor cells obtained from patients with coronary artery disease. European journal of clinical investigation 2009;39(5):359-67.

[28] Hoekstra M, van der Lans CA, Halvorsen B, Gullestad L, Kuiper J, Aukrust P, et al. The peripheral blood mononuclear cell microRNA signature of coronary artery disease. Biochemical and biophysical research communications 2010;394(3):792-7.

[29] Taurino C, Miller WH, McBride MW, McClure JD, Khanin R, Moreno MU, et al. Gene expression profiling in whole blood of patients with coronary artery disease. Clin Sci (Lond) 2010;119(8):335-43.

[30] Hulsmans M, Sinnaeve P, Van der Schueren B, Mathieu C, Janssens S, Holvoet P. Decreased miR-181a Expression in Monocytes of Obese Patients Is Associated with the Occurrence of Metabolic Syndrome and Coronary Artery Disease. The Journal of clinical endocrinology and metabolism 2012;97(7):E1213-8.

[31] Satoh M, Tabuchi T, Minami Y, Takahashi Y, Itoh T, Nakamura M. Expression of let-7i is associated with Toll-like receptor 4 signal in coronary artery disease: effect of statins on let-7i and Toll-like receptor 4 signal. Immunobiology 2012;217(5):533-9.

[32] Sondermeijer BM, Bakker A, Halliani A, de Ronde MW, Marquart AA, Tijsen AJ, et al. Platelets in patients with premature coronary artery disease exhibit upregulation of miRNA340* and miRNA624*. PloS one 2011;6(10):e25946.

[33] Zampetaki A, Kiechl S, Drozdov I, Willeit P, Mayr U, Prokopi M, et al. Plasma microRNA profiling reveals loss of endothelial miR-126 and other microRNAs in type 2 diabetes. Circulation research 2010;107(6):810-7.

[34] Balasubramanyam M, Aravind S, Gokulakrishnan K, Prabu P, Sathishkumar C, Ranjani H, et al. Impaired miR-146a expression links subclinical inflammation and insulin resistance in Type 2 diabetes. Molecular and cellular biochemistry 2011;351(1-2): 197-205.

[35] Meng S, Cao JT, Zhang B, Zhou Q, Shen CX, Wang CQ. Downregulation of microRNA-126 in endothelial progenitor cells from diabetes patients, impairs their functional properties, via target gene Spred-1. Journal of molecular and cellular cardiology 2012;53(1):64-72.

[36] Kong L, Zhu J, Han W, Jiang X, Xu M, Zhao Y, et al. Significance of serum microRNAs in pre-diabetes and newly diagnosed type 2 diabetes: a clinical study. Acta diabetologica 2011;48(1):61-9.

[37] Neal CS, Michael MZ, Pimlott LK, Yong TY, Li JY, Gleadle JM. Circulating microRNA expression is reduced in chronic kidney disease. Nephrology, dialysis, trans-

plantation : official publication of the European Dialysis and Transplant Association - European Renal Association 2011;26(11):3794-802.

[38] Vickers KC, Palmisano BT, Shoucri BM, Shamburek RD, Remaley AT. MicroRNAs are transported in plasma and delivered to recipient cells by high-density lipoproteins. Nature cell biology 2011;13(4):423-33.

[39] Feng B, Chen S, McArthur K, Wu Y, Sen S, Ding Q, et al. miR-146a-Mediated extracellular matrix protein production in chronic diabetes complications. Diabetes 2011;60(11):2975-84.

[40] Aikawa E, Aikawa M, Libby P, Figueiredo JL, Rusanescu G, Iwamoto Y, et al. Arterial and aortic valve calcification abolished by elastolytic cathepsin S deficiency in chronic renal disease. Circulation 2009;119(13):1785-94.

[41] Krupa A, Jenkins R, Luo DD, Lewis A, Phillips A, Fraser D. Loss of MicroRNA-192 promotes fibrogenesis in diabetic nephropathy. Journal of the American Society of Nephrology : JASN 2010;21(3):438-47.

[42] Wang B, Komers R, Carew R, Winbanks CE, Xu B, Herman-Edelstein M, et al. Suppression of microRNA-29 expression by TGF-beta1 promotes collagen expression and renal fibrosis. Journal of the American Society of Nephrology : JASN 2012;23(2): 252-65.

[43] Wang Q, Wang Y, Minto AW, Wang J, Shi Q, Li X, et al. MicroRNA-377 is up-regulated and can lead to increased fibronectin production in diabetic nephropathy. FASEB journal : official publication of the Federation of American Societies for Experimental Biology 2008;22(12):4126-35.

[44] Nigam V, Sievers HH, Jensen BC, Sier HA, Simpson PC, Srivastava D, et al. Altered microRNAs in bicuspid aortic valve: a comparison between stenotic and insufficient valves. The Journal of heart valve disease 2010;19(4):459-65.

[45] Yanagawa B, Lovren F, Pan Y, Garg V, Quan A, Tang G, et al. miRNA-141 is a novel regulator of BMP-2-mediated calcification in aortic stenosis. The Journal of thoracic and cardiovascular surgery 2012.

[46] Nakasa T, Shibuya H, Nagata Y, Niimoto T, Ochi M. The inhibitory effect of microRNA-146a expression on bone destruction in collagen-induced arthritis. Arthritis and rheumatism 2011;63(6):1582-90.

[47] Ichii O, Otsuka S, Sasaki N, Namiki Y, Hashimoto Y, Kon Y. Altered expression of microRNA miR-146a correlates with the development of chronic renal inflammation. Kidney international 2012;81(3):280-92.

[48] Donners MM, Wolfs IM, Stoger LJ, van der Vorst EP, Pottgens CC, Heymans S, et al. Hematopoietic miR155 deficiency enhances atherosclerosis and decreases plaque stability in hyperlipidemic mice. PloS one 2012;7(4):e35877.

[49] Zhu N, Zhang D, Chen S, Liu X, Lin L, Huang X, et al. Endothelial enriched microRNAs regulate angiotensin II-induced endothelial inflammation and migration. Atherosclerosis 2011;215(2):286-93.

[50] Jia G, Stormont RM, Gangahar DM, Agrawal DK. Role of Matrix Gla Protein in Angiotensin II-Induced Exacerbation of Vascular Stiffness. American journal of physiology Heart and circulatory physiology 2012.

[51] O'Brien KD, Shavelle DM, Caulfield MT, McDonald TO, Olin-Lewis K, Otto CM, et al. Association of angiotensin-converting enzyme with low-density lipoprotein in aortic valvular lesions and in human plasma. Circulation 2002;106(17):2224-30.

[52] Armstrong ZB, Boughner DR, Drangova M, Rogers KA. Angiotensin II type 1 receptor blocker inhibits arterial calcification in a pre-clinical model. Cardiovascular research 2011;90(1):165-70.

[53] Shavelle DM, Takasu J, Budoff MJ, Mao S, Zhao XQ, O'Brien KD. HMG CoA reductase inhibitor (statin) and aortic valve calcium. Lancet 2002;359(9312):1125-6.

[54] Taipaleenmaki H, Bjerre Hokland L, Chen L, Kauppinen S, Kassem M. Mechanisms in endocrinology: micro-RNAs: targets for enhancing osteoblast differentiation and bone formation. European journal of endocrinology / European Federation of Endocrine Societies 2012;166(3):359-71.

[55] New SE, Aikawa E. Molecular imaging insights into early inflammatory stages of arterial and aortic valve calcification. Circulation research 2011;108(11):1381-91.

[56] Hjortnaes J, Butcher J, Figueiredo JL, Riccio M, Kohler RH, Kozloff KM, et al. Arterial and aortic valve calcification inversely correlates with osteoporotic bone remodelling: a role for inflammation. European heart journal 2010;31(16):1975-84.

[57] Geng Y, Hsu JJ, Lu J, Ting TC, Miyazaki M, Demer LL, et al. Role of cellular cholesterol metabolism in vascular cell calcification. The Journal of biological chemistry 2011;286(38):33701-6.

[58] Rajamannan NM, Subramaniam M, Rickard D, Stock SR, Donovan J, Springett M, et al. Human aortic valve calcification is associated with an osteoblast phenotype. Circulation 2003;107(17):2181-4.

[59] Fadini GP, Rattazzi M, Matsumoto T, Asahara T, Khosla S. Emerging Role of Circulating Calcifying Cells in the Bone-Vascular Axis. Circulation 2012;125(22):2772-81.

[60] Doehring LC, Heeger C, Aherrahrou Z, Kaczmarek PM, Erdmann J, Schunkert H, et al. Myeloid CD34+CD13+ precursor cells transdifferentiate into chondrocyte-like cells in atherosclerotic intimal calcification. The American journal of pathology 2010;177(1):473-80.

[61] Naik V, Leaf EM, Hu JH, Yang HY, Nguyen NB, Giachelli CM, et al. Sources of cells that contribute to atherosclerotic intimal calcification: an in vivo genetic fate mapping study. Cardiovascular research 2012;94(3):545-54.

[62] Elia L, Quintavalle M, Zhang J, Contu R, Cossu L, Latronico MV, et al. The knockout of miR-143 and -145 alters smooth muscle cell maintenance and vascular homeostasis in mice: correlates with human disease. Cell death and differentiation 2009;16(12): 1590-8.

[63] Cordes KR, Sheehy NT, White MP, Berry EC, Morton SU, Muth AN, et al. miR-145 and miR-143 regulate smooth muscle cell fate and plasticity. Nature 2009;460(7256): 705-10.

[64] Boettger T, Beetz N, Kostin S, Schneider J, Kruger M, Hein L, et al. Acquisition of the contractile phenotype by murine arterial smooth muscle cells depends on the Mir143/145 gene cluster. The Journal of clinical investigation 2009;119(9):2634-47.

[65] Ji R, Cheng Y, Yue J, Yang J, Liu X, Chen H, et al. MicroRNA expression signature and antisense-mediated depletion reveal an essential role of MicroRNA in vascular neointimal lesion formation. Circulation research 2007;100(11):1579-88.

[66] Cheng Y, Liu X, Yang J, Lin Y, Xu DZ, Lu Q, et al. MicroRNA-145, a novel smooth muscle cell phenotypic marker and modulator, controls vascular neointimal lesion formation. Circulation research 2009;105(2):158-66.

[67] Steitz SA, Speer MY, Curinga G, Yang HY, Haynes P, Aebersold R, et al. Smooth muscle cell phenotypic transition associated with calcification: upregulation of Cbfa1 and downregulation of smooth muscle lineage markers. Circulation research 2001;89(12):1147-54.

[68] Yoshida T, Yamashita M, Hayashi M. Kruppel-like factor 4 contributes to high phosphate-induced phenotypic switching of vascular smooth muscle cells into osteogenic cells. The Journal of biological chemistry 2012.

[69] Xin M, Small EM, Sutherland LB, Qi X, McAnally J, Plato CF, et al. MicroRNAs miR-143 and miR-145 modulate cytoskeletal dynamics and responsiveness of smooth muscle cells to injury. Genes & development 2009;23(18):2166-78.

[70] Torella D, Iaconetti C, Catalucci D, Ellison GM, Leone A, Waring CD, et al. MicroRNA-133 controls vascular smooth muscle cell phenotypic switch in vitro and vascular remodeling in vivo. Circulation research 2011;109(8):880-93.

[71] Li Z, Hassan MQ, Volinia S, van Wijnen AJ, Stein JL, Croce CM, et al. A microRNA signature for a BMP2-induced osteoblast lineage commitment program. Proceedings of the National Academy of Sciences of the United States of America 2008;105(37): 13906-11.

[72] Komori T. Regulation of bone development and extracellular matrix protein genes by RUNX2. Cell and tissue research 2010;339(1):189-95.

[73] Byon CH, Javed A, Dai Q, Kappes JC, Clemens TL, Darley-Usmar VM, et al. Oxidative stress induces vascular calcification through modulation of the osteogenic transcription factor Runx2 by AKT signaling. The Journal of biological chemistry 2008;283(22):15319-27.

[74] Sun Y, Byon C, Yuan K, Chen J, Mao X, Heath JM, et al. Smooth Muscle Cell-Specific Runx2 Deficiency InhibitsVascular Calcification. Circulation research 2012.

[75] Speer MY, Li X, Hiremath PG, Giachelli CM. Runx2/Cbfa1, but not loss of myocardin, is required for smooth muscle cell lineage reprogramming toward osteochondrogenesis. Journal of cellular biochemistry 2010;110(4):935-47.

[76] Miller JD, Weiss RM, Serrano KM, Castaneda LE, Brooks RM, Zimmerman K, et al. Evidence for active regulation of pro-osteogenic signaling in advanced aortic valve disease. Arteriosclerosis, thrombosis, and vascular biology 2010;30(12):2482-6.

[77] Zhang Y, Xie RL, Croce CM, Stein JL, Lian JB, van Wijnen AJ, et al. A program of microRNAs controls osteogenic lineage progression by targeting transcription factor Runx2. Proceedings of the National Academy of Sciences of the United States of America 2011;108(24):9863-8.

[78] Lim K, Lu TS, Molostvov G, Lee C, Lam FT, Zehnder D, et al. Vascular Klotho deficiency potentiates the development of human artery calcification and mediates resistance to fibroblast growth factor 23. Circulation 2012;125(18):2243-55.

[79] Gui T, Zhou G, Sun Y, Shimokado A, Itoh S, Oikawa K, et al. MicroRNAs that target Ca(2+) transporters are involved in vascular smooth muscle cell calcification. Laboratory investigation; a journal of technical methods and pathology 2012.

[80] Cui RR, Li SJ, Liu LJ, Yi L, Liang QH, Zhu X, et al. MicroRNA-204 Regulates Vascular Smooth Muscle Cell Calcification in vitro and in vivo. Cardiovascular research 2012.

[81] Shanahan CM, Crouthamel MH, Kapustin A, Giachelli CM. Arterial calcification in chronic kidney disease: key roles for calcium and phosphate. Circulation research 2011;109(6):697-711.

[82] Mizuno Y, Yagi K, Tokuzawa Y, Kanesaki-Yatsuka Y, Suda T, Katagiri T, et al. miR-125b inhibits osteoblastic differentiation by down-regulation of cell proliferation. Biochemical and biophysical research communications 2008;368(2):267-72.

[83] Goettsch C, Rauner M, Pacyna N, Hempel U, Bornstein SR, Hofbauer LC. miR-125b regulates calcification of vascular smooth muscle cells. The American journal of pathology 2011;179(4):1594-600.

[84] Albinsson S, Suarez Y, Skoura A, Offermanns S, Miano JM, Sessa WC. MicroRNAs are necessary for vascular smooth muscle growth, differentiation, and function. Arteriosclerosis, thrombosis, and vascular biology 2010;30(6):1118-26.

[85] Bostrom KI, Rajamannan NM, Towler DA. The regulation of valvular and vascular sclerosis by osteogenic morphogens. Circulation research 2011;109(5):564-77.

[86] Bostrom K, Watson KE, Horn S, Wortham C, Herman IM, Demer LL. Bone morphogenetic protein expression in human atherosclerotic lesions. The Journal of clinical investigation 1993;91(4):1800-9.

[87] Dhore CR, Cleutjens JP, Lutgens E, Cleutjens KB, Geusens PP, Kitslaar PJ, et al. Differential expression of bone matrix regulatory proteins in human atherosclerotic plaques. Arteriosclerosis, thrombosis, and vascular biology 2001;21(12):1998-2003.

[88] Seya K, Yu Z, Kanemaru K, Daitoku K, Akemoto Y, Shibuya H, et al. Contribution of bone morphogenetic protein-2 to aortic valve calcification in aged rat. Journal of pharmacological sciences 2011;115(1):8-14.

[89] Itoh T, Nozawa Y, Akao Y. MicroRNA-141 and -200a are involved in bone morphogenetic protein-2-induced mouse pre-osteoblast differentiation by targeting distal-less homeobox 5. The Journal of biological chemistry 2009;284(29):19272-9.

[90] Monroe DG, McGee-Lawrence ME, Oursler MJ, Westendorf JJ. Update on Wnt signaling in bone cell biology and bone disease. Gene 2012;492(1):1-18.

[91] Miller JD, Chu Y, Brooks RM, Richenbacher WE, Pena-Silva R, Heistad DD. Dysregulation of antioxidant mechanisms contributes to increased oxidative stress in calcific aortic valvular stenosis in humans. Journal of the American College of Cardiology 2008;52(10):843-50.

[92] Al-Aly Z, Shao JS, Lai CF, Huang E, Cai J, Behrmann A, et al. Aortic Msx2-Wnt calcification cascade is regulated by TNF-alpha-dependent signals in diabetic Ldlr-/- mice. Arteriosclerosis, thrombosis, and vascular biology 2007;27(12):2589-96.

[93] Cheng SL, Shao JS, Halstead LR, Distelhorst K, Sierra O, Towler DA. Activation of vascular smooth muscle parathyroid hormone receptor inhibits Wnt/beta-catenin signaling and aortic fibrosis in diabetic arteriosclerosis. Circulation research 2010;107(2): 271-82.

[94] Faverman L, Mikhaylova L, Malmquist J, Nurminskaya M. Extracellular transglutaminase 2 activates beta-catenin signaling in calcifying vascular smooth muscle cells. FEBS letters 2008;582(10):1552-7.

[95] Glinka A, Wu W, Delius H, Monaghan AP, Blumenstock C, Niehrs C. Dickkopf-1 is a member of a new family of secreted proteins and functions in head induction. Nature 1998;391(6665):357-62.

[96] Mukhopadhyay M, Shtrom S, Rodriguez-Esteban C, Chen L, Tsukui T, Gomer L, et al. Dickkopf1 is required for embryonic head induction and limb morphogenesis in the mouse. Developmental cell 2001;1(3):423-34.

[97] Thambiah S, Roplekar R, Manghat P, Fogelman I, Fraser WD, Goldsmith D, et al. Circulating sclerostin and Dickkopf-1 (DKK1) in predialysis chronic kidney disease

(CKD): relationship with bone density and arterial stiffness. Calcified tissue international 2012;90(6):473-80.

[98] Beazley KE, Deasey S, Lima F, Nurminskaya MV. Transglutaminase 2-mediated activation of beta-catenin signaling has a critical role in warfarin-induced vascular calcification. Arteriosclerosis, thrombosis, and vascular biology 2012;32(1):123-30.

[99] Bai XY, Ma Y, Ding R, Fu B, Shi S, Chen XM. miR-335 and miR-34a Promote renal senescence by suppressing mitochondrial antioxidative enzymes. Journal of the American Society of Nephrology : JASN 2011;22(7):1252-61.

[100] Boon RA, Seeger T, Heydt S, Fischer A, Hergenreider E, Horrevoets AJ, et al. MicroRNA-29 in aortic dilation: implications for aneurysm formation. Circulation research 2011;109(10):1115-9.

[101] Zhang J, Tu Q, Bonewald LF, He X, Stein G, Lian J, et al. Effects of miR-335-5p in modulating osteogenic differentiation by specifically downregulating Wnt antagonist DKK1. Journal of bone and mineral research : the official journal of the American Society for Bone and Mineral Research 2011;26(8):1953-63.

[102] Kapinas K, Kessler C, Ricks T, Gronowicz G, Delany AM. miR-29 modulates Wnt signaling in human osteoblasts through a positive feedback loop. The Journal of biological chemistry 2010;285(33):25221-31.

[103] Kapinas K, Kessler CB, Delany AM. miR-29 suppression of osteonectin in osteoblasts: regulation during differentiation and by canonical Wnt signaling. Journal of cellular biochemistry 2009;108(1):216-24.

[104] Jones JA, Stroud RE, O'Quinn EC, Black LE, Barth JL, Elefteriades JA, et al. Selective microRNA suppression in human thoracic aneurysms: relationship of miR-29a to aortic size and proteolytic induction. Circulation Cardiovascular genetics 2011;4(6): 605-13.

[105] Chen NX, O'Neill KD, Chen X, Kiattisunthorn K, Gattone VH, Moe SM. Activation of arterial matrix metalloproteinases leads to vascular calcification in chronic kidney disease. American journal of nephrology 2011;34(3):211-9.

[106] Freeman RV, Otto CM. Spectrum of calcific aortic valve disease: pathogenesis, disease progression, and treatment strategies. Circulation 2005;111(24):3316-26.

[107] Mohammadpour AH, Shamsara J, Nazemi S, Ghadirzadeh S, Shahsavand S, Rezamani M. Evaluation of RANKL/OPG Serum Concentration Ratio as a New Biomarker for Coronary Artery Calcification: A Pilot Study. Thrombosis 2012;2012:306263.

[108] Kiechl S, Schett G, Schwaiger J, Seppi K, Eder P, Egger G, et al. Soluble receptor activator of nuclear factor-kappa B ligand and risk for cardiovascular disease. Circulation 2007;116(4):385-91.

[109] Dombkowski AA, Sultana Z, Craig DB, Jamil H. In silico analysis of combinatorial microRNA activity reveals target genes and pathways associated with breast cancer metastasis. Cancer informatics 2011;10:13-29.

[110] Mizoguchi F, Izu Y, Hayata T, Hemmi H, Nakashima K, Nakamura T, et al. Osteoclast-specific Dicer gene deficiency suppresses osteoclastic bone resorption. Journal of cellular biochemistry 2010;109(5):866-75.

[111] Wang K, Zhang S, Weber J, Baxter D, Galas DJ. Export of microRNAs and microRNA-protective protein by mammalian cells. Nucleic acids research 2010;38(20):7248-59.

[112] Arroyo JD, Chevillet JR, Kroh EM, Ruf IK, Pritchard CC, Gibson DF, et al. Argonaute2 complexes carry a population of circulating microRNAs independent of vesicles in human plasma. Proceedings of the National Academy of Sciences of the United States of America 2011;108(12):5003-8.

[113] Turchinovich A, Weiz L, Langheinz A, Burwinkel B. Characterization of extracellular circulating microRNA. Nucleic acids research 2011;39(16):7223-33.

[114] Diehl P, Fricke A, Sander L, Stamm J, Bassler N, Htun N, et al. Microparticles: major transport vehicles for distinct microRNAs in circulation. Cardiovascular research 2012;93(4):633-44.

[115] Pigati L, Yaddanapudi SC, Iyengar R, Kim DJ, Hearn SA, Danforth D, et al. Selective release of microRNA species from normal and malignant mammary epithelial cells. PloS one 2010;5(10):e13515.

[116] Chen TS, Lai RC, Lee MM, Choo AB, Lee CN, Lim SK. Mesenchymal stem cell secretes microparticles enriched in pre-microRNAs. Nucleic acids research 2010;38(1):215-24.

[117] Kosaka N, Iguchi H, Yoshioka Y, Takeshita F, Matsuki Y, Ochiya T. Secretory mechanisms and intercellular transfer of microRNAs in living cells. The Journal of biological chemistry 2010;285(23):17442-52.

[118] Hergenreider E, Heydt S, Treguer K, Boettger T, Horrevoets AJ, Zeiher AM, et al. Atheroprotective communication between endothelial cells and smooth muscle cells through miRNAs. Nature cell biology 2012;14(3):249-56.

[119] Creemers EE, Tijsen AJ, Pinto YM. Circulating microRNAs: novel biomarkers and extracellular communicators in cardiovascular disease? Circulation research 2012;110(3):483-95.

[120] Valadi H, Ekstrom K, Bossios A, Sjostrand M, Lee JJ, Lotvall JO. Exosome-mediated transfer of mRNAs and microRNAs is a novel mechanism of genetic exchange between cells. Nature cell biology 2007;9(6):654-9.

[121] Zernecke A, Bidzhekov K, Noels H, Shagdarsuren E, Gan L, Denecke B, et al. Delivery of microRNA-126 by apoptotic bodies induces CXCL12-dependent vascular protection. Science signaling 2009;2(100):ra81.

[122] Meckes DG, Jr., Raab-Traub N. Microvesicles and viral infection. Journal of virology 2011;85(24):12844-54.

[123] Wuthier RE, Lipscomb GF. Matrix vesicles: structure, composition, formation and function in calcification. Frontiers in bioscience : a journal and virtual library 2011;16:2812-902.

[124] Reynolds JL, Joannides AJ, Skepper JN, McNair R, Schurgers LJ, Proudfoot D, et al. Human vascular smooth muscle cells undergo vesicle-mediated calcification in response to changes in extracellular calcium and phosphate concentrations: a potential mechanism for accelerated vascular calcification in ESRD. Journal of the American Society of Nephrology : JASN 2004;15(11):2857-67.

[125] Chen NX, O'Neill KD, Chen X, Moe SM. Annexin-mediated matrix vesicle calcification in vascular smooth muscle cells. Journal of bone and mineral research : the official journal of the American Society for Bone and Mineral Research 2008;23(11): 1798-805.

[126] Kapustin AN, Davies JD, Reynolds JL, McNair R, Jones GT, Sidibe A, et al. Calcium regulates key components of vascular smooth muscle cell-derived matrix vesicles to enhance mineralization. Circulation research 2011;109(1):e1-12.

[127] New SE, Marchini JF, Aikawa M, Shanahan CM, Croce K, Aikawa E. Novel Role of Macrophage-derived Matrix Vesicles in Arterial Microcalcification Circulation 2011;124(21 Supplement):A10866.

[128] Sage AP, Lu J, Tintut Y, Demer LL. Hyperphosphatemia-induced nanocrystals upregulate the expression of bone morphogenetic protein-2 and osteopontin genes in mouse smooth muscle cells in vitro. Kidney international 2011;79(4):414-22.

[129] Naves M, Rodriguez-Garcia M, Diaz-Lopez JB, Gomez-Alonso C, Cannata-Andia JB. Progression of vascular calcifications is associated with greater bone loss and increased bone fractures. Osteoporosis international : a journal established as result of cooperation between the European Foundation for Osteoporosis and the National Osteoporosis Foundation of the USA 2008;19(8):1161-6.

[130] Jensky NE, Hyder JA, Allison MA, Wong N, Aboyans V, Blumenthal RS, et al. The association of bone density and calcified atherosclerosis is stronger in women without dyslipidemia: the multi-ethnic study of atherosclerosis. Journal of bone and mineral research : the official journal of the American Society for Bone and Mineral Research 2011;26(11):2702-9.

[131] Wang Y, Li L, Moore BT, Peng XH, Fang X, Lappe JM, et al. MiR-133a in human circulating monocytes: a potential biomarker associated with postmenopausal osteoporosis. PloS one 2012;7(4):e34641.

[132] Li H, Xie H, Liu W, Hu R, Huang B, Tan YF, et al. A novel microRNA targeting HDAC5 regulates osteoblast differentiation in mice and contributes to primary osteoporosis in humans. The Journal of clinical investigation 2009;119(12):3666-77.

[133] Paccou J, Brazier M, Mentaverri R, Kamel S, Fardellone P, Massy ZA. Vascular calcification in rheumatoid arthritis: Prevalence, pathophysiological aspects and potential targets. Atherosclerosis 2012.

[134] Pauley KM, Satoh M, Chan AL, Bubb MR, Reeves WH, Chan EK. Upregulated miR-146a expression in peripheral blood mononuclear cells from rheumatoid arthritis patients. Arthritis research & therapy 2008;10(4):R101.

Section 3

Genetics, Proteomics and Metabolomics of Calcific Aortic Valve Disease

Chapter 6

Proteomics and Metabolomics in Aortic Stenosis: Studying Healthy Valves for a Better Understanding of the Disease

L. Mourino-Alvarez, C.M. Laborde and M.G. Barderas

Additional information is available at the end of the chapter

http://dx.doi.org/10.5772/55589

1. Introduction

1.1. Aortic stenosis

Aortic stenosis is characterized by the abnormal narrowing of the aortic valve (AV) opening, producing a blockage of the blood flow from the left ventricle into the aorta. Two different types of aortic stenosis can be distinguished. In congenital aortic stenosis an inherited abnormal formation of the AV exists. Otherwise, in acquired aortic stenosis external causes such as rheumatic fever or valve degeneration occur. Calcific aortic stenosis (AS) is the most common valvular disease in elder population and remain the main cause of aortic valve replacement in developed countries [1].

AS progresses from a primary stage of aortic sclerosis, with thickening and stiffness of the AV, to severe calcific stenosis. Its most common symptoms are dyspnea, angina and syncope, which predict the rapid deterioration of left ventricular function, the development of heart failure and, if the pathology progresses, the patient's death. Therefore, the appearance of any of these symptoms is considered as an indication for the treatment of this pathology. In these cases, surgery is recommended to replace the AV since there is not treatment to delay the progression of the disease.

Classically, this disease has been considered as a consequence of the aging process of the valve. However, recent studies have provided evidences that inflammation plays a key role in the physiopathology of AS as well as classical cardiovascular risk factors such as hypertension, hypercholesterolemia, diabetes, smoking, age or sex [2]. Degeneration of the valve begins with an endothelial dysfunction in the aortic side as a result of the abovementioned risk factors. Low density lipoproteins (LDLs) are accumulated in the subendothelial space of the valve, where they are oxidized, resulting in the activation of the endothelial cells. These cells express adhesion and chemotactic molecules, which attract inflammatory cells such as monocytes and T lymphocytes. Monocytes extravasate to the fibrous layer and differentiate into macrophages, which capture oxidized lipoproteins and become foam cells. Proinflammatory cytokines released by both cell types induce phenotypic differentiation of a subset of myofibroblasts to osteoblasts, which leads to the subsequent formation of calcium nodules [3]. These numerous similarities suggest a common relationship between atherosclerosis and AS.

1.2. Proteomic and metabolomic study of healthy valves

A complete knowledge of the structures involved in a disease it is important to understand its development. Previously, healthy tissue such as vasculature and myocardial have been succesfully studied to better understand the molecular mechanisms involved in vascular develepment and angiogenesis as well as biochemical changes that occur during physiological ageing [4, 5].

Histologically, AV consists of three layers: fibrosa, spongiosa and ventricularis. The fibrosa is located in the aortic side of the leaflets and it is mainly composed of fibroblasts and collagen fibers. The spongiosa is located below and it is formed by fibroblasts, mesenchymal cells and a polysaccharides-rich matrix. The ventricularis, found in the ventricular side of the leaflet, is made up of elastic fibers radially distributed. The AV is externally covered by several layers of endothelial cells. Collagen is responsible for the mechanical integrity of the valve, the spongiosa serves as a shock absorber and elastic fibers contract cusps during systole [3, 6].

However, it is also essential to perform studies at the molecular level of the tissue, looking for the discovery of tissue- and disease-specific markers. For this purpose, proteomic and metabolomic analyses can be ideally used since they allow the unbias analysis of hundreds or thousands of molecules at a time, detecting and identifying which molecules are present. In contrast to genomics and transcriptomics, proteomics and metabolomics study dynamic protein products, low molecular weight compounds and their interactions, which have a direct effect on the phenotype of the tissue (Figure 1).

Descriptive proteomics is a methodology that enables unbiased large-scale study of the set of all proteins in a biologic system at any given time. Thus, the expression, localization, interaction, structural domains and activity of these proteins, including splice isoforms and post-translational modifications (PTMs), can be studied [7]. Metabolomics is the study of a complete metabolome or a single group of particular metabolites, which are small molecules that participate in general metabolic reactions and that are required for the maintenance, growth and normal function of a cell [8]. The study of healthy valves through proteomic and metabolomic approaches and the subsequent integration of data, can provide molecular level information of the metabolic pathways that are more active in that tissue and will help to understand the mechanisms of physiological/pathological processes in aortic stenosis valves. This makes it easier the search for potential markers for early diagnosis of the disease, thus being able to predict which people may develop aortic stenosis in the future.

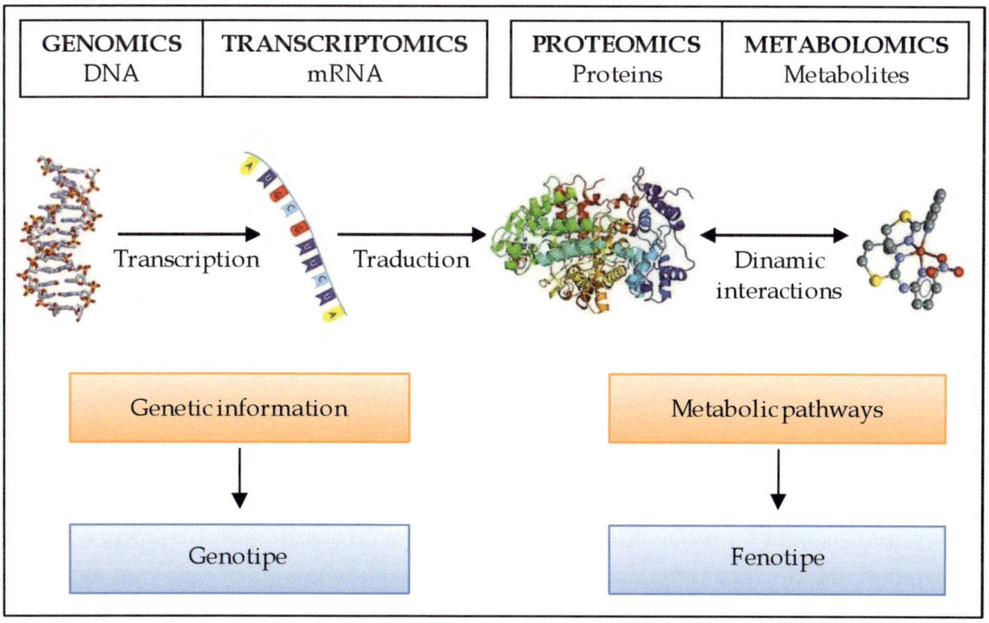

Figure 1. Dynamic study of the physiophatology of a disease through "-omics" technologies.

2. Proteomics

Proteomics is the large-scale study of the proteins content in a given sample (ie. biofluid or tissue) [9]. Since proteins are the final product of genes expression, proteomics constitutes a powerful tool for the study of biological systems thanks to proteome reflects the current state of the organism and it varies according to its functional situation [10]. These studies can be performed through a wide variety of techniques and methodologies, depending on the sample and the experimental design. In the case of descriptive proteomics, in which the most usually is the study of very complex samples, it is essential to perform certain steps to facilitate the study: 1) sample preparation, 2) protein separation and 3) analysis by mass spectrometry.

2.1. Sample preparation

Preparation of the samples prior to the analysis using proteomic techniques is an essential step for obtaining robust and reproducible data. Between the large number of standardized protocols, the selected one must be carefully chosen to suit the sample to be analyzed, as well as for the proteins of interest. In the case of the AV an effective and suitable protocol has been previously described [11] (Figure 2). Briefly, within 2 hours after surgery, valves were washed in PBS and then ground into a powder in liquid N2 with a mortar. 0.2 g of this powder was resuspended in 400 μl of protein extraction buffer (Tris 10 mM [pH 7.5], 500 mM NaCl, 0.1% Triton x-100, 1% β-mercaptoethanol, 1 mM PMSF) and then centrifuged to precipitate membranes and tissue debris [12]. Supernatant containing most of the soluble proteins was collected and pellet was solubilized in 7M urea, 2M thiourea, 4% CHAPS prior to another centrifugation [13, 14]. This second supernatant, which was rich in hydrophobic proteins, was also collected and stored at -20°. Depending on which is the fraction of interest, supernatants can be analyzed together or separately. Because of the nature of the extraction buffers, sample must be processed to eliminate interference substances with the downstream analyses. Samples must be filtered by centrifugation and dialyzed against Tris 2mM. Before proteomic analyses it is also recommended the use of the commercial kit 2D-Clean-Up (GE Healthcare), which precipitates proteins while leaving interfering substances, such as detergents, salts, lipids, phenolics, and nucleic acids, in solution. The pellet can then be solubilized in a proper buffer for further analyses.

Instead of solubilized the proteins of whole tissue, histology sections or specific cell types can be used for isolate different structures of the tissue as regions, cells or even subcellular fractions by means of laser microdissection (LMD) [15]. It consists in cutting microscopically selected tissue by laser using different systems [16]: 1) selected regions are transferred onto a film or to a special cap; 2) selected regions can be catapulted into a collection tube and 3) cut samples fall down into the lid of a collection tube by gravitation. The collected tissue has to be lysed and prepared for downstream analyses. The main disadvantage of this methodology in combination with proteomics is the scarce amount of protein that can be obtain, since the laser cannot be applied for a long time in order to avoid protein degradation. However, mass spectrometers have exponentially improved their sensitivity, so there are several interesting studies combining LMD and Proteomics in other cardiovascular tissues samples [17-20]. The application of LMD to the analysis of the AV tissue could provide specific data from the different layers/structures in the tissue, as well as from the behavior of the different cells in the tissue.

2.2. Protein separation

For complex mixtures, it is important to separate proteins according to their different characteristic to increase the efficiency of the study. For this purpose, the most usually used techniques are 2-dimensional electrophoresis (2-DE), off-gel fractionation, and 2-dimensional liquid chromatography (LC) [21-23] (Figure 3).

2.2.1. 2-Dimensional electrophoresis

This method stands out for its high applicability to a wide range of biological samples. In this case, a good protein separation can be reached through two simple steps: isoelectric focusing (IEF) and sodium dodecyl sulfate polyacrylamide gel electrophoresis (SDS-PAGE) [24, 25]. During the first phase, the protein mixture is separated on a pH gradient according to their isoelectric point (pI) using commercial strips covered by an acrylamide gel. To perform this separation, proteins are completely solubilized in a special buffer containing urea, a nonionic detergent (CHAPS) to prevent clustering, a reducing agent (DTT) to break the disulfide bonds and a mixture of ampholytes to minimize aggregations by charge interaction. In the second step, proteins are separated in a second dimension depending on their molecular mass and a two-dimensional protein spot map is obtained that can be visualized through different staining

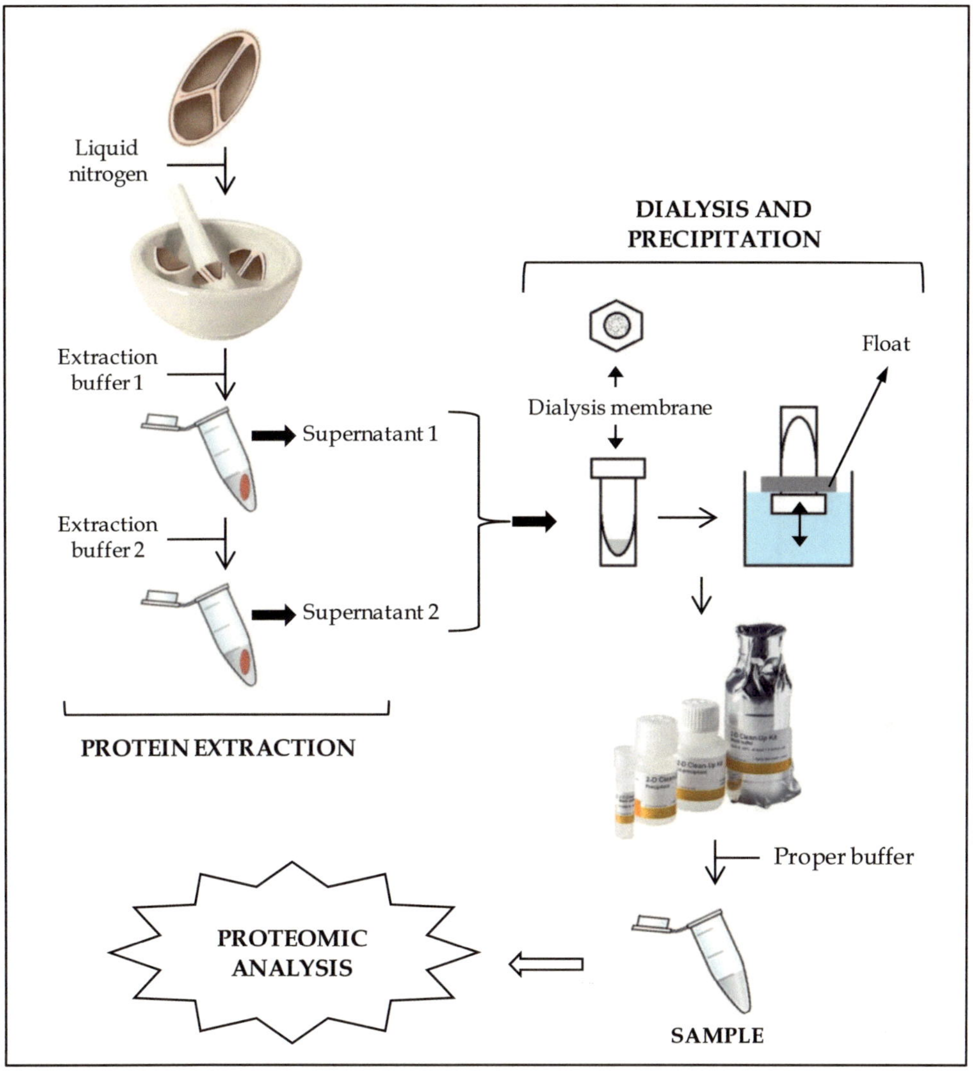

Figure 2. Protocol of aortic valve preparation for proteomic analyses

techniques as Coomassie blue, silver staining and Sypro Ruby [26]. Stained gels are scanned and digitalized using different computer programs to obtain an image of the gel and spots of interest will be identified by mass spectrometry techniques. There are three protein groups which are problematic: highly alkaline, extremely high and low molecular sizes and membrane-bound proteins. However, improving protein solubilization, pre-fractionation of protein groups of interest prior to 2DE, or adjustments to the 2-DE regime enhance separation of these more difficult-to-resolve proteins. The main advantage of 2-DE is that it delivers a map of intact proteins, which reflects changes in protein expression level, isoforms or post-translational modifications [27].

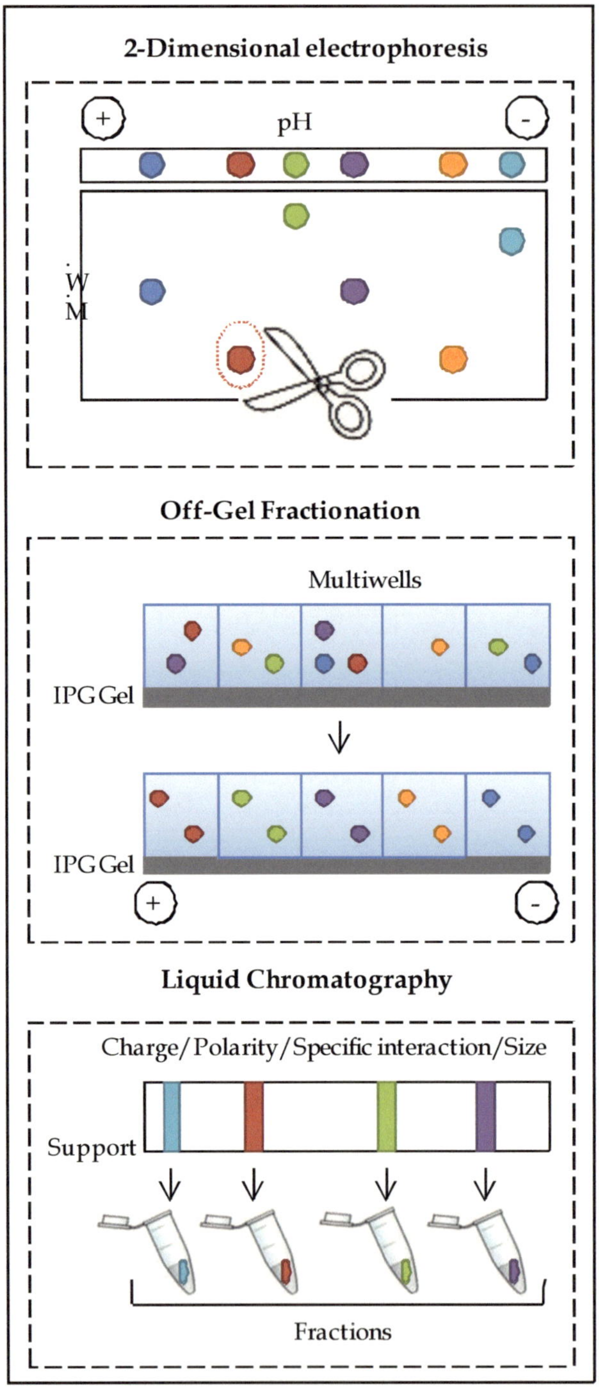

Figure 3. Most common used protein separation techniques

2.2.2. *Off-gel fractionation*

There is another protein fractionation technique which is based on off-gel IEF, where the proteins are separated according to their pI in a multiwell device. This separation is based on immobilized pH gradient (IPG) strips and permits to separate peptides and proteins according to their pI, but is realized in solution without the need of carrier ampholytes or buffers [28, 29]. The main advantage of this technique is that the fractions can be directly recovered in solution for further analysis and directly digested if necessary [28, 30]

2.2.3. *Liquid chromatography*

Liquid chromatography (LC) is a fractionation technique that can be applied to separate a wide range of molecules such as proteins or peptides according to their physical and/or chemical properties. Different types of chromatographic support can be distinguished: ion exchange (separation based on protein or peptide charge), reverse phase (according to their polarity), affinity (based on a highly specific interaction such as that between antigen and antibody, enzyme and substrate, or receptor and ligand) and molecular exclusion (depending on size). LC can be used before or after 2-DE [31-33] and can be directly coupled to a mass spectrometer for further identification [34, 35]. To increase the resolution of proteomics analyses, it is recommended the use several consecutive chromatographic methods. In this sense a combination of ion exchange and reverse phase chromatography allows a two-dimensional separation with the advantage that the second column can be directly coupled to MS, which enhances the automatization of the proteomic methodology. With this idea, multidimensional protein identification technology (MudPIT) has been developed. It consists of a column with two chromatographic supports in tandem: a cation exchange support in the proximal area followed by a reverse phase in the distal one. This method enables the two-dimensional LC using high-performance LC (HPLC) coupled to a mass spectrometer with electrospray ionization (ESI) source in an automated manner [36, 37]. This approach is more sensitivity and reproducibility than gel-based methodologies and allows the analyses of smaller quantities each time because of the development of new equipments which are able to work with sample volumes of the order of microliters and nanoliters. LC together with mass spectrometry has been successfully employed in a previous work in which the proteome of the coronary artery was described [17].

2.3. Protein analyses by mass spectrometry

Once our sample is separated, these fractions or spots must be analyzed to identify the different proteins. Since the development of matrix-assisted laser desorption ionization (MALDI) and ESI, two ionization methods that allows the analysis of proteins and peptides using MS, this technique have become indispensable for protein identification [38-40]. Mass spectrometers consist of three essential elements: ionization source, mass analyzer and detector (Figure 4). The ionization source ionizes and vaporizes the sample. Different ionization sources are MALDI, ESI or surface-enhanced laser desorption/ionization (SELDI) [41-43]. ESI allows the identification of many volatile and thermolabile compounds of a wide range of molecular weight with high sensitivity. MALDI and SELDI are very similar methods but they are used for low and high complex mixtures, respectively [44]. The mass analyzer separates the ions according to their relation m/z. There are also different types of mass analyzer, such as quadrupole (Q), time of flight (TOF), ion trap (IT), Fourier transform ion cyclotron resonance (FT-ICR) and Orbitrap. The ion stream reaches to the detector and it is transformed into an electrical signal. These signals are then integrated by a computer system which generates a mass spectrum which represents the abundance of the different generated ions.

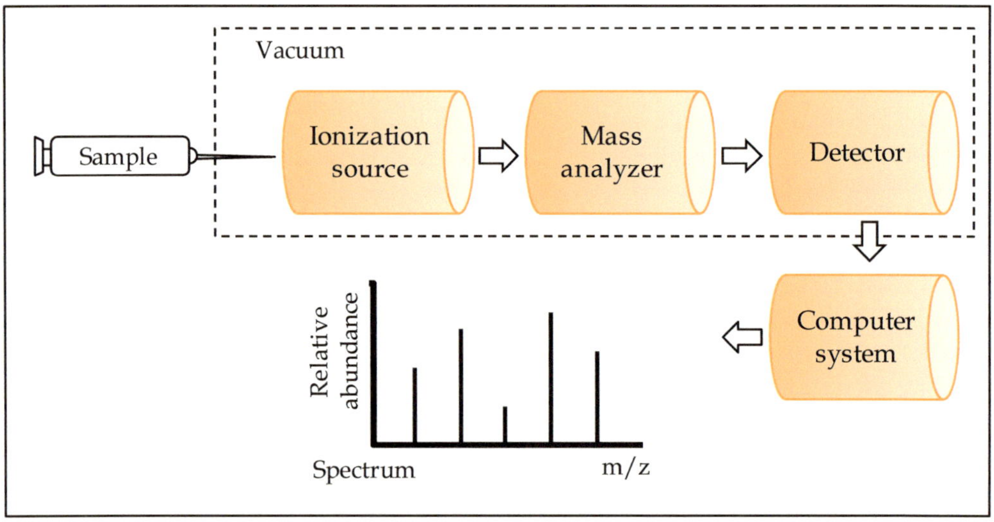

Figure 4. Different elements of a mass spectrometer

There are two different ways to identify the molecules included in a complex mix using MS: peptide mass fingerprinting (PMF) and tandem mass spectrometry (MS/MS or MS2). Briefly, identification based on PMF identifies proteins according to the peptides generated after digestion with specific endoproteases, usually trypsine. Experimentally obtained peptide masses are compared to theoretical peptide masses of proteins stored in databases through mass search engines such as MASCOT (Matrix Science Ltd.) [45], MS-Fit [46] or Profound [47, 48]. These samples usually come from gel bands, 2-DE spots or LC fractions with low complexity and are analyzed through MALDI-TOF or ESI-TOF [48, 49]. In the case of MS/MS, two mass analyzers are used in tandem. The first one allows the measurement of the m/z values of the peptides and the second one, after the fragmentation of some peptides, allows the measurement of the m/z values of these fragments. Thus, a partial or even total sequence of the peptide can be obtained. Most usually used mass spectrometer for this purpose are MALDI-TOF-TOF (for low complex mixtures) and ESI coupled to different analyzers (Q3, Q-TOF, IT, Q-Q-LIT, FT y Orbitrap).

2.4. Tissue sections analysis: MALDI imaging mass spectrometry

MALDI imaging mass spectrometry (IMS) is a powerful tool for investigating the distribution of proteins and small molecules present in thin tissue sections. This technique generates molecular profiles and two-dimensional ion density maps of peptide and protein signals directly from the surface of these sections [50]. For this analyses, it is indispensable a correct sample preparation in terms of chemical and structural integrity [51]. Preparation methods must avoid delocalization and degradation of the analytes so it is important to take into account several parameters such as treatment of tissue immediately after sample procurement, sectioning, sample transfer to the MALDI target plate, matrix application, and tissue storage after sectioning [52]. It is advisable the used of fresh tissue sections though sometimes it is necessary embedding the sample in gelatine or agarose to facilitate its manipulation [53-55]. One of the important aspects of tissue profiling is the comparison of histological features obtained from stained sections using light microscopy with molecular images obtained by mass spectrometry [56]. Previously, this was accomplished using two separate adjacent sections, one for histology and one for MALDI-IMS [57, 58]. However, visual registration between both sections it is difficult because of differences in tissue architecture. Ideally, histology and protein profiling should be performed on the same tissue section. For this reason, several commonly used histological dyes have been tested for compatibility with MS analysis. It was found that hematoxilin and eosin interfered with MS but, on the other hand, cresyl violet and methylene blue, between others, do not compromise mass spectra quality [56]. This methodology allows the study of the entire tissue, maintaining its structure, so MS analysis can be focused on specific morphological regions of interest.

3. Metabolomics

Metabolomics is the study of the set of final products and by-products of many metabolic pathways, called metabolites, which exist in humans and other living systems [8]. In order to perform a descriptive analysis of healthy valves, an untargeted approach, not focused on a specific group of metabolites, is the most recommended methodology. This method, also called metabolomic fingerprinting, permits to detect the largest number of metabolites optimizing different experimental conditions such as sample preparation and chromatographic and MS parameters. This approach usually compromises the sensitivity and specificity for identification of individual metabolites [59, 60]. Additionally, metabolomic fingerprinting involves less up-front method development when compared with targeted approaches but requires an exhaustive analysis due to the large number of identified metabolites. As well as in proteomics analyses, there are three main steps when performing a metabolomic study: [1] sample preparation; [2] metabolite detection and [3] data analysis.

3.1. Sample preparation

Optimization of sample-preparation protocol is extremely important in metabolomic studies because it affects both metabolite profile and quality data, leading to possible erroneous conclusions [61, 62]. An ideal sample-preparation method for metabolomic fingerprinting should have the following characteristics [1] non-selective to ensure adequate metabolite coverage; [2] simple and fast, with the minimum number of steps possible to minimize metabolite loss and/or degradation of the sample and enable high-throughput; [3] reproducible and [4] incorporate a metabolism-quenching step (low temperatures, addition of acid, or fast heating) to represent true metabolome composition at the time of sampling (Figure 5) [63]. For tissue metabolomics, the protocol includes a previous step of manual homogenization at low temperatures follow by a quenching step in liquid nitrogen [64]. Although the tissue disruption technique can altered the precision and metabolite coverage, the selection of the extraction solvent have a stronger effect on the number of extracted metabolites [65]. Several aqueous and organic solvents can be used, such us methanol [66, 67], methanol/water [68], isopropanol/acetonitrile/water [69], acetonitrile/methanol/water [70], acidic acetonitrile/water [71] or methanol/acetonitrile/acetone [72] between others. However, there is no an established protocol for aortic valve so it is important the development of an adequate method before metabolic fingerprinting.

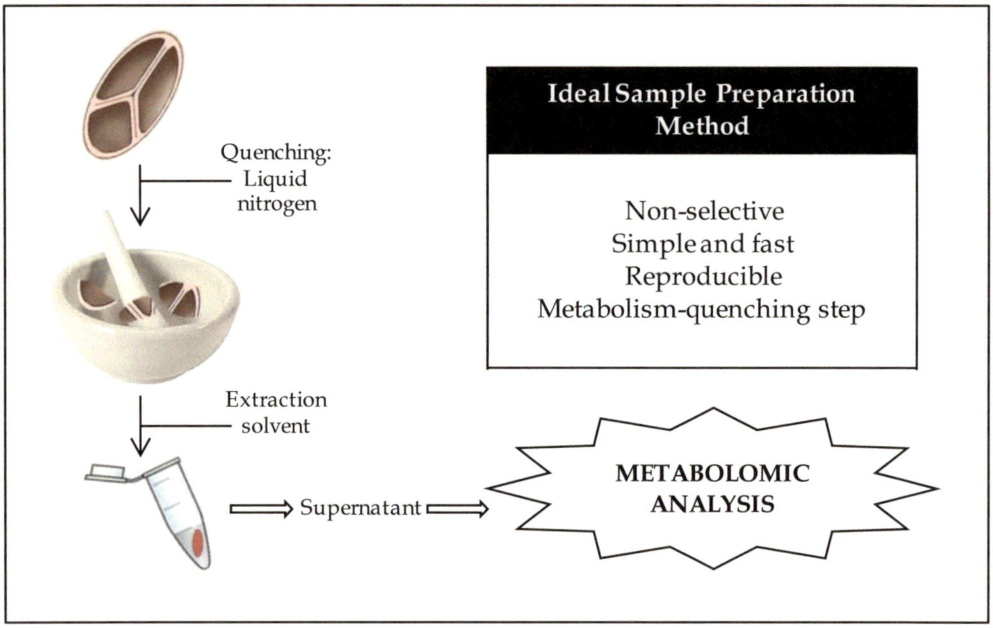

Figure 5. Protocol of tissue preparation for metabolomic analyses.

3.2. Metabolite detection

There is a great variability of metabolites in terms of polarity, solubility, and volatility with a wide dynamic range of concentration in biological samples. Therefore it is necessary to combine different chromatographic platforms for covering the largest range of metabolite possible. The two main platforms used in metabolomics analysis are nuclear magnetic resonance (NMR) and MS, usually coupled with a separation method for metabolites (LC or gas chromatography (GC)-MS) [73, 74]. The platform of choice will depend on the physico-chemical characteristics of the metabolites of interest. As it is explained below, CG-MS is a high-quality technique for analyzing hydrophobic compounds while LC-MS permits to determine a larger number of metabolites. Finally, NMR shows superior capability for determining the structure of unknown metabolites. Therefore, each platform has inherent advantages and disadvantages for the metabolomic analysis of different compounds and only through their combined use the best understanding of the physiopathology of AV will be achieved (Table 1).

Advantages	PLATFORM	Disadvantages
Minimal sample preparation Non-destructive Reproducible Structural information	NMR	Sensitivity Spectral resolution
No derivatization required Variety of metabolites	LC-MS	No comprehensive spectral libraries
Sensitivity Robust Reproducible Comprehensive spectral libraries	CG-MS	Derivatization required Limited mass range

Table 1. Comparison of the most common analytical methods used for metabolomics

3.2.1. Nuclear magnetic resonance

NMR is a spectroscopic analysis technique that exploits the specific magnetic spin or resonance frequency of the protons within atomic nuclei of specific molecules. When nuclei in a magnetic field are exposed to a radiofrequency pulse their protons temporarily move to a higher energy state, and then release a characteristic radiowave when they return to their normal energy state [75]. The resulting NMR spectrum is a collection of characteristic peaks and intensities of each compound that allow its identification [76]. NMR requires minimal sample preparation, it is a nondestructive and very reproducible technique and provides structural information of metabolites. These particular advantages confers NMR superior ability for the identification of unknown metabolites and constitutes a valuable approach for identification of unknown metabolites [77]. However, NMR is limited in terms of sensitivity and spectral resolution so it is not a good technology to identify metabolites that are found in low concentration [78].

NMR also allows the analyses of intact tissue using a technique called high-resolution magic angle spinning (HRMAS) NMR. The sample is spun at high speed about an axis at an angle of 54°44′(the so-called "magic angle") [79]. This rapid spinning at this precise angle has the effect of reducing dipolar coupling effects and narrowing of the broad lines found in this tissue. HRMAS-NMR has been applied successfully to analyze different intact cells and tissues [80-85], so it seems to be a powerful tool for the analyses of aortic valve tissue.

3.2.2. Mass spectrometry

As well as in proteomic studies, MS uses m/z value to identify metabolites. When coupled with chromatographic methods, MS can analyze a wide number of metabolites with enhanced sensitivity. The two main strategies for metabolite separation are LC (for nonvolatile compounds in solution) or GC (for volatile samples or when the expected compounds can be easily made volatile by derivatization). LC-MS using ESI as ionization source is the most currently used platform for metabolomic studies since it permits the analysis of a wider variety of metabolites than GC-MS [86, 87]. Also, derivatization step prior the analysis is no necessary reducing losses of compounds during the sample preparation. Single quadrupole, ion trap and TOF analyzers are the most commonly used mass analyzers. GC-MS is a first-rate choice for the analysis of volatile compounds such as fatty acids and organic acids [88]. In most cases, it is necessary a prior step for chemical derivatization of non-volatile and thermally stable metabolites. The two more used derivatization reagents include BSTFA (N, O-Bis (trimethylsilyl) trifluoroacetamide) and MSTFA (N-Methyl-N-(trimethylsilyl) trifluoroacetamide) [89-91]. Advantages of GC include higher resolution and more robust and reproducible retention times than LC, besides the existence of mass spectral libraries, which facilitates the identification process.

In the course of the study of the physiopathology of AS the better comprehension of implicated and altered biochemical pathways will be acquired through the metabolomic study of biological samples, specially plasma and tissue. For this purpose NMR and MS represent the two most valuable techniques for metabolite identification thus the information that both techniques provide will suppose a cornerstone for the study of this disease.

3.3. Identification and data analysis

The data processing challenges in metabolomics are quite unique and often require specialized (and/or expensive) data analysis software and a complete knowledge of cheminformatics, bioinformatics and statistics for a correct interpretation of data. Ideally, data analysis softwares must be able to remove noise from the spectra, properly identify which metabolite generates every chromatographic peak and make a correct alignment of the peaks corresponding to the same compound in several successive samples [92, 93].

There are several commercial softwares available free such as MSFacts, MetAlign or MetaboAnalyst which automatically import, reformat, align, correct the baseline, and export large chromatographic data sets to allow more rapid visualization of metabolomics data [94, 95]. However, most companies usually generate data that can be only read with own softwares which use mass spectral libraries for peak detection, identification and integration [96].

4. Towards a global understanding of physiology

The large number of genomes, including human, that have been mapped and the knowledge of the genetic code, have increased the interest in other –OMICS technologies, such as proteomics and metabolomics. Both proteomics and metabolomics differ from genomics in terms of complexity and dynamic variability. Proteome and metabolome are constantly changing according to the genome and the environment, therefore the ultimate phenotype of cell, organ, and organism is reflected in proteomic and metabolomic profiles. This variability, enhanced by the using of different methodologies and equipments, usually impedes obtaining reliable and reproducible results when comparing patients and healthy controls. The study of a large number of healthy valves using a standardized protocol may provide useful information about the heterogeneity of its profiles. Thus, different profiles could be assigned to different states such as sex, age or risk factors. This way, the creation of a protein atlas unmasking the expression and localization of proteins coupled to metabolomic results would function as a global knowledgebase with valuable information about normal cellular function [97, 98]. All these information can be storage in conventional web-based databases, in order to obtain a reference material to be used in further studies, when studying different valve diseases, helping to deepen the understanding of the beginning and development of the disease. It would also be possible to find some variation involving metabolic predisposition to develop the disease in the future. This will exponentially increase the possibilities to discover potential therapeutic targets and will open the door to develop a personalized medicine in this disease.

The major challenge of generating a complete database of AV tissue is obtaining enough biological material to be described, since it is not an easily accessible specimen. It is necessary a complex coordination of basic research activities, facilities and infrastructures, as well as the creation of an integrated and multidisciplinary environment with the participation of several different specialists in cardiovascular diseases, i.e. basic researchers, cardiologists, surgeons, pathologists, epidemiologists, patients, patient advocacy groups, funding agencies and industrial partners. Issues related to sample collection, handling and storage, standardization of protocols, common references, number of patients, availability of normal controls, access to bio-banks, tissue arrays, clinical information, follow-up clinical data, computational and statistical analysis, as well as ethical considerations are critical, and must be carefully considered and dealt with from the beginning [99]. With such a big collaborating work, there will be a more effective translation of basic discoveries into clinical applications.

No matter how much ambitious and complete the descriptive study is, it is essential integration of the results through a system biology approach. This consists of placing proteins and molecules from experimental analysis in the context of a network of biological interactions, such as gene–gene, gene–protein or protein–protein interactions, followed by different 'guilt-by-association' analyses [100]. Usually, these networks are deduced from previously published interactions or from computational prediction models. Different tools exist to perform these analyses, most of them based on Cytoscape Web, a freely available network visualization tool for integrating biomolecular interaction networks with high-throughput expression data and other molecular states into a unified conceptual framework [101-103]. Using an integrative approach, we can obtain a more holistic picture of the molecular mechanisms that occurs in normal aortic valves.

5. Conclusion

The study of healthy valves through proteomic and metabolomic approaches and the subsequent integration of data can provide molecular level information of the metabolic pathways that are more active in AV. The characterization of physiological proteins and metabolites in this tissue and the creation of a complete database with the results from the descriptive studies, may serve as a reference material for further studies. This would facilitate the searching for potential markers for early diagnosis of the disease, thus being able to predict which people may develop aortic stenosis in the future.

Acknowledgements

This work was supported by grants from the Instituto de Salud Carlos III (FIS PI070537, PI11/02239), Fondos Feder-Redes temáticas de Investigación Cooperativa en Salud (RD06/0014/1015), grants from Fundación para la Investigación Sanitaria de Castilla-La Mancha (FISCAM PI2008-08, PI2008-28, PI2008-52).

Author details

L. Mourino-Alvarez[1], C.M. Laborde[1,2] and M.G. Barderas[1,3]

1 Department of Vascular Physiopathology, Hospital Nacional de Paraplejicos, SESCAM, Toledo, Spain

2 Laboratory of Biochemistry, Hospital Nacional de Paraplejicos, SESCAM, Toledo, Spain

3 Proteomic Unit, Hospital Nacional de Paraplejicos, SESCAM, Toledo, Spain

References

[1] Goldbarg SH, Elmariah S, Miller MA, Fuster V. Insights Into Degenerative Aortic Valve Disease. J Am Coll Cardiol. 2007;50(13):1205-13.

[2] Helske S, Kupari M, Lindstedt KA, Kovanen PT. Aortic valve stenosis: an active atheroinflammatory process. Curr Opin Lipidol. 2007;18(5):483-91 10.1097/MOL. 0b013e3282a66099.

[3] Freeman RV, Otto CM. Spectrum of calcific aortic valve disease: Pathogenesis , disease progression, and treatment strategies. Circulation. 2005 June 21, 2005;111(24): 3316-26.

[4] Li Y, Yu J, Wang Y, Griffin NM, Long F, Shore S, et al. Enhancing Identifications of Lipid-embedded Proteins by Mass Spectrometry for Improved Mapping of Endothelial Plasma Membranes in Vivo. Mol Cell Proteomics. 2009 June 1, 2009;8(6):1219-35.

[5] Grant JE, Bradshaw AD, Schwacke JH, Baicu CF, Zile MR, Schey KL. Quantification of Protein Expression Changes in the Aging Left Ventricle of Rattus norvegicus. J Proteome Res. 2009 2012/10/08;8(9):4252-63.

[6] Schoen FJ. Evolving Concepts of Cardiac Valve Dynamics. Circulation. 2008 October 28, 2008;118(18):1864-80.

[7] Anderson N, Anderson N. Proteome and proteomics: new technologies, new concepts, and new words. Electrophoresis. 1998;Aug;19(11):1853-61.

[8] Pasikanti KK, Ho PC, Chan ECY. Gas chromatography/mass spectrometry in metabolic profiling of biological fluids. J Chromatogr B. 2008;871(2):202-11.

[9] Pandey A, Mann M. Proteomics to study genes and genomes. Nature. 2000;405(6788): 837-46.

[10] Marshall T, Williams KM. Proteomics and its impact upon biomedical science. British journal of biomedical science. 2002;59(1):47-64.

[11] Gil-Dones F, Martin-Rojas T, Lopez-Almodovar LF, Cuesta Fdl, Darde VM, Alvarez-Llamas G, et al. Valvular Aortic Stenosis: A Proteomic Insight. Clin Med Insights Cardiol. 2010;4;4:1-7.

[12] Barderas MG, Wigdorovitz A, Merelo F, Beitia F, Alonso C, Borca MV, et al. Serodiagnosis of African swine fever using the recombinant protein p30 expressed in insect larvae. J Virol Methods. 2000;89(1-2):129-36.

[13] Gonzalez-Barderas M, Gallego-Delgado J, Mas S, Duran MC, Lázaro A, Hernandez-Merida S, et al. Isolation of circulating human monocytes with high purity for proteomic analysis. Proteomics. 2004;4(2):432-7.

[14] Duran MC, Mas S, Martin-Ventura JL, Meilhac O, Michel JB, Gallego-Delgado J, et al. Proteomic analysis of human vessels: Application to atherosclerotic plaques. Proteomics. 2003;3(6):973-8.

[15] Emmert-Buck M, Bonner R, Smith P, Chuaqui R, Zhuang Z, Goldstein S, et al. Laser capture microdissection Science. 1996;274(5289):998-1001.

[16] Rabien A. Laser microdissection. Methods Mol Biol. 2010;576:39-47.

[17] Bagnato C, Thumar J, Mayya V, Hwang S-I, Zebroski H, Claffey KP, et al. Proteomics Analysis of Human Coronary Atherosclerotic Plaque. Mol Cell Proteomics. 2007 June 2007;6(6):1088-102.

[18] De la Cuesta F, Alvarez-Llamas G, Maroto AS, Donado A, Juarez-Tosina R, Rodriguez-Padial L, et al. An optimum method designed for 2-D DIGE analysis of human arterial intima and media layers isolated by laser microdissection. Proteomics Clin Appl. 2009;Oct;3(10):1174-84.

[19] de la Cuesta F, Alvarez-Llamas G, Maroto AS, Donado A, Zubiri I, Posada M, et al. A proteomic focus on the alterations occurring at the human atherosclerotic coronary intima. Mol Cell Proteomics. [Article]. 2011 Apr;10(4):13.

[20] De Souza AI, McGregor E, Dunn MJ, Rose ML. Preparation of human heart for laser microdissection and proteomics. Proteomics. 2004;4(3):578-86.

[21] Waller LN, Shores K, Knapp DR. Shotgun Proteomic Analysis of Cerebrospinal Fluid Using Off-Gel Electrophoresis as the First-Dimension Separation. J Proteome Res. 2008 2012/10/08;7(10):4577-84.

[22] Nägele E, Vollmer M, Hörth P, Vad C. 2D-LC/MS techniques for the identification of proteins in highly complex mixtures. Expert Rev Proteomics. 2004 2012/10/08;1(1): 37-46.

[23] Hey J, Posch A, Cohen A, Liu N, Harbers A. Fractionation of complex protein mixtures by liquid-phase isoelectric focusing. Methods Mol Biol. 2008;424:225-39.

[24] Görg A, Obermaier C, Boguth G, Harder A, Scheibe B, Wildgruber R, et al. The current state of two-dimensional electrophoresis with immobilized pH gradients. Electrophoresis. 2000;21(6):1037-53.

[25] Gygi SP, Corthals GL, Zhang Y, Rochon Y, Aebersold R. Evaluation of two-dimensional gel electrophoresis-based proteome analysis technology. Proc Natl Acad Sci U S A. 2000 August 15, 2000;97(17):9390-5.

[26] Chevalier F, Rofidal V, Rossignol M. Visible and fluorescent staining of two-dimensional gels. Methods Mol Biol. 2007;355:145-56.

[27] Görg A, Weiss W, Dunn MJ. Current two-dimensional electrophoresis technology for proteomics. Proteomics. 2004;4(12):3665-85.

[28] Michel PE, Reymond F, Arnaud IL, Josserand J, Girault HH, Rossier JS. Protein fractionation in a multicompartment device using Off-Gel™ isoelectric focusing. Electrophoresis. 2003;24(1-2):3-11.

[29] Heller M, Michel PE, Morier P, Crettaz D, Wenz C, Tissot J-D, et al. Two-stage Off-Gel™ isoelectric focusing: Protein followed by peptide fractionation and application to proteome analysis of human plasma. Electrophoresis. 2005;26(6):1174-88.

[30] Hörth P, Miller CA, Preckel T, Wenz C. Efficient Fractionation and Improved Protein Identification by Peptide OFFGEL Electrophoresis. Mol Cell Proteomics. 2006 October 2006;5(10):1968-74.

[31] Medzihradszky K, Leffler H, Baldwin M, Burlingame A. Protein identification by in-gel digestion, high-performance liquid chromatography, and mass spectrometry: Peptide analysis by complementary ionization techniques. J Am Soc Mass Spectrom. 2001;12(2):215-21.

[32] Pieper R, Gatlin C, Makusky A, Russo P, Schatz C, Miller S, et al. The human serum proteome: display of nearly 3700 chromatographically separated protein spots on

http://dx.doi.org/10.5772/55589

two-dimensional electrophoresis gels and identification of 325 distinct proteins. Proteomics. 2003;Jul;3(7):1345-64.

[33] Badock V, Steinhusen U, Bommert K, Otto A. Prefractionation of protein samples for proteome analysis using reversed-phase high-performance liquid chromatography. Electrophoresis. 2001;Aug;22(14):2856-64.

[34] Issaq HJ. The role of separation science in proteomics research. Electrophoresis. 2001;22(17):3629-38.

[35] Lesley SA. High-Throughput Proteomics: Protein Expression and Purification in the Postgenomic World. Protein Expr Purif. 2001;22(2):159-64.

[36] Washburn M, Wolters D, 3rd YJ. Large-scale analysis of the yeast proteome by multidimensional protein identification technology. Nat Biotechnol. 2001;Mar;19(3):242-7.

[37] Delahunty C, 3rd YJ. MudPIT: multidimensional protein identification technology. Biotechniques. 2007;43(5):563, 5, 7 passim.

[38] Domon B, Aebersold R. Mass spectrometry and protein analysis. Science. 2006;312(5771):212-7.

[39] Karas M, Hillenkamp F. Laser desorption ionization of proteins with molecular masses exceeding 10,000 daltons. Anal Chem. 1988;60(20):2299-301.

[40] Fenn J, Mann M, Menq C, Wong S, Whitehouse C. Electrospray for mass spectrometry of large biomolecules. Science. 1989;246(4926):64-71.

[41] Kinter M, Sherman NE. Fundamental Mass Spectrometry. Protein Sequencing and Identification Using Tandem Mass Spectrometry: John Wiley & Sons, Inc.; 2005. p. 29-63.

[42] Merchant M, Weinberger SR. Recent advancements in surface-enhanced laser desorption/ionization-time of flight-mass spectrometry. ELECTROPHORESIS. 2000;21(6):1164-77.

[43] Issaq HJ, Veenstra TD, Conrads TP, Felschow D. The SELDI-TOF MS Approach to Proteomics: Protein Profiling and Biomarker Identification. Biochem Biophys Res Commun. 2002;292(3):587-92.

[44] Issaq HJ, Conrads TP, Prieto DA, Tirumalai R, D.Veenstra T. SELDI-TOF MS for Di agnostic Proteomics. Anal Chem. 2003 2012/10/16;75(7):148 A-55 A.

[45] Perkins DN, Pappin DJC, Creasy DM, Cottrell JS. Probability-based protein identification by searching sequence databases using mass spectrometry data. ELECTROPHORESIS. 1999;20(18):3551-67.

[46] Clauser K, Baker P, Burlingame A. Role of accurate mass measurement (+/- 10 ppm) in protein identification strategies employing MS or MS/MS and database searching. Anal Chem. 1999;71(14):2871-82.

[47] Zhang W, Chait B. ProFound: an expert system for protein identification using mass spectrometric peptide mapping information. Anal Chem. 2000;72(11):2482-9.

[48] Aebersold R, Goodlett D. Mass spectrometry in proteomics. Chem Rev. 2001;101(2): 269-95.

[49] Aebersold R, Mann M. Mass spectrometry-based proteomics. Nature. 2003;422(6928): 198-207.

[50] Chaurand P, Stoeckli M, Caprioli RM. Direct Profiling of Proteins in Biological Tissue Sections by MALDI Mass Spectrometry. Anal Chem. 1999 2012/09/05;71(23):5263-70.

[51] McDonnell LA, Heeren RMA. Imaging mass spectrometry. Mass Spectrom Rev. 2007;26(4):606-43.

[52] Caldwell RL, Caprioli RM. Tissue Profiling by Mass Spectrometry. Mol Cell Proteomics. 2005 April 1, 2005;4(4):394-401.

[53] Altelaar AFM, van Minnen J, Jiménez CR, Heeren RMA, Piersma SR. Direct Molecular Imaging of Lymnaea stagnalis Nervous Tissue at Subcellular Spatial Resolution by Mass Spectrometry. Anal Chem. 2004 2012/10/08;77(3):735-41.

[54] Kruse R, Sweedler J. Spatial profiling invertebrate ganglia using MALDI MS. J Am Soc Mass Spectrom. 2003;14(7):752-9.

[55] Schwartz SA, Reyzer ML, Caprioli RM. Direct tissue analysis using matrix-assisted laser desorption/ionization mass spectrometry: practical aspects of sample preparation. J Mass Spectrom. 2003;38(7):699-708.

[56] Chaurand P, Schwartz SA, Billheimer D, Xu BJ, Crecelius A, Caprioli RM. Integrating Histology and Imaging Mass Spectrometry. Analytical Chemistry. 2004 2012/09/05;76(4):1145-55.

[57] Fournier I, Day R, Salzet M. Direct analysis of neuropeptides by in situ MALDI-TOF mass spectrometry in the rat brain. Neuro Endocrinol Lett. 2003;24(1-2):9-14.

[58] Yanagisawa K, Shyr Y, Xu BJ, Massion PP, Larsen PH, White BC, et al. Proteomic patterns of tumour subsets in non-small-cell lung cancer. Lancet. 2003;362(9382):433-9.

[59] Garcia DE, Baidoo EE, Benke PI, Pingitore F, Tang YJ, Villa S, et al. Separation and mass spectrometry in microbial metabolomics. Curr Opin Microbiol. 2008;11(3):233-9.

[60] Nordstrom A, Want E, Northen T, Lehtio J, Siuzdak G. Multiple Ionization Mass Spectrometry Strategy Used To Reveal the Complexity of Metabolomics. Anal Chem. 2007 2012/10/08;80(2):421-9.

[61] Bruce SJ, Tavazzi I, Parisod Vr, Rezzi S, Kochhar S, Guy PA. Investigation of Human Blood Plasma Sample Preparation for Performing Metabolomics Using Ultrahigh Performance Liquid Chromatography/Mass Spectrometry. Anal Chem. 2009 2012/10/08;81(9):3285-96.

[62] Duportet X, Aggio R, Carneiro S, Villas-Bôas S. The biological interpretation of metabolomic data can be misled by the extraction method used. Metabolomics. 2012;8(3):410-21.

[63] Vuckovic D. Current trends and challenges in sample preparation for global metabolomics using liquid chromatography–mass spectrometry. Anal Bioanal Chem. 2012;403(6):1523-48.

[64] Rammouz RE, Létisse F, Durand S, Portais J-C, Moussa ZW, Fernandez X. Analysis of skeletal muscle metabolome: Evaluation of extraction methods for targeted metabolite quantification using liquid chromatography tandem mass spectrometry. Anal Biochem. 2010;398(2):169-77.

[65] Geier FM, Want EJ, Leroi AM, Bundy JG. Cross-Platform Comparison of Caenorhabditis elegans Tissue Extraction Strategies for Comprehensive Metabolome Coverage. Anal Chem. 2011 2012/10/08;83(10):3730-6.

[66] Xu Y, Cheung W, Winder CL, Dunn WB, Goodacre R. Metabolic profiling of meat: assessment of pork hygiene and contamination with Salmonella typhimurium. Analyst. 2011;136(3):508-14.

[67] Ji B, Ernest B, Gooding J, Das S, Saxton A, Simon J, et al. Transcriptomic and metabolomic profiling of chicken adipose tissue in response to insulin neutralization and fasting. BMC Genomics. 2012;13(1):441.

[68] Koek M, van der Kloet F, Kleemann R, Koistra T, Verheij E, Hankemeier T. Semi-automated non-target processing in GC × GC-MS metabolomics analysis: applicability for biomedical studies. Metabolomics. 2011;7(1):1-14.

[69] Budczies J, Denkert C, Muller B, Brockmoller S, Klauschen F, Gyorffy B, et al. Remodeling of central metabolism in invasive breast cancer compared to normal breast tissue - a GC-TOFMS based metabolomics study. BMC Genomics. 2012;13(1):334.

[70] Ellinger JJ, Miller DC, Lewis IA, Markley JL. Semiautomated Device for Batch Extraction of Metabolites from Tissue Samples. Analytical Chemistry. 2012 2012/09/07;84(4): 1809-12.

[71] Hallows WC, Yu W, Smith BC, Devires MK, Ellinger JJ, Someya S, et al. Sirt3 Promotes the Urea Cycle and Fatty Acid Oxidation during Dietary Restriction. Mol Cell. 2011;41(2):139-49.

[72] Tan G, Lou Z, Liao W, Zhu Z, Dong X, Zhang W, et al. Potential Biomarkers in Mouse Myocardium of Doxorubicin-Induced Cardiomyopathy: A Metabonomic Method and Its Application. PLoS ONE. 2011;6(11):e27683.

[73] Dunn WB, Bailey NJC, Johnson HE. Measuring the metabolome: current analytical technologies. Analyst. 2005;130(5):606-25.

[74] Issaq HJ, Abbott E, Veenstra TD. Utility of separation science in metabolomic studies. J Sep Sci. 2008;31(11):1936-47.

[75] Trock BJ. Application of metabolomics to prostate cancer. Urol Oncol. 2011;29(5): 572-81.

[76] Nicholson J, Wilson I. Opinion: understanding 'global' systems biology: metabonomics and the continuum of metabolism. Nat Rev Drug Discov. 2003;2(8):668-76.

[77] Raamsdonk LM, Teusink B, Broadhurst D, Zhang N, Hayes A. A functional genomics strategy that uses metabolome data to reveal the phenotype of silent mutations. Nat Biotechnol. 2001;19:45.

[78] Pan Z, Raftery D. Comparing and combining NMR spectroscopy and mass spectrometry in metabolomics. Anal Bioanal Chem. 2007;387(2):525-7.

[79] Martínez-Bisbal M, Esteve V, Martínez-Granados B, Celda B. Magnetic resonance microscopy contribution to interpret high-resolution magic angle spinning metabolomic data of human tumor tissue. J Biomed Biotechnol. 2011;2011.

[80] Cheng LL, Ma MJ, Becerra L, Ptak T, Tracey I, Lackner A, et al. Quantitative neuropathology by high resolution magic angle spinning proton magneticâ€‰resonanceâ€ ‰spectroscopy. Proc Natl Acad Sci U S A. 1997 June 10, 1997;94(12):6408-13.

[81] Hu JZ, Rommereim DN, Minard KR, Woodstock A, Harrer BJ, Wind RA, et al. Metabolomics in Lung Inflammation:A High-Resolution 1H NMR Study of Mice Exposedto Silica Dust. Toxicol Mech Methods. 2008;18(5):385-98.

[82] Bollard ME, Murray AJ, Clarke K, Nicholson JK, Griffin JL. A study of metabolic compartmentation in the rat heart and cardiac mitochondria using high-resolution magic angle spinning 1H NMR spectroscopy. FEBS letters. 2003;553(1):73-8.

[83] Tate AR, Foxall PJD, Holmes E, Moka D, Spraul M, Nicholson JK, et al. Distinction between normal and renal cell carcinoma kidney cortical biopsy samples using pattern recognition of 1H magic angle spinning (MAS) NMR spectra. NMR Biomed. 2000;13(2):64-71.

[84] Righi V, Mucci A, Schenetti L, Tosi MR, Grigioni WF, Corti B, et al. Ex vivo HR-MAS Magnetic Resonance Spectroscopy of Normal and Malignant Human Renal Tissues. Anticancer Res. 2007 September-October 2007;27(5A):3195-204.

[85] Chen J-H, Wu YV, DeCarolis P, O'Connor R, Somberg CJ, Singer S. Resolution of creatine and phosphocreatine 1H signals in isolated human skeletal muscle using HR-MAS 1H NMR. Magn Reson Med. 2008;59(6):1221-4.

[86] Grandori R, Santambrogio C, Brocca S, Invernizzi G, Lotti M. Electrospray-ionization mass spectrometry as a tool for fast screening of protein structural properties. Biotechnol J. 2009;4(1):73-87.

[87] Ho C, Lam C, Chan M, Cheung R, Law L, Lit L, et al. Electrospray ionisation mass spectrometry: principles and clinical applications. Clin Biochem Rev. 2003;24(1):3-12.

[88] Kuhara T. Noninvasive human metabolome analysis for differential diagnosis of inborn errors of metabolism. J Chromatogr B. 2007;855(1):42-50.

[89] Chen M, Zhao L, Jia W. Metabonomic Study on the Biochemical Profiles of A Hydrocortisone-Induced Animal Model. J Proteome Res. 2005 2012/10/08;4(6):2391-6.

[90] Dettmer K, Aronov PA, Hammock BD. Mass spectrometry-based metabolomics. Mass Spectrom Rev. 2007;26(1):51-78.

[91] Lee SH, Woo HM, Jung BH, Lee J, Kwon OS, Pyo HS, et al. Metabolomic Approach To Evaluate the Toxicological Effects of Nonylphenol with Rat Urine. Anal Chem. 2007 2012/10/08;79(16):6102-10.

[92] Issaq HJ, Van QN, Waybright TJ, Muschik GM, Veenstra TD. Analytical and statistical approaches to metabolomics research. J Sep Sci. 2009;32(13):2183-99.

[93] Lange E, Tautenhahn R, Neumann S, Gropl C. Critical assessment of alignment procedures for LC-MS proteomics and metabolomics measurements. BMC Bioinformatics. 2008;9(1):375.

[94] Hansen MAE, Villas-Bôas SG, Roessner U, Smedsgaard J, Nielsen J. Data Analysis. Metabolome Analysis: John Wiley & Sons, Inc.; 2006. p. 146-87.

[95] Duran AL, Yang J, Wang L, Sumner LW. Metabolomics spectral formatting, alignment and conversion tools (MSFACTs). Bioinformatics. 2003 November 22, 2003;19(17):2283-93.

[96] Sturm M, Bertsch A, Gropl C, Hildebrandt A, Hussong R, Lange E, et al. OpenMS - An open-source software framework for mass spectrometry. BMC Bioinformatics. 2008;9(1):163.

[97] Teraishi T, Miura K. Toward an in situ phospho-protein atlas: phospho- and site-specific antibody-based spatio-temporally systematized detection of phosphorylated proteins in vivo. BioEssays. 2009;31(8):831-42.

[98] Persson A, Hober S, Uhlen M. A human protein atlas based on antibody proteomics. Curr Opin Mol Ther. 2006;8(3):185-90.

[99] Celis JE, Moreira JMA, Gromova I, Cabezon T, Ralfkiaer U, Guldberg P, et al. Towards discovery-driven translational research in breast cancer. FEBS J. 2005;272(1): 2-15.

[100] Merico D, Gfeller D, Bader G. How to visually interpret biological data using networks. Nat Biotechnol. 2009;Oct;27(10):921-4.

[101] Shannon P, Markiel A, Ozier O, Baliga NS, Wang JT, Ramage D, et al. Cytoscape: a software environment for integrated models of biomolecular interaction networks. Genome Res. 2003 November 1, 2003;13(11):2498-504.

[102] Cline MS, Smoot M, Cerami E, Kuchinsky A, Landys N, Workman C, et al. Integration of biological networks and gene expression data using Cytoscape. Nat Protoc. 2007;2(10):2366-82.

[103] Smoot ME, Ono K, Ruscheinski J, Wang P-L, Ideker T. Cytoscape 2.8: new features for data integration and network visualization. Bioinformatics. 2011 February 1, 2011;27(3):431-2.

Chapter 7

Genetics of Bicuspid Aortic Valve and Calcific Aortic Valve Disease

Robert B. Hinton

Additional information is available at the end of the chapter

http://dx.doi.org/10.5772/55506

1. The clinical taxonomy: Malformation vs. disease

Aortic valve malformation is a spectrum including Bicuspid Aortic Valve. Aortic valve malformation has been appreciated since the Renaissance when artists advanced our understanding of anatomy and specifically, Leonardo da Vinci illustrated and described variants of aortic valve morphology [1]. Aortic valve malformation is the most common cardiovascular malformation (CVM), and bicuspid aortic valve (BAV, MIM#109730) is the most common type of aortic valve malformation. BAV is present at birth and is characterized by two rather than three cusps. The incidence of BAV is 1-2% in the general population and affects an estimated 3 million people [2,3]. BAV itself is subclinical and the valve is typically functional, making BAV an endophenotype. Two patterns of BAV morphology are commonly observed: ~70% of isolated cases have fusion of the right and left (RL) coronary cusps with the remainder consisting almost entirely of those with fusion of the right and non (RN) coronary cusps [4,5]. Rarely, cases have shown fusion of the left and non (LN) coronary cusps. In addition to BAV subtypes, there is a spectrum of aortic valve malformation (Figure 1), ranging from various types of unicuspid to quadricuspid aortic valves with the three BAV morphology patterns and a thickened tricommissural aortic valve representing intermediate phenotypes [7]. Presently, it remains unclear to what degree these variations of malformation represent true differences.

Calcific Aortic Valve Disease is a growing public health problem. Aortic valve disease is defined by abnormal valve function. Valve disease may manifest as *stenosis*, an obstruction to normal forward blood flow, or *insufficiency*, a defective closure resulting in backward blood flow. Valve disease tends to progress. Ultimately, ventricular function can be compromised. Aortic valve stenosis is the most common manifestation of CAVD and classically presents as angina, syncope and heart failure. The diagnosis can be made clinically and confirmed by echocardiography, which quantifies the severity, and, over time, the progression of disease [8].

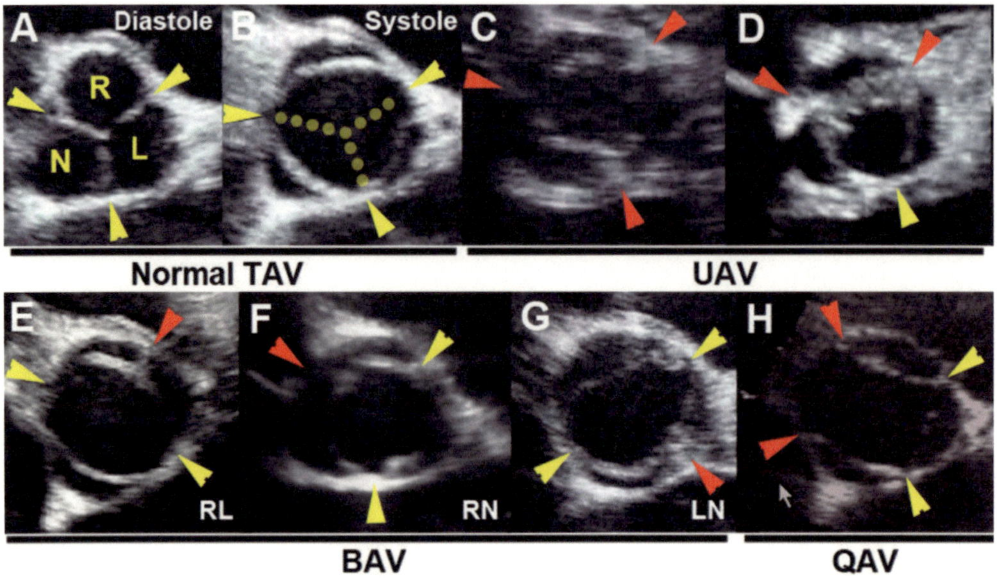

Figure 1. Phenotype definition: spectrum of aortic valve malformation. Aortic valve malformation Parasternal short axis echocardiographic views at the base of the heart showing the aortic valve en face (A-H). Normal tricommissural aortic valve (TAV) morphology is demonstrated in diastole (A) and systole (B). Distinct morphologies are based on fusion patterns of the commissures (dotted lines, B) as they relate to the right (R), left (L) and non (N) coronary sinuses of Valsalva (A). Aortic valve malformation ranges from unicuspid (UAV) to bicuspid (BAV) to a thickened tricuspid (not shown) to quadricuspid (QAV) morphology. Three normal commissures are demonstrated in panel A, and normal opening of the commissures results in complete cusp separation to the wall of the aorta at the sinotubular junction (yellow arrowheads). UAV manifests as either partial fusion of all three commissures (red arrowheads, C) or complete fusion of both the RN and RL commissures (D). Bicuspid aortic valve (BAV) may manifest as fusion of the RL (E), RN (F), and rarely LN (G) commissures. Rarely, a quadricuspid aortic valve (QAV, H) is identified. Adapted from [6].

Histopathology from diseased valves explanted at the time of surgery from patients with CAVD demonstrates large nodules of overt calcification, in addition to cell-matrix abnormalities (Figure 2). Research efforts have focused on the valve cusp, and as a result the valve annulus has been largely overlooked [4,7,9]. Human studies investigating valve disease have suggested that the base of the valve cusp and valve annulus regions is the origin of disease processes, including both sclerosis and calcification [10,11]. Greater than 2.5% of the population has AVD, causing more than 25,000 deaths annually in the US [12,13]. The actual direct cost for valve disease in the US alone has been estimated at 1 billion dollars per year [14]. Taken together, the public health impact and burden to society of CAVD is significant and underappreciated. The majority of valve disease at any age has an underlying valve malformation suggesting a genetic basis [15]. Aging is an independent risk factor for CAVD, resulting in a higher prevalence of disease as the population achieves greater longevity [16,17]. Aortic valve sclerosis, a marker of cardiovascular risk, and to a lesser extent valve disease, is present in more than 25% of the aged [18]. Therapy for CAVD remains primarily surgical and is restricted to late stage disease. Aortic valve replacement is the second most frequent cardiovascular surgical procedure [3,9], and the need for re-intervention is common [19]. Bioprosthetic replacement approaches are effective, but not durable [20,21]. Because there is a lack of

http://dx.doi.org/10.5772/55506

pharmacologic treatments for CAVD, the indications for surgical intervention dominate the clinical landscape. Early disease processes and progression remain poorly understood, and there are presently no pharmacologic based treatment options for CAVD.

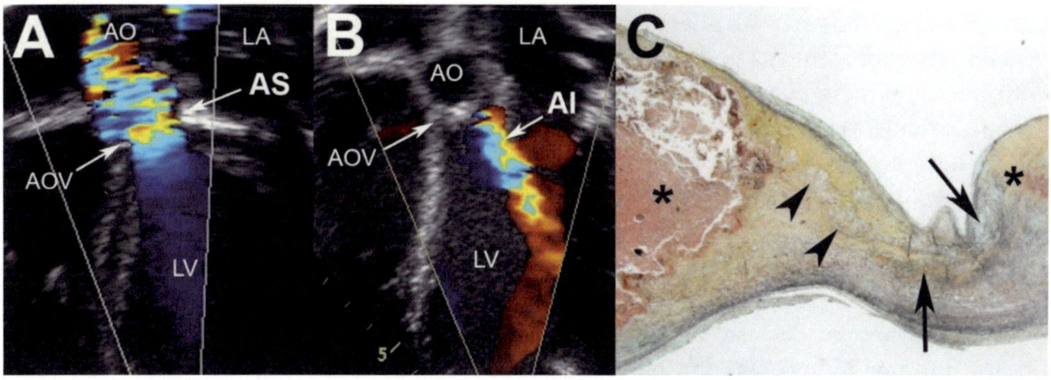

Figure 2. Phenotype definition: types of aortic valve disease. Color Doppler echocardiographic apical four chamber images demonstrate the two basic types of aortic valve disease. Aortic valve disease is characterized by a dysfunctional valve and is classified as stenosis (obstruction, A) and/or insufficiency (incompetence, B). Aortic stenosis (AS) and aortic insufficiency (AI) result in hemodynamic perturbations that lead to clinical disease states. Advanced calcific aortic valve disease is typically characterized by stenosis, and histopathology identifies gross calcific nodules in the fibrosa layer of the cusp (asterisks, C), clusters of cartilage like interstitial cells (arrowheads, C), and marked heterogeneity of extracellular matrix abnormalities (arrows, C). AO aorta; AOV aortic valve; LA left atrium; LV left ventricle.

Bicuspid Aortic Valve is an independent risk factor for Calcific Aortic Valve Disease. BAV is an established risk factor for CAVD [3,7,13]. The majority of CAVD cases at any age have an underlying BAV, and longitudinal studies in young adults with BAV have shown that >20% ultimately require surgical intervention [15,22,23]. In addition, those CAVD patients with an underlying BAV tend to develop calcification a decade earlier than those with normal aortic valve morphology [24]. Recently, a National Heart Lung and Blood Institute Executive Statement on CAVD identified a critical need to identify "clinical risk factors for the distinct phases of initiation and progression of AVD" [25], where standard cardiac risk factors including sclerosis have not yet been applicable. There has been avid interest and conflicting reports regarding the potential use of BAV morphology as a specific predictor of CAVD. Fernandes et al identified an association between RN BAV and AVD in a pediatric population, while Tzemos et al found no association in an adult population [5,22]. Exploring AVD in a pediatric population allows for examination of the disease process free from the confounding effects of cardiovascular comorbidities. Risk factors for AVD in children are poorly understood [23], but recently Calloway et al. reported that children with RN BAV and adults with RL BAV were more likely to develop AVD, suggesting BAV morphology may have predictive value for the time course of AVD [26]. It is unclear if AVD in children, which is not characterized by calcification, represents a different genetic type of disease or one end of a spectrum of the same disease.

Careful clinical phenotyping is critical for research, especially genetic discovery. Phenotype definition and stratification are necessary to advance our understanding of CAVD, especially in the context of genetic discovery. In addition to distinguishing malformation from disease, CAVD phenotyping needs to be detailed and comprehensive using all aspects of the clinical taxonomy, even those currently considered clinically inconsequential. The first step of any human genetic research study is to clearly and precisely define the phenotype. Studies that use too broad or too narrow a phenotype definition may fail to find association with an existing genetic variant or identify a pathologic one. Thus, identification of the phenotype most aligned with the underlying genetic etiology is essential for successful identification of associated genetic variants, a concept recently described as "deep phenotyping" [27]. Cardiovascular risk factors have been established for a variety of cardiovascular diseases, including substantial overlap for CAVD and coronary artery disease (CAD) or atherosclerosis [16,28,29]. While these disease processes often co-occur, as evidenced by the high frequency of concurrent coronary artery bypass grafting and aortic valve replacement surgery, only a small proportion of CAVD patients have CAD [30]. Likewise, there is an increased incidence of CAVD in patients with other cardiovascular disease, including systemic hypertension and chronic kidney disease [31,32]. Substantial investigation has established the adverse effects of common comorbid cardiovascular diseases on the progression of AVD; however, increasing attention on the underlying genetic and developmental processes will identify early mechanisms that incite disease processes. Emerging evidence suggests that both specific genetic factors and clinical cardiac risks may be necessary for disease initiation and progression.

Phenotype definition must expand to include non-clinical paradigms. Like many diseases, especially cardiovascular diseases, the clinical taxonomy of CAVD is based on anatomy and physiology. Classification schemes are organized with clinical standard of care, particularly surgical intervention, in mind [33,34]. The gold standard for diagnosis of cardiovascular diseases is imaging, such as echocardiography or magnetic resonance, modalities that define anatomy and physiology. While these approaches have been clinically useful, there is substantial phenotypic heterogeneity of unclear significance, including for example, the distinction between malformation and disease. Expanding phenotype to include an improved understanding of embryologic patterns underlying malformation will provide insight into pathogenesis [35-37]. Increasingly, combinations of phenotypes long held to be independent from a clinical perspective are now understood to be related from an etiologic perspective, challenging classic notions of disease classification. Molecular insights may inform new pharmacologic treatments the same way imaging informs surgical decision-making. Ultimately, identifying the genetic causes of disease will require reconciling clinical and molecular taxonomies of disease.

2. The genetic basis of BAV and CAVD

BAV has a strong genetic basis, but the precise causes remain unknown. Heritability estimates the proportion of a disease attributable to genetics. BAV heritability estimates are high, ranging from 75 to 89%, indicating that major genetic factors contribute to the develop-

http://dx.doi.org/10.5772/55506

ment of BAV [38]. Pedigree and segregation analyses have consistently identified autosomal dominant inheritance with reduced penetrance and complex inheritance underlying BAV [38-41], acknowledging that BAV is subclinical and therefore may be underestimated. Interestingly, while BAV is highly heritable, AVD is not, suggesting the phenotypic variability of CAVD is determined largely by non-genetic factors [26]. Consistent with these human observations, an established hamster model of BAV also shows the same characteristics of complex inheritance [42,43]. An additional quantitative measure of familial risk is recurrence risk. The recurrence risk of a disease measures the proportion of relatives who have the disease. BAV recurrence risk in siblings has been estimated to be approximately 9% [44], identifying further evidence of a genetic basis. Linkage analysis determines whether susceptibility variant segregates with disease in families. Previous studies have supported a strong underlying genetic basis for isolated nonsyndromic BAV, including family-based studies that have identified numerous loci [44-46]. Combined, these loci harbor hundreds of genes that may contribute to BAV. Multiple loci identify BAV as a genetically heterogeneous trait. Missense mutations in *NOTCH1* have been identified in a small proportion of nonsyndromic CAVD patients with BAV [47,48]. NOTCH1 is an intriguing biological candidate gene. In animal systems, Notch loss of function recapitulates the AVD phenotype, and actively regulates the maladaptive development of associated calcification, further supporting a mechanistic role [49-51]. In addition, a recent report described copy number variants (CNVs) in 10% of left-sided CVM cases, including BAV and aortic stenosis, potentially identifying new causes and/or modifiers of CAVD [52]. Association studies have not been used for BAV due to the large number of cases required to perform analyses (typically at least 1000), but combined linkage-association may be an excellent approach for discovery to leverage the strengths of each method. It is unclear how whole exome sequencing will impact discovery, but combining the various new tools for discovery promises to yield increasing insight into the genetic basis of BAV and CAVD.

BAV is a congenital malformation, a defect in cardiac development. Malformations present at birth often have strong genetic causes, if not monogenic etiology. Primary cardiac development occurs in humans from 2-8 weeks gestation, and semilunar valve (including the aortic valve) formation occurs in the seventh and eighth weeks. The heart is the first organ to form and continued survival of the organism is dependent on the circulation. The primitive heart tube is composed of a myocardial cell layer surrounding an endothelial cell layer. The formation of endocardial cushions is the first event of valve development. Endocardial cushion formation is accomplished by an early epithelial to mesenchymal transition (EMT) that generates a progenitor cell population embedded in a loosely organized extracellular matrix (ECM), followed by a late ECM remodeling stage that results in mature cusp organization (ventricularis, spongiosa, fibrosa) and valve interstitial cells [35-37]. Early defects in this process result in embryonic lethality, but late defects result in viable malformation and disease [53], hypothetically making the mechanisms of late developmental defects more applicable to human disease. It remains unknown why there are uneven frequencies of the different BAV types, but several developmental hypotheses have been proposed including a neural crest contribution that is not necessary but when present results in fusion of the right and left coronary cusps [42]. Further, the relatively rare unicuspid morphology underlies the majority of cases of critical aortic stenosis in the newborn and is associated with hypoplastic left heart syndrome (HLHS), suggesting genetic ("severe" malformation) and environmental (flow perturbations) factors combine to result in disease manifestation [15,54,55]. Elucidation of the genetic basis of both BAV and CAVD will result in a reconciled classification system that integrates the molecular basis of cardiac development with the pathologic basis of disease in a clinically meaningful manner.

Genetic factors contributing to CAVD are numerous and relatively small. Common complex traits are generally the result of numerous factors, each with a small additive effect and none necessary or sufficient to cause disease [56]. Coronary artery disease (CAD) and systemic hypertension (HTN) are well-described examples of this type of trait. While there is unequivocal evidence that BAV with CAVD is a complex trait, it is not nearly as common as CAD or HTN, and is more strongly linked to developmental processes, therefore it is likely that BAV/CAVD is an "intermediate" phenotype between the "rare single-gene" and "common complex" diseases. Importantly, this suggests that it is more likely to discover clinically useful patterns of variants associated with CAVD. Clinically, CAVD, CAD and HTN are considered discrete disease states, but there is a preponderance of epidemiologic and molecular evidence suggesting some pathogenesis is shared. Therefore, variants that have been identified studying individuals with CAD and HTN may inform risk assessment in patients with CAVD. Just as some clinical cardiovascular risk factors are common to all cardiovascular disease states, some genetic variants may pertain to predisposition of any cardiovascular disease depending on the aggregate risk (Figure 3). For example, the 10q24 locus has been identified in probands from BAV, CAD, HTN, thoracic aortic aneurysm (TAA) and intracranial aneurysm families [44, 57-60], suggesting the gene(s) in this region plays a role in each of these related cardiovascular phenotypes and therefore may be a general cardiovascular risk variant. It remains unclear whether a specified number of general cardiovascular risk variants are sufficient to cause any one disease, or more intuitively both *specific* and *general* disease variants are necessary.

CAVD is a latent phenotype, an injury or defect in valve maintenance. Typically, aortic valve disease does not manifest until the fourth or fifth decade of life and often does not progress to require surgical intervention until a decade later. How can developmental defects be functional for so long, only to fail in adulthood? The prevailing view is that individuals with a genetic predisposition for CAVD require an additional "second" insult to trigger disease initiation and progression that otherwise would not have occurred. While many of the genes that have been implicated in CAVD effect valve development [61,62], they may have additional distinct roles in valve maintenance [63], that is, how the tissue responds over time to the hemodynamic demands of constant motion and changing physiology. Similarly, there are genes that do not have a role in valve development but may be necessary for valve homeostasis [35,63]. Indeed, CAVD has been labeled a "degenerative" condition for decades, and age-related "wear and tear" contributes to valve failure. For example, elastic fiber degradation occurs with advanced age and predisposes the individual to inflammation, which may contribute to CAVD acceleration in later life [64,65]. Equally important, however, are comorbid conditions such as CAD that may serve to be an injury, or second hit, in vulnerable aortic valve tissue. For example, in an individual with genetic variants predisposing specifically for CAVD, the presence of CAD

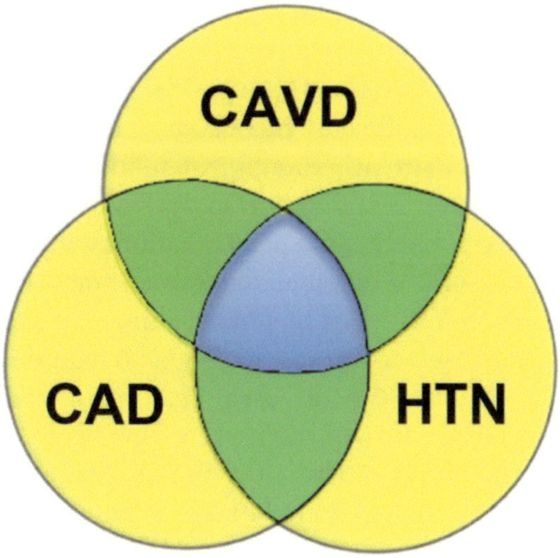

Figure 3. Shared predisposing genetic risk variants in common cardiovascular diseases. Cardiovascular diseases characterized by complex inheritance may have genetic variants specific to the clinical disease state, e.g., CAVD, CAD, HTN (yellow), as well as nonspecific genetic variants that may contribute to two (green) or three (blue) different cardiovascular diseases.

may initiate additional disease processes that incite CAVD (e.g. endothelial dysfunction). Taken together, a nonspecific cardiovascular insult in the context of a specific genetic predisposition for BAV may be necessary and sufficient for the manifestation of CAVD. As the genetic and developmental basis of valve malformation and disease is elucidated, opportunities for novel medical therapies will emerge and potentially preclude or delay the need for surgery. Defining regulation of valve tissue maintenance and homeostasis will provide exciting opportunities for cell-based or molecular therapies for valve disease.

Complex inheritance is characterized by a liability threshold. Polygenic conditions are characterized by a fixed number of susceptibility genes and a liability threshold, whereby a variety of combinations of predisposing variants may reach a specified level (e.g., 3 risk variants) to cause in combination the phenotype. In general, the importance of genetic modifiers and epigenetics is rapidly emerging, but little is known about these factors in the context of BAV/CAVD. Different BAV morphologies may reflect different combinations of shared genetic variants that carry different clinical risks, e.g. CAVD, thoracic aortic aneurysm and dissection, or associated CVM. It has been shown for example that RN BAV morphology is associated with a higher risk of developing valve disease and experiencing a cardiac event [5,22]. Together, patterns of predisposing genetic variants, which may be reflected in part by anatomical subtleties such as BAV morphology, may translate to variations in clinical disease states, suggesting major modifiers play a significant role in phenotype definition. Identifying these patterns may impact care, for example by facilitating the ability to consistently predict natural history [66,67].

3. The molecular taxonomy: Genes, pathways, and proteins

Genetic syndromes provide important biologic insights. Turner syndrome is associated with BAV and aorta abnormalities, and is the only monosomy compatible with life despite the fact that the vast majority of cases result in early spontaneous abortion. Turner syndrome can occur for a variety of reasons, including nondisjunction and mosaicism, and the exact genetic abnormality correlates with the severity of the malformations with 45,X more likely mosaicism less likely to have associated CVM. While there have been some studies examining possible maternal effects in nonsyndromic CVM [68], similar studies in Turner syndrome have not identified genomic imprinting in general or specifically with regard to BAV [69]. Interestingly, BAV morphology was RL in over 95% of cases, nearly uniform and significantly more disproportionate than the general ratio [70], suggesting a genotype-phenotype relationship of potential clinical significance. This is consistent with the observation that RL BAV is more commonly associated with aortic coarctation [5]. Little is known about long-term outcomes, e.g. the prevalence of CAVD requiring surgical aortic valve replacement or associated thoracic aneurysm that dissects, and there is not a mouse model to date that recapitulates the cardiac phenotype, but involvement of one of the sex chromosomes provides novel ways to explore specific genetic factors contributing to BAV.

The classic connective tissue disorders, Marfan and Ehlers-Danlos syndromes, caused by mutations in the FIBRILLIN-1 and COLLAGEN Type 3 genes respectively, are well-known to effect the aortic valve. While there is clearly reduced penetrance for BAV in these groups, there is a significantly increased incidence for BAV in both conditions of 10-30% [71,72]. Additional genetic syndromes that affect the connective tissue include Williams syndrome and osteogenesis imperfecta, caused by mutations in the ELASTIN and COLLAGEN Type 1 genes respectively, which also have an increased incidence of valve malformation and disease [73,74]. In addition, there are a number of genetic syndromes that are associated with BAV, often in the context of complex CVM. These include aneuploidies such as deletion 4p, deletion 10p, deletion 11q (Jacobsen syndrome), trisomy 18 (Edwards syndrome), deletion 20p12 (Alagille syndrome), as well as other genetic syndromes, including Adams-Oliver syndrome and Kabuki syndrome [75,76]. Trisomy 18 is a particularly interesting entity that is associated with polyvalvular disease, an unusual type of valve disease that is characterized by malformation, including BAV, and dysplasia of the valves, a poorly understood process that does not have a clear association with CAVD but challenges the malformation-disease distinction [77]. In addition, BAV is often one of multiple CVMs in the same individual and the patterns of co-occurrence can inform cause [78]. Taken together, there is a multitude of ways that valve tissue can be affected, and a molecular understanding of these conditions will inform CAVD.

Developmental signaling pathways identify basic regulatory factors in valvulogenesis. From a cardiac development perspective, there are three transcription factors that are considered the master regulators of basic heart development, NKX2.5, GATA4 and TBX5. Loss of function mutations in each of these genes has been associated with various forms of CVM [79-83]. While none of these genes has been associated with BAV, the Nkx2.5 mutant mouse is characterized by a variety of CVMs including BAV [84], suggesting like NOTCH1, NKX2.5

http://dx.doi.org/10.5772/55506

may account for a very small proportion of cases of BAV and therefore may contribute to the pathogenesis underlying CAVD. As the focus has shifted from early to late (post endothelial-mesenchymal transition) regulatory factors, the role of additional factors, such as Notch and Wnt have been studied in the context of ECM stratification in the mature cups [53,63,85]. The progression of CAVD includes activation of osteogenic gene regulatory pathways and calcification, generally localized to the fibrosa layer [25,86-88]. Atherosclerotic mechanisms have been implicated in valve calcification, and there are overlapping risk factors for CAVD and CAD as described above, suggesting endothelial injury and inflammation play a key role in disease progression [17,87,89]. However, it remains unclear if these are inciting causal factors or exacerbating factors. TGFB signaling dysregulation has been associated with CAVD and cardiovascular disease progression, especially as it pertains to fibrosis and inflammation [90-92]. During human aortic valve calcification, expression of several genes associated with osteogenesis, including *Runx2, osteocalcin, osteopontin, alkaline phophatase,* and *bone sialoprotein,* is induced [93-97]. There is increasing evidence that CAVD recapitulates gene regulatory interactions characteristic of osteogenesis.

The molecular basis of aberrant calcification is poorly understood. While physiologic mineralization in the context of bone development and maintenance has been used successfully as a paradigm to study aberrant calcification in CAVD [86,98], less is known about the genetic basis of disease phenotypes characterized by aberrant calcification. Vascular calcification and the calcification that can occur in advanced CAD has been studied extensively and forms some of the basis for the prevailing view that CAD and CAVD are related disease states. Using a rare genetic disease, alkaptonuria, Hannoush et al identified a metabolic link between vascular calcification and advanced CAVD in a cohort of nearly one hundred patients [99]. Importantly, CAVD in this population was present and advanced, often requiring surgery, independent of standard cardiac risk factors, suggesting a primary link in pathogenesis not related to common comorbidities. In vitro, studies have focused on vascular smooth muscle's role in calcification, especially in the context of clinical comorbidities of CAVD such as CAD and HTN, as well as the context of pathways regulating the associated inflammation and the renin-angiotensin system [92,100]. While vascular smooth muscle cells are not present in valve tissue, there are subsets of VICs that have smooth muscle cell-like properties [101,102] and the expression of smooth muscle actin is considered a marker of activated VICs, the cells implicated in CAVD progression [103].

Understanding valve tissue homeostasis or maintenance will require proteomics. Focusing on valve injury or defects in valve homeostasis or maintenance requires increasing attention to processes downstream from the transcriptional regulation that dominates cardiac development paradigms of CAVD. Proteomics is one emerging field that provides a compelling strategy to address the challenges of dynamic post-translational biology in valve tissue and will undoubtedly have significant impact on our understanding of healthy valve maintenance and CAVD pathogenesis [104]. Proteomics involves a sophisticated technical approach that requires in vitro validation and substantial bioinformatics support. Angel et al. have demonstrated a number of seminal observations by defining the semilunar valve proteome in the adult mouse using MALDI mass spectrometry [105,106]. Specifically, this rigorous and unbiased approach has yielded the identification and characterization of global protein expression and protein-protein networking provides a specific cell-matrix definition of valve maintenance that can be used further to explore the impact of aging, physiologic hemodynamic stresses due to constant motion, and systemic pathologic insults on specific signaling and metabolic dynamics. Importantly, this study provides proof of concept in mouse that will allow the approach to leverage the power of targeted mutagenesis [107]. Despite the difficulty of obtaining healthy controls, early observations have been made in human valve disease specimens, that when compared with control tissue, demonstrate misexpression of critical matrix proteins, including specific lipoproteins, inflammatory proteins, and proteases [108]. One study has focused this approach on VICs exposed to pro-calcific stimuli and has shown that specific chaperone proteins alter transport and cytoskeletal organization, providing insight into both valve homeostasis and CAVD [109]. Taken together, proteomics promises to generate novel insight into disease progression as well as potentially develop a new clinical tool that uses novel global proteomic analyses in plasma as a noninvasive comprehensive biomarker panel.

Dysregulation of structural proteins and remodeling enzymes is a common pathway. Normal valve function requires coordinated movement of complex structures. Gross and Kugel proposed nomenclature for valve tissue organization in 1931 that is now well established [110]. The mature valve structure is made up of highly organized ECM that is compartmentalized into three layers, the fibrosa, spongiosa, and ventricularis [9,53,111]. The annulus, composed primarily of fibrous collagens, provides a buttress for dispersion of forces, and tethering of the cusp in a crown-shape for tissue stabilization [112,113]. Studies examining ECM in valve tissue have focused by convention on structural properties, specifically durability (collagens) and flexibility (proteoglycans and elastic fibers). However, several studies have shown that ECM components reciprocally regulate growth factors and signaling pathways, in addition to causing architectural abnormalities, suggesting a primary rather than secondary role in pathogenesis [Reviewed in 53]. Studies in mouse models lacking ECM components critical for the mature aortic valve structure, including proteoglycans, collagens and elastic fiber components, demonstrate that the expression and organization of diverse ECM components are essential to the formation and structural integrity of the valves during development and after birth [114-123]. Further, mouse studies have shown that age and dietary manipulation can lead to ECM changes and CAVD [124-126].

During valve remodeling, the VICs regulate expression and organization of the valve ECM [127,128]. Additional ECM remodeling enzymes such as matrix metalloproteases (MMPs) and cathepsins also are expressed during valve maturation [128,129]. VICs from developing valves are highly synthetic, and extensive remodeling is required to achieve the mature organization [127,130]. In normal adult valves, the VICs are largely quiescent with little or no cell proliferation and maintain baseline levels of ECM gene expression necessary for valve homeostasis [103]. ECM enzyme dysregulation is established in the valve disease literature [131-135]. The elastin insufficient mouse demonstrates cartilage-like nodules in the valve annulus reminiscent of calcific nodules [119,136]. MMP misexpression malformation and more disease, suggesting malformation processes are due in part to remodeling defects and malformation and disease processes are shared [136]. Similar nodules are seen in the aortic valve annulus of the Adamts9 null mouse [137], confirming the importance of ECM remodeling enzymes. Elastolysis and associated elastic fiber fragments have been implicated as a trigger for myofibroblast mediated calcification [138,139]. Loss of balance between elastases and elastase inhibitors has been identified as one fundamental cause of elastolysis [140]. Interestingly, previous studies have shown that different elastic fiber fragments have different biologic functions, for example, some fragments induce calcification while others are chemo-attractants for endothelial cells [141,142].

The extracellular matrix is an interface between genetics and the environment. The heart valves function essentially to maintain unobstructed unidirectional blood flow. Valve structure-function relationships provide important insight in understanding mechanisms of valve homeostasis as well as developmental and disease processes. Valve ECM composition and biomechanics reflect underlying hemodynamics. There are three basic loading states that affect valve tissue during the cardiac cycle: flexure, shear and tension. Flexure occurs when the valve is actively opening or closing, shear occurs when blood is passing through the open valve, and tension occurs when the valve is closed [143]. Shear, compressive, and longitudinal stresses contribute to valve deformation, or displacement of the valve tissue during the constant motion of the cardiac cycle [144]. Valve tissue has exceptionally high strain because the tissue cycles to a completely unloaded state with each heart beat [145]. The heart beats more than 100,000 times per day handling approximately 5 liters of blood per minute. Over the average lifetime, there are greater than 3 billion heartbeats, or cardiac cycles. The long held appreciation of age-related degeneration and latent valve disease may in fact represent subtle defects in valve tissue maintenance.

CAVD is characterized by VIC activation, which in turn results in increased ECM and increased remodeling enzyme gene expression [103,127,128], and hemodynamic factors may activate VICs and therefore contribute to pathology. VIC activation is apparent by induction of myofibroblast markers, such as vimentin, smooth muscle actin, and embryonic non-muscle myosin heavy chain [129]. Some VICs have been shown to be dynamic and play an active role in ECM maintenance, as well as potentially regeneration and repair, and these VICs are progenitor cells with smooth muscle like properties [101,102,103,123,146,147]. Recently, two studies have demonstrated the complex interaction between developmental programs that predispose tissue to disease and shear stresses that trigger inflammation [148,149], providing examples of how these factors when combined may cause AVD. Research efforts are beginning to reconcile developmental and biomechanical considerations in an effort to more closely examine CAVD in vivo. A better understanding of hemodynamic-induced cell-matrix perturbations may inform the search for durable valve bioprostheses [150].

4. National Heart Lung and Blood Institute's research agenda for CAVD

New research agenda emphasizes genetics and development. Recently, the National Heart Lung and Blood Institute Aortic Stenosis Working Group defined a comprehensive research agenda for CAVD [25]. There are nine research priorities outlined in the statement that are summarized in Table 1. These priorities emphasize the identification of genetic factors that inform etiology, risk, and pharmacologic response, pointing to the clinical impact of these efforts being new diagnostic tests, biomarkers that may improve surveillance, and panels that may inform response to specific drugs. In addition, there is an emphasis on identifying genotype-phenotype relationships focusing on BAV. Improved understanding of valve biology, especially as it pertains to genetic predispositions for CAVD, is critical and will facilitate the identification of specific mechanisms involved in disease initiation and progression. The identification of molecular developmental processes and animal models of CAVD in vivo are needed to establish early pathogenesis and the effectiveness of new pharmacologic treatments for disease. In addition, genetic information will be increasingly important in the assessment of clinical studies that aim to refine clinical risk factors and identify new diagnostic and risk stratification tests.

1. Identify genetic, anatomic, and clinical risk factors for the distinct phases of initiation and progression of CAVD to identify individuals at higher risk, to determine interactions between risk factors, and to determine whether the severity of AS is a risk factor for surgical AV replacement.
2. Develop high-resolution and high-sensitivity imaging modalities that can identify early and subclinical CAVD, including molecular imaging and other innovative imaging approaches.
3. Understand the pathogenesis and pathophysiology of BAV, especially to establish correlations between phenotype and genotype, and to clarify the key features of this disease process that potentiate calcification.
4. Understand the basic valve biology (e.g., early events, mechanisms, and regulatory effects) of CAVD, including signaling pathways and the roles of valve interstitial and endothelial cells and the autocrine and paracrine signaling between them, the extracellular matrix and matrix stiffness, the role of age-related changes in both valve cells and extracellular matrix, the interacting mechanisms of cardiovascular calcification and physiological bone mineralization, and micro-scale mechanotransduction and macro-scale hemodynamics.
5. Develop and validate suitable multi-scale in vitro, ex vivo, and animal models. Improved models are needed that realistically duplicate the conditions in which human CAVD develops.
6. Identify the relationship between calcification of the AV and bone and the reciprocal regulation of these processes.
7. Encourage, promote, or establish tissue banks that make valve tissue from surgery, pathology, and autopsy unsuitable or unneeded for transplantation, with and without CAVD, available for research.
8. Conduct clinical studies specific to CAVD to determine the feasibility of earlier pharmacological intervention in aortic AV sclerosis versus stenosis.
9. Determine the risk factors and optimal timing of surgical valve replacement in view of the current state of the data defining the biological mechanisms of CAVD.

Table 1. Current NHLBI Research Agenda for CAVD. Reproduced from [25].

There is an increasing need for networks and biorepositories. The current paradigm in translational human genetics research involves discovery (the identification of sequence variation associated with disease), mechanistic investigation (definition of pathogenesis), and finally development of new clinical approaches (application). Findings from human genetic studies are being taken into the laboratory where increasingly sophisticated animal models are providing the basis to define pathogenesis in a variety of diseases. The elucidation of pathogenesis subsequently results in the development of new diagnostic and therapeutic strategies, which can then be taken back to the patient. Taken together, this is referred to as the "bedside to bench to bedside" approach to disease and has led to numerous initiatives aiming to realize "translational" research goals, e.g., the NHLBI's Bench to Bassinet Program supporting excellence in pediatric cardiovascular translational research (http://www.bench-tobassinet.com), including CVMs such as BAV. Given the incidence of BAV and the sample size required to use new genetic discovery tools, it is necessary to combine cohorts. Genetic information is also impacting the understanding of pharmacology as it relates to drug indications and drug responses further facilitating improved care. Taken together, genetic information provides an impetus to shift the focus of medicine from treatment of end stage disease to strategies emphasizing primary prevention and early intervention.

Given some of the specific research priorities, for example the need to immortalize valve interstitial cell (VIC) lines, it will be important both to design biorepositories that are specifically built for cardiovascular disease needs and to organize virtual biobanks that can leverage combined resources from multiple centers. In effect, this will maximize translational impact and return on investment. The organization of biorepositories has advanced considerably in recent years, and significant strides have been made by international groups to coordinate resources. For example, the mission of the International Society for Biological and Environmental Repositories (ISBER) is to address technical, legal, ethical and managerial issues relevant to the governance of wide ranging biorepositories (http://www.isber.org) [151]. Several institutions have initiated biorepositories that include blood and tissue from CAVD patients. Virtual repositories, or multiple repositories that coordinate efforts to leverage sample size considerations, are becoming operational and the current funding climate is accelerating development of special rules to optimize tissue utility [152]. Funding bodies at the government and foundation levels need to recognize valve disease as a significant public health problem and establish valve specific funding opportunities. Further, valve biology and CAVD specific symposia are needed at large conferences, such as the American Heart Association.

5. Comprehensive counseling and genetic testing increasingly impact clinical care

A detailed family history remains a powerful tool and genetic testing will advance its impact. A detailed family history refers to questioning multiple individuals within a family and requires specific demographic information (e.g., age at disease onset) and documentation of disease and other pertinent health issues by medical record review [153]. The results of a detailed family history may warrant referral to a cardiovascular genetics service. A detailed family history is a powerful tool and can help establish a diagnosis and initiate comprehensive care in a timely fashion [154-158]. There are significant barriers to the optimal use of family history information, primarily a lack of awareness on the family's part and considerable time restrictions on the health care professional's part. Studies have shown that a majority of people do not know their family history and do not appreciate its relevance in medical management, and consequently the potential impact of family history information is diminished [159]. In an effort to increase family history awareness, tools have been developed and are available to the general public to generate and maintain a detailed family history. For example, the Health and Human Services Family History Initiative has designed a publicly available, web-based program providing a means to generate and maintain a detailed family history [160]. Genetics has transformed the use of family history information and has led to the reemergence of the detailed genetic family history. Detailed family history information is necessary for the optimal use of genetic screening and testing and this translates to the essential need of genetic counselors embedded in cardiology clinics.

Genetic testing is anticipated for BAV and CAVD. As the etiology of BAV is defined and the complex genetics of CAVD is elucidated, a variety of variants associated with BAV and CAVD will be identified, including variants associated with etiology as well as variants associated with specific types of subsequent risk. All variants pertaining to CAVD will have to be organized based on utility. Once a significant proportion of cases can be diagnosed using genetic testing, clinical testing may be warranted. Presently, there are no CLIA (Clinical Laboratory Improvement Amendments) approved tests for the diagnosis or stratification of BAV or CAVD. NOTCH1 screening is of too little yield to justify testing (<2%), but may be included in larger panels of tests at a future time. Presently, there is no diagnostic utility for genetic testing for BAV or CAVD, but given the rate of discovery and the various technological advances being made, it would appear that this will occur in the near term. It is imperative that cardiologists understand the indications and limitations of clinical genetic testing [161,162]. However, genetic testing is being used for various clinical management reasons, and several of these uses have cardiovascular applications. For example, sequence variants in CYP2C9 and VKORC1 are associated with an increased bleeding risk and drug resistance, respectively, in patients taking warfarin [163,164]. Because CAVD patients often require valve replacement, and mechanical prostheses require anticoagulation, this particular example may be directly useful for CAVD patients. Ultimately, diagnostic panels of genetic variants that identify cause, and may provide insight regarding natural history, and additional management panels that identify disease-specific risks may inform clinical decision-making. Taken together, panels of genetic variants may be used in a manner similar to newborn screening, becoming an important part of the working information for every patient.

The opportunities and challenges of genotype definition in the clinic. Genotype definition will empower individuals and families to further control their health, extending the paradigm shift that occurred when the medical field embraced preventive medicine [165]. Increasing genetic information in the clinic creates new opportunities to improve cardiovascular health. However, this development also creates new challenges, including ethical and legal issues that challenge the existing regulatory landscape and directly impact application in the clinic [166]. For example, the meaning of a negative test often will not be clear, in addition to the ambiguity variants of unknown significance present. Despite the passage of the Genetic Information Nondiscrimination Act (GINA), a law that protects the public from insurance companies using genetic information for underwriting purposes, there are increasing concerns about privacy issues. Public education, including physician awareness, will be critical to facilitate the anticipated clinical uses of genetic information. Genetic testing will play an increasing role in the clinical management of BAV and CAVD patients. Ultimately, genotype definition may be able to identify those patients with BAV that are at risk (or not at risk) of developing CAVD or other associated problems, impacting clinical management decisions. As more is learned about the genetic basis of BAV and CAVD, the yield of clinical genetic testing will be sufficient to warrant routine diagnostic testing. As the genotypes associated with BAV and CAVD are defined, there will be a need to expand Consensus Guidelines for BAV to include full consideration of genetic information, especially overlapping silent and/or latent disease processes. Clinical applications of genetic variant panels will potentially include refined diagnosis, risk stratification (early intervention, timing of surgery), pharmacogenomics (which drug, what dose, risk of adverse effects), and screening strategies for relatives.

The clinical implications of genotype definition: examples. Because CAVD remains essentially a surgical problem, early clinical impact may be realized first in surgical considerations. For example, the pulmonary artery dimension is increased in BAV patients [167,168], consistent with previously reported histopathologic abnormalities in the pulmonary artery of BAV patients [169]. This may be clinically relevant in BAV patients who require aortic valve replacement and may be candidates for the Ross procedure (autologous pulmonary valve placed in the aortic position). Some patients with apparently isolated CAVD undergoing surgical repair may be at risk for subsequently developing TAA, a not uncommon scenario that may be predicted by genotyping. McKellar et al recently described aorta complications in 1,286 aortic valve replacement patients with a median 12 year follow up, and reported that 10% demonstrate progressive aortic enlargement and only a minority of these lead to dissection or require further surgery [170]. However, in those patients, prophylactic replacement of the aorta would be warranted and would fundamentally change the overall approach to this group of patients. In addition, stratifying by genotype CAVD patients into those with and those without aorta abnormalities potentially informs type of surgical approach as well [171,172]. The ability to identify those patients at risk before the first surgery may substantially impact clinical decision-making, including for example a selective approach to combined valve and aorta replacement.

Genotype phenotype information will have important implications for clinical surveillance. For example, current recommendations for functional BAV patients include screening echocardiograms every 5 years for all first-degree relatives [13]. Recently it was shown that surveillance may be modified by morphology such that pediatric patients with RN morphology are screened every 2 years because they are at higher risk of developing new AVD, while individuals with RL BAV could be monitored less aggressively in early childhood as the risk of having AVD at this time is relatively low [26]. Family members of BAV patients may be at risk for TAA or other cardiovascular disease (even if they don't have BAV), underscoring the importance of thoughtful monitoring. Since CAVD is a latent phenotype, continued surveillance is required. Since some individuals with BAV have progressive CAVD and others never develop disease, there is reason to think that genetic insights will clarify this phenomenon. Overall, refined screening strategies promise to provide opportunities for improved care.

Ultimately, genetic information will inform the identification of new pharmacologic based therapies for CAVD [173]. Genetics research in CAVD will lead to further basic research in animal models that can define the early pathogenesis and natural history of disease and therefore identify new therapeutic targets. This paradigm will have increasing significance as bioinformatics approaches overcome the challenges of extraordinary amounts of data. There has been considerable interest in applying CAD treatment paradigms to valve disease. However, while statin therapy showed early in vitro evidence of a potentially beneficial effect, a large clinical trial demonstrated that statin therapy does not positively impact either aortic valve disease progression or the need for surgery [174]. Recently, a strategy to use pediatric valve disease patients as a means to identify early genetic aspects of CAVD has been advanced because this population provides insight into the disease process that is not confounded by the common comorbidities of adulthood, such as CAD and HTN [127,175]. Increasingly, developmental paradigms will inform the search for etiology, new treatments and better bioprostheses. New therapies are likely to emerge from molecular biology fields, and innovative approaches to studying the genetic basis of CAVD will be needed to realize this goal.

Author details

Robert B. Hinton

Address all correspondence to: robert.hinton@cchmc.org

The Heart Institute, Division of Cardiology, Cincinnati Children's Hospital Medical Center, USA

References

[1] Clayton M. Leonardo's anatomy years. Nature 2012;484:314-316.

[2] Hoffman JI, Kaplan S. The incidence of congenital heart disease. J Am Coll Cardiol 2002;39:1890-1900.

[3] Roger VL, Go AS, Lloyd-Jones DM, Adams RJ, Berry JD, Brown TM, Carnethon MR, Dai S, De Simone G, Ford ES, Fox CS, Fullerton HJ, Gillespie C, Greenlund KJ, Hailpern SM, Heit JA, Ho M, Howard VJ, Kissela BM, Kittner SJ, Lackland DT, Lichtman JH, Lisabeth LD, Makuc DM, Marcus GM, Marelli A. Heart disease and stroke statis-

tics--2011 update: A report from the American Heart Association. Circulation 2011;123:e18-e209.

[4] Roberts WC. The congenitally bicuspid aortic valve. A study of 85 autopsy cases. Am J Cardiol 1970;26:72-83.

[5] Fernandes SM, Sanders SP, Khairy P, Jenkins KJ, Gauvreau K, Lang P, Simonds H, Colan SD. Morphology of bicuspid aortic valve in children and adolescents. J Am Coll Cardiol 2004;44:1648-1651.

[6] Hinton RB. Bicuspid aortic valve and thoracic aortic aneurysm: three patient populations, two disease phenotypes, and one shared genotype. Cardiol Res Pract 2012;2012:926975.

[7] Ward C. Clinical significance of the bicuspid aortic valve. Heart 2000;83:81-85.

[8] Otto CM. Valvular aortic stenosis: disease severity and timing of intervention. J Am Coll Cardiol 2006;47:2141-2151.

[9] Schoen FJ. Evolving concepts of cardiac valve dynamics: the continuum of development, functional structure, pathobiology, and tissue engineering. Circulation 2008;118:1864-1880.

[10] Otto CM, Kuusisto J, Reichenbach DD, Gown AM, O'Brien KD. Characterization of the early lesion of 'degenerative' valvular aortic stenosis. Histological and immunohistochemical studies. Circulation 1994;90:844-853.

[11] Thubrikar MJ, Aouad J, Nolan SP. Patterns of calcific deposits in operatively excised stenotic or purely regurgitant aortic valves and their relation to mechanical stress. Am J Cardiol 1986;58:304-308.

[12] Nkomo VT, Gardin JM, Skelton TN, Gottdiener JS, Scott CG, Enriquez-Sarano M. Burden of valvular heart diseases: a population-based study. Lancet 2006;368:1005-1011.

[13] Bonow RO, Carabello BA, Chatterjee K, de Leon AC Jr, Faxon DP, Freed MD, Gaasch WH, Lytle BW, Nishimura RA, O'Gara PT, O'Rourke RA, Otto CM, Shah PM, Shanewise JS. Focused update incorporated into the ACC/AHA 2006 guidelines for the management of patients with valvular heart disease: a report of the American College of Cardiology/American Heart Association Task Force on Practice Guidelines. Circulation 2008;118:e523-661.

[14] Rajamannan NM, Gersh B, Bonow RO. Calcific aortic stenosis: from bench to the bedside--emerging clinical and cellular concepts. Heart 2003;89:801-805.

[15] Roberts WC, Ko JM. Frequency by decades of unicuspid, bicuspid, and tricuspid aortic valves in adults having isolated aortic valve replacement for aortic stenosis, with or without associated aortic regurgitation. Circulation 2005;111:920-925.

[16] Stewart BF, Siscovick D, Lind BK, Gardin JM, Gottdiener JS, Smith VE, Kitzman DW, Otto CM. Clinical factors associated with calcific aortic valve disease. Cardiovascular Health Study. J Am Coll Cardiol 1997;29:630-634.

[17] Owens DS, Katz R, Takasu J, Kronmal R, Budoff MJ, O'Brien KD. Incidence and progression of aortic valve calcium in the Multi-ethnic Study of Atherosclerosis (MESA). Am J Cardiol 2010;105:701-708.

[18] Otto CM, Lind BK, Kitzman DW, Gersh BJ, Siscovick DS. Association of aortic-valve sclerosis with cardiovascular mortality and morbidity in the elderly. N Engl J Med 1999;341:142-147.

[19] Keane JF, Driscoll DJ, Gersony WM, Hayes CJ, Kidd L, O'Fallon WM, Pieroni DR, Wolfe RR, Weidman WH. Second natural history study of congenital heart defects: Results of treatment of patients with aortic valvar stenosis. Circulation 1993;87:I16-27.

[20] Schoen FJ. Mechanisms of function and disease of natural and replacement heart valves. Annu Rev Pathol 2012;7:161-183.

[21] Gallegos RP. Selection of Prosthetic Heart Valves. Curr Treat Options Cardiovasc Med 2006;8:443-452.

[22] Tzemos N, Therrien J, Yip J, Thanassoulis G, Tremblay S, Jamorski MT, Webb GD, Siu SC. Outcomes in adults with bicuspid aortic valves. JAMA 2008;300:1317-1325.

[23] Mahle WT, Sutherland JL, Frias PA. Outcome of Isolated Bicuspid Aortic Valve in Childhood. J Pediatr 2010;157:445-449.

[24] Collins MJ, Butany J, Borger MA, Strauss BH, David TE. Implications of a congenitally abnormal valve: a study of 1025 consecutively excised aortic valves. J. Clin. Pathol 2008;61:530-536.

[25] Rajamannan NM, Evans FJ, Aikawa E, Grande-Allen KJ, Demer LL, Heistad DD, Simmons CA, Masters KS, Mathieu P, O'Brien KD, Schoen FJ, Towler DA, Yoganathan AP, Otto CM. Calcific aortic valve disease: not simply a degenerative process: A review and agenda for research from the National Heart and Lung and Blood Institute Aortic Stenosis Working Group. Executive summary: Calcific aortic valve disease. Circulation 2011;124:1783-1791.

[26] Calloway TJ, Martin LJ, Zhang X, Tandon A, Benson DW, Hinton RB. Risk factors for aortic valve disease in bicuspid aortic valve: a family-based study. Am J Med Genet A 2011;155:1015-1020.

[27] Lanktree MB, Hassell RG, Lahiry P, Hegele RA. Phenomics: expanding the role of clinical evaluation in genomic studies. J Investig Med 2010;58:700-706.

[28] Rajamannan NM. Calcific aortic stenosis: lessons learned from experimental and clinical studies. Arterioscler Thromb Vasc Biol 2009;29:162-168.

[29] Mohler ER, Sheridan MJ, Nichols R, Harvey WP, Waller BF. Development and progression of aortic valve stenosis: atherosclerosis risk factors--a causal relationship? A clinical morphologic study. Clin Cardiol 1991;14:995-999.

[30] Rapp AH, Hillis LD, Lange RA, Cigarroa JE. Prevalence of coronary artery disease in patients with aortic stenosis with and without angina pectoris. Am J Cardiol 2001;87:1216-1217.

[31] Aronow WS, Schwartz KS, Koenigsberg M. Correlation of serum lipids, calcium, and phosophorus, diabetes mellitus and history of systemic hypertension with presence or absence of calcified or thickened aortic cusps or root in elderly patients. Am J Cardiol 1987;59:998-999.

[32] Piers LH, Touw HRW, Gansevoort R, Franssen CFM, Oudkerk M, Zijlstra F, Tio RA. Relation of aortic valve and coronary artery calcium in patients with chronic kidney disease to the stage and etiology of the renal disease. Am J Cardiol 2009;103:1473-1477.

[33] Botto LD, Lin AE, Riehle-Colarusso T, Malik S, Correa A. Seeking causes: Classifying and evaluating congenital heart defects in etiologic studies. Birth Defects Res A Clin Mol Teratol 2007;79:714-727.

[34] Luo AK, Jefferson BK, Garcia MJ, Ginsburg GS, Topol EJ. Challenges in the phenotypic characterisation of patients in genetic studies of coronary artery disease. J Med Genet 2007;44:161-165.

[35] Markwald RR, Norris RA, Moreno-Rodriguez R, Levine RA. Developmental basis of adult cardiovascular diseases: valvular heart diseases. Ann N Y Acad Sci 2010;1188:177-183.

[36] Bruneau BG. The developmental genetics of congenital heart disease. Nature 2008;451:943-948.

[37] Schoen FJ. Evolving concepts of cardiac valve dynamics: the continuum of development, functional structure, pathobiology, and tissue engineering. Circulation 2008;118:1864-1880.

[38] Cripe L, Andelfinger G, Martin LJ, Shooner K, Benson DW. Bicuspid aortic valve is heritable. J Am Coll Cardiol 2004;44:138-143.

[39] Loscalzo ML, Goh DL, Loeys B, Kent KC, Spevak PJ, Dietz HC. Familial thoracic aortic dilation and bicommissural aortic valve: a prospective analysis of natural history and inheritance. Am J Med Genet A 2007;143A:1960-1967.

[40] Huntington K, Hunter AG, Chan KL. A prospective study to assess the frequency of familial clustering of congenital bicuspid aortic valve. J Am Coll Cardiol 1997;30:1809-1812.

[41] McBride KL, Marengo L, Canfield M, Langlois P, Fixler D, Belmont JW. Epidemiology of noncomplex left ventricular outflow tract obstruction malformations (aortic

valve stenosis, coarctation of the aorta, hypoplastic left heart syndrome) in Texas, 1999-2001. Birth Defects Res A Clin Mol Teratol 2005;73:555-561.

[42] Fernandez B, Duran AC, Fernandez-Gallego T, Fernández MC, Such M, Arqué JM, Sans-Coma V. Bicuspid aortic valves with different spatial orientations of the leaflets are distinct etiological entities. J Am Coll Cardiol 2009;54:2312-2318.

[43] Sans-Coma V, Carmen Fernández M, Fernández B, Durán AC, Anderson RH, Arqué JM. Genetically alike Syrian hamsters display both bifoliate and trifoliate aortic valves. J Anat 2012;220:92-101.

[44] Hinton RB, Martin LJ, Rame-Gowda S, Tabangin ME, Cripe LH, Benson DW. Hypoplastic left heart syndrome links to chromosomes 10q and 6q and is genetically related to bicuspid aortic valve. J Am Coll Cardiol 2009;53:1065-1071.

[45] Martin LJ, Ramachandran V, Cripe LH, Hinton RB, Andelfinger G, Tabangin M, Shooner K, Keddache M, Benson DW. Evidence in favor of linkage to human chromosomal regions 18q, 5q and 13q for bicuspid aortic valve and associated cardiovascular malformations. Hum Genet 2007;121:275-284.

[46] McBride KL, Zender GA, Fitzgerald-Butt SM, Koehler D, Menesses-Diaz A, Fernbach S, Lee K, Towbin JA, Leal S, Belmont JW. Linkage analysis of left ventricular outflow tract malformations (aortic valve stenosis, coarctation of the aorta, and hypoplastic left heart syndrome). Eur J Hum Genet 2009;17:811-819.

[47] Garg V, Muth AN, Ransom JF, Schluterman MK, Barnes R, King IN, Grossfeld PD, Srivastava D. Mutations in NOTCH1 cause aortic valve disease. Nature 2005;437:270-274.

[48] Mohamed SA, Aherrahrou Z, Liptau H, Erasmi AW, Hagemann C, Wrobel S, Borzym K, Schunkert H, Sievers HH, Erdmann J. Novel missense mutations (p.T596M and p.P1797H) in NOTCH1 in patients with bicuspid aortic valve. Biochem Biophys Res Commun 2006;345:1460-1465.

[49] Nus M, MacGrogan D, Martínez-Poveda B, Benito Y, Casanova JC, Fernández-Avilés F, Bermejo J, de la Pompa JL. Diet-induced aortic valve disease in mice haploinsufficient for the Notch pathway effector RBPJK/CSL. Arterioscler Thromb Vasc Biol 2011;31:1580-1588.

[50] Acharya A, Hans CP, Koenig SN, Nichols HA, Galindo CL, Garner HR, Merrill WH, Hinton RB, Garg V. Inhibitory role of Notch1 in calcific aortic valve disease. PLoS One 2011;6:e27743.

[51] Nigam V, Srivastava D. Notch1 represses osteogenic pathways in aortic valve cells. J Mol Cell Cardiol 2009;47:828-834.

[52] Hitz MP, Lemieux-Perreault LP, Marshall C, Feroz-Zada Y, Davies R, Yang SW, Lionel AC, D'Amours G, Lemyre E, Cullum R, Bigras JL, Thibeault M, Chetaille P, Montpetit A, Khairy P, Overduin B, Klaassen S, Hoodless P, Nemer M, Stewart AF,

Boerkoel C, Scherer SW, Richter A, Dubé MP, Andelfinger G. Rare copy number variants contribute to congenital left-sided heart disease. PLoS Genet 2012;8(9):e1002903.

[53] Hinton RB, Yutzey KE. Heart Valve Structure and Function in Development and Disease. Annual Review of Physiology 2011;73:29-46.

[54] Hinton RB, Jr., Martin LJ, Tabangin ME, Mazwi ML, Cripe LH, Benson DW. Hypoplastic left heart syndrome is heritable. J Am Coll Cardiol 2007;50:1590-1595.

[55] Novaro GM, Mishra M, Griffin BP. Incidence and echocardiographic features of congenital unicuspid aortic valve in an adult population. J Heart Valve Dis 2003;12:674-678.

[56] Kathiresan S, Srivastava D. Genetics of human cardiovascular disease. Cell 2012;148:1242-1257.

[57] Guo DC, Papke CL, Tran-Fadulu V, Regalado ES, Avidan N, Johnson RJ, Kim DH, Pannu H, Willing MC, Sparks E, Pyeritz RE, Singh MN, Dalman RL, Grotta JC, Marian AJ, Boerwinkle EA, Frazier LQ, LeMaire SA, Coselli JS, Estrera AL, Safi HJ, Veeraraghavan S, Muzny DM, Wheeler DA, Willerson JT, Yu RK, Shete SS, Scherer SE, Raman CS, Buja LM, Milewicz DM. Mutations in smooth muscle alpha-actin (ACTA2) cause coronary artery disease, stroke, and Moyamoya disease, along with thoracic aortic disease. Am J Hum Genet 2009;84:617-627.

[58] Takeuchi F, Isono M, Katsuya T, Yamamoto K, Yokota M, Sugiyama T, Nabika T, Fujioka A, Ohnaka K, Asano H, Yamori Y, Yamaguchi S, Kobayashi S, Takayanagi R, Ogihara T, Kato N. Blood pressure and hypertension are associated with 7 loci in the Japanese population. Circulation 2010;121:2302-2309.

[59] Schunkert H, König IR, Kathiresan S, Reilly MP, Assimes TL, Holm H, Preuss M, Stewart AF, Barbalic M, Gieger C, Absher D, Aherrahrou Z, Allayee H, Altshuler D, Anand SS, Andersen K, Anderson JL, Ardissino D, Ball SG, Balmforth AJ, Barnes TA, Becker DM, Becker LC, Berger K, Bis JC, Boekholdt SM, Boerwinkle E, Braund PS, Brown MJ, Burnett MS, Buysschaert I; Cardiogenics, Carlquist JF, Chen L, Cichon S, Codd V, Davies RW, Dedoussis G, Dehghan A, Demissie S, Devaney JM, Diemert P, Do R, Doering A, Eifert S, Mokhtari NE, Ellis SG, Elosua R, Engert JC, Epstein SE, de Faire U, Fischer M, Folsom AR, Freyer J, Gigante B, Girelli D, Gretarsdottir S, Gudnason V, Gulcher JR, Halperin E, Hammond N, Hazen SL, Hofman A, Horne BD, Illig T, Iribarren C, Jones GT, Jukema JW, Kaiser MA, Kaplan LM, Kastelein JJ, Khaw KT, Knowles JW, Kolovou G, Kong A, Laaksonen R, Lambrechts D, Leander K, Lettre G, Li M, Lieb W, Loley C, Lotery AJ, Mannucci PM, Maouche S, Martinelli N, McKeown PP, Meisinger C, Meitinger T, Melander O, Merlini PA, Mooser V, Morgan T, Mühleisen TW, Muhlestein JB, Münzel T, Musunuru K, Nahrstaedt J, Nelson CP, Nöthen MM, Olivieri O, Patel RS, Patterson CC, Peters A, Peyvandi F, Qu L, Quyyumi AA, Rader DJ, Rallidis LS, Rice C, Rosendaal FR, Rubin D, Salomaa V, Sampietro ML, Sandhu MS, Schadt E, Schäfer A, Schillert A, Schreiber S, Schrezenmeir J, Schwartz SM, Siscovick DS, Sivananthan M, Sivapalaratnam S, Smith A, Smith TB, Snoep JD,

Soranzo N, Spertus JA, Stark K, Stirrups K, Stoll M, Tang WH, Tennstedt S, Thorgeirsson G, Thorleifsson G, Tomaszewski M, Uitterlinden AG, van Rij AM, Voight BF, Wareham NJ, Wells GA, Wichmann HE, Wild PS, Willenborg C, Witteman JC, Wright BJ, Ye S, Zeller T, Ziegler A, Cambien F, Goodall AH, Cupples LA, Quertermous T, März W, Hengstenberg C, Blankenberg S, Ouwehand WH, Hall AS, Deloukas P, Thompson JR, Stefansson K, Roberts R, Thorsteinsdottir U, O'Donnell CJ, McPherson R, Erdmann J; CARDIoGRAM Consortium, Samani NJ. Large-scale association analysis identifies 13 new susceptibility loci for coronary artery disease. Nat Genet 2011;43:333-338.

[60] Yasuno K, Bilguvar K, Bijlenga P, Low SK, Krischek B, Auburger G, Simon M, Krex D, Arlier Z, Nayak N, Ruigrok YM, Niemelä M, Tajima A, von und zu Fraunberg M, Dóczi T, Wirjatijasa F, Hata A, Blasco J, Oszvald A, Kasuya H, Zilani G, Schoch B, Singh P, Stüer C, Risselada R, Beck J, Sola T, Ricciardi F, Aromaa A, Illig T, Schreiber S, van Duijn CM, van den Berg LH, Perret C, Proust C, Roder C, Ozturk AK, Gaál E, Berg D, Geisen C, Friedrich CM, Summers P, Frangi AF, State MW, Wichmann HE, Breteler MM, Wijmenga C, Mane S, Peltonen L, Elio V, Sturkenboom MC, Lawford P, Byrne J, Macho J, Sandalcioglu EI, Meyer B, Raabe A, Steinmetz H, Rüfenacht D, Jääskeläinen JE, Hernesniemi J, Rinkel GJ, Zembutsu H, Inoue I, Palotie A, Cambien F, Nakamura Y, Lifton RP, Günel M. Genome-wide association study of intracranial aneurysm identifies three new risk loci. Nat Genet 2010;42:420-425.

[61] Armstrong EJ, Bischoff J. Heart valve development: endothelial cell signaling and differentiation. Circ Res 2004;95:459-470.

[62] Olson EN. Gene regulatory networks in the evolution and development of the heart. Science 2006;313:1922-1927.

[63] Combs MD, Yutzey KE. Heart valve development: regulatory networks in development and disease. Circ Res 2009;105:408-421.

[64] Antonicelli F, Bellon G, Debelle L, Hornbeck W. Elastin-elastases and Inflamm-Aging. Current Topics in Dev Biol 2007;79:99-138.

[65] Stephens EH, de Jonge N, McNeill MP, Durst CA, Grande-Allen KJ. Age-related changes in material behavior of porcine mitral and aortic valves and correlation to matrix composition. Tissue Eng Part A 2010;16:867-878.

[66] Michelena HI, Desjardins VA, Avierinos JF, Russo A, Nkomo VT, Sundt TM, Pellikka PA, Tajik AJ, Enriquez-Sarano M. Natural history of asymptomatic patients with normally functioning or minimally dysfunctional bicuspid aortic valve in the community. Circulation 2008;117:2776-2784.

[67] Beroukhim RS, Kruzick TL, Taylor AL, Gao D, Yetman AT. Progression of aortic dilation in children with a functionally normal bicuspid aortic valve. Am J Cardiol 2006;98:828-830.

[68] Whittemore R, Hobbins JC, Engle MA. Pregnancy and its outcome in women with and without surgical treatment of congenital heart disease. Am J Cardiol 1982;50:641-651.

[69] Bondy CA, Matura LA, Wooten N, Troendle J, Zinn AR, Bakalov VK. The physical phenotype of girls and women with Turner syndrome is not X-imprinted. Hum Genet 2007;121:469-474.

[70] Sachdev V, Matura LA, Sidenko S, Ho VB, Arai AE, Rosing DR, Bondy CA. Aortic valve disease in Turner syndrome. J Am Coll Cardiol 2008;51:1904-1909.

[71] Roberts WC, Honig HS. The spectrum of cardiovascular disease in the Marfan syndrome: a clinico-morphologic study of 18 necropsy patients and comparison to 151 previously reported necropsy patients. Am Heart J 1982;104:115-135.

[72] Atzinger CL, Meyer RA, Khoury PR, Gao Z, Tinkle BT. Cross-sectional and longitudinal assessment of aortic root dilation and valvular anomalies in hypermobile and classic Ehlers-Danlos syndrome. J Pediatr 2011;158:826-830.

[73] Eronen M, Peippo M, Hiippala A, Raatikka M, Arvio M, Johansson R, Kahkonen M. Cardiovascular manifestations in 75 patients with Williams syndrome. J Med Genet 2002;39:554-558.

[74] Radunovic Z, Wekre LL, Diep LM, Steine K. Cardiovascular abnormalities in adults with osteogenesis imperfecta. Am Heart J 2011;161:523-529.

[75] Pierpont ME, Basson CT, Benson DW, Gelb BD, Giglia TM, Goldmuntz E, McGee G, Sable CA, Srivastava D, Webb CL. Genetic basis for congenital heart defects: current knowledge: a scientific statement from the American Heart Association Congenital Cardiac Defects Committee, Council on Cardiovascular Disease in the Young: endorsed by the American Academy of Pediatrics. Circulation 2007;115:3015-3038.

[76] Goldmuntz E, Lin AE. Genetics of Congenital heart defects. In: Moss and Adams' Heart Disease in Infants, Children and Adolescents, 7th edition (Editors: Allen HD, Driscoll DJ, Feltes TF, Shaddy RE). p 545-572.

[77] Bharati S, Lev M. Congenital polyvalvular disease. Circulation 1973;47:575-586.

[78] Duran AC, Frescura C, Sans-Coma V, Angelini A, Basso C, Thiene G. Bicuspid aortic valves in hearts with other congenital heart disease. J Heart Valve Dis 1995;4:581-590.

[79] Schott JJ, Benson DW, Basson CT, Pease W, Silberbach GM, Moak JP, Maron BJ, Seidman CE, Seidman JG. Congenital heart disease caused by mutations in the transcription factor NKX2-5. Science 1998;281:108-111.

[80] McElhinney DB, Geiger E, Blinder J, Benson DW, Goldmuntz E. NKX2.5 mutations in patients with congenital heart disease. J Am Coll Cardiol 2003;42:1650-1655.

[81] Garg V, Kathiriya IS, Barnes R, Schluterman MK, King IN, Butler CA, Rothrock CR, Eapen RS, Hirayama-Yamada K, Joo K, Matsuoka R, Cohen JC, Srivastava D. GATA4

mutations cause human congenital heart defects and reveal an interaction with TBX5. Nature 2003;424:443-447.

[82] Rajagopal SK, Ma Q, Obler D, Shen J, Manichaikul A, Tomita-Mitchell A, Boardman K, Briggs C, Garg V, Srivastava D, Goldmuntz E, Broman KW, Benson DW, Smoot LB, Pu WT. Spectrum of heart disease associated with murine and human GATA4 mutation. J Mol Cell Cardiol 2007;43:677-685.

[83] Basson CT, Cowley GS, Solomon SD, Weissman B, Poznanski AK, Traill TA, Seidman JG, Seidman CE. The clinical and genetic spectrum of the Holt-Oram syndrome (heart-hand syndrome). N Engl J Med 1994;330:885-891.

[84] Biben C, Weber R, Kesteven S, Stanley E, McDonald L, Elliott DA, Barnett L, Köentgen F, Robb L, Feneley M, Harvey RP. Cardiac septal and valvular dysmorphogenesis in mice heterozygous for mutations in the homeobox gene Nkx2-5. Circ Res 2000;87:888-895.

[85] Jain R, Engleka KA, Rentschler SL, Manderfield LJ, Li L, Yuan L, Epstein JA. Cardiac neural crest orchestrates remodeling and functional maturation of mouse semilunar valves. J Clin Invest 2011;121:422-430.

[86] Miller JD, Weiss RM, Heistad DD. Calcific aortic valve stenosis: Methods, models, and mechanisms. Circ. Res 2011;108:1392-1412.

[87] Bostrom K, Rajamannan NM, Towler DA. The regulation of valvular and vascular sclerosis by osteogenic morphogens. Circ. Res 2011;109:564-577.

[88] Simmons CA, Grant GR, Manduchi E, Davies PF. Spatial heterogeneity of endothelial phenotypes correlates with side-specific vulnerability to calcification in normal porcine aortic valves. Circ Res 2005;96:792-799.

[89] Hans CP, Koenig SN, Huang N, Cheng J, Beceiro S, Guggilam A, Kuivaniemi H, Partida-Sánchez S, Garg V. Inhibition of notch1 signaling reduces abdominal aortic aneurysm in mice by attenuating macrophage-mediated inflammation. Arterioscler Thromb Vasc Biol 2012;32:3012-3023.

[90] Jian B, Narula N, Li QY, Mohler ER 3rd, Levy RJ. Progression of aortic valve stenosis: TGF-beta1 is present in calcified aortic valve cusps and promotes aortic valve interstitial cell calcification via apoptosis. Ann Thorac Surg 2003;75:457-465.

[91] Chen JH, Chen WL, Sider KL, Yip CY, Simmons CA. β-catenin mediates mechanically regulated, transforming growth factor-β1-induced myofibroblast differentiation of aortic valve interstitial cells. Arterioscler Thromb Vasc Biol 2011;31:590-597.

[92] Xu S, Liu AC, Gotlieb AI. Common pathogenic features of atherosclerosis and calcific aortic stenosis: role of transforming growth factor-beta. Cardiovasc Pathol 2010;19:236-247.

[93] Caira FC, Stock SR, Gleason TG, McGee EC, Huang J, Bonow RO, Spelsberg TC, McCarthy PM, Rahimtoola SH, Rajamannan NM. Human degenerative valve disease is

associated with up-regulation of low-density lipoprotein-related protein 5 receptor-mediated bone formation. J Am Coll Cardiol 2006;47:1707-1712.

[94] Rajamannan NM, Subramaniam M, Rickard DJ, Stock SR, Donovan J, Springett M, Orszulak T, Fullerton DA, Tajik AJ, Bonow RO, Spelsberg TC. Human aortic valve calcification is associated with an osteoblast phenotype. Circulation 2003;107:2181-2184.

[95] Rajamannan NM, Nealis TB, Subramaniam M, Pandya S, Stock SR, Ignatiev CI, Sebo TJ, Rosengart TK, Edwards WD, McCarthy PM, Bonow RO, Spelsberg TC. Calcified rheumatic valve neoangiogenesis is associated with vascular endothelial growth factor expression and osteoblast-like bone formation. Circulation 2005;111:3296-3301.

[96] Mohler ER, Gannon F, Reynolds C, Zimmerman R, Keane MG, Kaplan FS. Bone formation and inflammation in cardiac valves. Circulation 2001;103:1522-1528.

[97] Steiner I, Kasparová P, Kohout A, Dominik J. Bone formation in cardiac valves: a histopathological study of 128 cases. Virchows Arch 2007;450:653-657.

[98] Lincoln J, Lange AW, Yutzey KE. Hearts and bones: shared regulatory mechanisms in heart valve, cartilage, tendon, and bone development. Dev Biol 2006;294:292-302.

[99] Hannoush H, Introne WJ, Chen MY, Lee SJ, O'Brien K, Suwannarat P, Kayser MA, Gahl WA, Sachdev V. Aortic stenosis and vascular calcifications in alkaptonuria. Mol Genet Metab 2012;105:198-202.

[100] Aikawa E, Aikawa M, Libby P, Figueiredo JL, Rusanescu G, Iwamoto Y, Fukuda D, Kohler RH, Shi GP, Jaffer FA, Weissleder R. Arterial and aortic valve calcification abolished by elastolytic cathepsin S deficiency in chronic renal disease. Circulation 2009;119:1785-1794.

[101] Filip DA, Radu A, Simionescu M. Interstitial cells of the heart valves possess characteristics similar to smooth muscle cells. Circ Res 1986;59:310-320.

[102] Walker GA, Masters KS, Shah DN, Anseth KS, Leinwand LA. Valvular myofibroblast activation by transforming growth factor-beta: implications for pathological extracellular matrix remodeling in heart valve disease. Circ Res 2004;95:253-260.

[103] Liu AC, Joag VR, Gotlieb AI. The emerging role of valve interstitial cell phenotypes in regulating heart valve pathobiology. Am J Pathol 2007;171:1407-18.

[104] Zerkowski HR, Grussenmeyer T, Matt P, Grapow M, Engelhardt S, Lefkovits I. Proteomics strategies in cardiovascular research. J Proteome Res 2004;3:200-208.

[105] Chaurand P, Cornett DS, Angel PM, Caprioli RM. From whole-body sections down to cellular level, multiscale imaging of phospholipids by MALDI mass spectrometry. Mol Cell Proteomics 2011;10:O110.004259.

[106] Angel PM, Nusinow D, Brown CB, Violette K, Barnett JV, Zhang B, Baldwin HS, Caprioli RM. Networked-based characterization of extracellular matrix proteins from adult mouse pulmonary and aortic valves. J Proteome Res 2011;10: 812-823.

[107] Yutzey KE, Robbins J. Principles of genetic murine models for cardiac disease. Circulation 2007;115:792-799.

[108] Martín-Rojas T, Gil-Dones F, Lopez-Almodovar LF, Padial LR, Vivanco F, Barderas MG. Proteomic profile of human aortic stenosis: insights into the degenerative process. J Proteome Res 2012;11:1537-1550.

[109] Bertacco E, Millioni R, Arrigoni G, Faggin E, Iop L, Puato M, Pinna LA, Tessari P, Pauletto P, Rattazzi M. Proteomic analysis of clonal interstitial aortic valve cells acquiring a pro-calcific profile. J Proteome Res 2010;9:5913-5921.

[110] Gross L, Kugel MA. Topographic anatomy and histology of the valves in the human heart. Am J Path 1931;7:445-456.

[111] Misfeld M, Sievers HH. Heart valve macro- and microstructure. Philos Trans R Soc Lond B Biol Sci 2007;362:1421-1436.

[112] Anderson RH. Clinical anatomy of the aortic root. Heart 2000;84:670-673.

[113] Yacoub MH, Kilner PJ, Birks EJ, Misfeld M. The aortic outflow and root: a tale of dynamism and crosstalk. Ann Thorac Surg 1999;68:S37-43.

[114] Mjaatvedt CH, Yamamura H, Capehart AA, Turner D, Markwald RR. The Cspg2 gene, disrupted in the hdf mutant, is required for right cardiac chamber and endocardial cushion formation. Dev Biol 1998;202:56-66.

[115] George EL, Georges-Labouesse EN, Patel-King RS, Rayburn H, Hynes RO. Defects in mesoderm, neural tube and vascular development in mouse embryos lacking fibronectin. Development 1993;119:1079-1091.

[116] Löhler J, Timpl R, Jaenisch R. Embryonic lethal mutation in mouse collagen I gene causes rupture of blood vessels and is associated with erythropoietic and mesenchymal cell death. Cell 1984;38:597-607.

[117] Liu X, Wu H, Byrne M, Krane S, Jaenisch R. Type III collagen is crucial for collagen I fibrillogenesis and for normal cardiovascular development. Proc Natl Acad Sci U S A 1997;94:1852-1856.

[118] Ng CM, Cheng A, Myers LA, Martinez-Murillo F, Jie C, Bedja D, Gabrielson KL, Hausladen JMW, Mecham RP, Judge DP, Dietz HC. TGF-b-dependent pathogenesis of mitral valve prolapse in a mouse model of Marfan syndrome. J Clin Invest 2004;114:1586-1592.

[119] Hinton RB, Adelman-Brown J, Witt S, Krishnamurthy VK, Osinska H, Sakthivel B, James JF, Li DY, Narmoneva DA, Mecham RP, Benson DW. Elastin haploinsufficien-

cy results in progressive aortic valve malformation and latent valve disease in a mouse model. Circ Res 2010;107:549-557.

[120] Cheek JD, Wirrig EE, Alfieri CM, James JF, Yutzey KE. Differential activation of valvulogenic, chondrogenic, and osteogenic pathways in mouse models of myxomatous and calcific aortic valve disease. J Mol Cell Cardiol 2012;52:689-700.

[121] Snider P, Hinton RB, Moreno-Rodriguez R, Wang J, Rogers R, Lindsley A, Li F, Ingram DA, Menick D, Field L, Firulli AB, Molkentin JD, Markwald RR, Conway SJ. Periostin is required for maturation and extracellular matrix stabilization of noncardiomyocyte lineages of the heart. Circ Res 2008;102:752-760.

[122] Lincoln J, Florer JB, Deutsch GH, Wenstrup RJ, Yutzey KE. ColVa1 and ColXIa1 are required for ventricular chamber morphogenesis and heart valve development. Dev Dyn 2006;235:3295-3305.

[123] Schroeder JA, Jackson LF, Lee DC, Camenisch TD. Form and function of developing heart valves: coordination by extracellular matrix and growth factor signaling. J Mol Med 2003;81:392-403.

[124] Drolet MC, Roussel E, Deshaies Y, Couet J, Arsenault M. A high fat/high carbohydrate diet induces aortic valve disease in C57BL/6J mice. J Am Coll Cardiol 2006;47:850-855.

[125] Weiss RM, Ohashi M, Miller JD, Young SG, Heistad DD. Calcific aortic valve stenosis in old hypercholesterolemic mice. Circulation 2006;114:2065-2069.

[126] Towler DA, Bidder M, Latifi T, Coleman T, Semenkovich CF. Diet-induced diabetes activates an osteogenic gene regulatory program in the aortas of low density lipoprotein receptor-deficient mice. J Biol Chem 1998;273:30427-30434.

[127] Hinton RB, Lincoln J, Deutsch GH, Osinska H, Manning PB, Benson DW, Yutzey KE. Extracellular matrix remodeling and organization in developing and diseased aortic valves. Circ Res 2006;98:1431-1438.

[128] Aikawa E, Whittaker P, Farber M, Mendelson K, Padera RF, Aikawa M, Schoen FJ. Human semilunar cardiac valve remodeling by activated cells from fetus to adult. Circulation 2006;113:1344-1352.

[129] Rabkin E, Aikawa M, Stone JR, Fukumoto Y, Libby P, Schoen FJ. Activated interstitial myofibroblasts express catabolic enzymes and mediate matrix remodeling in myxomatous heart valves. Circulation 2001;104:2525-2532.

[130] Lincoln J, Alfieri CM, Yutzey KE. Development of heart valve leaflets and supporting apparatus in chicken and mouse embryos. Dev Dyn 2004;230:239-250.

[131] Fedak PW, de Sa MP, Verma S, Nili N, Kazemian P, Butany J, Strauss BH, Weisel RD, David TE. Vascular matrix remodeling in patients with bicuspid aortic valve malfor-

mations: implications for aortic dilatation. J Thorac Cardiovasc Surg. 2003;126:797-806.

[132] Fondard O, Detaint D, Lung B, Choqueux C, Adle-Biassette H, Jarraya M, Hvass U, Couetil JP, Henin D, Michel JB, Vahanian A, Jacob MP. Extracellular matrix remodelling in human aortic valve disease: the role of matrix metalloproteinases and their tissue inhibitors. Eur Heart J 2005;26:1333-1341.

[133] Dreger SA, Taylor PM, Allen SP, Yacoub MH. Profile and localization of matrix metalloproteinases (MMPs) and their tissue inhibitors (TIMPs) in human heart valves. J Heart Valve Dis 2002;11:875-880.

[134] Edep ME, Shirani J, Wolf P, Brown DL. Matrix metalloproteinase expression in nonrheumatic aortic stenosis. Cardiovasc Pathol 2000;9:281-286.

[135] Jian B, Jones PL, Li Q, Mohler ER 3rd, Schoen FJ, Levy RJ. Matrix metalloproteinase-2 is associated with tenascin-C in calcific aortic stenosis. Am J Pathol 2001;159:321-327.

[136] Krishnamurthy VK, Opoka AM, Kern CB, Guilak F, Narmoneva DA, Hinton RB. Maladaptive matrix remodeling and regional biomechanical dysfunction in a mouse model of aortic valve disease. Matrix Biol 2012;31:197-205.

[137] Kern CB, Wessels A, McGarity J, Dixon LJ, Alston E, Argraves WS, Geeting D, Nelson CM, Menick DR, Apte SS. Reduced versican cleavage due to Adamts9 haploinsufficiency is associated with cardiac and aortic anomalies. Matrix Biol 2010;29:304-316.

[138] Perrotta I, Russo E, Camastra C, Filice G, Di Mizio G, Colosimo F, Ricci P, Tripepi S, Amorosi A, Triumbari F, Donato G. New evidence for a critical role of elastin in calcification of native heart valves: immunohistochemical and ultrastructural study with literature review. Histopathology 2011;59:504-513.

[139] Aikawa E, Aikawa M, Libby P, Figueiredo JL, Rusanescu G, Iwamoto Y, Fukuda D, Kohler RH, Shi GP, Jaffer FA, Weissleder R. Arterial and aortic valve calcification abolished by elastolytic cathepsin S deficiency in chronic renal disease. Circulation 2009;119:1785-1794.

[140] Jacob MP. Extracellular matrix remodeling and matrix metalloproteinases in the vascular wall during aging and in pathological conditions. Biomed Pharmacother 2003;57:195-202.

[141] Long MM, King VJ, Prasad KU, Freeman BA, Urry DW. Elastin repeat peptides as chemoattractants for bovine aortic endothelial cells. J Cell Physiol 1989;140:512-518.

[142] Hollinger JO, Schmitz JP, Yaskovich R, Long MM, Prasad KU, Urry DW. A synthetic polypentapeptide of elastin for initiating calcification. Calcif Tissue Int 1988;42:231-236.

[143] Sacks MS, David Merryman W, Schmidt DE. On the biomechanics of heart valve function. J Biomech 2009;42:1804-1824.

[144] Grande KJ, Cochran RP, Reinhall PG, Kunzelman KS. Stress variations in the human aortic root and valve: the role of anatomic asymmetry. Ann Biomed Eng 1998;26:534-545.

[145] Sacks MS, Yoganathan AP. Heart valve function: a biomechanical perspective. Philos Trans R Soc Lond B Biol Sci 2007;362:1369-1391.

[146] Visconti RP, Ebihara Y, LaRue AC, Fleming PA, McQuinn TC, Masuya M, Minamiguchi H, Markwald RR, Ogawa M, Drake CJ. An in vivo analysis of hematopoietic stem cell potential: hematopoietic origin of cardiac valve interstitial cells. Circ Res 2006;98:690-6.

[147] Li C, Xu S, Gotlieb AI. The response to valve injury. A paradigm to understand the pathogenesis of heart valve disease. Cardiovasc Pathol 2011;20:183-90.

[148] Hakuno D, Kimura N, Yoshioka M, Mukai M, Kimura T, Okada Y, Yozu R, Shukunami C, Hiraki Y, Kudo A, Ogawa S, Fukuda K. Periostin advances atherosclerotic and rheumatic cardiac valve degeneration by inducing angiogenesis and MMP production in humans and rodents. J Clin Invest 2010;120:2292-306.

[149] Woo KV, Qu X, Babaev VR, Linton MF, Guzman RJ, Fazio S, Baldwin HS. Tie1 attenuation reduces murine atherosclerosis in a dose-dependent and shear stress-specific manner. J Clin Invest. 2011;121:1624-35.

[150] Schoen FJ. Mechanisms of function and disease of natural and replacement heart valves. Annu Rev Pathol. 2012;7:161-83.

[151] Campbell LD, Betsou F, Garcia DL, Giri JG, Pitt KE, Pugh RS, Sexton KC, Skubitz APN, Somiari SB, Astrin J, Baker S, Barr TJ, Benson E, Cada M, Campbell L, Hugo A, Froes J, Campos M, Carpentieri D, Clement O, Coppola D, De Souza Y, Fearn P, Feil K, Garcia D, Giri J, Grizzle WE, Groover K, Harding K, Kaercher E, Kessler J, Loud S, Maynor H, McCluskey K, Meagher K, Michels C, Miranda L, Muller-Cohn J, Muller R, O'Sullivan J, Pitt K, Pugh R, Ravid R, Sexton K, Silva RLA, Simione F, Skubitz A, Somiari S, van der Horst F, Welch G, Zaayenga A. 2012 Best Practices for Repositories: Collection, Storage, Retrieval, and Distribution of Biological Materials for Research. Biopreserv Biobank 2012;10:79-161.

[152] McCarty CA, Chisholm RL, Chute CG, Kullo IJ, Jarvik GP, Larson EB, Li R, Masys DR, Ritchie MD, Roden DM, Struewing JP, Wolf WA; eMERGE Team. The eMERGE Network: a consortium of biorepositories linked to electronic medical records data for conducting genomic studies. BMC Med Genomics 2011;4:13.

[153] Bennett R. The Practical Guide to the Genetic Family History. Wiley-Liss, Inc, 1999.

[154] Yoon PW, Scheuner MT, Peterson-Oehlke KL, Gwinn M, Faucett A, Khoury MJ. Can family history be used as a tool for public health and preventive medicine? Genet Med 2002;4:304-10.

[155] Williams RR, Hunt SC, Heiss G, Province MA, Bensen JT, Higgins M, Chamberlain RM, Ware J, Hopkins PN. Usefulness of cardiovascular family history data for population-based preventive medicine and medical research (the Health Family Tree Study and the NHLBI Family Heart Study). Am J Cardiol 2001;87:129-35.

[156] Greendale K, Pyeritz RE. Empowering primary care health professionals in medical genetics: how soon? How fast? How far? Am J Med Genet 2001;106:223-232.

[157] Hinton RB. The family history: reemergence of an established tool. Crit Care Nurs Clin North Am 2008;20:149-58.

[158] O'Neill SM, Rubinstein WS, Wang C, Yoon PW, Acheson LS, Rothrock N, Starzyk EJ, Beaumont JL, Galliher JM, Ruffin MT 4th; Family Healthware Impact Trial group. Familial risk for common diseases in primary care: the Family Healthware Impact Trial. Am J Prev Med 2009;36:506-14.

[159] Collins FS, Bochm K. Avoiding casualties in the genetic revolution: the urgent need to educate physicians about genetics. Acad Med 1999;74:48-49.

[160] Guttmacher AE, Collins FS, Carmona RH. The family history--more important than ever. N Engl J Med 2004;351:2333-2336.

[161] Robin NH, Tabereaux PB, Benza R, Korf BR. Genetic testing in cardiovascular disease. J Am Coll Cardiol 2007;50:727-737.

[162] Rogowski WH, Grosse SD, Khoury MJ. Challenges of translating genetic tests into clinical and public health practice. Nat Rev Genet 2009;10:489-495.

[163] Aithal GP, Day CP, Kesteven PJ, Daly AK. Association of polymorphisms in the cytochrome P450 CYP2C9 with warfarin dose requirement and risk of bleeding complications. Lancet 1999;353:717-719.

[164] Rost S, Fregin A, Ivaskevicius V, Conzelmann E, Hörtnagel K, Pelz HJ, Lappegard K, Seifried E, Scharrer I, Tuddenham EG, Müller CR, Strom TM, Oldenburg J. Mutations in VKORC1 cause warfarin resistance and multiple coagulation factor deficiency type 2. Nature 2004;427:537-541.

[165] Rose G. Strategy of prevention: lessons from cardiovascular disease. Br Med J 1981;282:1847-1851.

[166] Ashley EA, Hershberger RE, Caleshu C, Ellinor PT, Garcia JG, Herrington DM, Ho CY, Johnson JA, Kittner SJ, Macrae CA, Mudd-Martin G, Rader DJ, Roden DM, Scholes D, Sellke FW, Towbin JA, Van Eyk J, Worrall BB; American Heart Association Advocacy Coordinating Committee. Genetics and cardiovascular disease: a policy statement from the American Heart Association. Circulation 2012;126:142-157.

[167] Loscalzo ML, Goh DL, Loeys B, Kent KC, Spevak PJ, Dietz HC. Familial thoracic aortic dilation and bicommissural aortic valve: a prospective analysis of natural history and inheritance. Am J Med Genet A 2007;143A:1960-1967.

[168] Martin LJ, Hinton RB, Zhang X, Cripe LH, Benson DW. Aorta Measurements are Heritable and Influenced by Bicuspid Aortic Valve. Front Genet 2011;2:61.

[169] de Sa M, Moshkovitz Y, Butany J, David TE. Histologic abnormalities of the ascending aorta and pulmonary trunk in patients with bicuspid aortic valve disease: clinical relevance to the Ross procedure. J Thorac Cardiovasc Surg 1999;118:588-594.

[170] McKellar SH, Michelena HI, Li Z, Scharr HV, Sundt TM. Long-Term Risk of Aortic Events Following Aortic Valve Replacement in Patients with Bicuspid Aortic Valves. Am J Cardiol 2010;106:1626-1633.

[171] David TE, Armstrong S, Ivanov J, Feindel CM, Omran A, Webb G. Results of aortic valve-sparing operations. J Thorac Cardiovasc Surg 2001;122:39-46.

[172] Bethea BT, Fitton TP, Alejo DE, Barreiro CJ, Cattaneo SM, Dietz HC, Spevak PJ, Lima JA, Gott VL, Cameron DE. Results of aortic valve-sparing operations: experience with remodeling and reimplantation procedures in 65 patients. Ann Thorac Surg 2004;78:767-772.

[173] Conti R, Veenstra DL, Armstrong K, Lesko LJ, Grosse SD. Personalized medicine and genomics: challenges and opportunities in assessing effectiveness, cost-effectiveness, and future research priorities. Med Decis Making 2010;30:328-340.

[174] Rossebo AB, Pedersen TR, Boman K, Brudi P, Chambers JB, Egstrup K, Gerdts E, Gohlke-Barwolf C, Holme I, Kesaniemi YA, Malbecq W, Nienaber CA, Ray S, Skjaerpe T, Wachtell K, Willenheimer R. Intensive lipid lowering with simvastatin and ezetimibe in aortic stenosis. N Engl J Med 2008;359:1343-1356.

[175] Wirrig EE, Hinton RB, Yutzey KE. Differential expression of cartilage and bone-related proteins in pediatric and adult diseased aortic valves. J Mol Cell Cardiol 2011;50, 561-569.

Section 4

New Strategies in Heart Valve Tissue Engineering and Regenerative Medicine

Chapter 8

The Immune Response in *In Situ* Tissue Engineering of Aortic Heart Valves

S. L. M. van Loon, A. I. P. M. Smits, A. Driessen-Mol,
F. P. T. Baaijens and C. V. C. Bouten

Additional information is available at the end of the chapter

http://dx.doi.org/10.5772/54354

1. Introduction

The gold standard for treatment of advanced heart valve disease is surgical heart valve replacement. None of the currently available mechanical and bioprosthetic heart valve substitutes resembles normal heart valve function. While mechanical heart valves offer excellent durability, they require life-long anticoagulation to control thromboembolism, which inherently leads to an increased risk of hemorrhage complications. Bioprosthetic valves on the other hand, retain a more physiological blood flow pattern, but these valves are prone to calcification and structural deterioration, limiting their lifespan. For both types of replacement valves, the main limitation is that they are non-living prostheses, incapable of adapting to changes in the hemodynamic environment. It was shown that a living autograft implanted in the aortic position (the Ross procedure) improves long-term clinical outcome compared to a non-living homograft [1]. This illustrates the importance of the regulatory and adaptive properties of a living valve substitute. Tissue engineered aortic valves can provide such an autologous, viable valve with the potential to grow, adapt, and regenerate within the hemodynamic environment. Evidently, the pediatric and young adult population would benefit most from such a tissue engineered aortic valve. The valve's ability to grow as the recipient grows and matures, eliminates the need for repetitive surgeries. [2-7].

Foundational principle of regenerative medicine is restoring the native tissue structure and function by providing a microenvironment necessary to promote tissue regeneration. Tissue engineering scaffolds are biomaterials designed to create this microenvironment and to promote tissue regeneration [8]. The traditional tissue engineering paradigm for creating trileaflet heart valves consists of harvesting autologous cells from the patient, expanding the cells *in vitro,* and subsequently seeding the cells into a biodegradable scaffold. The cell-scaffold constructs are conditioned in a bioreactor to promote extracellular matrix formation (ECM), while the scaffold is degraded [9]. Although this approach leads to an autologous, living heart valve, the *in vitro* process is a very costly and time consuming procedure. Therefore, a novel approach emerged from this, in which the *in vitro* phase is completely omitted, the so-called *in situ* tissue engineering, or 'guided tissue regeneration' (figure 1). This approach relies on the body's natural regenerative potential and uses the human body as a bioreactor [4]. Key to this process is the use of a functional scaffold, capable of host cell repopulation and subsequent *in situ* tissue remodeling. After implantation, cells will colonize the scaffold to form tissue, while the scaffold withstands physiological stresses and strains from its hemodynamic environment and may gradually degrade [2,4]. Clearly, these characteristics put more stringent demands on the biomaterial used, as it should provide both mechanical strength and the cellular niche, balancing between material degradation and tissue formation. The scaffold can be biological or synthetic or a combination of both (a hybrid scaffold), loaded with bioactive components and/or cells to provide stimuli for favorable host cell repopulation, differentiation and tissue formation. The *in situ* approach allows for the minimization of risks and costs associated with cell and tissue culture, while providing off-the-shelf availability.

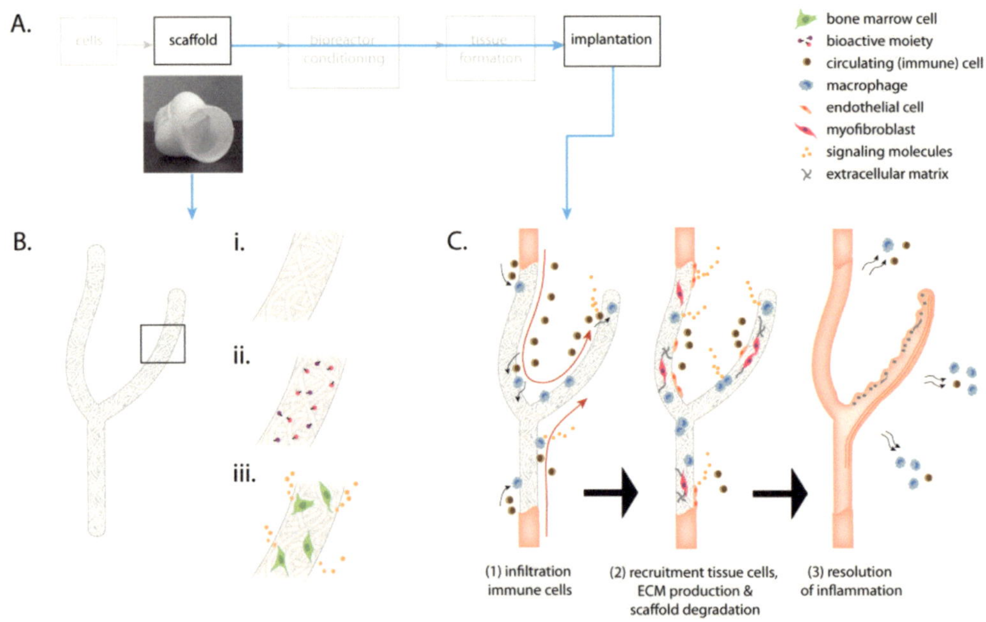

Figure 1. (A) The *in situ* tissue engineering paradigm in which the scaffold is directly implanted, omitting lengthy *in vitro* conditioning phases. (B) The scaffold consists of the bare biomaterial (*i*), which may harbor incorporated bioactive moieties (*ii*) and/or cells (e.g. bone marrow stromal cells) seeded directly prior to implantation (*iii*). (C) Hypothesized mechanism of *in situ* heart valve tissue engineering: after implantation, the scaffold will trigger the host immune response, leading to recruitment of various immune cells and macrophage infiltration. The infiltrated cells secrete cytokines and growth factors to attract additional immune cells, as well as tissue cells, originating from surrounding tissue and/or circulating (progenitor) cells. Endothelial cells cover the blood-scaffold interface and activated myofibroblasts migrate into the scaffold to produce extracellular matrix. Scaffold degradation correlates to a decrease in pro-inflammatory stimuli, eventually leading to resolution of inflammation. Ideally, the valve remodels into the physiological three-layered structure with endothelial cells covering the blood-contact area and quiescent myofibroblasts as valve interstitial-like cells populating the spongiosa layer. Illustration by Anthal Smits.

The *in situ* tissue engineering approach is heavily reliable on the wound healing response. Both the injury incurred during the implantation process and the host inflammatory response to the implanted biomaterial and its degradation products, influence the local microenvironment created by the scaffold. The biomaterial intensifies the inflammatory response by inducing a foreign body response (FBR), propagated by infiltrating immune cells [10,11]. This response is characterized by the presence of macrophages and their fusion into multinucleated giant cells associated with chronic inflammation arising from the persistent presence of a foreign body. The FBR, especially inflammation, may drive valve calcification. However, inflammation is not merely a detrimental response to biomaterial scaffolds. Rather, it can be considered as a natural agent of tissue remodeling, orchestrated by various cell types and potent signaling molecules. By unraveling the inflammatory response towards the foreign biomaterial and the triggers for pathological outcome, targets may be identified to control the inflammatory response through modifications of the biomaterial. The goal is to develop strategies that harness the beneficial aspects of the inflammatory response, while limiting its potential deleterious effects by modulating the inflammatory response towards regeneration.

This chapter deals with the use of biomaterials for *in situ* heart valve tissue engineering and the immune response to the implanted biomaterial. The FBR to biomaterials is discussed, leading to biomaterial design approaches directed to immunomodulation towards tissue regeneration, identifying pitfalls as well as current research challenges for this innovative technology.

2. Biomaterial scaffolds

Biomaterials are materials that interact with the body and its cells. As such, they are central to many strategies for regenerative medicine. They are employed as vehicles for transplanting (progenitor) cells, timed and localized delivery of bioactive moieties, and/or as 3D scaffolds for tissue engineering. Scaffolds are biomaterials designed to create a microenvironment that promotes regeneration. Besides creating and maintaining a defined space for tissue growth, biomaterial scaffolds also provide mechanical stability, and support cell adhesion and migration. Ideally, a scaffold for tissue engineering should be bioresorbable, biocompatible and have a highly porous macrostructure necessary for cell growth, nutrient supply, and waste removal [2,3,6,8,12]. By engineering the proper cellular niche, such scaffolds can provide an environment suitable to modify host responses and direct cell survival, migration, proliferation, differentiation, as well as matrix formation and remodeling. The premise is that in order to unlock the full potential of the cells, at least some aspects of the native 3D tissue environment associated with their renewal, differentiation and organization needs to be mimicked in the applied scaffold materials [3].

2.1. Biomaterial scaffold use in *in situ* heart valve tissue engineering

Trileaflet heart valves are sophisticated tissues with an anisotropic three-layered structure, optimized to withstand the repetitive hemodynamic loads it is subjected to. A human heart valve opens and closes approximately 100.000 times per day, resulting in cyclic changes in the shape, dimensions, and stress of its leaflets and supporting structures. Furthermore, rather than being a purely passive structure, heart valves consist of active components that allow them to adapt to changes in the hemodynamic environment to a certain degree. This puts stringent demands on biomaterial scaffolds used for heart valve tissue engineering, in particular on the mechanical properties. The hemodynamic environment requires a strong biomaterial bearing the repetitive and substantial mechanical stresses applied, especially in the aortic position. This calls for excellent elastic and fatigue properties of the scaffold. A successful tissue engineered heart valve must not only accommodate the resulting deformations, but also have ongoing strength, flexibility, and durability, beginning at the instant of implantation and continuing throughout the lifetime of the recipient [2]. For the *in situ* tissue engineering approach, this means the scaffold has to maintain valve functionality while ECM is formed and remodeled and the biomaterial is degraded *in situ*. In contrast, for the traditional *in vitro* tissue engineering approach the load-bearing function of the biomaterial is overtaken by ECM *in vitro*, prior to implantation. This balance between scaffold resorption and synthesis of new matrix by the host's cells is one of the main challenges in designing scaffolds for *in situ* tissue engineering [4].

2.1.1. Biological scaffolds

The ECM is the natural scaffold for tissue and organ morphogenesis, maintenance, and reconstruction following injury, and is associated with constructive tissue remodeling [12]. The ECM proteins are potent regulators of cell adhesion and activation, and provide a 3D scaffold for cellular organization and migration. They provide mechanical support and store and mobilize signaling molecules. The fibrous ECM structure is provided by collagen, elastin, and fibrin, while non-fibrous proteins as fibronectin and laminin are domains for cell-matrix interactions. This protein scaffold is embedded in a gelatinous matrix composed of glycosaminoglycans (GAGs) and proteoglycans. It serves as a lubricant and as a reservoir for signaling molecules, regulating their distribution and mode of action serving cell-matrix interactions, and activation of enzymes and mediators [11]. Hence, ECM serves as a native modulator of cell activity, also in immune responses and tissue repair. The 3D organization of its components and the complexity of the composition distinguish the native ECM from synthetic scaffolds [4,12,13]. Consequently, the use of a decellularized valve is currently the predominant choice as scaffold material for application in *in situ* engineering of heart valves.

In contrast to cross-linked bioprostheses, decellularized xenografts or homografts allow for infiltration of host cells and matrix remodeling, which may render an autologous, living replacement valve in time. Upon decellularization, the xenograft or homograft is depleted of cells and cellular components. The decellularized matrix possesses a native-like geometry and structure with mechanical properties and physiological hemodynamics similar to its native counterpart [3,4,14]. Signaling components present in the matrix provide natural cues to dictate cell adhesion, proliferation, and growth. With respect to biocompatibility, it is crucial to remove all cellular components, without harming or altering the matrix properties by the decellularization treatment [15]. The method of decellularization strongly determines the degree of preservation of matrix integrity, as well as the efficiency of cell removal. Various decellularization techniques are being studied in an effort to suppress the immunogenic potential of such biological matrices while retaining matrix integrity [2,4,5,7,14]. Results from studies on recellularization of decellularized homografts and xenografts in animal models are controversial, as reviewed elsewhere [2-4,7,16]. In decellularized aortic valves, residual devitalized cells and their epitopes are primary initiators of valve calcification leading to failure of this bioprosthetic valve [7,17]. It is suggested that inflammation inhibitory factors, naturally present in the ECM, are lost due to the decellularization treatment, accounting for the activation of granulocytes and the initiation of the immune response [4]. Furthermore, xenografts are associated with the risk of immunogenic reactions or disease transmission and availability of homografts is limited. To overcome these issues, recent studies have suggested the use of homologous decellularized tissue engineered heart valves. For this, heart valves were engineered *in vitro* using adult saphenous vein cells seeded onto a synthetic polyglycolic acid (PGA)/poly-4-hydroxybutyrate (P4HB) scaffold. After conditioning the cell-scaffold construct in an *in vitro* bioreactor, the tissue engineered valve was decellularized and used as a starter matrix for subsequent recellularization and remodeling *in situ* [18].

An alternative, natural resorbable scaffold material suitable for *in situ* tissue engineering and studied extensively is small intestine submucosa (SIS) [2,3,13]. SIS consists almost entirely of acellular collagen so there is no need for these substrates to undergo extensive decellularization procedures, making it an attractive alternative to decellularized matrices [3]. The success of SIS has been attributed to its intrinsic ECM proteins, cytokines, and growth factors, showing rapid remodeling by the host tissue and exhibiting good vascularization and tissue growth without excessive inflammation and FBR [2]. With respect to heart valve tissue engineering, complete valvular replacements from SIS have been produced demonstrating remodeling potential *in vivo* [19]. As for all animal derived materials, a disadvantage of using SIS is the risk of transferring zoonoses and its availability may be a limiting factor when homograft material is used [3,14]. Further studies should clarify the underlying mechanisms involved before translating the use of decellularized matrices as heart valve scaffolds to human clinic.

2.1.2. Synthetic scaffolds

Synthetic scaffolds have the advantage that they can be tailored to demands, offering precise control of various aspects, such as mechanical properties, chemical properties, degradation rate, as well as the immunogenic potential [7,8]. However, this level of control comes at a price in the sense that multi-disciplinary in-depth knowledge is required to engineer a scaffold appropriate for *in situ* tissue engineering. Engineering of synthetic scaffolds is a discipline that spans multiple length-scales. On the macroscale, a scaffold should exhibit mechanical properties appropriate to fulfill its function. The 3D architecture affects the global mechanical properties of the scaffold, but additionally, on the microscale, it influences cell infiltration and organization (e.g. by contact guidance). Apart from the global mechanical properties of a scaffold, the local mechanical properties, such as material surface stiffness, determine the stimuli experienced by the cells. Surface chemistry (e.g. hydrophobicity/hydrophilicity) has a major effect on cell- and protein-biomaterial interactions and with state-of-the art incorporation of bioactive or even bioresponsive molecules, scaffold engineering has advanced down to the nanoscale [3]. This emphasizes that not only the choice of biomaterial but also the method of processing is of key importance in scaffold development.

Synthetic biodegradable materials, such as PGA, P4HB, polylactic acid (PLA), polycaprolactone (PCL) and copolymers, are the main biocompatible materials of choice, varying in their rates of degradation and manufacturing possibilities [2-4,6,7,14]. Their degradation rate can be tailored by varying their copolymer ratio [3]. Fast-degrading scaffolds such as PGA/P4HB have been used extensively as scaffolds for *in vitro* tissue engineering procedures of heart valves [9,20,21]. Whereas the use of synthetic scaffolds in traditional *in vitro* tissue engineering is abundant, experience with the use of synthetic scaffolds for *in situ* tissue engineering of heart valves is rather limited. However, recent studies applying synthetic scaffolds for small-caliber blood vessels demonstrate the ground-breaking potential of such scaffolds for endogenous regeneration. Small-diameter nanofibrous PCL grafts showed fast endothelialization and ECM formation in the systemic circulation of a rat model [22]. Vascular grafts composed of a nonwoven PGA mesh with a PCL/Poly-L-lactic acid (PLLA) copolymer, seeded with bone marrow stromal cells, demonstrated regeneration of mature blood vessels *in situ* via an inflammation-mediated response in a mouse model [23], as well as in clinical trials [24]. To improve mechanotransduction from the biomaterial to the cells, Wu *et al.* employed a fast degrading elastomeric graft, consisting of poly(glycerol sebacate) (PGS), resulting in fast *in situ* regeneration of neoarteries with mechanical properties and functionality similar to the native vascular tissue [25]. Alternatively, Yokota *et al.* developed a hybrid scaffold consisting of a collagen sponge with layered PGA and PLLA, resulting in regeneration of the canine carotid artery [26]. Although these results demonstrate the great potential of synthetic or hybrid scaffolds for *in situ* tissue engineering, translating these results to heart valves is not trivial due to the complexity of mechanical loads and high-demanding function of the heart valve. Furthermore, slow and/or incomplete polymer degradation may result in excessive chronic inflammation, possibly leading to fibrosis and hampered valve function.

Despite these challenges to overcome, synthetic scaffolds have the potential to offer a strong cost-effective off-the-shelf alternative for heart valve replacements, yielding them very interesting for future clinical application.

2.2. Modulating the immune response

Independent of the biomaterial, the injury incurred during the implantation process will trigger an immune response, due to the disruption of host tissue and induction of cell damage. However, the extent of the inflammatory response evoked is dependent on location, implantation procedure, and biocompatibility of the biomaterial [14,27]. The natural human host response to the scaffold is an excellent target to modulate and control cell and tissue fate. Valvular regeneration is hypothesized to start with a rapid infiltration of the scaffold by monocytes. These monocytes differentiate into macrophages and attract progenitor cells that differentiate into tissue-producing cells. In addition, the macrophages themselves may differentiate into tissue-producing cells. Next, clearance of the macrophages occurs and extracellular matrix is formed and remodeled toward the natural heart valve matrix architecture with quiescent cells. Detailed understanding of this response will provide guidelines to achieve cell and tissue homeostasis, while preventing adverse tissue development (e.g. fibrosis) by mitigating early cellular responses. As the nature of the infiltrating cells in the scaffold and their differentiation is believed to tune the balance of later stage tissue formation towards regeneration or fibrosis, controlling the endogenous production or presentation to the cells of key regulating cytokines in these early processes is essential. Thus, insights in the sequential cell influx and cytokine production and their role in cell differentiation/polarization and tissue formation, will allow the development of optimized scaffolds for *in situ* heart valve tissue engineering applications.

3. The immune response to biomaterials

The defensive response of the human body to invasion by disease-causing entities is referred to as the immune response. In general, its main function is to resolve the infection, restore the tissue damage and reestablish a state of homeostasis. The ideal response is rapid and destructive when necessary, yet specific and self limiting [28]. The immune response consists of two stages: the innate response and the adaptive response (figure 2). The innate immune response refers to the antigen-nonspecific defense mechanism that a host uses immediately or within several hours after exposure to a pathogen or other foreign entity, e.g. a biomaterial. The response is aimed at the recognition and removal of the entity, inhibiting infection and inducing a state of inflammation. When the innate immune response is outrun by a continuing infection and antigen is drained to regional lymph nodes, the adaptive immune response is triggered. Adaptive immunity is antigen-specific, generating responses that are tailored to maximally eliminate pathogens and cells displaying non-self antigens. A key feature of adaptive immunity is the development of immunological memory, in which specific antibodies are generated [29,30]. Synthetic biomaterials are thought not to initiate an adaptive response because they are typically not immunogenic. However, cells and mechanisms involved in the initiation of an adaptive immune response have been found at sites of synthetic implants, suggesting the involvement of an adaptive response in the immune response to biomaterials [11]. In *in situ* tissue engineering, an immune response is inevitable and its beneficial aspects, i.e. dead cell removal and initiation of wound healing, must be harnessed while the potential deleterious effects, i.e. excessive inflammation and fibrosis, must be limited.

3.1. The acute and chronic inflammatory response

The classification 'acute' or 'chronic' is primarily defined by the duration of the inflammatory response and the type of cells infiltrating in response to pro-inflammatory signals [27]. As part of the innate immune response, the acute inflammatory response occurs in the first days after implantation and is characterized by the presence of blood-derived polymorphonuclear leukocytes (PMNs, or granulocytes), predominantly neutrophils. The infiltrating cells cause a state of inflammation to develop within the tissue, generally described by the local accumulation of fluid accompanied by warming (*calor*), pain (*dolor*), reddening (*rubor*), swelling (*tumor*), and functional changes (*functio laesa*). These cells secrete reactive oxygen intermediates (ROIs) and inflammatory cytokines, including interleukin-1β (IL-1β), tumor necrosis factor-α (TNF-α), and interferon-γ (IFN-γ), which orchestrate the character and degree of the subsequent immune response [31]. Their actions can, besides eliminating the pathogen or other foreign entity, also cause secondary damage to the surrounding tissue. Controlling the numbers and types of immune cells at the implant site has the potential to reduce secondary tissue damage and promote regeneration [8].

The inflammatory response prolonging within subsequent weeks, months or even years after implantation is referred to as the chronic inflammatory response. Ideally, the chronic phase of the inflammatory response is avoided through adequate and quick elimination of the disease-causing entity during the acute phase. Chronic inflammation develops as inflammatory stimuli persist at the implant site, with macrophages representing the driving force in continuing the inflammatory response, mediating prolonged expression of cytokines, i.e. IL-1β and TNF-α [11]. Implantation of a biomaterial can intensify the inflammatory response by inducing a FBR, propagated by the infiltrating macrophages, which influences subsequent wound healing.

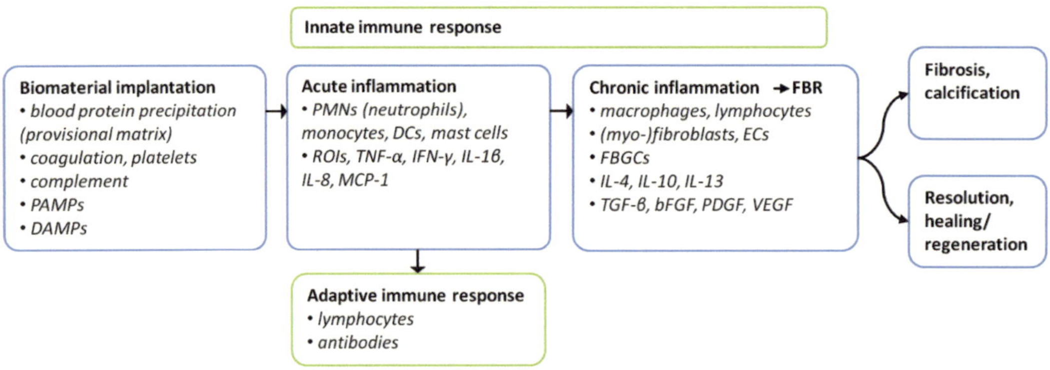

Figure 2. Overview of the immune response to a biomaterial; pathogen-associated molecular patterns (PAMPs), damage-associated molecular patterns (DAMPs), polymorphonuclear leukocytes (PMNs), dendritic cells (DCs), reactive oxygen intermediates (ROIs), tumor necrosis factor-α (TNF-α), interferon-γ (IFN-γ), interleukin-1β (IL-1β), monocyte chemotactic protein-1 (MCP-1], foreign body response (FBR), endothelial cells (ECs), foreign body giant cells (FBGCs), transforming growth factor-β (TGF-β), basic fibroblast growth factor (bFGF), platelet-derived growth factor (PDGF), vascular endothelial growth factor (VEGF).

3.2. Mediators of the immune response

The complete process from innate immune response to wound healing is tuned by a broad spectrum of cytokines and growth factors. Cytokines are a large family of proteins, peptides and glycoproteins, recognized as intercellular signaling immunomodulators [27]. Cytokines are produced by cells and affect the behavior of other cells by binding to specific receptors on their target cells. The term chemokine refers to a specific class of cytokines that is involved in guiding leukocytes to sites where their functions are needed, and as such, have a central role in inflammatory processes. This migration of cells to the site of interest via unidirectional movement towards an increasing gradient of a chemical signal is called chemotaxis [27,30].

Chemokines are not only involved in orchestrating cellular migration in inflammation and wound healing, but also play roles in hematopoiesis, angiogenesis, and tumor metastasis [10].

The secreted chemical mediators usually have a very short half-life due to their high susceptibility to proteolytic degradation. Local linkage to the ECM protects them from enzymatic cleavage, while others may become inactive when bound and can only act when released by matrix proteolysis [11]. Hereby, chemical mediators and ECM proteins collaborate in creating a distinct cellular niche that regulates tissue regeneration.

3.3. Initiation of the innate immune response

Implantation of a biomaterial scaffold typically leads to thrombus formation and initiation of an acute immune response by activation of the coagulation system, complement system, fibrinolytic system, and platelets. Interaction of the biomaterial with blood leads to protein deposition on the biomaterial surface forming a provisional matrix, which affects subsequent leukocyte adhesion interactions [8]. Synthetic polymers, their degradation products and/or the associated provisional matrix activate the complement cascade, marking the biomaterial as being foreign. Phagocytic cells are recruited to the implant by the chemokines released from the provisional matrix and surrounding cells. These phagocytic cells adhere to the matrix surface and further enhance secretion of inflammatory products.

3.3.1. Blood protein precipitation

Upon contact with blood, the blood-biomaterial interaction leads to adsorption of blood proteins, dependent on the biomaterial surface properties [10,11,29,31,32]. The adsorption of endogenous proteins from blood or interstitial fluid onto the surface of the biomaterial, rather than the biomaterial itself, dictates the immune cell response to implanted biomaterials [27]. All other host components, including leukocytes, encounter and/or interact with this surface as an adhesion substrate. It serves as a provisional matrix, which may also contain a milieu of cytokines, chemokines, or other bioactive agents. This provisional matrix furnishes structural, biochemical, and cellular components to the processes of wound healing and FBR. It can be seen as a naturally derived, biodegradable sustained release system in which bioactive moieties are released to control subsequent phases of wound healing [10].

The precipitation of proteins from blood and tissue occurring immediately after implantation determines the activation of the coagulation cascade, the complement system, platelets and immune cells. The proteins guide their interplay, leading to the formation of the provisional matrix and to the onset of the immune response [11,29]. The adsorbed protein layer includes complement activation fragments, immunoglobulin G (IgG), fibrinogen, fibronectin, and vitronectin. Fibrinogen and fibronectin bind a large number of extracellular macromolecules as well as cell surface proteins, providing a matrix for cell proliferation and organization [33]. Whereas complement and fibrinogen mainly contribute to the activation of inflammatory cells, fibronectin and vitronectin are critical in regulating the inflammatory response to biomaterials [11]. The composition of the protein layer changes over time, described as the Vroman effect [10,29]. Adsorbed proteins may desorb rapidly and, therefore, present time-dependent variations in the type and level of proteins which cells encounter. The highest mobility proteins of the blood serum generally arrive first, e.g. albumin and globulin, and are later replaced by less motile proteins that have a higher affinity for the biomaterial surface, e.g. fibronectin and factor XII.

Complement receptors function as a non-specific aid in detection and removal of foreign materials. Activation of the complement system leads to subsequent reactions in host defense and functions as one of the players in the tight cross-talk between the different cascade systems, platelets, and leukocytes, inducing clotting and inflammation. The complement system is activated by the coating of the implant with complement activation fragments within the provisional matrix, and through release of anaphylatoxins, i.e. C3a and C5a, which are chemo-attractants for leukocyte infiltration and cause leukocyte activation [32,34]. Upon complement activation, proteases in the system cleave specific proteins to release cytokines, e.g. TNF-α, IL-1β, IL-6, and IL-8, and initiate an amplifying cascade of further cleavages. Furthermore, it contributes to the onset of the inflammatory response by triggering degranulation of mast cells, attraction and activation of PMNs and monocytes, induction of ROI-release by PMNs, supporting platelet adhesion and activation, and promotion of tissue factor expression by monocytes and PMNs on biomaterial surfaces [11]. Destruction of host cells is prevented by the presence of membrane-bound complement regulatory proteins, e.g. CD46, CD55, and CD59 [29].

Blood coagulation on biomaterials requires the combination of contact activation by factor XII, platelet adhesion and their activation by thrombin. This leads to the cleavage of fibrinogen to fibrin and subsequent clot formation. Platelet adhesion and activation, through adsorbed IgG and fibrinogen, mediates neutrophil reactive oxygen generation and monocyte tissue factor expression, leading to neutrophil and monocyte adhesion [29]. Platelets trapped in the fibrin clot, as well as fibroblasts and leukocytes themselves are major resources of chemo-attractants at the site of implantation, initiating and modulating inflammatory reactions and immune responses [35,36].

Cell adhesion and activation on biomaterials primarily occurs through interaction of adhesion receptors with the adsorbed proteins. The major adhesion receptors of leukocytes are represented by integrins, which regulate aggregation, immune functions, cell migration, matrix deposition, and wound contraction [33]. Surface integrin molecules allow cells to migrate through the ECM and mediate signal transduction between the cell and its environment, enabling the cell to respond to its environment. Integrin molecule engagement on leukocytes promotes leukocyte survival, activation, and differentiation [29]. Ligands for integrin receptor binding and cellular adhesion are provided by the adsorbed proteins, including fibrinogen, IgG, iC3b, fibronectin, and vitronectin [10].

3.3.2. Pattern recognition

Besides recognition of biomaterials through adhesion receptors, i.e. integrins, immune cells are activated by another type of receptor-ligand interaction that is based on pattern recognition. A class of molecules classically defined as pathogen-associated molecular pattern (PAMP) molecules, alerts the innate immune system and triggers defensive immune

http://dx.doi.org/10.5772/54354

responses. PAMPs include lipopolysaccharide (LPS), viral RNA and bacterial peptidoglycans, which interact with dedicated receptors on immune cells, the pattern recognition receptors (PRRs) [8,11,28,29,35,37,38]. These receptors are specialized in the recognition of microbial components that are chemically distinct from the host's endogenous molecules [39]. PRRs include transmembrane Toll-like receptors (TLRs), cytoplasmic NOD-like receptors (NLRs), and cytoplasmic C-type lectin receptors (CLRs) [28,37]. The TLR family is a well-known family of PRRs, in which each member recognizes a specific set of molecular patterns. For example, TLR2 and TLR4 recognize damaged ECM by binding breakdown products of hyaluronan cleaved in tissue damage, while TLR7, TLR8, and TLR9 recognize host RNA and DNA [28]. TLRs are expressed on e.g. platelets, macrophages, dendritic cells (DCs), neutrophils, and endothelial cells [36,37]. Tissue-resident macrophages and DCs, both functioning as antigen-presenting cells (APCs), are most influential in early PRR-signaling and are the primary inducers of an inflammatory reaction [28,39].

An inflammatory response can, besides initiation by PAMPs, also be initiated by several endogenous molecules interacting with signaling receptors. These innate danger signals are described as endokines or alarmins, but are also known as damage-associated molecular patterns (DAMPs) [11,35,38,40]. These signals have immunostimulatory effects and include an array of structurally diverse, multifunctional host proteins that are rapidly released during infection or tissue damage, e.g. after biomaterial implantation. The resulting necrotic cell death leads to the release of cytoplasmic and nuclear components that contain DAMPs, recognized by PRRs expressed by leukocytes. In addition, proteases and hydrolases released from dead cells modify extracellular components to generate mediators (e.g. complement fragments) or other DAMPs (e.g. ECM fragments), which can activate leukocytes [39]. DAMPs have intranuclear, intracellular and/or extracellular functions in mobilizing and activating receptor-expressing cells engaged in host defense and tissue repair, e.g. macrophages and DCs. One of the members of the DAMP family is the group of high-mobility-group box (HMGB) proteins, which are chromosomal proteins helping in transcription, replication, recombination, and DNA repair. HMGB-1 is one of the best known proteins within this family and is released by necrotic cells, cytolytic cells, and cells stimulated by pro-inflammatory stimuli. It was shown to have extracellular activity as a chemokine, attracting neutrophils and mononuclear inflammatory cells [28,39,40]. Other members of the DAMP family include interleukins, heat-shock proteins, defensins, eosinophil-derived neurotoxin, macrophage-/PMN-derived cathelicidins, and nucleosomes. Injury-related TLR-ligands are small hyaluronan fragments, fibrinogen, and fibronectin, of which the latter two are present in the adsorbed protein layer on a biomaterial surface [28].

Induction of inflammation through pattern recognition leads to activation of the receptor expressing cell. When a ligand has bound to a PRR, activation signals are sent out, which initiate signaling pathways leading to the activation of transcription factors, notably nuclear factor κB (NF-κB). This factor migrates into the nucleus and mediates gene transcription and production of inflammatory mediators, such as chemokines, adhesion molecules, growth factors, and pro-inflammatory cytokines, especially TNF-α, and IL-1, which themselves also mediate activation of NF-κB [37]. Many molecules with important functions in immunity and repair mediate their effects through activation of the NF-κB pathway. Transcriptional control of inflammation by NF-κB during the immune response has emerged as one of the most important signaling cascades in the regulation of the inflammatory response [35].

3.4. Cell recruitment in the acute inflammatory response

The acute inflammatory response is driven by fast acting leukocytes, mostly neutrophils and macrophages, as the primary defense against nonspecific infecting entities [11,27]. After implantation of a biomaterial, inherently causing cell damage, these immune cells are activated through the engagement of their integrins and PRRs with the protein-coated biomaterial surface. The activation of immune cells leads to the initiation of inflammatory cytokine production and subsequent chemokine recruitment of more immune cells, i.e. PMNs, monocytes, and macrophages, but also endothelial cells and fibroblasts to the site of implantation [28,35]. Activation of PMNs includes a phagocytic response and degranulation, which subsequently leads to biomaterial degradation and potential damaging of the surrounding tissue, prolonging the inflammatory response [11].

During the inflammatory response, macrophages and lymphocytes predominantly synthesize and release immunoregulatory cytokines, e.g. IL-1β, IL-6, and TNF-α, and chemokines, e.g. IL-8, monocyte chemotactic protein-1 (MCP-1), and macrophage inflammatory protein-1β (MIP-1β). These are potent chemo-attractants and activation factors for inflammatory effector cells such as PMNs, monocytes, macrophages, immature DCs, natural killer (NK) cells, and lymphocytes. Changes in cellularly released chemical factors mediate additional cell recruitment and activity [27]. The increasing influx of mononuclear cells over time is balanced by a decreased infiltration of PMNs, leading to a decrease in PMN activation signals followed by their apoptosis and engulfment by macrophages. Within two days after implantation PMNs typically disappear from the site [11].

3.4.1. Neutrophils

Neutrophils are the most dominant cell type among the PMNs present in the acute inflammatory response. They are phagocytic leukocytes containing granules and are activated by pro-inflammatory cytokines, such as IL-1β, TNF-α, and IFN-γ [35]. The life span of a neutrophil inside the blood stream is 12 hours, but increases to 24-48 hours upon activation outside the vasculature [27,39]. Crucial mediators for neutrophil recruitment in acute inflammation are chemokines and their receptors, e.g. IL-8 [35]. The primary function of IL-8 is induction of the chemotaxis of neutrophils, with their arrival at the site within hours after injury, followed by a later influx of monocytes [38].

Neutrophils eradicate foreign entities by immediate phagocytosis, a process by which solid particles are uptaken by the cell. After phagocytosis of the biomaterial, neutrophils die, and are, together with other material debris, cleared by resident macrophages [27]. This uptake promotes anti-inflammatory lipoxin production by the macrophage, which down-regulates further neutrophil recruitment and activity, while promoting monocyte migration [39]. When neutrophils detect TNF-α, but do not directly encounter any exogeneous particles, they mobilize and release their granules into the extracellular space, a process called degranulation, to create an inhospitable environment for nearby foreign entities [28]. The granules of neutrophils are loaded with proteases, which, together with the production of ROIs and reactive nitrogen intermediates (RNIs), leads to the denaturation of proteins, disruption of lipids, and damaging of DNA [28,39]. Upon degranulation, the neutrophil reorganizes its surrounding microenvironment and promotes the recruitment of additional immune responsive cells, mainly monocytes, but also generates secondary damage to the host tissue and cells [8,28]. Therefore, neutrophil activation has to be tightly controlled to avoid excessive tissue damage while enabling the rapid recruitment of monocytes [39].

3.4.2. Monocytes

After neutrophils, monocytes enter the site of implantation and subsequently mature into tissue macrophages or DCs. Bone marrow precursors give rise to the monocytes in the blood, which circulate for a few days before they migrate into the tissue and mature [41]. Monocytes are recruited by cytokines and chemotactic factors, released by resident macrophages and neutrophils [27]. In general, monocytes reach maximum numbers 24-36 hours after injury [37]. There is a guided movement of monocytes in response to chemokines and other chemo-attractants [10]. MCP-1, also known as C-C chemokine ligand 2 (CCL2), binds to C-C chemokine receptor 2 (CCR2) and mediates monocyte recruitment [42]. Although expression of CCR2 is restricted to only a few cell types including monocytes, most (if not all) nucleated cells express MCP-1 in response to activation by pro-inflammatory cytokines or stimulation of innate immune receptors. A hypothesis on the mechanism of action of MCP-1 in monocyte recruitment from the bone marrow is that MCP-1 dimerizes and associates with tissue GAGs, creating a gradient which guides monocytes toward the site of infection or inflammation [42].

In the blood, monocytes are not a homogeneous population of cells. Human monocytes are divided into subsets according to their surface expression of CD14 and CD16 [39,42]. CD14 is a PRR that can recognize and bind various structures from invading microbes (e.g. LPS), while CD16 is a receptor binding IgG antibodies [41]. $CD14^{++}CD16^{-}$ monocytes are the most prevalent monocyte subset present in the blood (~85% of total monocytes) and express CCR2 [43]. The $CD16^{+}$ monocyte population comprises two subsets, $CD14^{++}CD16^{+}$ and $CD14^{+}CD16^{++}$ monocytes [41,42]. There appears to be a developmental relationship between these different subtypes in that, during the course of an inflammatory reaction, the $CD14^{++}CD16^{-}$ monocytes first develop into $CD14^{++}CD16^{+}$ monocytes to then become $CD14^{+}CD16^{++}$ monocytes. Hence, $CD14^{+}CD16^{++}$ monocytes may represent a more mature subset [41]. The precise role of the different monocyte subsets in initiating immune responses remains unclear, although $CD14^{++}CD16^{-}$ monocytes are believed to contribute more effectively to pathogen clearance while $CD14^{+}CD16^{++}$ monocytes show a patrolling role and account for more vigorous production of pro-inflammatory cytokines [39,42].

At the site of implantation, monocytes become activated and develop into DCs or mature tissue macrophages, undergoing a phenotypic change. This process is directed by mediators present in the microenvironment, such as cytokine receptors, TLRs, and complement receptors, which are crucial for the proper adaptation of cell function to the specific requirements at the site.

[11,35]. For example, TLR-activated monocytes produce IL-10, which has a central role in preventing excessive inflammation [38]. Additionally, there is substantial debate about whether specific monocyte populations give rise to specific tissue macrophages [39,44]. It has been suggested that monocytes continue maturing in the blood and can be recruited to the tissue at various points during this maturation continuum. The point at which they leave the blood may define their function [42].

3.4.3. Dendritic cells

Dendritic cells (DCs), monocytes, and macrophages are closely related, as blood monocytes can differentiate into macrophages and DCs and, in their turn, DCs can differentiate into macrophages [41]. The main function of DCs is to function as APCs, processing foreign material and presenting it on its surface to other immune cells, e.g. T-lymphocytes (T cells) [45]. They act as messengers between the innate and adaptive immune response, initiating the T-cell response [29]. Besides their presence as resident cells in tissues, they are also found in the blood, circulating in an immature state. Upon activation, DCs migrate to the lymph nodes and interact with lymphocytes to initiate and modulate the adaptive immune response [30].

By triggering receptors and signaling cascades of the pathogen recognition system, biomaterials activate DCs through the adherent protein layer [11,29]. DC maturation is promoted or inhibited depending on which PRR is engaged, leading to immunity or tolerance, respectively. Immunogenic DCs may prolong the immune response to biomaterials and delay wound healing, while tolerogenic DCs are capable of down-regulating the immune cells and resolve inflammation [11]. Activated immunogenic DCs promote T-cell proliferation and secrete pro-inflammatory cytokines, e.g. IL-1β, IL-6, IL-12, and TNF-α, which further amplify DC maturation by autocrine stimulation. The immature and semi-mature tolerogenic DCs are promoters of tolerance and secrete e.g. IL-10 and TGF-β [45]. Besides PRR engagement, integrin signaling due to binding of DCs to ECM proteins on the biomaterial, may act as an alternative mechanism of DC maturation and activation and should be taken into account in the strategy of modulating immune responses to biomaterials.

3.4.4. Mast cells

Mast cells are a leukocyte subset represented in most tissues and are best known for their role in allergy. However, they play an important protective role as well, being intimately involved in host defense and wound healing. In the innate immune response, they are an important source of pro-inflammatory mediators and cytokines, containing many granules that are rich in histamine, and producing prostaglandins and cytokines that promote inflammation [35]. Together with tissue-resident macrophages and DCs, mast cells are responsible for the recruitment of inflammatory cells in the innate immune response, i.e. chemotaxis of PMNs and monocytes through secretion of e.g. IL-1β, TNF-α, and MCP-1 [11,28,29]. Besides functioning in host defense mechanisms, mast cells participate more generally in the orchestration of inflammatory responses, e.g. through IL-10 secretion, and tissue remodeling, through secretion of proteases and anti-inflammatory cytokines, such as IL-4 [46]. They express a large set of receptors allowing them to respond to a large variety of stimuli, with activation of specific

http://dx.doi.org/10.5772/54354

receptors leading to specific actions. Therefore, mast cell functions are highly dependent on the physiological context, as small differences in the mast cell environment may yield variant or even opposite actions [46].

3.5. The chronic inflammatory response

Once neutrophils, monocytes and macrophages have entered the site of injury or infection in the acute phase of the response, they collaborate to remove the foreign entity [39]. The transition of the acute inflammatory response to the chronic inflammatory response is signified by the departure of the PMNs and infiltration of more macrophages and lymphocytes, which give rise to new tissue formation [8,10,31].

3.5.1. Macrophages

Generally, when the acute phase of inflammation has not sufficed to clear the source of infection within the first 2 days after implantation, macrophages become the dominating force in the persisting inflammatory response. Macrophages are recruited by many of the same signals as neutrophils but have a longer life span. Tissue-resident macrophages have a life span up to months [27,28]. The primary role of macrophages is to function as a common guardian cell of which the main function in homeostasis is to clear the interstitial environment of extraneous cellular material through phagocytosis [44]. Macrophages are professional phagocytes with extraordinary synthetic and secretory capacities and exert key controlling influences on wound healing and fibrosis responses [31].

A resting macrophage is activated by microbial products, immune complexes, chemical mediators, certain ECM proteins, and T-cell-derived cytokines. An adherent macrophage on a biomaterial is activated to initiate phagocytosis and cytokine secretion, hereby directing the inflammatory and wound healing response to the biomaterial [10]. Several of the key biomaterial-dependent chemokines and cytokines (e.g. IL-1β, IL-6, IL-8, and TNF-α) have the potential to induce multiple autocrine and paracrine effects in the chronic inflammatory and wound healing phases, as well as a time-dependent switch in cytokine secretion from acute to chronic phase phenotype [31]. Uptake of apoptotic neutrophils can stimulate macrophages to release mediators that suppress the inflammatory response, e.g. TGF-β, IL-10 and prostaglandin E_2 (PGE_2) [39]. In bridging the innate and adaptive immune response, macrophages can fuse to become multinucleated giant cells and act as APCs to activate leukocytes which are responsible for the adaptive immune response, e.g. through expression of co-stimulatory molecules that are essential for T-cell activation [27,37].

Beside their function as phagocytes and APCs, it is assumed that macrophages play a prominent role in a successful wound healing response through the synthesis of growth factors such as TGF-β, basic fibroblast growth factor (bFGF), platelet-derived growth factor (PDGF), and vascular endothelial growth factor (VEGF), which promote cell proliferation and synthesis of ECM molecules by resident cells [10,35]. TGF-β is a potential stimulator of ECM production, promoting both fibronectin and collagen synthesis in fibroblasts, and decreasing collagen breakdown. With respect to angiogenesis, bFGF is probably one of the major growth factor families involved, being strongly mitogenic for endothelial cells, directing their migration and proliferation. PDGF recruits neutrophils and monocytes, stimulates the activation of macrophages, and induces expression of TGF-β [33]. Production of VEGF by cells present in the damaged microenvironment is induced by both IL-1β and IL-10, stimulating vasculogenesis and angiogenesis [38].

3.5.2. *Macrophage phenotypes*

Macrophages show remarkable plasticity, which allows them to efficiently respond to environmental signals and change their phenotype concordantly. The different macrophage phenotypes are identified and distinguished according to markers present at the cell surface and profiles of cytokine and gene expression. Both the acute and the chronic inflammatory response can markedly alter the physiology of macrophages [44]. Furthermore, surface topology and molecular organization of biomaterials affects macrophages, and the cell-surface interaction can change quantity and identity of secreted pro-inflammatory cytokines and chemokines, gene expression patterns, and downstream remodeling events [47].

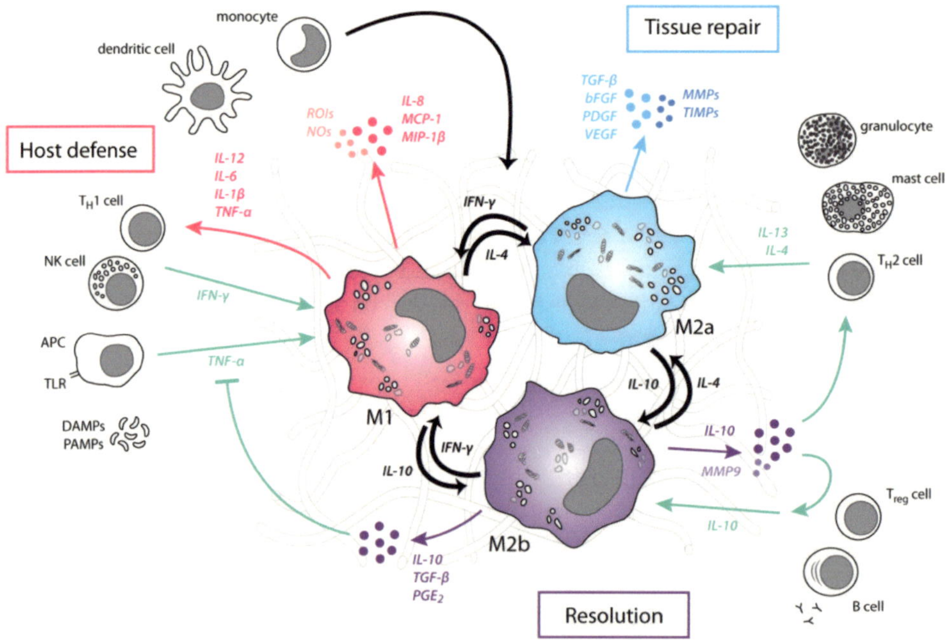

Figure 3. Schematic representation of macrophage plasticity. Macrophages can adapt their phenotype in response to environmental cues provided via paracrine or autocrine signaling. Illustrated are extremities within the continuous spectrum of macrophage polarization states ('M1', 'M2a', 'M2b') (adapted from [11,44]). Illustration by Anthal Smits.

Two main macrophage phenotypes have been suggested, classified as "M1" and "M2", mirroring the T helper 1 (T_H1) and T helper 2 (T_H2) cell polarization [48,49] (figure 3). The pro-inflammatory, cytotoxic macrophage phenotype, signified as M1, is characterized by the promotion of pathogen killing and is associated with classic signs of inflammation. These classically activated macrophages are involved in killing intracellular pathogens, up-regulation of pro-inflammatory cytokines, inhibition of anti-inflammatory cytokines, and synthesis of oxygen and nitrogen radicals, making them a crucial part of host defense [10,11,44,45,47]. Their activation is stimulated by pro-inflammatory cytokines, e.g. IFN-γ (released by T_H1 cells or NK cells), TNF-α (released by APCs), IL-1β, IL-6, and IL-12, but also by PAMPs, DAMPs, hypoxia, and abnormal matrix, such as pathological collagen deposition [11,29]. Activated M1 macrophages also secrete pro-inflammatory cytokines themselves, i.e. TNF-α, IL-1, IL-6, IL-12, and IL-23, inducing T_H1 cell responses [45]. Furthermore, they produce low levels of anti-inflammatory IL-10 [29,48]. Macrophages activated by a biomaterial are typically of the M1 phenotype and can promote the invasion of additional inflammatory cells by secreting chemokines such as IL-8, MCP-1, and MIP-1β. They also secrete degradative enzymes and display high phagocytic activity [11]. Via the production of a variety of enzymes that degrade ECM components, such as matrix metalloproteinases (MMPs), collagenase, and elastase, M1 macrophages are crucial in matrix destruction and tissue reorganization, allowing them to quickly migrate through injured tissues [45]. However, prolonged activation of M1 macrophages can lead to tissue damage.

Immuno-regulation, tissue repair, and constructive tissue regeneration are promoted by the anti-inflammatory macrophage phenotype, signified as M2. These macrophages inhibit pro-inflammatory cytokine secretion, promote anti-inflammatory cytokine secretion, and up-regulate mannose receptors which are necessary for FBGC-formation and play a role in matrix remodeling [10,47]. This alternative macrophage activation is stimulated by the release of IL-4 and IL-13 by T_H2 cells, cytokines (e.g. IL-10, TGF-β), glucocorticoids, and apoptotic cells [29,35,50]. In contrast to M1 macrophages, M2 macrophages typically produce high levels of IL-10 and low levels of IL-12, leading to T_H2 cell responses [45,48]. These macrophages show reparative actions by promoting angiogenesis, production of pro-fibrogenic factors resulting in enhanced fibrinogenic activity of fibroblasts, over-expression of certain ECM proteins, and differential secretion of MMPs and tissue inhibitors of metalloproteinases (TIMPs) [10,49].

The M2 phenotype can be divided into two subsets, i.e. wound healing (M2a) and regulatory (M2b) macrophages (figure 3) [11,44]. Wound healing macrophages are mainly triggered by IL-4, released by mast cells, granulocytes, or T_H2 cells, which down-regulates pro-inflammatory cytokine secretion by the macrophage. These macrophages promote wound healing processes by contributing to the production of ECM proteins, such as fibronectin, and by the activation of fibroblasts [11]. Although M2a macrophages exert anti-inflammatory activities, they are not capable of down-regulating immune responses. Regulatory macrophages are triggered by a variety of signals, e.g. IL-10, apoptotic cells, immune complexes, and glucocorticoids. Their main task is to limit inflammation and to dampen the immune response, restoring homeostasis while limiting the development of fibrosis [11,49]. They achieve this by releasing high levels of IL-10, which is a very potent immune-suppressive cytokine acting through inhibition of IL-6 signaling and NF-κB activation [38].

Macrophages seem to retain their plasticity and respond to environmental signals. The activation of stimulus-specific transcription factors is likely to dictate the functionalized polarization of macrophages through effects on inducible gene promoters with specific features, translating signals in the microenvironment of the macrophage into a polarized phenotype [51]. The progression from an inflammatory macrophage phenotype (M1) toward a more regenerative/anti-inflammatory macrophage phenotype (M2a/b) correlates with a change in cytokine secretion profile by T helper cells changing from type 1 (T_H1) to type 2 (T_H2), promoting resolution of the inflammation [8]. The phenotype of a macrophage population can change over time but a single biochemical marker to distinguish between populations has not been identified [44]. It is suggested that macrophages possess a continuum of phenotypes for distinct biological functions, showing overlap of biomarkers and functions for M1 and M2 macrophages [45]. The primary three macrophage phenotypes suggested here, i.e. pro-inflammatory, wound healing, and regulatory, can blend into a continuum of secondary phenotypes that serve a wide variety of functions [44]. It is also unknown whether uncommitted macrophages are recruited to the site of scaffold remodeling and subsequently stimulated to differentiate locally or whether phenotype-committed macrophages are selectively recruited to sites of remodeling, depending on the antigens or substrates that are present [47]. The molecular determinants that precisely control macrophage plasticity, e.g. switching between polarization states, are to a large extend unknown, which makes targeting transcription factors for modulatory aims a challenge [51].

3.5.3. Lymphocytes

In the chronic phase of the inflammatory response, lymphocytes appear at the site of inflammation together with macrophages [31]. Lymphocytes play a role in the adaptive immune response, involving major histocompatibility complex (MHC) class I and class II molecules, expressed on the surface of APCs, and recognized by receptors and co-receptors on T cells. In general, MHC class I molecules present peptide antigens derived from pathogens that replicate intracellularly and whose proteins are present in the cytosol of the cell, to cytotoxic $CD8^+$ T cells. MHC class II molecules present peptides obtained from pathogens and their products that are present in the extracellular milieu and have been taken up into the endocytic vesicles of phagocytic cells, to helper $CD4^+$ T cells. The $CD4^+$ T_H1 cells and cytolytic $CD8^+$ T cells migrate to the infected tissue, where they activate macrophages to kill antigen-bearing pathogens. This response is referred to as the cell-mediated immune response. On the other hand, $CD4^+$ T_H2 cells and B-lymphocytes (B cells) perform their functions in the lymphoid tissues, where T_H2 cells activate B cells to produce antibodies against target antigens, called the humoral immune response [29,30].

Accumulation of T cells is associated with the expression of MCP-1 few days after injury, with production of the chemokines interferon-γ-inducible protein-10 (IP-10), and monokine induced by interferon-γ (MIG), of which macrophages appear to be a major source [35]. T cells become activated via interactions with APCs, i.e. macrophages, DCs, and B cells, which present processed antigens bound to MHC molecules on their cell surfaces. Additional co-stimulatory interactions with specific molecules on APCs are required upon lymphocyte activation, i.e. interaction between CD80 or CD86 on the APC and CD28 on the T-cell surface [30]. Characteristics of activation include expression of specific cell surface markers and production

http://dx.doi.org/10.5772/54354

of the classic activation cytokines IL-2 and IFN-γ [31]. T cells will undergo clonal expansion by proliferation and up- or down-regulation of their effector function. When T cells are activated but not co-stimulated, they become anergic, a mechanism for suppression of inappropriate immune reactivity. Via this mechanism, cells that may have been inappropriately activated, undergo apoptosis, and are removed by macrophages. For example, anti-inflammatory IL-10 induces antigen specific anergy of T helper cells, helping in the prevention of excessive inflammation [31].

Macrophages and lymphocytes are capable of activating each other through direct and indirect mechanisms [31]. Activated T cells induce production of pro-inflammatory cytokines IL-1β, TNF-α, and IL-6, and chemokines IL-8, MCP-1, and MIP-1β by macrophages in a contact-dependent manner. T cells promote the adhesion of macrophages to biomaterials and their subsequent fusion, as well as biomaterial-dependent cytokine production, having consequences for the biocompatibility of the biomaterial [31]. NK cells, a lymphocyte subset next to T and B cells, are potential sources of IL-4 and IL-13 and may promote the FBR by inducing macrophage fusion into FBGCs [31].

3.6. Inflammatory resolution and wound healing

After the inflammatory stimulus has been eliminated, the ongoing inflammatory response must be resolved to avoid excessive tissue damage and to initiate the healing process. During the resolution of inflammation, further infiltration of leukocytes is prevented and removal of debris from the inflamed site is promoted, thereby restoring tissue homeostasis [39]. The process of resolution is an active process requiring signals that turn off neutrophil infiltration and, at the same time, promote the uptake and clearance of apoptotic cells and debris. Lipid mediators, e.g. lipoxins and resolvins, seem to have a key role in this process, and the resolution of inflammation is accompanied by an active switch in the types of lipid mediator found at the inflamed site [28,39]. During the inflammatory response, prostaglandins and cytokines that amplify inflammation are generated by various cell types, including neutrophils, monocytes, and macrophages. Following this, PGE_2 and prostaglandin D2 (PGD_2) gradually promote the synthesis of anti-inflammatory and pro-resolving mediators, such as lipoxins. Another mechanism of inflammatory resolution is inactivation of chemokines through cleavage by MMPs, terminating inflammatory cell influx [39].

The initiation of wound healing is generally marked by the arrival of fibroblasts for the production of ECM proteins, and of endothelial cells for angiogenesis. They occur within the 3 to 5 days of monocyte invasion and activation of resident macrophages, resulting in the formation of granulation tissue [27]. Granulation tissue formation is a wound healing response in which fibroblasts and endothelial cells recruited by macrophages, invade and proliferate within the inflamed tissue in an attempt to establish structure and homeostasis at the local inflammation site [11,27]. Granulation tissue consists of a dense population of macrophages, fibroblasts, and neovasculature embedded within a loose matrix of fibronectin, collagen, and hyaluronic acid, serving as an intermediary substrate [31,33]. Fibroblasts are mesenchyme-derived cells with their primary function being to produce and remodel the local ECM, providing scaffolding and framework to repair the wound [3]. The persistent presence of macrophages within the granulation tissue ensures constant remodeling of the tissue matrix and constant recruitment of fibroblasts and endothelial cells [27].

The outcome of tissue regeneration or scar formation, i.e. fibrosis, is dependent on the duration of the chronic response that contributes to cytokine production and formation of granulation tissue [8]. Fibrosis is the excessive deposition of matrix components that results in destruction of normal tissue architecture and compromised tissue function and arises from a continuous injuring stimulus, excessive synthesis or decreased degradation [33]. Synthetic and degradative functions of fibroblasts are controlled and regulated by signals from the matrix, as well as leukocyte cytokines and growth factors, wherein macrophages and their phenotype play an important role [27,52].

4. The foreign body response to biomaterials

The implantation of a biomaterial can intensify the inflammatory response by inducing a foreign body response (FBR). The FBR at the tissue-material interface is composed of macrophages and foreign body giant cells (FBGCs) and forms the end-stage response of the inflammatory and wound healing responses following implantation of a medical device, prosthesis, or biomaterial [10,29]. Typically, within 2-4 weeks the foreign material is encapsulated within an almost avascular, fibrous connective tissue, depending on the porosity of the biomaterial [52]. The FBR is characterized by the presence of macrophages and FBGCs together with the components of granulation tissue. Macrophages and FBGCs are believed to exert critical effects on both tissue and implanted material, e.g. degradation, and chemokine and cytokine production [31].

4.1. Macrophage fusion

Macrophages develop integrins, which play a major role in the adhesion of macrophages to a biomaterial and in the IL-4-induced macrophage fusion to form FBGCs [10]. Macrophage-integrin binding to the protein layer on the biomaterial surface provides intracellular signals that can modulate macrophage behavior, such as cytoskeletal rearrangements and the formation of adhesion structures, called podosomes. There is extensive interplay between intracellular signaling molecules activated by integrin binding and cytoskeletal proteins. Disruption of the adhesion signals promotes anoikis, i.e. apoptosis induced by cell detachment from its supportive matrix. A hypothesis is that macrophage fusion to form FBGCs is an escape mechanism to avoid apoptosis [10].

Macrophages adhere to the surface of an implanted biomaterial when they are unable to phagocytose the material due to a large material-to-cell size ratio. Phagocytosis of large, non-degradable implanted materials usually does not occur due to the size disparity. When the particle size in phagocytosis >5 μm, frustrated phagocytosis may occur instead, a process in which ROIs are secreted aimed to degrade the biomaterial [10,29]. Macrophages fuse with other macrophages to form multinucleated FBGCs, associated with chronic inflammation arising from the persistent presence of a foreign body. These multinucleated cells are characteristic of granulomatous inflammation and show abundant chromatin with scattered nuclei in an irregular pattern [31]. The fusion of macrophages to form FBGCs serves to prolong the life span of these frustrated macrophages, allowing continued release of cytokines and growth factors [27].

Lymphocytes also seem to play a critical role in the FBR. They have been observed to associate with adherent macrophages and FBGCs, and enhance macrophage adhesion and fusion, while the presence of macrophages stimulates lymphocytes to proliferate [31]. Dependent on the biomaterial, next to macrophages, lymphocytes themselves also produce inflammatory mediators [10,31]. Lymphocytes enhance adherent macrophage and FBGC activation in terms of inflammatory cytokine production via paracrine (indirect) and juxtacrine (direct) means [10]. T cells have been demonstrated to promote macrophage adhesion and fusion via paracrine effects, however, close association of lymphocytes and macrophages also suggests direct signaling which has been shown to dominate at later time points of their interaction [11].

4.2. Macrophage phenotype in fusion

The phenotype of the macrophages involved has been shown to play an important role in biomaterial scaffold remodeling [10,11,52]. The fusion of adherent macrophages to FBGCs is typically associated with a phenotype switch of the macrophages over time, going from a more pro-inflammatory activation state (M1) to a more anti-inflammatory activation state (M2). M1 versus M2 macrophage activation has led to morphological variants of multinucleated giant cells *in vitro* [10]. The M2 activation cytokines IL-4 and IL-13 promote macrophage fusion and the formation of large FBGCs with randomly arranged nuclei and high degrees of cytoplasmic spreading, while the M1 activation cytokine IFN-γ induces more limited degrees of macrophage fusion with resultant Langerhans-type giant cells. However, the activation state of fusing macrophages is neither M1-like, nor M2-like but rather an in-between state in the continuous spectrum of macrophage polarization. This suggests that biomaterial activation is unique in the process of inflammation [10,11].

The fusion of M2-activated macrophages into FBGCs is stimulated by IL-4 and IL-13, assumed to be secreted by activated T cells [11]. The precise origins of FBGC-inducing cytokines at the implant site remain unclear, with T_H2 cells, NK cells, eosinophils, basophils, and mast cells as possible candidates [31]. Both IL-4 and IL-13 were found to up-regulate mannose receptors on fusing macrophages, which mediate endo- and phagocytosis, with localization of the receptor at the fusion interface [10]. MCP-1 is also involved in FBGC formation though not by recruiting cells but rather by guiding macrophage chemotaxis toward each other [10,11].

Biomaterial-adherent macrophages and FBGCs seem to show combined action of biomaterial degradation and down-modulation of pro-inflammatory mediators. Perhaps the presence of macrophage fusion and FBGC formation on biomaterial surfaces represents host down-modulation of pro-inflammatory cytokine production, possibly via phagocytic removal of macrophages actively releasing these cytokines [31]. Next to promoting M2 phenotype and macrophage fusion, IL-4 prevents apoptosis of biomaterial-adherent macrophages by inducing shedding of TNF-α receptor I, preventing this TNF-α-mediated process [11].

4.3. Biomaterial degradation and fibrosis

Macrophages and FBGCs mediate biomaterial degradation by concentrating phagocytic and oxidative activities at the interface between the cell and the biomaterial. During frustrated phagocytosis, macrophages and FBGCs release degradative mediators such as ROIs, degradative enzymes, and acid into the privileged zone between the cell membrane and the biomaterial surface such that immediate buffering or inhibition of these mediators is delayed or reduced [10]. In this process the phagocytic activity of macrophages decreases, while their degradative capacity increases [11].

FBGCs have the potential to be responsive to cellular signals via cell surface receptor expression as well as actively participate in the inflammatory response through the production of cytokines [10]. They produce anti-inflammatory cytokines, e.g. IL-10, which may be counter-regulated by the proteolytic and pro-oxidant microenvironment. Additionally, FBGCs are thought to release pro-fibrotic factors, e.g. TGF-β and PDGF, which trigger the action of fibroblasts and endothelial cells. Continuous action of FBGCs is assumed to result in prolonged fibroblast activation and excessive biomaterial-associated matrix deposition, leading to impaired wound healing and excessive fibrosis [11]. Therefore, FBGC formation has appeared to be an undesirable phenomenon with a negative impact on biocompatibility, producing cytokines that bias wound healing cells toward a fibrogenic phenotype [31]. Efforts in the design of the biomaterial for *in situ* tissue engineering of heart valves should enhance the biocompatibility, limiting macrophage fusion into FBGCs. Surface chemistry-dependent modulation of the protein layer may enable different receptor binding and signaling in the immune cells leading to altered cellular responses, promoting wound healing while sustaining implant function [11].

5. Modulating the immune response

The implantation of any biomaterial initiates an immune response. However, the extent and severity of this response can be modulated by adapting scaffold properties. As described in the previous sections, the immune response is a multi-phased cascade involving many different components. The combined effect of these components will determine the end-stage outcome of the immune response, ranging from pathological fibrotic repair to fully functional regeneration of the original tissue. By interfering with specific elements within this inflammatory cascade, the downstream outcome can be drastically affected, for better or for worse. In this plane of intersection, immuno-modulating scaffolds for *in situ* tissue engineered heart valves are being developed. The development of such a 'smart' scaffold bridges multiple length-scales and is dependent on a multitude of scaffold features. Biological scaffolds inherently come with a natural architecture and a cocktail of signaling components, which would be difficult to replicate with a synthetic counterpart. Synthetic scaffolds, on the other hand, offer a more dedicated control of individual elements in comparison to biological scaffolds. Either scaffold type can be modified within its own framework. There is a legion of possibilities to modify scaffolds over various interdependent scales, ranging from tuning biomaterial surface chemistry, scaffold architecture and mechanical properties, to the incorporation of bioactives and targeting of specific cell types. Apart from the scaffold itself, the implantation procedure contributes to the immune response. The method of implantation affects the degree of inflammation [27], and as such should be taken into account in scaffold design.

5.1. Biomaterial surface engineering

Biocompatibility and thrombogeneity are particularly important during the onset of the immune response. Immediately after implantation, blood proteins precipitate onto the biomaterial surface, creating an inflammatory milieu that determines the activation of the complement and coagulation cascades. Biomaterial surface chemistry influences the proteins that adsorb, which mediates subsequent interactions with immune cells and may lead to their activation [8]. Factors that affect the amount, composition, and conformation of proteins within the initial layer include the hydrophobicity/hydrophilicity of a surface, as well as its charge and the distribution of charged groups [32]. Incorporation of anti-fouling properties into the biomaterial surface has proven an efficient method to block non-specific protein binding and promote specific biomolecule-binding. This is typically achieved by modifications with hydrophilic polymers, such as poly(ethylene glycol) (PEG), that act as molecular spacers and create a hydrophilic microenvironment that can resist non-specific protein adsorption and cell binding [53].

Biomaterial surface topography and micron-scale architecture can modulate the cell-scaffold interactions that influence immune cell activation, alignment, infiltration, and fusion. Variations in surface roughness and topography affect cell adhesion, morphology, and cytokine secretion. The cell-surface interaction can change quantity and identity of secreted pro-inflammatory cytokines and chemokines, the gene expression pattern, and downstream remodeling events [11,47]. For example, one of the key cellular immune response mechanisms which can be targeted for control of biocompatibility is the mechanism for macrophage adhesion [31,54]. Macrophage fusion on biomaterial surfaces is material dependent, indicating that the surface must have an appropriate array of adsorbed proteins in order for adherent cells to adopt the necessary phenotype to fuse into FBGCs [10]. Furthermore, surface roughness of electrospun fibers has been shown to affect blood activation [55], illustrating the importance of appropriate surface engineering, in particular in the early phases of inflammation.

5.2. Scaffold architecture

Cell infiltration into the scaffold is one of the prerequisites for succesful tissue regeneration. It was shown that early infiltration of immune cells determines the degree of downstream ECM production and remodeling [56]. Cell infiltration is primarily determined by the scaffold architecture, or microstructure. Decellularized homograft/xenograft valves have shown limited cell infiltration, resulting in poor tissue remodeling and even degeneration. In contrast, decellularized *in vitro* tissue-engineered valves have shown fast repopulation with host cells and tissue remodeling following a distinct demarcation line. It has been suggested that this critical difference in cell infiltration is due to a lack of the dense, native-like microstructural arrangement in tissue-engineered valves, as opposed to native valves [57].

For synthetic scaffolds, the importance of scaffold architecture is even more evident. In contrast to natural ECM, cells are typically unable to rapidly break down synthetic biomaterials in order to migrate. Therefore, cell infiltration into a synthetic scaffold is generally dependent on the available pore size, or void space [58,59]. Apart from overall cell infiltration, the pore size can also affect cell phenotype. For example, pore size has shown to be an important factor in the degree of macrophage fusion and material encapsulation. Porous implants with uniform spherical pores of 30-40 μm were shown to elicit healing with minimal fibrosis, high vascularity, and a higher M2/M1 macrophage ratio [52]. It has to be noted however, that the optimal pore size is not generic and has to be tailored to the application.

Synthetic scaffolds for heart valve tissue engineering typically consist of nano- or microfibers, with a high surface area-to-volume ratio. This fibrous architecture dictates the behavior of infiltrating cells. In addition to the void space, the fiber diameter and inter-fiber distance determine cell adhesion, spreading and proliferation [60,61]. Fiber diameter has also shown to affect platelet adhesion and coagulation activation [55]. Fiber alignment guides cell orientation and migration via contact guidance. Furthermore, it was shown that fiber alignment enhanced cell infiltration into a nanofibrous PLLA scaffold [62]. Novel processing techniques to produce fibrous 3D scaffolds with adjustable void space and/or aligned fibers (e.g. low-temperature electrospinning [63]), enhance the degrees of freedom in scaffold modification via 3D architecture (figure 4). For complex structures, such as the aortic valve, multi-layered scaffolds might be required to achieve suitable local cues [59,64].

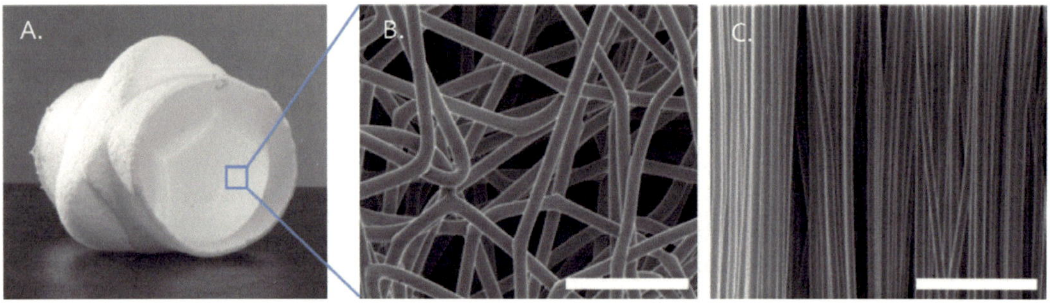

Figure 4. (A) Photograph of an electrospun poly(ε-caprolactone) heart valve demonstrating 3D valve architecture, and scanning electron micrographs of its microstructure showing either random (B) or aligned microfibers (C) (scalebar = 100 μm; images courtesy of M. Simonet and G. Argento).

5.3. Mechanical properties and degradation rate

Heart valve scaffolds require appropriate mechanical properties to endure the cyclic stresses and strains exerted by the hemodynamic environment. However, next to proper functioning in the hemodynamic environment, scaffold mechanical properties play an important role on the cellular level. The macromechanical properties are determined by the intrinsic material properties, the scaffold architecture and the degradation rate. The intrinsic material properties (e.g. stiffness) and the scaffold architecture (e.g. anisotropy) determine the local stresses and strains experienced by the cell. It is well recognized that mechanical conditioning is an important stimulus for ECM production and remodeling. It has been hypothesized that polymeric scaffolds can divert loads from the cells, so-called 'cell shielding', resulting in hampered ECM production. Furthermore, the scaffold or matrix stiffness can modulate the differentiation of cells into pathological phenotypes, e.g. osteoblastic or myofibroblastic, in response to mechanical and biochemical cues [5]. Therefore, efficient transduction of loads from the biomaterial to the cells is crucial. Elastomers typically exhibit adequate mechanotransduction properties, making them a favorable class of materials for application as synthetic scaffolds [25].

Mechanical integrity of the scaffold is dependent on the degradation rate of the material, or rather on the balance between material degradation and ECM production. Accelerated material degradation can result in mechanical instability and valve failure. On the other hand, long-term presence of the biomaterial results in prolonged macrophage activity. Macrophages typically persist at the implantation site until the biomaterial is completely resorbed. When uncontrolled, this may lead to excessive chronic inflammation resulting in fibrosis, calcification, and/or degeneration. Mineralization of synthetic or biologic scaffolds is end-stage pathology, generally irreversible and untreatable. This underlines the importance of timely degradation of the biomaterial. Apart from proper material selection, degradation rate of polymers is tunable by varying copolymer ratios [3]. Variations in degradation kinetics of materials are also employed for controlled delivery of bioactives, for example by introducing fast-degrading fibrin gel [65] or synthetic or biological microspheres [23,66] into the scaffold.

5.4. Incorporation of bioactives

Throughout the course of the immune response, signaling factors orchestrate the actions of the immune cells. By incorporating bioactive factors into the biomaterial scaffold, the cellular niche can be modulated locally. These biochemical factors can direct local cellular function, or promote recruitment of specific cell types via chemotaxis. Additionally, the crosstalk between immune cells and tissue cells can be enhanced, regulating the healing process [11]. Since these signaling factors play a role in a specific phase of the immune response, spatio-temporal control of growth factor or cytokine release has been the aim for many tissue engineering scaffolds. For example, long-term release of stromal cell-derived factor 1α (SDF-1α) from porous PLGA scaffolds has demonstrated to result in reduced numbers and degranulation of mast cells at the scaffold in a subcutaneous mouse model. This led to downstream alterations in the inflammatory cascade, jumpstarting regeneration with enhanced participation of progenitor cells, increased angiogenesis and decreased fibrosis [67]. De Visscher *et al.* developed heart valves constructed from photo-oxidized bovine pericardium, which were impregnated with SDF-1α in combination with fibronectin to improve the SDF-1α presentation to the cells. Implanted in the pulmonary position in sheep, these valves demonstrated improved homing of primitive cells and normal functioning at 5 months follow-up [68]. Other pro-angiogenic factors, such as VEGF, have shown to play a similar role in vascularization and endothelialization via recruitment of bone marrow-derived circulating cells, with an essential paracrine role for myeloid cells [69]. Injectable hydrogels featuring a sustained release of VEGF, either or not combined with PDGF, have shown to enhance angiogenesis [70,71]. Dual delivery of MCP-1 and VEGF was applied to promote early monocyte invasion as well as angiogenesis. This was shown to increase mature vessel formation via enhanced endothelial and smooth muscle cell recruitment and displayed a trend of macrophage polarization to the M2 type in a time- and dose-dependent manner [66]. MCP-1 has demonstrated to be a potent immune-modulatory factor, leading to successful remodeling and regeneration of a PCL/PLLA blood vessel graft in mice [23]. Decellularized porcine aortic valves coated with a fusion protein of fibronectin and hepatocyte growth factor (HGF) demonstrated modest acceleration of infiltration of tissue cells, particularly in the valve leaflet, after implantation in a dog model [72].

Single extracellular molecules can impact both pro-inflammatory and anti-inflammatory pathways in different cell types participating in the repair response [35]. The shift from pro-inflammatory to anti-inflammatory response is generally mediated by lipoxins, protectins, and resolvins, actively promoting resolution of infection and tissue repair. Lipoxins are arachidonic acid (AA) derivatives generated by lipoxygenases, and stop the influx of neutrophils, promote the uptake of apoptotic neutrophils by macrophages and recruit additional monocytes to help clear away dead cells and tissue debris [28,39]. Incorporation of such bioactive components may enhance the resolution of the inflammatory response, avoiding uncontrolled chronic inflammation. Resolution of inflammation is also mediated by glucocorticoids, which inhibit inflammatory cell activation by withdrawing the synthesis of inflammatory mediators, and promote resolution of inflammation by enhancing anti-inflammatory cytokine release [29,54]. Glucocorticoids have been shown to modulate the phenotype of infiltrating macrophages and lymphocytes and could thus be used locally to regulate the cellular response [54].

An alternative to incorporating specific signaling moieties into a scaffold is to preseed the scaffold with cells that act as natural signaling factories. Cells, typically bone marrow-derived mononuclear cells, harvested from the host are directly seeded into a scaffold, which is subsequently implanted in a single operation. Although the preseeded cells are cleared from the scaffold within several days after implantation, they mediate the immune response via paracrine signaling by secreting a natural cocktail of growth factors and cytokines. This approach has shown prosperous results in clinical trials using synthetic blood vessel grafts [24]. Furthermore, a similar approach using decellularized tissue-engineered heart valves has shown promising short-term results after 4 week implantation in the pulmonary position in non-human primates [73].

Apart from boosting selected signaling molecules, biomaterials can be designed to tether endogenously released factors to promote a regenerative microenvironment. Natural occurring GAGs have been identified to bind and modify inflammatory factors like interleukins and chemokines, e.g. IL-10 [11]. Subtle differences in GAG structure and/or sequence might be sensed by signaling molecules, guiding their interaction with the ECM and mediating their presentation to leukocytes [11]. In this way, physiological cytokine concentrations are ensured, reducing the risk of adverse side-effects. Heparan sulfate is well-recognized as a natural binding site for many growth factors and cytokines, a feature which has been exploited by developing heparin-mimetic peptide nanofibers that are capable of binding growth factors such as VEGF and HGF [74].

Clearly, the use of bioactives or on-the-fly harvestable cells is a powerful tool to create immune-modulating scaffolds. Methods using covalent immobilization of factors [65], microspheres with controlled degradation profiles [66] or hollow-fiber electrospinning techniques [59] enable optimized spatio-temporal control of one or multiple factors. Furthermore, advanced hydrogels have been developed to offer on-demand, remote-controlled release using a magnetic field [75]. With state-of-the-art supramolecular polymers it is possible to engineer cell-responsive substrates [76], offering truly 'smart' scaffolds that can interact with their environment to mediate the host response to the biomaterial.

5.5. Cell recruitment and differentiation

The inflammatory response is mainly driven by colonization of the scaffold by blood-derived cells. The nature of the infiltrating cells and their differentiation were demonstrated of pivotal importance to control the delicate balance between fibrotic or functional regenerated ECM production. Of all the cells involved in the immune response, several cell populations can be identified as target cells for *in situ* heart valve tissue engineering.

Macrophages are the predominant mediators throughout the entire immune response, making them an attractive therapeutic target [77]. Although, the precise nature of macrophage plasticity and polarization has yet to be illuminated, it has been shown that early macrophage phenotype determines the end-stage outcome in various biological matrices. In particular, an increased ratio of M2/M1 macrophages correlates to enhanced remodeling, which is likely mediated by differential attraction of secondary cells [78]. By promoting the M2 phenotype, either via specific recruitment or local polarization, the inflammatory response may instantly be directed towards healing instead of inflammation [48,52]. With the identification of multiple subtypes, it is likely that the various macrophage phenotypes play a critical role throughout the various stages of acute inflammation, the healing phase and the resolution of inflammation (figure 5).

ECM production and remodeling is governed by the attraction of secondary cells to the scaffold, consisting of mature (myo-)fibroblasts and endothelial cells, as well as various stem/progenitor cells, released into the circulation by the bone marrow. Furthermore, it has been suggested that adult valve interstitial cells are continuously replenished via circulating endothelial or mesenchymal cell precursors derived from the bone marrow and subsequently undergo endothelial-to-mesenchymal-transition (EndoMT) [5]. Circulating progenitors, such as endothelial progenitor cells (EPC), can have a significant influence on the inflammatory response [4,12,79]. EPC are hypothesized to be an important target cell for endothelialization. Rapid formation of an endothelium over a scaffold is desirable as it acts as a dynamic and selective barrier by maintaining a nonthrombogenic surface, controlling the transfer of molecules across the layer, and regulating immune and inflammatory reactions. The endothelial layer also interacts with underlying cells to regulate their growth and proliferation [12].

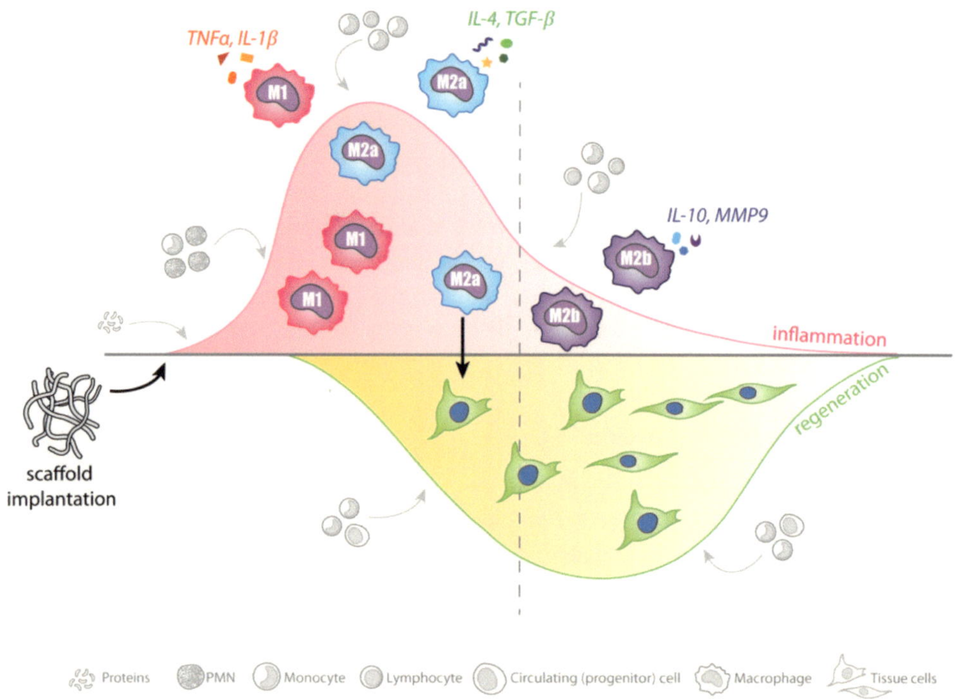

Figure 5. Hypothesized role of the various macrophage polarization states throughout the process of inflammation and tissue regeneration in response to scaffold implantation. Illustration by Anthal Smits.

Mesenchymal stem cells (MSCs) proliferate during the healing phase, directed by cytokines secreted by nearby cells, e.g. activated platelets and macrophages, and by ECM components such as collagen peptides and fibronectin [29]. MSCs produce an immunoprivileged environment by preventing the activation and proliferation of DCs, T cells, macrophages, and PMNs through direct cell-cell interactions and paracrine signaling [8]. Cells derived from immunoprivileged regions have been delivered to promote cell engraftment and protect grafts against autoimmune and allogeneic rejection. These cells secrete a range of factors, eg. TGF-β and IL-10, inducing regulatory T-cell differentiation/expansion, which enhances immuno-protection [8].

Recruitment and adhesion of target cell types can be achieved by offering binding domains on the scaffold, for example using supramolecular building blocks with cell-specific peptide sequences [76,79]. When combined with anti-fouling materials, such as PEG, this results in highly selective substrates.

5.6. Minimally invasive implantation methods

Independent of the biomaterial, the injury incurred during the implantation process will trigger an immune response, due to the disruption of host tissue and induction of cell damage. Besides substantial mortality and morbidity risks, invasive open heart surgery for heart valve replacement causes extensive tissue damage, giving rise to DAMPs, which prime the system for an enhanced immune response [29]. As an alternative, various transvascular, catheter-based techniques, as well as alternative minimally invasive surgical techniques, such as the transapical approach, have been developed [4,80,81]. This has implication for the scaffold design as the scaffold must be crimped and incorporated into a stent. Upon delivery at the valve annulus, the scaffold must also be able to expand properly, be held in place and instantly function within the hemodynamic environment. Transapical valve implantation of preseeded decellularized tissue engineered heart valves into both the aortic and pulmonary position has already proven feasible in pre-clinical models [82,83].

6. Challenges and pitfalls

In situ tissue engineering of heart valves represents a quick, cheap, and on-demand approach. Immunomodulatory scaffolds hold great promise for future application and commercialization. However, some priority challenges remain to be addressed in the translation from bench to bed.

6.1. ECM formation versus fibrosis

One of the main challenges for *in situ* tissue engineering is to stimulate functional ECM formation without inducing fibrosis. To maintain functionality of the valve, rapid ECM formation is required in order to overtake the load-bearing role of the degrading scaffold. However, cells and molecules that are stimulatory for ECM production have been designated as pro-fibrotic mediators. This poses a paradoxal challenge. Macrophage plasticity is a striking example. M2 macrophages have been identified as pro-wound healing cells, promoting ECM production by secretion of IL-4 and TGF-β. On the other hand, both IL-4 and TGF-β are strong inducers of fibrosis if not tightly regulated. Chemokines, such as MCP-1, have been identified as pro-fibrotic mediators by attracting fibrocytes and stimulation of M2 polarization [84,85]. On the other hand, MCP-1 inhibition leads to delayed or inhibited wound healing [86]. Fibrocytes are blood-borne mesenchymal stem cell progenitors with a fibroblast/myofibroblast-like phenotype ($CD34^+/CD45^+$/collagen type I^+) that similarly have been related to both ECM formation and fibrosis. The same holds for EndoMT-derived (myo-)fibroblasts. However, the local activation state of recruited myofibroblasts, rather than the source, determines their ECM remodeling activity. For example, TLR-signaling promotes fibroblasts to differentiate into collagen-producing myofibroblasts [84]. Valvular interstitial cells (VICs) in the adult valve have a quiescent myofibroblast-like phenotype. Regulating the activation state of colonizing myofibroblasts in the scaffold is pivotal in the prevention of fibrosis and obtaining a VIC-like population. The TGF-β pathway is one of the main players in this process. Furthermore, IL-10 has been shown to inhibit fibrosis in numerous animal models [84], underlining that timely resolution of inflammation is one of the main challenges for *in situ* tissue engineering.

6.2. Hemodynamic environment

In cardiovascular *in situ* tissue regeneration, the hemodynamic environment plays a key role by directing cell recruitment and cell differentiation. The mechanical load applied to the heart valves is a powerful regulator of cell phenotype, influencing many cell functions such as orientation, replication, growth factor production, and collagen synthesis [33]. In cardiovascular devices, apoptosis is often induced by shear stress arising from the blood flow [10]. Shear stress also has a significant effect on adhesion of circulating cells to the valve scaffold. Direct intimal binding of cells to the ventricular side of the leaflet is unlikely due to high shear forces during systole. In contrast, end-systolic and diastolic turbulations on the aortic side of the leaflet typically result in low shear stresses that allow for cell adhesion to the scaffold [4].

So far, the exact mechanism behind cell population of heart valve replacements with host cells remains elusive. For blood vessels, animal studies have identified trans-anastomotic ingrowth as the main source of host tissue cells in the scaffold [87]. However, this is most likely an animal model-dependent phenomenon, as it is known that trans-anastomotic ingrowth is very limited in humans [88]. Therefore, the use of humanized animal models or *in vitro* model systems [89] is indispensible in evaluating scaffold performance for future clinical applications.

6.3. Comorbidity and impaired wound healing

Little is known about the effect of the pathological status of a tissue, organ, or patient on the fate of a tissue engineered heart valve. It is reasonable to believe that the pre-existing pathology or existing risk factors would influence wound healing and long-term outcomes of valve implantation. One of the most complicated aspects of designing a replacement scaffold for diseased tissue would be the incorporation of measures which prevent the device from succumbing to the same fate as the diseased tissue it is replacing [12].

Impaired wound healing conditions include advanced age, diabetes mellitus (insulin resistance), vascular diseases (e.g. atherosclerosis), and obesity, in which adipose tissue functions as initiator of the chronic inflammatory response. Diabetic patients have significantly impaired wound healing as they are relatively immunocompromised and have higher blood glucose levels affecting leukocyte function [90]. Diabetes and advanced age are associated with delayed or impaired wound healing through a reduced ability to transition from an M1 to an M2 macrophage phenotype [52]. Malnutrition adversely affects wound healing by prolonging inflammation, inhibiting fibroblast function, and reducing angiogenesis and collagen deposition. For example, carbohydrates are needed for collagen synthesis, and ω-3-fatty acids are needed for modulation of the arachidonic acid pathway, resolving inflammation [90].

The patient's regenerative potential is dependent on age. The concentration of progenitor cells in human blood decreases with age [4]. Furthermore, aging typically leads to impaired angiogenesis and local immunity is altered due to lack of growth factors, increased neutrophil invasion and higher number of mature macrophages. Levels of TGF-β in wounds of elderly are, like fetal, markedly reduced, which is possibly related to reduced scarring with age [35]. Next to regeneration potential, the rate at which the scaffold degrades may also be age-specific due to variations in cell availability.

Any chronic disease which affects the cardio-respiratory system may adversely affect the supply of oxygen and other nutrients required for wound healing. Although hypoxia is one of the chemoattractants for neutrophils and macrophages, oxygen is needed for their optimal function and to allow phagocytosis. Oxygen is also essential for collagen deposition as it acts as a substrate in the hydroxylation of proline and lysine residues. Smoking affects oxygen partial pressures and causes more wound healing complications and it is likely that smoking may also affect immune function and collagen deposition [90].

The use of diseased cells or tissues in humanized animal models or *in vitro* model systems [89] may aid in gaining insight in the effects of comorbidities on valve regeneration.

6.4. Patient heterogeneity

In vivo remodeling of tissue engineered heart valves displays considerable variability among patients, owing to biological heterogeneity among individuals in physiological tissue remodeling potential [5]. This heterogeneity could be a result of mutations or polymorphisms in key proteins central to ECM synthesis and remodeling [2]. The goal is to understand and potentially control human variation in different facets of biomaterial-tissue interaction and the healing process by developing robust or even patient-tailored scaffolds.

To cope with patient-to-patient heterogeneity, an important issue in tissue engineering of aortic heart valves will be the real-time noninvasive and non-destructive assessment of mechanical properties both *in vitro* and *in vivo* to ensure tissue quality and function [5]. The challenge here is to find appropriate methodologies to evaluate the evolving structural remodeling and functionality, especially in a noninvasive manner so that the valve can be followed over time [5]. One way of approaching this issue is developing imaging modalities and discovering new biomarkers of inflammation which would help further understanding of inflammatory diseases and discerning events related to inflammation in heart valve tissue-engineered implants [12]. When applied to engineered heart valves, developed biomarkers should correlate directly with success and failure in order to generate outcome measurements, such as laboratory assays or imaging results that substitute for and reflect the mechanism of a significant clinical event or characteristic, e.g. stenosis, calcification, or infection [5]. An important consideration is whether calcification, the major pathologic process in valve degeneration, will be problematic. Evidence suggests that calcification may not be a major problem as long as the scaffold is ultimately resorbed and/or not intrinsically mineralizable, the interstitial cells are viable, and the ECM is capable of remodeling [5].

For the translation from bench to bed, there must be understanding of the mechanisms involved and development of biomarkers, assays and tools for the assessment of valve regeneration. Surrogate and true endpoints must be defined to characterize and assure the quality of the tissue constructs, and predict outcomes as early as possible [5]. Key targets for characterizing tissue-engineered constructs include tissue composition, cellular gene expression and phenotype, ECM, and other key effectors of tissue remodeling and tissue quality [5].

7. Conclusion

The complexity of the immune response poses a challenging environment for *in situ* tissue engineering of heart valves [46]. Clearly, a better understanding of the underlying pathways appears crucial for controlling the fate of implanted biomaterial scaffolds and modulating inflammatory reactions in such a way as to induce tissue regeneration and remodeling and prevent fibrosis and/or degeneration [12]. Remaining largely unknown are the specifications of the optimal components (i.e. cells, scaffold and potentially biological modulators) and process conditions (mechanical and metabolic) that will facilitate the formation of optimal substitute heart valve tissues, whose function best emulates the structure, function, and extended durability of a natural valve in vivo [5]. However, the prosperous results of synthetic and biological scaffolds so far demonstrate the ground-breaking potential of *in situ* tissue engineering for heart valves.

Acknowledgements

This work was supported by a grant from the Dutch government to the Netherlands Institute for Regenerative Medicine (NIRM, grant No. FES0908). This research forms part of the Project P1.01 iValve of the research program of the BioMedical Materials institute, co-funded by the Dutch Ministry of Economic Affairs, Agriculture and Innovation. The financial contribution of the Nederlandse Hartstichting is gratefully acknowledged.

Author details

S. L. M. van Loon, A. I. P. M. Smits, A. Driessen-Mol, F. P. T. Baaijens and C. V. C. Bouten*

*Address all correspondence to: C.V.C.Bouten@tue.nl

Department of Biomedical Engineering, Eindhoven University of Technology, MB, Eindhoven, The Netherlands

References

[1] El-Hamamsy I, Eryigit Z, Stevens LM, Sarang Z, George R, Clark L, et al. Long-term outcomes after autograft versus homograft aortic root replacement in adults with aortic valve disease: a randomised controlled trial. Lancet 2010 Aug 14;376(9740):524-31.

[2] Mendelson K, Schoen FJ. Heart valve tissue engineering: concepts, approaches, progress, and challenges. Ann Biomed Eng 2006 Dec;34(12):1799-819.

[3] Bouten CV, Dankers PY, Driessen-Mol A, Pedron S, Brizard AM, Baaijens FP. Substrates for cardiovascular tissue engineering. Adv Drug Deliv Rev 2011 Apr 30;63(4-5):221-41.

[4] Mol A, Smits AI, Bouten CV, Baaijens FP. Tissue engineering of heart valves: advances and current challenges. Expert Rev Med Devices 2009 May;6(3):259-75.

[5] Schoen FJ. Heart valve tissue engineering: quo vadis? Curr Opin Biotechnol 2011 Oct; 22(5):698-705.

[6] Sacks MS, Schoen FJ, Mayer JE. Bioengineering challenges for heart valve tissue engineering. Annu Rev Biomed Eng 2009;11:289-313.

[7] Breuer CK, Mettler BA, Anthony T, Sales VL, Schoen FJ, Mayer JE. Application of tissue-engineering principles toward the development of a semilunar heart valve substitute. Tissue Eng 2004 Nov;10(11-12):1725-36.

[8] Boehler RM, Graham JG, Shea LD. Tissue engineering tools for modulation of the immune response. Biotechniques 2011 Oct;51(4):239-40, 242, 244.

[9] Mol A, Driessen NJ, Rutten MC, Hoerstrup SP, Bouten CV, Baaijens FP. Tissue engineering of human heart valve leaflets: a novel bioreactor for a strain-based conditioning approach. Ann Biomed Eng 2005 Dec;33(12):1778-88.

[10] Anderson JM, Rodriguez A, Chang DT. Foreign body reaction to biomaterials. Semin Immunol 2008 Apr;20(2):86-100.

[11] Franz S, Rammelt S, Scharnweber D, Simon JC. Immune responses to implants - a review of the implications for the design of immunomodulatory biomaterials. Biomaterials 2011 Oct;32(28):6692-709.

[12] Simionescu A, Schulte JB, Fercana G, Simionescu DT. Inflammation in cardiovascular tissue engineering: the challenge to a promise: a minireview. Int J Inflam 2011;2011:958247.

[13] Badylak SF. The extracellular matrix as a biologic scaffold material. Biomaterials 2007 Sep;28(25):3587-93.

[14] Weber B, Emmert MY, Schoenauer R, Brokopp C, Baumgartner L, Hoerstrup SP. Tissue engineering on matrix: future of autologous tissue replacement. Semin Immunopathol 2011 May;33(3):307-15.

[15] Keane TJ, Londono R, Turner NJ, Badylak SF. Consequences of ineffective decellularization of biologic scaffolds on the host response. Biomaterials 2012 Feb;33(6):1771-81.

[16] Klopsch C, Steinhoff G. Tissue-engineered devices in cardiovascular surgery. Eur Surg Res 2012;49(1):44-52.

[17] Schoen FJ, Levy RJ. Calcification of tissue heart valve substitutes: progress toward understanding and prevention. Ann Thorac Surg 2005 Mar;79(3):1072-80.

[18] Dijkman PE, Driessen-Mol A, Frese L, Hoerstrup SP, Baaijens FP. Decellularized homologous tissue-engineered heart valves as off-the-shelf alternatives to xeno- and homografts. Biomaterials 2012 Jun;33(18):4545-54.

[19] White JK, Agnihotri AK, Titus JS, Torchiana DF. A stentless trileaflet valve from a sheet of decellularized porcine small intestinal submucosa. Ann Thorac Surg 2005 Aug;80(2): 704-7.

[20] Hoerstrup SP, Sodian R, Daebritz S, Wang J, Bacha EA, Martin DP, et al. Functional living trileaflet heart valves grown in vitro. Circulation 2000 Nov 7;102(19 Suppl 3):III44-III49.

[21] Schmidt D, Dijkman PE, Driessen-Mol A, Stenger R, Mariani C, Puolakka A, et al. Minimally-invasive implantation of living tissue engineered heart valves: a comprehensive approach from autologous vascular cells to stem cells. J Am Coll Cardiol 2010 Aug 3;56(6):510-20.

[22] Pektok E, Nottelet B, Tille JC, Gurny R, Kalangos A, Moeller M, et al. Degradation and healing characteristics of small-diameter poly(epsilon-caprolactone) vascular grafts in the rat systemic arterial circulation. Circulation 2008 Dec 9;118(24):2563-70.

[23] Roh JD, Sawh-Martinez R, Brennan MP, Jay SM, Devine L, Rao DA, et al. Tissue-engineered vascular grafts transform into mature blood vessels via an inflammation-mediated process of vascular remodeling. Proc Natl Acad Sci U S A 2010 Mar 9;107(10): 4669-74.

[24] Hibino N, McGillicuddy E, Matsumura G, Ichihara Y, Naito Y, Breuer C, et al. Late-term results of tissue-engineered vascular grafts in humans. J Thorac Cardiovasc Surg 2010 Feb;139(2):431-6, 436.

[25] Wu W, Allen RA, Wang Y. Fast-degrading elastomer enables rapid remodeling of a cell-free synthetic graft into a neoartery. Nat Med 2012 Jul;18(7):1148-53.

[26] Yokota T, Ichikawa H, Matsumiya G, Kuratani T, Sakaguchi T, Iwai S, et al. In situ tissue regeneration using a novel tissue-engineered, small-caliber vascular graft without cell seeding. J Thorac Cardiovasc Surg 2008 Oct;136(4):900-7.

[27] Gonzales-Simon A, Eniola-Adefeso O. Host Response to Biomaterials. In: Bhatia S, editor. Engineering Biomaterials for Regenerative Medicine. 1 ed. Cambridge: Springer New York; 2012. p. 143-59.

[28] Barton GM. A calculated response: control of inflammation by the innate immune system. J Clin Invest 2008 Feb;118(2):413-20.

[29] Norton LW, Babensee JE. Innate and Adaptive Immune Responses in Tissue Engineering. In: Meyer U, Handschel J, Wiesmann HP, Meyer T, editors. Fundamentals of Tissue Engineering and Regenerative Medicine. Springer Berlin Heidelberg; 2009. p. 721-47.

[30] Parham P. The Immune System. 2 ed. Garland Science; 2005.

[31] Anderson JM, McNally AK. Biocompatibility of implants: lymphocyte/macrophage interactions. Semin Immunopathol 2011 May;33(3):221-33.

[32] Ekdahl KN, Lambris JD, Elwing H, Ricklin D, Nilsson PH, Teramura Y, et al. Innate immunity activation on biomaterial surfaces: a mechanistic model and coping strategies. Adv Drug Deliv Rev 2011 Sep 16;63(12):1042-50.

[33] Mutsaers SE, Bishop JE, McGrouther G, Laurent GJ. Mechanisms of tissue repair: from wound healing to fibrosis. Int J Biochem Cell Biol 1997 Jan;29(1):5-17.

[34] Nilsson B, Ekdahl KN, Mollnes TE, Lambris JD. The role of complement in biomaterial-induced inflammation. Mol Immunol 2007 Jan;44(1-3):82-94.

[35] Eming SA, Hammerschmidt M, Krieg T, Roers A. Interrelation of immunity and tissue repair or regeneration. Semin Cell Dev Biol 2009 Jul;20(5):517-27.

[36] von Hundelshausen P, Weber C. Platelets as immune cells: bridging inflammation and cardiovascular disease. Circ Res 2007 Jan 5;100(1):27-40.

[37] Tsirogianni AK, Moutsopoulos NM, Moutsopoulos HM. Wound healing: immunological aspects. Injury 2006 Apr;37 Suppl 1:S5-12.

[38] Grimstad O, Sandanger O, Ryan L, Otterdal K, Damaas JK, Pukstad B, et al. Cellular sources and inducers of cytokines present in acute wound fluid. Wound Repair Regen 2011 May;19(3):337-47.

[39] Soehnlein O, Lindbom L. Phagocyte partnership during the onset and resolution of inflammation. Nat Rev Immunol 2010 Jun;10(6):427-39.

[40] Harris HE, Raucci A. Alarmin(g) news about danger: workshop on innate danger signals and HMGB1. EMBO Rep 2006 Aug;7(8):774-8.

[41] Ziegler-Heitbrock L, Ancuta P, Crowe S, Dalod M, Grau V, Hart DN, et al. Nomenclature of monocytes and dendritic cells in blood. Blood 2010 Oct 21;116(16):e74-e80.

[42] Shi C, Pamer EG. Monocyte recruitment during infection and inflammation. Nat Rev Immunol 2011 Nov;11(11):762-74.

[43] Shantsila E, Wrigley B, Tapp L, Apostolakis S, Montoro-Garcia S, Drayson MT, et al. Immunophenotypic characterization of human monocyte subsets: possible implications for cardiovascular disease pathophysiology. J Thromb Haemost 2011 May;9(5):1056-66.

[44] Mosser DM, Edwards JP. Exploring the full spectrum of macrophage activation. Nat Rev Immunol 2008 Dec;8(12):958-69.

[45] Kou PM, Babensee JE. Macrophage and dendritic cell phenotypic diversity in the context of biomaterials. J Biomed Mater Res A 2011 Jan;96(1):239-60.

[46] Beghdadi W, Madjene LC, Benhamou M, Charles N, Gautier G, Launay P, et al. Mast cells as cellular sensors in inflammation and immunity. Front Immunol 2011;2:37.

[47] Badylak SF, Valentin JE, Ravindra AK, McCabe GP, Stewart-Akers AM. Macrophage phenotype as a determinant of biologic scaffold remodeling. Tissue Eng Part A 2008 Nov;14(11):1835-42.

[48] Biswas SK, Chittezhath M, Shalova IN, Lim JY. Macrophage polarization and plasticity in health and disease. Immunol Res 2012 Sep;53(1-3):11-24.

[49] Murray PJ, Wynn TA. Protective and pathogenic functions of macrophage subsets. Nat Rev Immunol 2011 Nov;11(11):723-37.

[50] Gordon S, Martinez FO. Alternative activation of macrophages: mechanism and functions. Immunity 2010 May 28;32(5):593-604.

[51] Lawrence T, Natoli G. Transcriptional regulation of macrophage polarization: enabling diversity with identity. Nat Rev Immunol 2011 Nov;11(11):750-61.

[52] Brown BN, Ratner BD, Goodman SB, Amar S, Badylak SF. Macrophage polarization: an opportunity for improved outcomes in biomaterials and regenerative medicine. Biomaterials 2012 May;33(15):3792-802.

[53] Yu Q, Zhang Y, Wang H, Brash J, Chen H. Anti-fouling bioactive surfaces. Acta Biomater 2011 Apr;7(4):1550-7.

[54] Rolfe B, Mooney J, Zhang B, Jahnke S, Le S, Chau Y, et al. The Fibrotic Response to Implanted Biomaterials: Implications for Tissue Engineering. In: Eberli D, editor. Regenerative Medicine and Tissue Engineering - Cells and Biomaterials. InTech; 2011. p. 551-68.

[55] Milleret V, Hefti T, Hall H, Vogel V, Eberli D. Influence of the fiber diameter and surface roughness of electrospun vascular grafts on blood activation. Acta Biomater 2012 Jul 27.

[56] Hibino N, Yi T, Duncan DR, Rathore A, Dean E, Naito Y, et al. A critical role for macrophages in neovessel formation and the development of stenosis in tissue-engineered vascular grafts. FASEB J 2011 Dec;25(12):4253-63.

[57] Dijkman PE. Tissue-engineered heart valves for minimally invasive surgery. PhD thesis. Eindhoven University of Technology, The Netherlands; 2012.

[58] Balguid A, Mol A, van Marion MH, Bank RA, Bouten CV, Baaijens FP. Tailoring fiber diameter in electrospun poly(epsilon-caprolactone) scaffolds for optimal cellular infiltration in cardiovascular tissue engineering. Tissue Eng Part A 2009 Feb;15(2): 437-44.

[59] Szentivanyi A, Chakradeo T, Zernetsch H, Glasmacher B. Electrospun cellular microenvironments: Understanding controlled release and scaffold structure. Adv Drug Deliv Rev 2011 Apr 30;63(4-5):209-20.

[60] Li WJ, Cooper JA, Jr., Mauck RL, Tuan RS. Fabrication and characterization of six electrospun poly(alpha-hydroxy ester)-based fibrous scaffolds for tissue engineering applications. Acta Biomater 2006 Jul;2(4):377-85.

[61] Lowery JL, Datta N, Rutledge GC. Effect of fiber diameter, pore size and seeding method on growth of human dermal fibroblasts in electrospun poly(epsilon-caprolactone) fibrous mats. Biomaterials 2010 Jan;31(3):491-504.

[62] Kurpinski KT, Stephenson JT, Janairo RR, Lee H, Li S. The effect of fiber alignment and heparin coating on cell infiltration into nanofibrous PLLA scaffolds. Biomaterials 2010 May;31(13):3536-42.

[63] Simonet M, Driessen-Mol A, Baaijens FP, Bouten CV. Heart valve tissue regeneration. In: Bosworth L, Downes S, editors. Electrospinning for tissue regeneration.Cambridge: Woodhead Publishing Limited; 2011. p. 202-24.

[64] Pham QP, Sharma U, Mikos AG. Electrospun poly(epsilon-caprolactone) microfiber and multilayer nanofiber/microfiber scaffolds: characterization of scaffolds and measurement of cellular infiltration. Biomacromolecules 2006 Oct;7(10):2796-805.

[65] Chiu LL, Radisic M. Scaffolds with covalently immobilized VEGF and Angiopoietin-1 for vascularization of engineered tissues. Biomaterials 2010 Jan;31(2):226-41.

[66] Jay SM, Shepherd BR, Andrejecsk JW, Kyriakides TR, Pober JS, Saltzman WM. Dual delivery of VEGF and MCP-1 to support endothelial cell transplantation for therapeutic vascularization. Biomaterials 2010 Apr;31(11):3054-62.

[67] Thevenot PT, Nair AM, Shen J, Lotfi P, Ko CY, Tang L. The effect of incorporation of SDF-1alpha into PLGA scaffolds on stem cell recruitment and the inflammatory response. Biomaterials 2010 May;31(14):3997-4008.

[68] De Visscher G, Lebacq A, Mesure L, Blockx H, Vranken I, Plusquin R, et al. The remodeling of cardiovascular bioprostheses under influence of stem cell homing signal pathways. Biomaterials 2010 Jan;31(1):20-8.

[69] Grunewald M, Avraham I, Dor Y, Bachar-Lustig E, Itin A, Jung S, et al. VEGF-induced adult neovascularization: recruitment, retention, and role of accessory cells. Cell 2006 Jan 13;124(1):175-89.

[70] Silva EA, Mooney DJ. Spatiotemporal control of vascular endothelial growth factor delivery from injectable hydrogels enhances angiogenesis. J Thromb Haemost 2007 Mar;5(3):590-8.

[71] Sun Q, Silva EA, Wang A, Fritton JC, Mooney DJ, Schaffler MB, et al. Sustained release of multiple growth factors from injectable polymeric system as a novel therapeutic approach towards angiogenesis. Pharm Res 2010 Feb;27(2):264-71.

[72] Ota T, Sawa Y, Iwai S, Kitajima T, Ueda Y, Coppin C, et al. Fibronectin-hepatocyte growth factor enhances reendothelialization in tissue-engineered heart valve. Ann Thorac Surg 2005 Nov;80(5):1794-801.

[73] Weber B, Scherman J, Emmert MY, Gruenenfelder J, Verbeek R, Bracher M, et al. Injectable living marrow stromal cell-based autologous tissue engineered heart valves:

first experiences with a one-step intervention in primates. Eur Heart J 2011 Nov;32(22): 2830-40.

[74] Mammadov R, Mammadov B, Guler MO, Tekinay AB. Growth factor binding on heparin mimetic peptide nanofibers. Biomacromolecules 2012 Sep 10.

[75] Zhao X, Kim J, Cezar CA, Huebsch N, Lee K, Bouhadir K, et al. Active scaffolds for on-demand drug and cell delivery. Proc Natl Acad Sci U S A 2011 Jan 4;108(1):67-72.

[76] Dankers PY, Harmsen MC, Brouwer LA, van Luyn MJ, Meijer EW. A modular and supramolecular approach to bioactive scaffolds for tissue engineering. Nat Mater 2005 Jul;4(7):568-74.

[77] Koh TJ, DiPietro LA. Inflammation and wound healing: the role of the macrophage. Expert Rev Mol Med 2011;13:e23.

[78] Brown BN, Londono R, Tottey S, Zhang L, Kukla KA, Wolf MT, et al. Macrophage phenotype as a predictor of constructive remodeling following the implantation of biologically derived surgical mesh materials. Acta Biomater 2012 Mar;8(3):978-87.

[79] Fioretta ES, Fledderus JO, Burakowska-Meise EA, Baaijens FP, Verhaar MC, Bouten CV. Polymer-based scaffold designs for in situ vascular tissue engineering: controlling recruitment and differentiation behavior of endothelial colony forming cells. Macromol Biosci 2012 May;12(5):577-90.

[80] Lutter G, Ardehali R, Cremer J, Bonhoeffer P. Percutaneous valve replacement: current state and future prospects. Ann Thorac Surg 2004 Dec;78(6):2199-206.

[81] Walther T, Dewey T, Borger MA, Kempfert J, Linke A, Becht R, et al. Transapical aortic valve implantation: step by step. Ann Thorac Surg 2009 Jan;87(1):276-83.

[82] Emmert MY, Weber B, Behr L, Frauenfelder T, Brokopp CE, Grunenfelder J, et al. Transapical aortic implantation of autologous marrow stromal cell-based tissue-engineered heart valves: first experiences in the systemic circulation. JACC Cardiovasc Interv 2011 Jul;4(7):822-3.

[83] Emmert MY, Weber B, Wolint P, Behr L, Sammut S, Frauenfelder T, et al. Stem cell-based transcatheter aortic valve implantation: first experiences in a pre-clinical model. JACC Cardiovasc Interv 2012 Aug;5(8):874-83.

[84] Wynn TA. Cellular and molecular mechanisms of fibrosis. J Pathol 2008 Jan;214(2): 199-210.

[85] Sun L, Louie MC, Vannella KM, Wilke CA, LeVine AM, Moore BB, et al. New concepts of IL-10-induced lung fibrosis: fibrocyte recruitment and M2 activation in a CCL2/ CCR2 axis. Am J Physiol Lung Cell Mol Physiol 2011 Mar;300(3):L341-L353.

[86] Low QE, Drugea IA, Duffner LA, Quinn DG, Cook DN, Rollins BJ, et al. Wound healing in MIP-1alpha(-/-) and MCP-1(-/-) mice. Am J Pathol 2001 Aug;159(2):457-63.

[87] Hibino N, Villalona G, Pietris N, Duncan DR, Schoffner A, Roh JD, et al. Tissue-engineered vascular grafts form neovessels that arise from regeneration of the adjacent blood vessel. FASEB J 2011 Aug;25(8):2731-9.

[88] Zilla P, Bezuidenhout D, Human P. Prosthetic vascular grafts: wrong models, wrong questions and no healing. Biomaterials 2007 Dec;28(34):5009-27.

[89] Smits AI, Driessen-Mol A, Bouten CV, Baaijens FP. A mesofluidics-based test platform for systematic development of scaffolds for in situ cardiovascular tissue engineering. Tissue Eng Part C Methods 2012 Jun;18(6):475-85.

[90] Young A, McNaught CE. The physiology of wound healing. Surgery (Oxford) 2011 Oct; 29(10):475-9.

Chapter 9

Cutting-Edge Regenerative Medicine Technologies for the Treatment of Heart Valve Calcification

Laura Iop and Gino Gerosa

Additional information is available at the end of the chapter

http://dx.doi.org/10.5772/55327

1. Introduction

An early attempt of designing a valvular device was made already in 1513 by Leonardo da Vinci, who depicted the appearance of a prosthetic aortic valve to be reproduced in glass material [1].

The first real manufacture of valve substitutes goes back to the '50s of the previous century, when the application in heterotopic position of an aortic mechanical valve by Hufnagel and colleagues triggered the beginning of the surgical therapeutic era of valvulopathies [2]. It was however the contribution of Harken, Starr and Edwards to demonstrate the feasibility of orthotopic valve replacement with these early devices [3]. Since then, several mechanical and bioprosthetic replacements have been proposed as valve substitutes. Still, these solutions are not meeting important prerequisites.

Heart valve tissue engineering and, later, tissue-guided regeneration have been proposed to overcome the limitations associated to current valve substitutes. Principles, preclinical and clinical models of each approach are discussed in this chapter, together to the diverse improving strategies for the final achievement of viable and functional aortic valve substitutes.

2. Tissue engineering

The different drawbacks related to commercial replacement devices compromise their durability once in the patient and have shift the attention of cardiac surgeons and biomedical engineers towards a new therapeutic concept: heart valve tissue engineering. The first general definition of this approach has been proposed by Langer and Vacanti, as the *in vitro* creation of a viable tissue by combining separate elements, i.e. cells plus an extracellular matrix (ECM), properly conditioned to attain the correct mature function [4]. This universal paradigm has to be applied also to the reconstruction of the valve tissue. The rationale is to achieve the ability to construct *in vitro* a valve with adequate biomechanical properties, good hemodynamic performance, vital competence, growth/remodelling permissiveness and lack of inflammatory/immunological reactions. Such researches have required the synergistic application of different scientific disciplines, from cell biology to engineering and surgery. *In vitro* valve creation is commonly pursued via two different methods diverging for the starter matrix.

2.1. Biomaterial scaffolds

2.1.1. Polymeric materials

The choice of the ECM scaffold is not only a distinction parameter among diverse approaches, but also essential for the successful realization of tissue-engineered heart valves (TEHVs). ECM is able to establish the necessary 3D configuration and guides cell attachment and structural development of the new tissue.

Synthetic materials have often represented the privileged option in TEHV formulations. Biopolymers as aliphatic polyesters, polyhydroxyalcanoates or different polyurethane compounds have been preferentially employed, providing scaffolds with controllable chemo-physical characteristics as reproducibility, porousness and biodegradability rate. The chosen biomaterials have to respond to important requirements, as good cell-affinity and adequate structural architecture able to sustain the organ mechanics. To enable cell adhesion and spreading in the selected biopolymeric mesh, the modulation of porousness until 90% achievement is recommended [5].

In particular, most of these materials offer a further regenerative advantage also thanks to the good immunotolerance induced in the host body. In fact, after an initial guiding effect, the non-natural material is progressively degraded by colonizing cells, which in turn operate a new matrix synthesis. The process results in a newly produced tissue of completely autologous origin.

First generation polymeric heart valves were designed to overcome the poor durability and excessive wear shown by Teflon fabric-composed substitutes. These more rigid valves, with caged-ball or low-profile design, were based either on metals, like titanium or stellite 21, or on silicone with fixed fabric sewing rings. While metallic devices mostly presented difficulties in the insertion phase, elastomeric ball valves demonstrated less stability in the mid/long-term evaluation [6]. Polyurethanes were lately proposed for their relatively good haemodynamic behaviour especially in contact with blood cells and indeed for their easy manipulable chemical structure [7,8].

Again, biostability represented the major drawback associated to these elastomers together to the high calcification potential: polyester, polyether and polycarbonate urethanes were sequentially suggested for valve fabrication with minor biodegradation, but still insufficient stability [9]. The introduction of further chemical groups and other modifications in the polymer segments has been carried out and is still under study to improve the durability of polyurethane-based devices *in vivo* [8, 10]. In particular, when modified with polyhedral oligomeric silsesquioxanes (POSS), polycarbonate urethane-composed polymeric substitutes offer improved biological and hydrodynamic functioning in respect to bioprosthetic valves [11].

Shinoka et al. firstly reported in 1995 the application of aliphatic polyesters in TEHV formulation. The constructs were composed of polyglactin, polyglycolic acid (PGA) or polylactic acid (PLA) [12-14]. The scarce pliability of these biomaterials did not allow, however, a perfect shape modelling [15]. Conversely, polyhydroxyalcanoates, as polyhydroxyoctanoate (PHA) mixed or not with poly-4-hydroxybutyrate (PH4B), have demonstrated better thermoplastic proficiencies: a polyester group combined with bacterial-derived hydroxyacids is the chemical composition of these last polymers [16,17].

Polystyrene/polyisobutylene compounds were also developed for cardiovascular structure fabrication, showing superior resistance to the high environmental heart valve stresses [18].

Novel promising biopolymers are currently tested to better mimic chemo-physical properties of native heart valves: *inter alia*, polyvinyl alcohol-bacterial cellulose-based hydrogels can be opportunely modelled for a broad range of tuneable mechanical properties [19].

Contemporary procedures for polymeric aortic heart valve fabrication must rely on optimal tricuspid design, used as template for successive valve production. Multiple dip-coatings into poorly concentrated polymeric solutions have as major drawback inhomogeneous tissue thickness.

Another manufacturing technique combines the use of solvent and thermal treatment to properly shape polymeric films in a desired arrangement. Tri-dimensional models, additionally created through direct laser 'recording' in photo-sensitive polymers, act as blueprint for successive casting of hot biopolymers, which will assume the chosen conformation during chilling [20]. Similarly, injection systems assisted by hot/cold baths can be applied to the same aim [21].

2.1.2. Decellularized extracellular matrices

Despite the evident ability of these biopolymers to undergo cell remodelling, a proper mature, cell-operated tissue architectural reconstitution might require a chemo-mechanical stimulation for a long time. Often, to the best of their biostability and mechanical behaviour, biopolymeric heart valves do not develop a trilaminate structure and remarkably, the elastin network in leaflet layer *ventricularis* and wall *media* can be inconsistently achieved.

On this account, another research stream inside the heart valve tissue engineering approach prefers the usage of animal-derived decellularized scaffolds. A suitable decellularization procedure allows the removal of xenogeneic cells, maintaining all the fibre composition and distribution of the natural ECM. In addition, as further advantage in respect to commonly produced bioprostheses, the treatment with glutaraldehyde can be skipped following the absence of xenogeneic cells. The avoidance of this cytotoxic agent enables remodelling processes to occur by providing a cell-friendly milieu, where viable engrafting elements are able to accomplish synthetic and contractile functions with extracellular matrix continuous remodelling.

Cell-freed natural matrices can be realised by means of several methods: trypsin-based enzymatic and detergent decellularization procedures are only two examples of the proposed treatments. Most decellularizing protocols take advantage of a combined mechanical and chemical tissue handling to ease cell removal.

Grauss and colleagues interestingly compared various protocols currently applied to decellularize porcine aortic heart valves and verified that the combination of trypsin and Triton X-100, an anionic detergent, could be able to provoke a loss of matrix integrity [22]. Not only the enzymatic treatment with trypsin can induce elastin defragmentation, but also the use of sodium dodecyl sulphate can end out with a similar deleterious effect [23]. Conversely, the adoption of sodium cholate- and deoxycholate-based methods allows the achievement of fully nude matrices, able to be cell-recolonized *in vitro* and/or *in vivo* even for clinical implantation [23-28].

Besides native heart valves, another natural tissue has been regarded with attention for the production of animal-derived acellular scaffolds. Pericardium has been extensively applied in bioprosthetic manufacturing thanks to its biocompatible, mechanical and biological properties, entirely suitable for long-lasting heart valve substitutes. More often of bovine origin, this tissue partially differs from a native heart valve for its low cellularity and extremely compacted ECM, raising the question on which decellularization process can best convey the optimal outcome [29]. With regards to this tissue, the comparative analysis developed by Yang et al. revealed a superior decellularizing and preserving effect of enzymatic/detergent treatment or trypsin alone on Triton X100/sodium-deoxycholate-based extraction.

Sodium cholate demonstrates instead a less aggressive behaviour towards the pericardial tissue providing analogous results to its application on native semilunar heart valves [30].

Together to the elimination of xenogeneic cells, a variable depletion in the glycosaminoglycan (GAG) content is usually observed after decellularization procedure. GAGs play a significant viscoelastic role by mitigating valve stress during flexion: their highly hydrophilic nature allows, in fact, the hydration of the *spongiosa* layer in this cycle phase. Indeed, several biological processes appear to be modulated by GAGs, therefore their loss has profound consequences in the mechanical behaviour and in the cellular functions of successively repopulated scaffolds [31]. Associated to GAG content is also the hydrated state of the tissue: a reduction in hydration following decellularization can induce collapse of collagen fibres and introduces a less suitable environment for colonizing cells [32], 33].

While GAG and water preservation is pivotal, an opposite decellularizing effect is expected as far as DNA/RNA content. Similar to cell membrane residues, the phosphate groups of the nucleic acid backbone behave as powerful calcification triggers [34]. Aspecific endonucleases are often applied as efficient tools for the complete removal of nucleic acid debris [25-26].

Extracting processes should be hence developed ad hoc depending on the specific tissue to use as starter matrix, otherwise adversely affecting the original mechanical and bioactive properties of the natural ECM.

In addition, the realization of viable constructs must not be regardless of detergent scaffold retention. Incomplete washout of detergents could induce the creation of a toxic microenvironment for engrafting cells. *In vitro* evaluations should be critically performed in respect to each decellularization procedure currently applied [unpublished data, 35, 36].

2.2. Cells

Cells embody the second key-component of a TEHV: it is this element that provides viability to the ECM and consequently permits its remodelling and maturation towards a functional organ. Furthermore, the use of cell elements of allogeneic or autologous source can prevent from non-self reactions towards synthetic biomaterials or decellularized natural tissues.

2.2.1. Differentiated cells

For a similar selection principle operated by those researchers preferring the more committed animal-derived matrix, endothelial cells, fibroblasts, myofibroblasts and/or smooth muscle cells isolated from vascular or valve conduits have been extensively utilized to seed nude matrices and obtain both endothelial coverage with antithrombotic activity and tissue repopulation [24, 37].

Endothelial cells (ECs) were first applied in the '90s to test the feasibility of endothelialisation on Biomer and Mitrathane thromboresistant polyurethane ureas in response to physiological shear stress [38]. Commonly harvested from cardiovascular structures, as adult saphenous or more immature umbilical veins, endothelial cells were also seeded onto bioprosthetic heart valves to increase their low thrombogenic properties [39]. In an analogous fashion, a previous endothelial coverage on harshly decellularized native tissues can avert *in vivo* thromboembolic events, related to basal membrane damage/loss resulting in collagen fibres exposure.

More frequently, ECs were employed in combination to other cell elements, as for example myo/fibroblasts. A sequential seeding of fibroblasts and ECs was demonstrated effective in the *in vitro* creation of tissue-engineered valve constructs endowed with appropriate cell topography [40]. However, the district of fibroblast cell origin is able to significantly affect the degree of recellularization with better outcome associated to the usage of arterial myofibroblasts rather than of dermal fibroblasts [41, 42].

Valve fibroblasts, known as valve interstitial cells (VICs) for their cusp origin, have been successfully employed as sole repopulating cell population, exhibiting unmodified proliferative and synthetic abilities once engrafted in decellularized scaffolds [24].

While dissimilar to VICs, smooth muscle cells of vascular derivation (vSMCs) can be chemically manipulated with epidermal growth factor (EGF), platelet-derived growth factor (PDGF) and transforming growth factor beta-1 (TGF-beta1) for a phenotypic switch towards leaflet cells [43].

2.2.2. *Stem cells and progenitors*

Marrow stromal cells, umbilical cord myofibroblasts and progenitor cells, chorionic villi-derived cells and placenta or amniotic fluid progenitors share not only the potential to transdifferentiate in valve phenotypes after appropriate stimulation, but are also associated to several positive aspects, making them particularly attractive for bioengineering applications [25, 44-46].

Stem and progenitor cells are now of relatively safe isolation from foetal and neonatal tissues, such as amniotic fluid, chorionic villi or umbilical cord. Most of them demonstrate mesenchymal properties, potentiated by higher cell plasticity in relation to their immature state. The embryonic-like phenotype, possessed by these early precursors, can be 'frozen' in cell banks at its genuine isolation state without further differentiation/maturation and loss of stemness [45, 47-51].

While neonatal progenitor cells can be cryopreserved at birth in view of a future use, adult bone marrow-derived cells, and especially their mesenchymal compartment, can be easily harvested from the same cardiopathic patient for a fully autologous TEHV or even employed for the creation of allogeneic constructs [25], with no risk of cell rejection thanks to their beneficial immunomodulatory properties [52, 53]. MSCs reside virtually in all post-natal body departments, as for example adipose tissue or dermis [54, 55]. MSCs obtained from bone marrow (BM-MSCs) offer some advantages over other stem or progenitor cells in terms of their prospects for use in routine clinical practice, i.e. relatively simple protocols for their isolation, storage and *in vitro* expansion and a surprising phenotypic resemblance to valve cells [56, 57]. Indeed, their phenotypic convertibility into ECs, fibroblasts/myofibroblasts and SMCs might allow in a single step-seeding procedure to reconstruct the cell geographic distribution typical of valve cusps [25, 47, 58-60]. hBM-MSCs display a repertoire of molecules that may be relevant to their adhesion and penetration in synthetic or decellularized scaffolds, including b1-integrin (which plays a pivotal role by mediating cell–ECM interactions), CD54, CD105 and CD44 (which act cooperatively in cell homing via binding to hyaluronan, the major non-protein glycosaminoglycan of the ECM) [25].

Another cell type with attractive potential for heart valve tissue engineering is the equally rare, but more easily harvestable circulating fraction of endothelial progenitor cells (EPCs). Commonly isolated from the peripheral blood with a simple venous drawing (i.e. umbilical vein), these progenitors have a high proliferation activity and can commit to transform into a mesenchymal phenotype, reminiscent of the endothelial-mesenchyme transition during embryonic valve development [61-63].

2.2.3. *Bioreactors*

Scaffolds and cells do not represent alone sufficient components for a successful TEHV, but conditioning is indispensable to achieve a perfect maturation of the construct prior to implantation. This last step in manufacturing a viable valve can be guaranteed by the use of bioreactors able to submit it to physiological pressures and flow [64, 65]. Besides mechanical stimulation, the addition of specific chemicals can further train tissue-engineered valve constructs towards their proper functionality [66].

Firstly developed devices were very simple systems based on common or modified petri supports, in which TEHVs could be statically cultured.

The introduction of a dynamic conditioning was hence operated to improve cell engraftment and differentiation through the assemblage of two chambers: one for lodging the valvular construct, the other mimicking ventricular function. Connected to an air pump, the ventricle-like compartment can exert defined hydrodynamic settings in terms of flow and pressure. Diaphragms of different materials, as for example silicone, separate the two chambers and are displaced periodically by air influx [16].

The small size of the device has been primarily regarded for ensuring long-term culturing in defined temperature/gaseous environment. A compact system can, in fact, easily fit in an incubator, where CO_2 saturation, humidity and temperature are already set for cell culture [16]. To this aim, the implementation with gas sensors directly placed in the device can result in a superior chemical control of CO_2, N_2, O_2, glucose and lactate [67, 68].

Single specific mechanical stresses were successively applied to better induce tissue maturation and, furthermost, to activate endothelial-mesenchymal transformation. Laminar flow-, flexure- and cyclic strain-based stimulations could have profound effects on mechanical stiffness, collagen synthesis and alignment in the tissue-engineered valve [69-71].

A three-chamber bioreactor was developed by Sierad et al. in 2010 to respect previously indicated criteria and other important conditions, as easy valve mounting, physiological stimulation (transvalvular pressures, pulsatile forces, flow rate, frequency, stroke rate and shear stresses) and full control over parameters. Absence of toxic or degradable fabrication materials, maximum visibility, together to ease of sterilization and waste removal, further increase the yield of repeatable results. Compliance and reservoir tanks with sterile filters for gas exchange, one-way and resistance valves, pressure transducers, a web-cam and a ventilator pump complement this efficient system [72].

2.2.4. *In Vitro applications*

The reconstruction of a heart valve tissue in a plate dish was first endeavoured by the Bostonian teams of R. Langer, J.P. Vacanti and J.E. Jr Mayer, who published in 1995 the results of this pioneering work [12]. Vascular cells, outgrown from ovine neonatal femoral artery explants, were divided into two populations by LDL selection. LDL-negative SMCs/fibroblasts and LDL-positive ECs were sequentially seeded onto polyglycolic acid/polyglatin scaffolds in a 2-week-long procedure. Later, different cells and polymers were combined in the most efficient valve tissue combinations [41, 73, 74]. The introduction of PHAs, PH4B/PHAs and pulsatile flow conditioning in a bioreactor for heart valve construction allowed the attainment of more pliable scaffolds. After dynamic seeding, cells demonstrated to be actively involved in GAG and collagen synthesis, leading to an autologous replacement of the polymeric mesh [16, 75, 76]. PH4B/PHA became, in particular, the most promising scaffold for several successful TEHV approaches relying on diverse stem cells [44, 45, 49, 77-79].

Elastomeric poly(glycerol sebacate) scaffolds treated with multiple coating strategies based on ECM-derived proteins allowed adhesion and transdifferentiation of EPCs [61, 80].

In respect to the application of bioabsorbable polymers, the other TEHV modality, founded on natural ECMs, was experimented some years later. After the development of various decellularizing treatments, the combination with differentiated cells, as ECs and VICs, was able to generate directly *in vitro* by static conditioning surrogates of early heart valve tissues [24, 81]. As well as polymeric TEHVs, cell-repopulated decellularized ECMs were positively remodelled after dynamic stimulation with proper mechanical signals. In this case, actually, also elastin content was demonstrated to increase [82-84].

The usage of stem cells as cell source for the engineering of plain ECMs led to even better *in vitro* outcomes. Multipotent differentiation potential of human bone marrow MSCs can represent the ideal characteristic for complete repopulation of natural valve matrices. MSC engrafting ability was evaluated on decellularized porcine and human scaffolds. In both considered interactions, stem cells were able to adhere, spread within the ECM and transdifferentiate towards typical valve phenotypes (ECs, VICs). Collagen, GAG and elastin synthesis was indeed activated in engrafted cells, which tend to distribute similarly to the original valve cell topography. It was, however, the homotypic combination to better favour MSC-to-SMC conversion in the *ventricularis* layer [25].

3. Tissue regeneration

TEHV is not the sole approach investigated to obtain new viable valve devices: tissue-guided regeneration has been proposed as an alternative method for *in vivo* direct tissue reconstruction, by exploiting ECM instructive abilities. Once eliminated the allogeneic or xenogeneic cell component through decellularizing treatment, the fibre mesh still maintains biomechanical proficiency assuring in vivo prompt restoration of hydrodynamic performance. Furthermore, in the body, conceived as physiological bioreactor, naked natural scaffolds recruit recipient's cells thanks to their chemo-attractant properties. Positive aspects associated with this option should be identified in the possibility to construct autologous-like tissues, by skipping difficultly controllable procedures of cell seeding and chemo-mechanical stimulation *in vitro*.

Among the first experimental evidences, biomaterials, as patches of pure type I collagen, have been successfully introduced in the therapy of ischemic myocardium: once applied to the diseased tissue, the collagen sponge attracts progenitors and less undifferentiated cells, which in turn or alone are able to fully colonize it and start a cardiovascular transdifferentiation [85]. It is noteworthy to remember that these patches, either synthetic or cell-purified from biological tissues, have found FDA-approved applications as haemostatics or for skin reconstruction with excellent results [86].

A further surprising element for a positive consideration of this method has been given by Campbell and colleagues, who were able to obtain a tubular cell construct by implanting a polymeric tube in the animal peritoneal cavity. The newly formed tissue, pulled from the tube, had anatomical and histological resemblance to a quite mature blood vessel and it could be hence considered an optimal vascular substitute [87].

Also offering the opportunity to create tissue banks for ready-to-use devices at the moment of clinical need, the investigation on tissue-guided regenerated heart valves (TGRHVs) has particularly increased in recent years.

4. Preclinical and clinical applications of tissue engineering and tissue regeneration approaches

The preclinical proof-of-principle of TEHVs as valve substitutes has been demonstrated in the lamb model already with the polymeric bioconctructs firstly produced *in vitro* [12]. Vascular cell-repopulated polyglycolic acid/polyglactin matrices were implanted in the pulmonary position up to 21 days. Function assessment by Doppler echocardiography demonstrated no stenosis or regurgitation signs, even if a substantial leaflet thickness was reported.

Each subsequent modification in scaffold or cell types, as introduced by the same group, was generally tested *in vivo*, validating progressive functional improvements in transplanted lambs or sheep [41, 73, 74].

Further TEHVs applications in preclinical models were substantially based on the use of P4HB/PHA with few exceptions, as electrospun polydioxanone [88]. In combination with stem cells of various stromal origins, P4HB/PHA-formulated engineered tissues were evaluated in a long-term animal model, showing replacement of the exogenous matrix after nearly 8 weeks *in vivo* [16].

A MSC-engineered mesh of polyglycolic and polylactic acids was evaluated as autologous pulmonary valve replacement in juvenile sheep. The good performance of this *in vitro* generated construct could be appreciated in a long follow-up of 4 months with restoration of a native-like pulmonary heart valve [59].

Despite biomechanical stimulation induced optimal results in term of cell viability and differentiation almost independently from the cytotype utilised, combined polymer/cell-based efforts to obtain a valve substitute have usually failed in recreating the fibre arrangement of a native ECM. In fact, trilaminate distribution of collagens, GAGs and elastin has been reported only in few cases [88].

A finely organized ECM already exists in native heart valves and can be conserved after cell removal. After decellularization with trypsin/EDTA, heart valve conduits were seeded with ECs and myofibroblasts. Allogenically implanted in orthotopic position, they performed adequately. Ex vivo tissue analyses revealed surface endothelium reconstitution, myofibroblasts-mediated repopulation and ECM synthesis with no signs of inflammation and calcification [89].

Sole ECs were used to obtain *in vitro* endothelium coverage of ovine acellular scaffolds. After 6 months of *in vivo* evaluation, explanted tissues presented no calcifications as assessed by atomic absorption spectrometry [90].

Lutter et al. coated stented pulmonary valves with small interstinal submucosa, both pig-derived and decellularized. These scaffolds, dynamically seeded *in vitro* with ECs and myofibroblasts, were deployed in orthotopic position by means of transcatheter assistance. Valve performance and macroscopic appearance demonstrated to be normal during *in vivo* and post-mortem evaluation [91].

Despite rare reports of deleterious therapeutic effects associated to TEHVs' implantation in humans [92], clinical application of these substitutes, attained by combination of acellular scaffolds and ECs or EPCs, reached already more than 10 years of experience with proved function and absence of calcifications [93, 94].

Another modality of heart valve tissue engineering has been more recently proposed. It is realized by means of a one-phase intraoperative approach. The rational of such a strategy rises from the necessity of a ready-to-apply TEHV, when the surgical therapy has to be promptly adopted with no time for *in vitro* cell seeding and bioreactor conditioning. Weber and colleagues implanted such prepared TEHVs in the RVOT of non-human primates through minimally invasive, transapical procedures. These polymeric trileaflet heart valves have been just seeded with unselected autologous bone marrow cells before the crimping necessary for valve insertion. After one month, the completely remodelled valves were still functioning [95]. Similarly conceived TEHVs demonstrated patency also in the aortic position, being able to sustain the higher pressure regimen of the systemic circulation [96,97]. Another *in situ* TEHV delivery has been applied by Vincentelli et al, by injecting mesenchymal stem cells into a just deployed decellularized heart valve. As element of comparison, they used acellular scaffolds: these ones showed equal performance and reconstructed tissue [98]. However, these are no more TE-, but TGRHVs.

The first attempt of tissue-guided heart valve regeneration has been challenged by the extensive work of Konertz and colleagues, who, moving from the classical paradigm of tissue engineering, compared the two methods. Common for each approach is only the application of the same decellularizing detergent, deoxy-cholic acid. By using an allogeneic decellularized valve for the reconstruction of the right ventricular outflow tract in sheep, they ascertained there was no need to seed the scaffolds prior to implantation, after the good repopulation observed at six months [99]. Follow-up of the valve function revealed increase in the annulus diameter in response to animal growth [100]. As further step to the clinic, they developed a xenogeneic model again with substitution of the autologous pulmonary valve, transferred in aortic position during Ross intervention. They tested porcine decellularized valves, called Matrix P, in a pig-to-sheep interaction. By comparison to sheep cryopreserved allografts, decellularized porcine valves demonstrated better valvular performance, decreased calcific potential and feasible tissue regeneration [101]. Another group compared the haemodynamic function of valve allografts, either cryopreserved and/or decellularized, verifying a reduced calcification tendency in the sheep implanted with decellularized matrices [102].

Equivalently promising results have been reported for the implantation of Triton X100/sodium cholate-decellularized allogeneic valves in the longest preclinical follow-up ever realized for a TGRHV. Evaluated in Vietnamese minipigs as RVOT replacements in heterotopic position, these acellular, alpha-gal-free certified valve substitutes have demonstrated good haemodynamic performance with low transvalvular gradients in a 15-month-long *in vivo* observation.

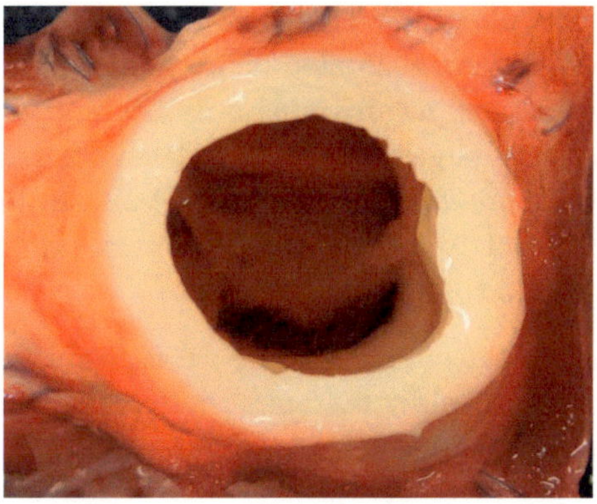

Figure 1. *In vivo* tissue-regenerated heart valve after 12 months of implantation in Vietnamese minipig

No calcification events could be appreciated within engrafted tissues by trans-thoracic echocardiography: these macroscopic observations found ex vivo confirmation by undetectable calcific foci after von Kossa staining. In addition, no inflammatory or immunogenic cells could be observed. A progressive repopulating process occurred in implanted valves: most tissues were endothelialised and engrafted by rare stem cells and numerous myo/fibroblasts, both highly proliferating and suggesting the onset of a smooth muscle cell conversion. Provision of oxygen and nutrients was again established by a dense capillary network and re-created vasa vasorum. Moreover, re-innervation aspects were also identified [26, 27].

Acellular allologous conduits were also favourably approved as aortic valve substitutes in a sheep model [103].

Few unfavourable outcomes with a TGRHV have been seldom disclosed. Two groups of heart valves, cryopreserved or decellularized and treated with an anticalcinosis devitalisation (digitonin and ethylenediaminetetraacetic acid), were tested in dogs by substituting an aorta fragment with the non-coronary sinus of the cusp allografts: albeit the lack of immune infiltrate in inserted decellularized specimens in contrast to cryopreserved ones, no engrafting of recipient 's cells was observed in both cases [104].

The reasons for such different findings should first be searched in the used decellularization procedure for TGRHV production.

Apart from animal studies, allologeneic TGR approaches were also applied in humans with optimal outcomes. Decellularized allogeneic valves, as obtained with the deoxycholic acid procedure, were evaluated in 68 patients in the medium term for RVOT reconstruction in Ross aortic valve substitution. Up to 4 years, Costa et al. observed very low mortality (1, 4 %), a good valve function, both comparable with the cryopreserved allografts used as control, and a progressive engraftment – even if discontinuous [105].

TGR has been further practised as an alternative RVOT replacement strategy for human paediatric and young patients with confident results in a follow-up of more than 5 years. Freedom from re-intervention, lower transvalvular gradients and adaptive dimensional modifications in response to somatic growth have been reported from *in vivo* early-term comparison with pulmonary allografts [106]. In a just slighter observational window, allogeneic pulmonary valves were evaluated in a multicentre study with 342 patients undergoing RVOT reconstruction: improvement in haemodynamic function was registered for implanted valves and suggested to be related to decreased tissue antigenicity [107]. After a 5-year follow-up in 48 patients, Burch et al. put the accent on the relevance of the economic burden, related to the use of decellularized cryopreserved allografts in respect to their untreated counterparts [108].

Although good reported outcomes open the route for a promising treatment of heart valve failure, it will be imperative to reconsider therapeutic effects in a longer clinical evaluation, by taking into account also socio-economic considerations.

A debated note is, however, represented by the clinical application of unseeded decellularized xenogeneic tissues as valvular replacement solutions. *In vivo* infiltration of tissue-engineered Matrix P heart valves by human cells, not related to inflammatory or immune system, was observed in some explanted specimens [109]. These relevancies were at the basis of the pure Matrix P adoption in the clinical arena. Although favourable performance and lack of xenogeneic tissue-mediated immune reactions have been demonstrated by the same valve-manufacturing group in respect to current RVOT substitutes [110, 111], controversial issues were evidenced after implantation of the same Matrix P valves in other studies [112, 113].

These reports, together with the dramatic results of the early failed Synergraft decellularized valves [114], should lower the speed in the human application of xenogeneic tissues-derived devices, moving a step backward to more robust human-like preclinical trials, as non-human primate animal models.

5. New insights on heart valve regenerative medicine

5.1. Immunogenicity of xenogeneic tissues

Allotransplantation has been widely consolidated as valid therapy to rescue a failed vital function, but the shortage of human cells, tissues and organs dramatically increases the waiting lists for replacement: in 2006, Eurotransplant referred almost 16.000 patients were attending to receive a substitute, while in the United States these ones were reaching the number of 90.000 [115]. The numerical entity of these registers is expected to sensitively grow during the near future. Surely, the employ of unlimitedly supplied, animal-derived organs could allow an immediate intervention to recover the lost function and in combination with bioengineering methodologies, might favour the achievement of human-like organs throughout strictly controlled fabrication procedures. So far, animal tissues fixed in glutaraldehyde have been the reserve to exploit at the time of clinical need. However, this should be no longer considered as viable route in accordance to vitality maintenance, above all for those organs that cannot perform a correct function in absence of a proper cell physiology. The use of non-human sources is accompanied by a major raising concern for a broad clinical application, i.e. the immunological barrier. For a donor-receiver mismatched allocombination, the most serious medical issue is the inability of accommodation and therefore the onset of chronic rejection, whose main manifestation, in the case of heart transplant, is graft vascular disease. This allotransplantation drawback is characterized by an unchanged gravity and entity in respect to 40 years ago, when this research line started to be investigated as possible treatment of end-stage pathologies [116].

A peculiar atherosclerotic process interests the heart transplant with few calcifications, but increased cellularity and extracellular matrix deposition at the entire intimal level with a concentric distribution [117].

A similar event occurs in the xenotransplantation approach, where an even more severe expression is attended. Furthermore, in addition to a chronic response, antibody-mediated hyperacute rejection represents a dramatic hurdle to early-term xenograft survival, when a trans-species interaction has to be considered. By developing in a time period from minutes to hours in the pig-to-primate combination, hyperacute rejection, commonly defined as HAR, is a typical humoral immune response in vascularized organs with deposition of xenoreactive natural antibodies and complement activation [118]. Pig-to-primate xenotransplantation has properly enabled to discover the progression of delayed immunological answer to the cardiac graft (DXR): besides a strong humoral activity, acute cellular infiltrates and endothelium activation seriously compromise the function of newly transplanted organ [119].

5.1.1. Alpha-gal and other xenoantigens

Not well known - and in the last years very debated- is the real immunological trigger able to cause the complete loss of the xenograft during time. Probably the prompts of this phenomenon are not to be found in a unique opponent, but in more factors, which alone or in cooperation provoke it. One of the most powerful antigens is definitely Galα1-3Galβ1-4GlcNAc, commonly identified as α-Gal. This oligosaccharide is a component of the glycoproteins and glycolipids, displayed on the surface of vascular endothelial cells in all mammals except apes, Old World monkeys and humans, unable to metabolize it for evolutionary gene silencing of the related enzyme α1-3-Galactosyltransferase [120, 121]. Reaching an expression concentration of at least 10^7 epitopes per pig cell, alpha-gal is recognized by human cells in a highly specific pattern soon after birth similarly to ABO antibodies. In fact, microorganisms colonizing or transiting through the intestinal flora express it on their surface and due also to the dietary use of animal-derived nourishment, 1% of serum circulating IgGs are specifically directed against this epitope with a quite pure protective role against parasite and viral attacks [122, 123]. Already at the end of the previous century, a restricted but well developed body of evidence considered alpha-gal as an immunogenic suspect, but it was only more recent the full demonstration of its causative role in HAR, by studying the pig-to-primate interaction

[124]. Other important observations have been made available with this research about the amount of natural anti-pig antibodies in humans and their specific subclasses. At least 85% of humoral anti-pig players are specific for alpha-gal and belong to IgG and IgM classes: more recurrently, IgMs tend to deposit on the graft endothelium [124-126]. Anti-Gal antibodies have been shown to contribute both to HAR and lately DXR, if an initial tolerance regimen has been introduced [127].

Hence, the issue is unquestionably alarming for new therapeutic approaches of biomedicine using xenogeneic biological materials.

In order to face this problem, different strategies have been developed just from the observation of the glyco-composition differences between pig and human cells. In the endothelium of both species, N-acetyllactosamine and sialic acid are expressed, but the human one –as previously mentioned- lacks alpha-gal and is characterized by the presence of ABH-Galβ1-4GlcNAcβ1-R (ABO system) and a supplementary sugar, NeuGca2-3Galβ1-4GlcNAcβ1-R (N-glycolylilneuraminic acid). Since the complete elimination of anti-Gal IgMs resulted in null complement-mediated cytotoxicity by human serum without side effects on the IgG counterpart, various methods to deplete the whole range of anti-alpha gal antibodies have been tested.

First xenotransplantation experiments have been started in the 1960s, when the existence of alpha-gal and its antibodies was still ignored, however a decrease in xenoreaction could be achieved by perfusing the recipient's blood in a donor-specific organ, such as the liver, possessing high immunoadsorbent ability. Analogously, other depletion procedures have ameliorated the survival of the xenogeneic tissue, even if still at the initial developmental phases: plasma exchange and plasma perfusion through column systems based on specific protein interaction or on immunoaffinity could extend implant durability, but rarely for more than one month due to failed establishment of accommodation.

A more direct method, independent from external devices, is the intravenous approach based on similar affinity principles. Infused antibodies precisely targeting idiotypes of anti-gal humoral effectors, immunoglobulin (IVIG) or even oligosaccharides behave as silencers, by blocking –at least quite completely- any possible immunological response against alpha-gal. In the case of IVIG, it has been postulated an indirect beneficial role through the acceleration of IgG physiological catabolism and inhibition of macrophage function [126].

A further procedure inducing an accommodation state can be identified in the suppression of anti-gal cell effectors, by full depletion of B-lymphocytes and plasma cells. Methods proposed for this purpose are irradiation, pharmacological therapy, anti-B cells specific antibodies (mAbs) and immunotoxins. The irradiation of the entire body with the clinically used dose of 300 cGy does not result in a lethal condition, but provokes a transient B-cell ablation, whose effects are therefore time-limited. The administration of mAbs underlies a more selective way of action and benefits from clinical experiences completed in the haemato-oncological field. Anti-CD20 mAbs, for instance, have been used to treat baboons for 4 weeks: at the end of this course, a complete deficiency in B cells could be maintained both in bone marrow and peripheral blood for at least 3 months. A combination of immunotoxins, such as ricin A and sapporin, and mAbs can promote better ablation results [126]. In the transplantation setting, a wide line of investigation has been directed to discover chemical agents able to perform immunosuppressive effects. Even in xenografting, this kind of therapy seems to have a supporting role for other strategies in order to induce accommodation.

Cyclophosphamide is one of the most common pharmacological agents with this task: in heart transplant, function prolongation induced by this drug is positive without doubt, but many risks are associated with its permanent use, as leukopenia [128].

Alkylating agents, as melphalan, or DNA polymerase blockers, as zidovudine, or even enzymatic inhibitors, as methotrexate, have been analogously experimented with different results. The first ones are particularly interesting because they are quite the unique to target plasma cells. Although reducing anti-alpha gal IgGs, suppressive effects of zidovudine are not so important in a prospective clinical use. Methotrexate, on the contrary, appears to be a valid agent if added to other B cell-destroying therapies. In new-born baboons, mycophenolate mofetil (MMF), an inhibitor of the purine synthesis, has allowed, as therapeutic adjuvant, to prolong the survival of transplanted porcine hearts of at least the double time in respect to non-treated animals [129]. These results in themselves could not seem particularly appealing if compared to the effects of other drugs, but MMF is able to offer a similar efficacy in the face of lack of side consequences and seems very promising for future uses on xenotransplanted patients.

A special mention should be addressed to a therapeutic approach based on a quite new soluble glycoconjugate, GAS914, in combination with different drugs (among which MMF too). GAS594 has demonstrated a constant proficiency in lowering the titres of anti-gal IgGs and IgMs, and hence prolonging durability of transgenic porcine hearts transplanted in cynomolgus monkeys [130].

All these methods search to abate the recipient's response to this carbohydrate, but generally a certain refractoriness does not allow a long permanence of the xenograft and consequently provokes the inability to maintain the organ function [126].

5.1.2. Animal humanization

Alpha-gal-induced rejection could be possibly avoided also throughout the modulation of the donor tissue, i.e. by bioengineering the animal donor for elimination of antigenicity sources. Gene engineering techniques enable to introduce human genes directly in the animal genome. So-generated porcine transgenic cell lines expressing human α1, 2-fucosyltransferase display in their cell membranes more universal donor O antigens than alpha-gal epitopes, therefore evoke decreased antibody reactivity [131]. Genetically induced human decay-accelerating factor (hDAF) expression in animal grafts plays an inhibitory role in the onset of HAR [132]. Nevertheless, more incisive approaches are gene knocking down or out of α1, 3-galactosyltransferase (Galt). When transplanted in heterotopic position into immunosuppressed baboons, Galt-KO porcine hearts could survive *in vivo* for at least 6 months with graft surviving at least HAR, but failing for later complications [133].

5.1.3. Decellularization strategies

Xenoantigens are commonly accepted to be cell-derived, so the removal of membranes, where these epitopes are displayed, should definitely circumvent xenoreactions. Such a perspective could particularly fit the case of engineered arterial vessels or heart valves, based on decellularized tissues. When the first human paediatric implantations of plain porcine heart valves, produced in an industrialized and controlled manner, were performed, a severe inflammatory/immune response provoked premature graft failure [114]. These dramatic events could be attributed to an incomplete cell removal: the same Authors imputed in residual alpha-Gal the responsibility of observed HAR occurrences and later, suggested the use of the detergent IGEPAL CA-630 for total extraction and correctly wash-out from treated heart valves [134].

More recently, clinical evaluations by Bloch et al. have revealed no IgG-mediated, but minor IgM-related responses towards decellularized valves in respect to common bioprostheses [111].

It is undeniably important to improve decellularization strategies for alpha-gal removal. *Ex vivo* investigations on bovine and porcine valve tissues revealed that alpha-Gal is not only expressed at the endothelial level of the leaflet surface coverage, but also by ECs lining the arterioles' vascular lumen at the cusp base [25]. Also some stromal cells in the *interstitium* display this antigen on their cell membrane [134].

Particular attention should be addressed to validate techniques used for alpha-gal revelation. The isolectin BSI-B4, commonly suggested in the literature as detector, gives consistent results only for fresh specimens, but displays an aspecific affinity when applied to decellularized leaflets. The affinity binding of BSI-B4 towards glucidic molecules contained in alpha-Gal epitopes is less stable than the link achieved by immunodetection with the highly specific antibody M86 [25].

For future applications in this field, implantable valve substitutes should be certified for alpha-gal subtraction. Furthermost, for the good manufacture practice of therapeutic strategies based on decellularized extracellular matrices, it would be of paramount importance to rely on specific assays able to quantitatively detect the residual amount of alpha-gal xenoantigens (i.e. M86-based alpha-gal ELISA test) [25, 135, 136].

5.1.4. Decellularized scaffolds obtained from tissue-engineered constructs

A completely new approach to overcome xenograft/allograft-related immunogenicity has been recently proposed, by drastically bypassing the use of non-human tissues. Dijkam et al. decellularized a previously tissue-engineered heart valve and demonstrated the feasibility of an *in vitro* regeneration guided by the acellular ECM. First, TEHVs were obtained by seeding vascular cells on poly-4-hydroxybutyrate/polyglycolic acid scaffolds and by dynamic conditioning. Then, cell removal was operated using a detergent-based treatment (Triton X100, sodium deoxycholate and EDTA), followed by endonuclease digestion. Decellularized matrices were consequently repopulated with MSCs and tested for haemodynamic performance through a simulated transapical implantation. Mechanical characteristics of acellular scaffolds were also evaluated. Considerably, obtained scaffolds could be conserved for up to 18 months without modifying their bioactivity and biomechanical properties [137].

While representing an absolutely novel therapeutic concept to solve immunologic issues, it is associated to some significant drawbacks. The procedure to generate such a fully biocompatible scaffold is quite long, complicated and depending on multiple conditionings.

By the way, by exploiting a controlled large-scale industrial production, it would be possible to manufacture off-the-shelf valve substitutes. The major limitation is represented, indeed, by the immature nature of fabricated scaffolds. As in other tissue engineering-based solutions, the synthesized ECM, rich in collagen and GAGs, risks to be deficient in resilience following the absence of an elastin network.

5.2. Mimicking aortic valve formation

5.2.1. Valve cell progenitors: Possible surrogates and gene engineering for their generation

In the development of cardiac valves, the endocardial cushions appear to be the primordial of the valvular leaflets and the membranous septa: they derive from regionalized expansions of extracellular matrix between cardiomyocyte sheets and endocardial cells of the cardiac tube. A subset of endothelial cells acquires specific abilities of delamination and invasion of the cardiac jelly, by assuming a typical mesenchymal phenotype, with high proliferative activity and able to remodel the cushions in definitive cusps. The work of Markwald and Colleagues about Endothelial-Mesenchymal Transition (EMT) first evidenced the involvement of soluble factors in the extracellular matrix and nevertheless a close myocardium-endothelium relationship, likely to emphasize the unique responsive property of endocardial cells to cardiomyocytes' mechanical and paracrine stimuli [138].

At the end of the developmental process, at least four are the cellular contributions which constitute the different valvular phenotypes: the myocardium, whose involvement is immediate in the formation of the atrioventricular valves; the endocardium, which undergoes an endothelial-mesenchymal transdifferentiation; the epicardium, contributing to the atrioventricular valves; and the neural crest cells, which migrate from the brachial arches to the distal outflow tract, participating to the aorto-pulmonary septation [139-141].

Excluding embryonic cells for ethical concerns, cells with EMT potentiality should be endowed with a certain degree of plasticity: as seen before, EPCs and MSCs, isolable from several tissue sources of various donor ages, could possess among other cell phenotypes these requisites and find, in fact, broad application in tissue engineering practices.

Not yet followed in heart valve manufacturing are two other modalities to achieve more committed valve cell lines. On one hand, it would be possible to introduce genome modifications in cells already applied in TEHVs to induce paracrine mechanisms able to foster cell differentiation. On this basis, VEGF-overexpressing stem cells transplanted in the ischemic myocardium induced an improvement in vascularization [142]. Indeed, MSCs engineered to express Akt did not only participate to the repair of the infarcted heart, but also improved cardiac function [143].

The other more attracting frontier in advanced TEHV formulations is represented by the conversion of adult somatic cells to pluripotent stem cells (iPSCs) mediated by gene engineering. Cellular reprogramming to pluripotency is induced by the ectopic expression of 4 factors, i.e. Klf-4, c-Myc, Oct4 and Sox2 [144], rendering these cells phenotypically similar to embryonic stem cells but for an ethically acceptable use. iPSC cardiovascular applications range from the modelling of congenital cardiac diseases to the heart restoration after myocardial infarction [145, 146]. iPSC-based tissue-engineered heart valves could represent new powerful tools for the therapy of valvulopathies both as replacement solutions and as *in vitro* 3D valvular disease models.

5.2.2. *Scaffold incorporation of growth factors*

The close observation of the molecular events undergoing in heart valve formation would give specific indications on which signals bioengineered constructs could benefit for their maturation.

Endocardial cells undergo a profound phenotypic switch loosing the initial morphology, specific surface molecule expression and ability of acetylated-low density lipoprotein uptake in favour of a contractile, invasive profile. Transforming growth factor 1 and 2 (TGF-beta1 and 2), vascular endothelial growth factor (VEGF), bone morphogenetic protein 2 (BMP-2), mitogen-activated protein kinase 3 (MEKK3) and Notch1 are known to activate and strictly regulate EMT by direct control of Wnt/beta-catenin pathway. In addition, other molecular pathways are involved in heart valve development and the high complexity of regulation can be appreciated in the following chart (Figure 2):

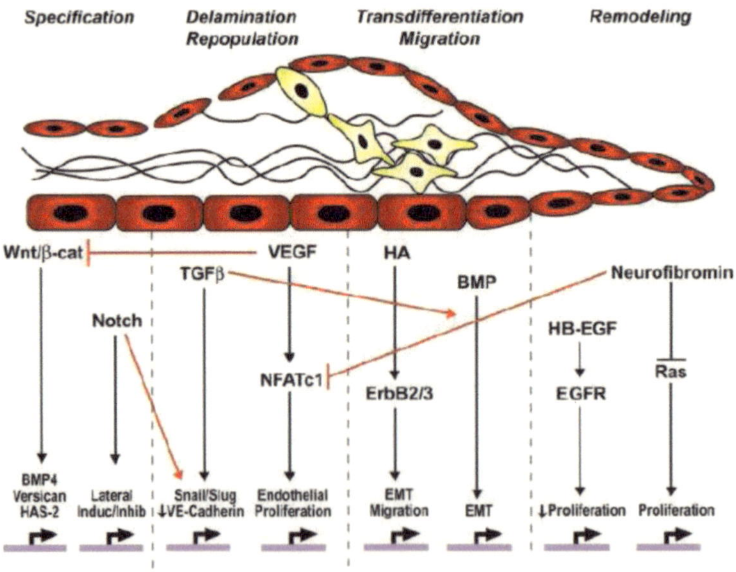

Figure 2. Valvulogenesis signalling complexity as proposed by Armstrong EJ and Bischoff J. From [147]

The pleiotropic factor VEGF is considered a specific mediator in EMT, favouring endothelial cell proliferation. Downstream of VEGF, the transcriptional factor NFATc1 has intranuclear expression: this is limited to the endocardium not activated in the EMT process during the temporal window of cushion development, while it is expressed by some valve endothelial cells in the post-natal life, leading to hypothesize their participation in the repopulation of the adult endothelium. Even RANKL (receptor activator of nuclear factor κB ligand) exercises a control role on NFATc1, by inhibiting VEGF-induced cell proliferation when the endocardial cushion is more mature [148]. Upstream of NFATc1, two elements, connexins and DSCR1 (Down Syndrome Critical Region 1) play their function via signalling pathways associated to calcium cellular gradients. In cardiomyocytes, DSCR1 seems to be overexpressed during the increase of the cytosolic calcium and acts as modulator of the calcineurin dephosphorilating activity on NFATc1, by preventing its translocation to the nucleus. Connexin 45-composed gap junctions might allow the calcium extracellular diffusion in the endocardial cushions after the VEGF-mediated activation of the calcium transients in endothelial subpopulations[147].

The transcriptional factor Notch1 rules osteogenic differentiation as well as valve development: its signalling in the endocardium might induce an increase of TGF-β2 expression in the myocardium, able to trigger EMT in endocardial cells through the cytosolic activation of Snail and Smad [149]. Activators of the TGF-β transduction pathway are even the bone morphogenetic proteins (BMPs), in particular BMP2, which causes powerful induction of Smad6 in the cusp endothelium [150, 151].

During EMT, PECAM down-regulation in endothelial cells is followed by smooth muscle actin hyper-regulation: Wnt/β-catenin pathway can be hence considered a link in between the mesenchymal activation and the populating process of the cardiac jelly with mesenchymal cells.

Beside these transduction pathways, it is equally important the integration of extracellular matrix signals, so called matrikines. ErbB proteins are involved in cell proliferation of cardiac cushions and their signalling is mediated by hyaluronic acid (HA), a highly hydrophilic glycosaminoglycan, which is able to extend the extracellular space and controls the ligand availability [147]. For both development and maintenance of mesenchymal cells in the valve leaflet, Sox9 is necessary by favouring cell proliferation and ECM correct alignment [152]. Recently, it has been recognized to the epicardium cell-secreted protein periostin a particular importance during the atrioventricular valve development in promoting differentiation of epicardial stem cells [153, 154].

New high-speed fluorescence microscopic technologies have allowed verifying the large interplay of different pathways in the development of the cusps and especially, they enabled a better understanding of the first events in valvulogenesis, arguing in favour of an invagination rather than a formation of endocardial cushions [155].

Recent gene expression studies revealed an up-regulation for α-SMA, Snail and β-catenin as well as acetyltransferase p300 (ATp300). Indeed, microRNA analysis identified a specific role for miR-125b in the down-regulation of p53 [156].

Growth factors involved in embryonic development have been incorporated as widely contemplated strategy in bone and joint regenerative medicine. In the heart valve field, this approach has not been frequently applied [157], until now preferring *in vitro* comparative investigations on cell stimulation with sole growth factors, as TGF-beta, VEGF and BMPs [158, 159].

5.2.3. EMT-inducing biomaterials

Heart valve development is a complex process where signalling molecules and specific extracellular matrix elements interact. In response to these several stimuli, endocardial and epicardial cells adhere to the surface of the cardiac cushions and start an endothelial-to-mesenchymal transition (EMT), leading to the formation of an elongated cusp structure [138].

The initial phase of valve formation depends on many extracellular matrix proteins [160]. The highly hydrophilic glycosaminoglycan HA is the major component of the endocardial cushions and its content is also elevated in the adult *spongiosa* layer, guaranteeing appeasement from the shocks provoked by the enormous pressure variations during the cardiac cycle. When seeded *in vitro* with VICs, hydrogels at various HA percentage have demonstrated to modulate ECM synthesis and induce also the production of elastin [161, 162].

Composite scaffolds of collagen and elastin have shown to reproduce the anisotropic spatial distribution of aortic ECM fibres and hence possess the potential to create heart valve replacements with a native-like microenvironment [163]. Mechanical strength properties of collagen have also been previously exploited in combination with HA, thus obtaining a cell-bioactive ECM milieu [164].

5.3. Biocompatibility indications

5.3.1. Biomimetic strategies

Functional endothelium together to resistant and flexible mechanical performance, mainly ensured by collagen and elastin, are critical components in the early clinical patency of a viable valve substitute. Starter matrices both for TEHV and TGRHV approaches should possess attractive properties towards cell elements facilitating their adhesion, penetration and further maturation. Most decellularized heart valves retain an intact basal membrane lamina, which represent the ideal microenvironment for endothelial cell attachment and spreading. This so-called contact guidance takes advantage of the specific nanotopography of the heart valve intimal ECM to increase cell bioaffinity. In order to recreate a valve-like microenvironment, surface functionalization with peptides, as laminin-extracted YIGSR (Tyr-Ile-Gly-Ser-Arg), selectively enhances endothelial cell adhesion and proliferation without thrombogenic effects [165]. Protein pre-coating of valve scaffolds with fibronectin or elastin-derived VAPG (Val-Ala-Pro-Gly) can enhance cell engrafting and differentiation [25, 80]. Self-assembling peptides containing YIGSR or VAPG create nanomatrix milieu mimicking the endothelium and resulting in increased endothelialisation and proliferation of vSMCs [166].

RGD and GRGDSP are both functional domains belonging to fibronectin. Stent biofunctionalisation with these cell adhesive ligands has been reported to result in controversial issues: while promoting endothelial cell adhesion and coverage, it favours platelet attachment [167-169]. Thus, the usage of these adhesive sequences should be cautious in perspective of thrombotic events.

Positive cell-affinity effects can be instead obtained by coating scaffold surfaces with fibrin, which however can be employed only as coating solution lacking of important mechanical assets [170, 171].

Particularly appealing is the application of peptides selected by phage display. This technology offers the possibility to create combinatorial peptide libraries, where still unknown cell recognition surface molecules can be discovered. A new peptide ligand, i.e. TPS, was identified through cell-SELEX system (Systematic Evolution of Ligands by EXponential enrichment) and covalently linked to methacrylic polymeric matrix to selectively capture endothelial cells [172].

In combination with natural materials, new matrices based on silk and chitosan, a polysaccharide found in Crustaceans, could consent the accomplishment of hybrid valve scaffolds, where endothelial cells can better adhere and proliferate [173].

5.3.2. Antimicrobial treatments

Although no infections have been recorded yet after implantation of porcine- or bovine-derived tissues, the risk of transmission of porcine retroviruses or Creutzfeldt-Jacob disease has not to be underestimated. In order to avoid new trans-species viral combinations, endonuclease treatments generally applied after decellularization could be therefore preventing in this sense. The use of foetal bovine serum in heart valve tissue engineering and cryopreservation is also controversial and its substitution with serum replacement should be introduced in good manufacture practice.

The first infective risk is primarily represented by bacterial/fungal contamination. Current antimicrobial treatments are based on cocktails of large spectrum antibiotics and antimycotics and are performed on decellularized scaffolds prior to further *in vitro* cell seeding or *in vivo* implantation. Synthetic biomaterials are mostly submitted to gaseous disinfection with plasma gas or ethylene oxide.

While UV rays have a low penetration power for disinfection, gamma-irradiation is effective in abrogating contaminations. However, even when combined with the radioprotective cryopreservant DMSO, it is able to induce deep damages on the ECM fibres with deleterious effects in the long-term performance of so-treated heart valve substitutes [174].

5.3.3. Cues for thrombosis and neointimal hyperplasia prevention

Scaffold modifications for antithrombogenicity have been developed using endothelial coverage, ECM peptides inducing endothelium formation or by engineering their surface with inhibitors of platelet function or anticoagulant agents [175].

As already discussed, a normal endothelium is protective from platelet adhesion and aggregation in the first phases after implantation. Achievable *in vitro* with endothelial cells and their circulating progenitors, endothelialisation has to occur on all surfaces contacting blood, otherwise uncovered regions can be platelet-attractive. The implementation of extracellular matrix with endothelial adhesive ligands, as YIGSR, can foster a complete endothelial coverage [165].

Other cell sources for non-thrombogenic surfaces are represented by MSCs, which offer high compatibility with blood cells and are lacking of the platelet selective surface ligand HSPG [176].

Besides its EC and SMC affinity, HA, similarly to other GAGs, is effective in the prevention of platelet adhesion [177].

Other molecules able to inhibit thrombotic formations are phosphorylcholine phospholipid and polyethylene glycol, which counteract the adsorption of serum proteins [178, 179].

Instead of its preventive blockage, protein adsorption can be opportunely manipulated with fibrinogen to circumvent further diffusion of other serum molecules: while some hydrophobic domains of the molecule are adsorbed, others are exposed creating fibrous conformations able to attract endothelial cells [180].

Nitric oxide (NO), a chemical compound normally produced by functional endothelial cells and owning antithrombogenic efficacy can be also derived from decomposition of diazeniumdiolates. The incorporation of these molecules in scaffolds is able to drastically reduce *in vivo* thrombi formation [165, 181]. NO performs a second function in preventing valve complications. In fact, it is able to directly down-regulate proliferation pathways in vSMCs, thus precluding neointimal hyperplasia [182, 183]. Upon NO treatment, the activity of the protein synthesis machinery is reduced in these cells, observing a drastic reduction in the production of collagen [182]. Local delivery of stable S-nitrosothiol groups, incorporated in different compounds of serum albumin, has demonstrated to significantly reduce both platelet aggregation and neointimal proliferation in animal models of vascular injury [184]. Other NO formulations were identified to ensure a sustained and controlled release of the endothelial-derived molecule. When applied to VICs from the porcine aortic valve, combinations of poly(L-lactic acid) (PLLA) matrix systems incorporating NO-delivering poly(lactic-co-glycolic acid) (PLGA) nanoparticles reduced intercellular adhesion molecule 1 signalling and increased cyclic guanosine monophosphate levels, demonstrating therefore NO antiinflammatory and anticalcific potentialities [185].

Among anticoagulants, heparin is the most employed drug in the clinical activity. Resembling the glycosaminoglycan heparin sulphate in its chemical composition, it exerts blocking effect on the coagulation cascade also when immobilized into a scaffold. However, its pharmaceutical validity in this setting is not so good as in its soluble form [186].

Limited activity shown by immobilized heparin is surpassed by hyrudin scaffold incorporation. When conjugated to several biomaterials, this chemical agent is able both *in vitro* and *in vivo* to quench thrombin and prevent its further activity [187, 188].

Neointimal hyperplasia represents another complication in the *in vivo* performance of new viable valve substitutes. Besides NO, other chemical agents are currently used to counteract vSMC proliferation at the basis of neointima development. Local delivery of growth factors involved in the apoptotic pathways of vSMCs has been reported to attenuate the phenomenon with efficiency extents depending on the local concentration of the cytokine at the injury site [190, 191]. In lieu of locally delivering specific growth factors, the oral administration of drugs stimulating their cell production could represent a more compliant therapy for treated patients [192].

Other blocking strategies have been developed by directly targeting oligonucleotides or receptor molecules involved in vSMC proliferation. The use of antisense strategies or humanized monoclonal antibodies contributes to abolish the expression of proteins needed for cell cycling [193-195].

As for the administration of growth factors, these approaches rely on a non-functional endothelium and on the local vector availability.

Nevertheless, even if not yet tested in other formulations than soluble particles, growth factor- and antisense-based approaches could show promising potential when incorporated in scaffolds for cardiovascular applications.

More specifically tackling tactics can be exercised throughout the usage of viral particles with vascular tropism. Attenuated herpes simplex virus 1, obtained by removing only $\gamma_1 34.5$ genes, originally demonstrated its efficacy in malignant cancer therapies. Indeed, its ability to infect dividing cells can be used together with its tropism to vSMCs as efficient antiproliferative agent. In particular, while showing no systemic toxicity and a persistent activity for at least 4 weeks, its infective state can be electively blocked by antiviral drugs [196].

TGF-beta 1 and PDGF-BB pathways are up-regulated in the genesis of intimal hyperplasia. These growth factors contribute to the recruitment of adventitial cells by neighbouring medial SMCs through a paracrine mechanism and are, therefore, perfect targets in a blockade strategy. Cell-selective adenoviral gene transfer of Smad7 or PDGF-beta receptor reduced adventitial cell migration and vascular remodelling after balloon injury [197, 198].

Notwithstanding the efficiency and the possibility of control related to these systems, the use of viral agents is still accompanied by ethical and safety concerns, which argue in favour of other therapeutic strategies.

Already evaluated in combination to biomaterials is another drug class, which has been firstly applied in the immunotransplantation field. Limus derivatives are a large family of compounds preventing either allograft rejections or restenosis after angioplasty. Conversely, systemic toxic effects, unspecific antiproliferation activity on ECs and SMCs, and variable efficacy associated with their usage *in vitro* or *in vivo* are at the basis of the reported controversial results [199-203].

5.3.4. Functionalization of decellularized extracellular matrices

While decellularized ECMs have demonstrated the ability of *in vivo* self-regeneration, their structural and functional properties can be improved by conditioning with synthetic biomaterials. The advantage of such strategies resides in the combination of uniform and mouldable artificial products with bioactive natural scaffolds. Nanotechnology approaches are currently under investigation for the stable introduction of adhesive sequences or for the entrapment of structure-mouldable peptides (unpublished data).

5.3.5.. Anticalcification approaches

From the observation of the pathological events occurring in vessel/valve deterioration, different anticalcification strategies have been developed. In the bioprosthetic valves, mineralization is strictly related to the presence of phospholipids (phosphatidil serine and phosphaditil choline) and phosphate backbone of degraded nucleic acids in the extracellular milieu of a no more vital tissue [204, 205]. These extracellular phosphate groups are perfect nucleation sources for mineral deposition. The progression and entity of calcification is dependent on many factors and surely, the lack of a cell-favoured homeostatic pathway, provoked by glutaraldehyde (GA) cytotoxicity, can be useful to accelerate the phenomenon of diffuse mineralization on ECM fibres.

A reduction in the mineral deposition has been attempted through addition of several GA-detoxifying approaches. Challenged alone with valvular cells or cross-linked to GA-fixed bioprostheses in simulated body fluid, procyanidines have demonstrated cell biocompatibility, dose-dependent inhibition of alkaline phosphatase cellular activity and consequently, of matrix mineralization [206].

Lipid extraction for the removal of cell membrane phospholipids has been pursued by applying solvents or detergents with special attention to the preservation of ECM fibres. In an *in vivo* model, the long chain aliphatic alcohol octanediol in 40% concentration has proven to be an efficient anticalcification agent for GA-treated bovine pericardium [207].

A more diluted octanediol is in the organic solvent used as buffer for genypin/glutaraldehyde fixation of bovine pericardial tissues, previously submitted to sodium dodecyl sulphate decellularization and/or successively treated with several amino acids or sodium bisulphite. In respect to GA-fixed samples, all these different genypin-based variants turned out in in decreased calcium/phosphorus content and conserved tissue stability by resistance to pronase enzymatic degradation [208]. However, despite the concomitant evaluation of decellularization, which could have partaken in the removal of alpha-gal epitopes, the levels of these xenoantigens were valuated only between genipin/GA- versus sole GA-fixations particularly [208].

Ethanol cross-linked to triglycidyl amine is also able to reduce GA-associated calcification both in rat subdermal and sheep models, however it is responsible of structural instability in treated tissues [209]. In another study by Sacks et al, triglycidyl epoxy-crosslinking without GA addition demonstrated improved biomechanics in respect to GA alone [210].

Amino acids, as glycine, phenylalanine or aspartic acid, are largely employed in anticalcification processes to potentiate the action of alcohols and metallocene dichlorides [211].

Detergent application, at the basis of most decellularizing techniques, exploits tensioactivity to eliminate membrane lipids, indistinctly from the presence of phosphate groups. Treatments with Triton X100 and sodium cholate, deoxycholic acid, N-lauroyl sarcosinate or sodium dodecyl sulphate, especially if combined with DNA/RNA nucleases, resulted in no calcific events both *in vitro*, in preclinical animal models and/or in the clinical stage [25-28, 102, 212].

Calcium and phosphorus signalling has been tackled via calcimimetics and biphoshonates by directly acting on calcifying cells. So far evaluated mainly in the renal district, calcimimetics, as R-568 and AMG 641, could in the future be incorporated in synthetic and natural matrices to selectively block parathyroid hormone pathway responsible for renal artery calcification [213]. Interestingly, another calcimimetic, cinacalcet, has been reported to reduce vascular calcification in the renal aorta of uremic rats in association with further encouraging outcomes on vascular remodelling and myocardial fibrosis [214].

Testified as possible medical therapy for calcific aortic stenosis, bisphosphonate molecules incorporated into polyurethane scaffolds induced resistance from calcification in 60 day-long rat subdermal tests and in 90 day-long evaluation in the circulation as pulmonary valve cusp [215].

5.4. *In vitro* and *in vivo* novel tissue technologies

5.4.1. Bio-electrospray

Further advances in cardiovascular regenerative medicine have recently been introduced to ease the achievement of intraoperative tissue-engineered organ units: bioelectrospray is emerging as a powerful tool both for the creation of specific nanotopographic surface and for homogeneous/spatial cell seeding or coating of valve scaffolds [216, 217].

5.4.2. Monoclonal antibodies and DNA aptamers

Monoclonal antibodies can be applied to selectively capture cell populations expressing specific cluster differentiation molecules: an increase in the attachment of endothelial or mesenchymal stem cells was achieved by coating scaffold surface with anti-CD34, anti-CD90 or anti-CD133 [218-220].

Aptamers, 70-90 nucleotide-long single strand oligos, can bind to specific molecules with high selectivity and affinity. Identified through combinatorial phage display technology, they were immobilized on the surface of polydimethylsiloxan or polytetrafluoroethylene patches pre-coated with the antithrombogenic PEG. The scaffold formulation was able to block serum protein adsorption and selectively recruit EPCs from the bloodstream [221]. EPC-attracting aptamer technology has also been applied with similar results in valve scaffolds [222].

5.4.3. Organ printing

Extremely fascinating in bioengineering is the possibility to fabricate complex living structures by organ printing. This approach contemplates different sequential steps for the realization of biological tissue and organ substitutes: computer-aided design (CAD), image processing, modelling with solids, free-form fabrication, designing, simulation and finally manufacturing [223]. Several applications of this technology have been proposed since 2001 [224] and are currently focusing also in the preparation of cardiovascular tissues [225, 226]. Until now, organ printing has been rendered useful in the heart valve field not for biofabrication, but for pre-operative planning and valve replacement simulation in complex interventions [227].

5.4.4. In body tissue architecture

Actually, the concept of in body tissue architecture finds limited exploitation in the development of heart valves substitutes. Interestingly, the Japanese group of Nakayama et al. has produced a trileaflet valved-shaped construct based on this technology. As in the case of Campbell et al. [87], the approach takes advantage of the normal biological response to a foreign material developed by the body, implanting silicon rods in the subcutaneous tissues. In a period of 4 weeks, these grafts are first 'embedded' by granulation-like tissue, then removed and fused each other for correct valvular shaping and reinserted to complete the cell covering. At the end of the process, the particular arrangement given by the researchers allows eliminating supporting artificial materials to attain a trileaflet valve conduit [228].

5.5. Implantation techniques: Classical cardio-surgical implant versus transapical and TAVI access

Open chest interventions have represented the main surgical modality for diseased heart valve treatment. The classic cardio-surgical implant generally implies median sternotomy and cardio-pulmonary bypass with cannulation of both venae cavae and aorta in hypothermic conditions. This technique is largely used for the implantation of bioengineered valves in animal model testing or in clinical valve substitutions [93].

Classic cardio-surgical valve substitution is for sure a life-saving procedure. However, its invasiveness results in infective risk and pain in the immediate post-intervention period. Additionally, in children the current lack for valve substitutes with somatic adaptation ability submits these paediatric patients to several re-do procedures until their adulthood.

Owing to the improvement in life expectancy, the elderly represent another cardiopathic population in need for re-intervention.

Catheter-assisted techniques are minimally invasive implantation approaches, experimented in animal models in 1965 and in humans in 2000 [229, 230]. The percutaneous trans-catheter implantation of an aortic valve prosthesis (TAVI) was firstly performed by Cribier et al. some years later [231]. In a TAVI device, a bioprosthetic aortic valve is mounted on an expandable stainless steel stent. It is then compressed to nearly one-third of its diameter through a crimping procedure and introduced in a catheter before its implantation in the patient. Once the correct position has been assessed by fluoroscopy imaging, the crimped valve is balloon- or self-expanded and tightly juxtaposed to the insufficient aortic valve. The procedure of trans-catheter aortic valve insertion in degenerated surgically implanted bioprostheses is particularly indicated for high surgical risk patients, since a minimal thoracotomy access is required instead of sternotomy and cardio-pulmonary bypass.

Through a catheter-assisted system, tissue-engineered heart valves were transapically implanted in sheep and non-human primates as pulmonary valve replacements following a minithoracotomy [95, 232]. Although performing during 2 month-long experimental evaluation, cusp thickening was reported in these poly-4-hydroxybutyrate coated nonwoven polyglycolic acid-based TEHVs [233].

A similar transapical approach was adopted by the same group for TEHV implantation in sheep systemic circulation. Haemodinamically evaluated up to 2 weeks, these tissue-engineered aortic replacements were found post-mortem in active remodelling, with merely collagen/GAG ECM synthesis and freedom from thrombotic formations or structural degenerations [97].

These intriguing experimental evidences demonstrate the feasibility of such an approach also for bioengineered valve substitutes. In addition, a transapically-delivered bioengineered TAVI could be a particularly beneficial option for patients with severe aortic valve calcification.

However, crimping/re-opening effects on cell survival, ECM microstructure and valve function should be further examined both *in vitro* and *in vivo* within a longer observational time. Decellularized scaffold-relying approaches could be especially influenced by this mounting-related shock with immediate and significant consequences on tissue hydration, GAG content and collagen/elastin fibre interplay.

5.6. Imaging tools

5.6.1. Two Photon-laser scanning confocal microscopy

More and more advanced optical visualization systems are offering sophisticated functions for non-invasive deeper penetration and dynamic evaluation of developing organs and bioengineered constructs. Cell adhesion and spreading in thick 3D structures can now be analysed until almost millimetre depth by means of 2 photon-laser scanning confocal microscopy (2P-LSCM). Differently from more common linear-based imaging, 2P-LSCM exploits the simultaneous adsorption of two near IR-photons to excite endogenous fluorophores, as tricarboxylic triamipiridinium elastin-derivates, without previous sectioning or staining. Besides elastin networks, it is possible to study collagen fibres through second harmonic generation in an adsorption-free process [234]. This unique imaging modality offers the unquestionable possibility to dynamically monitor relatively small living tissues without manipulation artefacts [235].

5.6.2. MRI

Another non-invasive imaging modality is magnetic resonance: widely applied in the clinical setting, it surpasses ionizing radiation-based echocardiography for the optimal spatio-temporal resolution [236]. *In vivo* performance of bioengineered heart valves can be constantly monitored by MRI with the feasibility of precise dimensional measurements [229, 237]. Cell passive loading of magnetic resonance nanoparticles *in vitro* allows for their dynamic tracing in implanted tissue-engineered constructs. Formulated in different diameter size (10-1.000 nm), most used MR nanoparticles, i.e. 50 nm-diameter superparamagnetic iron oxide (SPIO) ones, are cell-incorporated by endocytotic loading or up-taken in enhanced way by combination with protamine sulphate. Cell survival, motility and differentiation abilities have been reported to be not strongly influenced by SPIOs, thus perturbing mainly the magnetic field in the populated tissue [238].

5.6.3. μOCT, PET and SPECT

While MR technology allows qualitative and quantitative dynamic functional studies, detailed information on valve degeneration can be attained by means of tomography-based imaging [239]. With its 1-μm-axial resolution, micro-optical coherence tomography (μOCT) would be a particularly interesting tool in in bioengineering to elucidate cellular and subcellular events in the early tissue engraftment as well as in the initial onset of valve disease [240].

Positron emission and single photon emission computed tomography (respectively PET and SPECT) possess an inferior spatial resolution. As SPIOs, radionuclide-labelled cells can be obtained by means of passive loading. Cell tracking, however, will be strictly limited by the radioisotope half-life: among the commonly used radionuclides, the SPECT probe ^{111}In-Oxine has the longest detectable radioactivity of 2.8 days. Another limitation associated with SPECT is the necessity to load a relatively high amount of radioisotopes for quantitative evaluations, at the expense of cell viability. The more sensitive PET suffers instead of the shorter half-life of used probes [241]. On this account, PET and SPECT are not ideal to evaluate *in vivo* mid/long-term dynamic remodelling of bioengineered valves, but necessary to identify calcific degenerations [28].

5.7. Heart valve tissue banks

After the production of new valve substitutes, their storage and further capillary distribution are essential steps to the prompt realization of interventional therapies.

Off-the-shelf solutions must rely on appropriate conservation procedures, avoiding the use of cytotoxic fixatives able to compromise further *in vivo* remodelling/regeneration of TEHVs and TGRHVs.

Cryopreservation has been established as alternative storage technique to GA-fixation, when allografts started to be employed in clinic 50 years ago. Initially called homografts, pulmonary valves from cadaveric donors found large usage in the Ross procedure instead of the patient's own valve, eterotopically transposed for the replacement of the degenerated aortic root [242]. After isolation, donor tissues are examined to exclude lacerations and/or unsuitability sources and graded following macroscopic qualitative evaluation. Antimicrobial procedures are then performed to eliminate bacterial and fungal infective risks with constant control for effective microbe removal [243, 244]. Decontaminated tissues are immersed in cryopreserving solutions, usually based on cell culture medium added with a low percentage of the cryoprotectant dimethyl sulfoxide (DMSO). DMSO contributes to reduce hyperosmolarity shocks and ice crystal formation, which would induce deleterious effects on heart valve structure and mechanics. Tissues, introduced in highly resistant package, are then submitted to time- and condition-controlled cryofreezing and stored in vapour-phase nitrogen tanks for a maximum 5 years long period if unused.

On a constantly updated survey of the European Homograft Bank, nearly 4.500 cryopreserved valves on about 5.200 selected tissues were employed for complex valve malformations in children, women of child-bearing age with diseased cardiac valves, patients with anticoagulation contra-indication or patients with severe endocarditis [245].

While undoubtedly more immunotolerable than xenogeneic bioprostheses, their performance in the patients has a comparable endurance. Causes for this restricted durability have been firstly searched in the survival of populating cell elements. Strips of aortic valve cusps and walls were stimulated with vasoactive concentrations of potassium, 5-hydroxytryptamine, noradrenaline, endothelin-1 and prostaglandin F-(2alpha) to test cell contractility after cryopreservation: no significant differences were observed in comparison to fresh tissues [246]. Apoptotic studies revealed cell necrosis, related to ischemia rather than a cryopreservation-dependent activation of death program [247]. Indeed, albeit its cryoprotective action, DMSO is cytotoxic at physiologic temperature and could be responsible for cell death in unwell washed out thawed valves [248]. In addition, ultrastructural damage was reported as major source of scarce ECM stability.

Cryopreservation technique has already been tested as possible storage modality of tissue-engineered or *in vivo* regenerating decellularized valve substitutes: independent deep imaging analyses revealed however contrasting observations upon this treatment. Evaluations with transmission electron microscopy of cryopreserved/decellularized specimens found typical ECM pattern with no collagen swelling/shrinkage or clearly distorted/disrupted elastin fibres [25]. Two photon-laser scanning confocal microscopy on decellularized/cryopreserved valves demonstrated structural integrity of ECM fibres [249]. Cryopreservation detrimental effects were instead reported with the application of the same imaging technology by Schenke-Layland et al. [250]. The same group proposed vitrification as ECM preserving alternative to cryopreservation. Vitrification, defined by the Authors as 'ice-free cryopreservation', mainly differs from the standard method for the additional use of formamide and 1,2-propanediol. Vitrified porcine pulmonary valves showed better haemodynamic and biologic performance in comparison to cryopreserved tissues [251]. However, chemical compounds added to the cryopreserving medium could negatively affect cell viability.

5.8. Inflammation in heart valve regenerative medicine

5.8.1. Adverse effects of inflammation on cardiovascular tissue engineering/regeneration

The natural response of a body to an implanted tissue develops similarly to the healing process of a wound and analogously resolves at the graft acceptance. The implant is initially surrounded and infiltrated by a granulation tissue rich in inflammatory mononucleated cells, as monocytes and neutrophils acquiring *in situ* a mature, active phenotype. Debris removal and cytokine release, operated by macrophages, contribute to activate the last remodelling phases, depending on recruited fibroblasts and smooth muscle cells. A delicate balancing is involved in this rejecting/engrafting process. An intensification in the pro-inflammatory macrophage function, related to a not fully biocompatible synthetic or natural scaffold, provokes the onset of immunologic responses by enrolling further cells, as lymphocytes.

A related aspect is also the genesis of firstly cell calcification and hence extended ECM mineralization. Remained into incompletely decellularized tissues (especially of xenogeneic origin) or fruit of cell death activation (necrosis or apoptosis) in tissue-engineered constructs, cellular debris can, in fact, trigger inflammatory and/or immunologic response activation. Comparably to foam cells in atherosclerotic lesions, cell death of foreign body giant cells, i.e. fused collections of macrophages, generates apoptotic bodies. These latter, together to the similar ones or to the debris both released by dying construct cells, further propagate inflammation and generate a suitable microenvironment for calcium nucleation [252-254].

As previously mentioned, retention of xenoantigens and detergents could further increase the *in vivo* pro-inflammatory potential of decellularized matrix-based approaches [255]. Nevertheless, some unsuccessful results described for both TEHVs and TGRHVs, trusting on decellularized tissues, could hypothetically reside in the decellularization-induced exposure of previously masked epitopes or even in ECM micro-modifications, recognized as non-self by the immune system. A recent paper by Zhou and coll. discussed upon the effects of different decellularizing treatments on ECM preservation, thrombogenicity and immunogenicity, by *in vitro* direct human blood contact. While sodium deoxycholate-based decellularization induced no ECM disruption and complete decellularization, for all proposed methods, including sodium dodecyl sulphate, trypsin/EDTA or trypsin-detergent-nuclease, thrombotic and immunological responses were surely higher than those in glutaraldehyde-fixed specimens [256]. A confirmation about these findings is supported by another work published in the same year: through a quantitative approach based on immunoblotting technique, Arai and Orton were able to demonstrate the detection of soluble protein antigens still maintained in bovine pericardium and porcine heart valves after decellularization with sodium dodecyl sulphate and sodium deoxycholate [257].

The treatment based on Triton X100, sodium cholate and endonucleases, not evaluated in the previously cited studies, demonstrated to produce acellular heart valve substitutes, evoking *in vivo* null thrombogenic or inflammatory/immunogenic responses thanks to the complete alpha-gal elimination [26, 27, 135, 136].

So far, endothelialisation strategies represent - also in the clinical setting - the almost unique modalities to prevent thrombogenicity-related excessive inflammation in tissue-engineered heart valves approaches, especially when autologous endothelial cells are employed [93].

5.8.2. Favourable inflammatory events on cardiovascular tissue engineering/regeneration

Differently from any other cardiovascular tissue, as the adjacent myocardium and arterial wall, adult heart valve atrioventricular and semilunar leaflets possess a highly represented CD34-

positive interstitial population (Figure 3), as also evidenced in the work of Barth and colleagues [258]. The presence of CD34-expressing cells in these tissues reminds on almost two possible and equally valuable hypotheses on the role of these cytotypes in these districts. CD34 is a glycoprotein expressed on endothelial cells and on their circulating progenitors (EPCs). It is also identifiable on the surface of bone marrow-residing haematopoietic stem cells, which are known to be myeloid cell precursors of EPCs and of other cells, among which monocytes and macrophages (their tissue-activated form) [259]. Other inflammatory cell markers have been found positive even in uncompromised cusps of young donor's valve allografts (Figure 3) [260]. In particular, CD68-expressing macrophages are widespread both in semilunar and atrioventricular valve tissues, without the intensely site-concentrated cell distribution usually observed in pathological specimens.

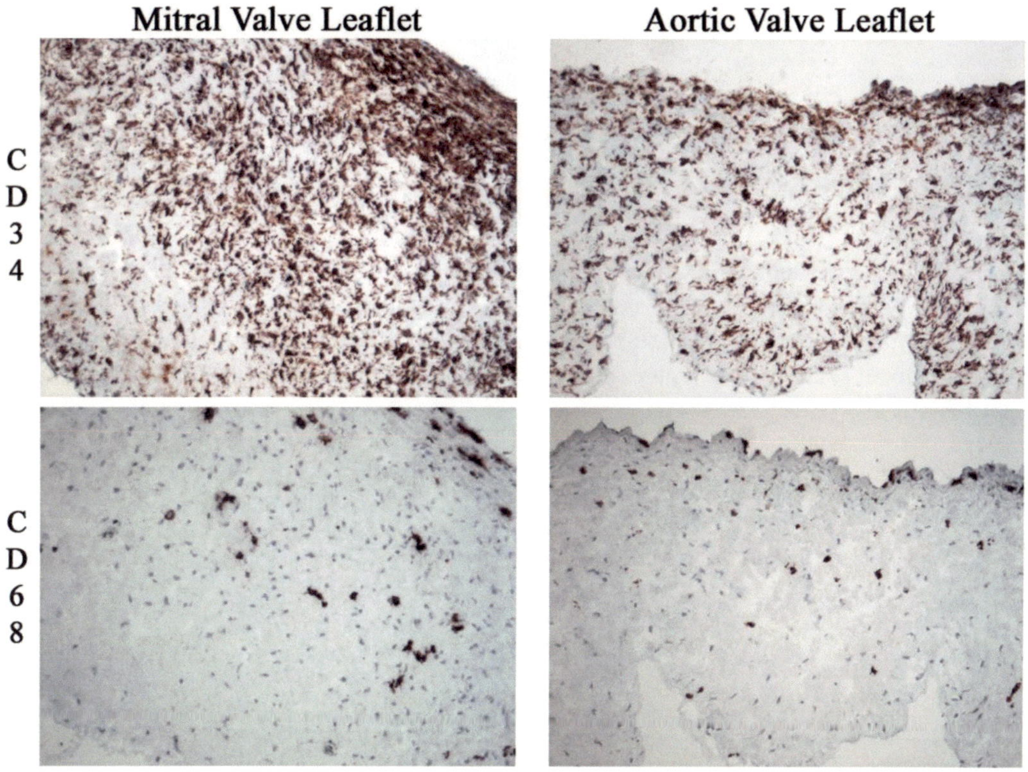

Figure 3. Hematopoietic cell markers expressed in the mitral and aortic valve leaflets of a 26 year-old donor allograft. CD34 is widely positive in all cusps tissues. CD68 expression is scattered and homogenously distributed in all leaflets, likely to identify a protective function, as that observable in the healthy myocardium. Magnification: 70x

The meaning of this presence in healthy tissues is not known, but it could be likely that the continuous mechanical stress imposed to the thin leaflets, together with the direct exposure to blood, needs a sentinel function exerted by macrophages and other cells.

Another interesting hypothesis rises from the observation of the double nature of the macrophage cell. In effect, a phenotype committed to tissue regeneration has been discovered besides the typical protective tasks played by these cells. For the similarity to T2 helper lymphocytes, these macrophages have been named M2 and can be characterized by the expression of interleukin-10 (IL-10) and mannose receptor (MR) [261]. In the analysed valve specimens, the immunodetection of CD68, a broad macrophage marker, is associated to the expression of MR and IL-10, as visible in Figure 4.

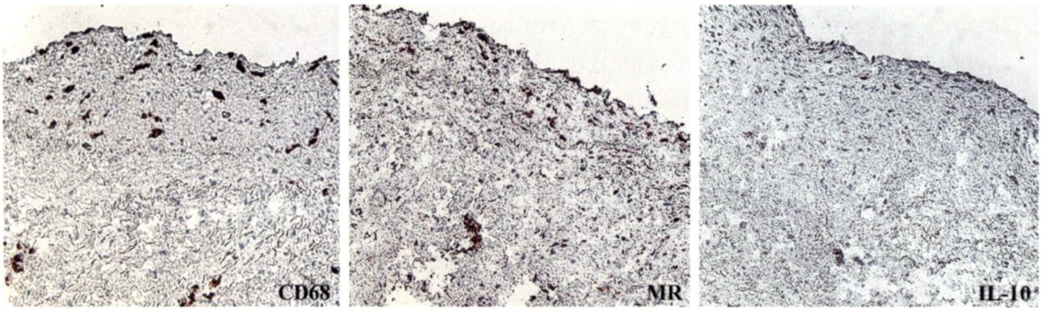

Figure 4. Evaluation of M2 macrophages in the mitral valve leaflet of a 26 year-old donor allograft. MR and IL-10 are likely to be expressed by the same CD68-positive cells. Magnification: 100x

This expression pattern of M2 macrophage typical markers is also preserved interspecies in mammals, further corroborating the notion of an evolutionarily conserved, constantly undergoing protection/regeneration process in the heart valve tissue. Porcine, bovine, sheep and non-human primate heart valves share, in fact, a similar cell distribution and localisation of CD68, MR and IL-10 markers (Figure 5).

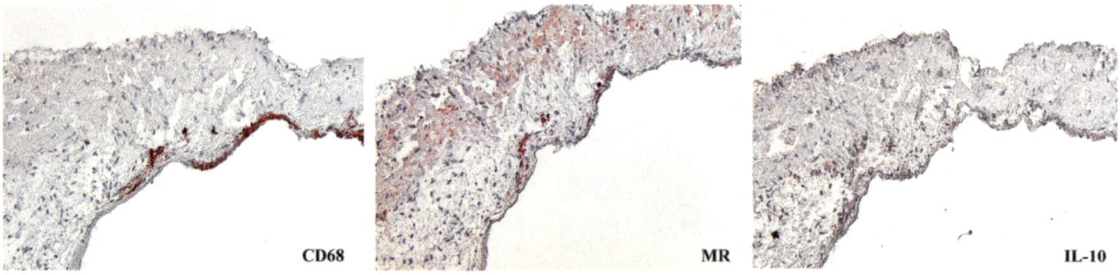

Figure 5. M2 macrophage pattern in the aortic valve leaflet of a Macaca fascicularis subject. Magnification: 50x

As further supportive remark, the extensive identification of stem cells with diverse lineages in heart valves evidences the unique regenerative properties endowed by these tissues [260].

Type 2 macrophages have been additionally found in the early post-implantation phases of bioengineered valve replacements and reported to remain in the implanted tissues until the construct scaffold has been completely replaced by an autologous matrix [262].

The engraftment of differently attainable biocompatible TEHVs and TGRHVs could be facilitated with the modulation of the M1/M2 ratio in favour of the second player: as often verified for other cardiovascular tissues [263], inflammatory responses could be mitigated through specific pharmaceutical treatments. While still at the sunrise of a possible clinical application in cardiovascular disease treatments, RNA interference (RNAi) technology could be an attenuator of inflammation, thanks to the selective silencing of targeted genes. Scaffold-mediated therapeutic delivery of RNAi could enable localize treatment of inflammation without secondary systemic effects [264].

Author details

Laura Iop* and Gino Gerosa

*Address all correspondence to: laura.iop@unipd.it

Department of Cardiac, Thoracic and Vascular Sciences School of Medicine, University of Padua, Padua, Italy

References

[1] Wells FC and Crowe T. Leonardo da Vinci as a paradigm for modern clinical research. J Thorac Cardiovasc Surg 2004;127(4): 929-4

[2] Hufnagel CA. Surgery of acquired diseases of the cardiac valves. GP. 1953;7(2):69-81

[3] Starr A, Edwards ML. Mitral replacement: clinical experience with a ball-valve prosthesis. Ann Surg 1961;154: 726-40

[4] Langer R, Vacanti JP. Tissue engineering. Science 1993;260: 920–6

[5] Agrawal CM, Ray RB. Biodegradable polymeric scaffolds for musculoskeletal tissue engineering. J Biomed Mater Res 2001;55: 141–150

[6] Braunwald NS. Performance of materials in vascular prosthetic devices: heart valves. Bull N Y Acad Med 1972;48(2): 357-61

[7] Wisman CB, Pierce WS, Donachy JH, Pae WE, Myers JL, Prophet GA. A polyurethane trileaflet cardiac valve prosthesis: in vitro and in vivo studies. Trans Am Soc Artif Intern Organs 1982;28: 164-8

[8] Bernacca GM, O'Connor B, Williams DF, Wheatley DJ. Hydrodynamic function of polyurethane prosthetic heart valves: influences of Young's modulus and leaflet thickness.Biomaterials2002;23(1): 45-50

[9] Kolff WJ, Yu LS. The return of elastomer valves. Ann Thorac Surg 1989;48(3 Suppl): S98-9

[10] Joshi RR, Frautschi JR, Phillips RE Jr, Levy RJ. Phosphonated polyurethanes that resist calcification.J Appl Biomater 1994;5(1): 65-77

[11] Rahmani B, Tzamtzis S, Ghanbari H, Burriesci G, Seifalian AM. Manufacturing and hydrodynamic assessment of a novel aortic valve made of a new nanocomposite polymer. J Biomech2012;45(7): 1205-11

[12] Shinoka T, Breuer CK, Tanel RE, Zund G, Miura T, Ma PX, Langer R, Vacanti JP, Mayer JE. Tissue engineering heart valves: valve leaflet replacement study in a lamb model. Ann Thorac Surg 1995;60(Suppl. 3): S513–6

[13] Shinoka T, Ma PX, Shum-Tim D, Breuer CK, Cusick RA, Zund G, Langer R, Vacanti JP, Mayer JE. Tissue engineered heart valves. Autologous valve leaflet replacement study in a lamb model. Circulation 1996;94(Suppl.): II164–8

[14] Shinoka T, Shum-Tim D, Ma PX, Tanel RE, Isogai N, Langer R, Vacanti JP, Mayer JE. Creation of viable pulmonary artery autografts through tissue engineering. J Thorac Cardiovasc Surg 1998;115: 536–546

[15] Schmidt D, Stock UA, Hoerstrup SP. Tissue engineering of heart valves using decellularized xenogeneic or polymeric starter matrices. Philos Trans R Soc Lond B Biol Sci 2007;362(1484): 1505-12

[16] Hoerstrup SP, Sodian R, Daebritz S, Wang J, Bacha EA, Martin DP, Moran AM, Guleserian KJ, Sperling JS, Kaushal S, Vacanti JP, Schoen FJ, Mayer JE Jr. Functional living trileaflet heart valves grown *in vitro*. Circulation 2000;102: III44–49

[17] Hoerstrup SP, Cummings Mrcs I, Lachat M, Schoen FJ, Jenni R, Leschka S, Neuenschwander S, Schmidt D, Mol A, Günter C, Gössi M, Genoni M, Zund G. Functional growth in tissue-engineered living, vascular grafts: follow-up at 100 weeks in a large animal model. Circulation 2006;114(1 Suppl): I159-66

[18] Yin W, Gallocher S, Pinchuk L, Schoephoerster RT, Jesty J, Bluestein D. Flow-induced platelet activation in a St. Jude mechanical heart valve, a trileaflet polymeric heart valve, and a St. Jude tissue valve.Artif Organs 2005;29(10): 826-31

[19] Mohammadi H. Nanocomposite biomaterial mimicking aortic heart valve leaflet mechanical behaviour. Proc Inst Mech Eng H 2011;225(7): 718-22

[20] Koroleva A, Gittard S, Schlie S, Deiwick A, Jockenhoevel S, Chichkov B. Fabrication of fibrin scaffolds with controlled microscale architecture by a two-photon polymerization-micromolding technique.Biofabrication 2012;4(1): 015001

[21] Ghanbari H, Viatge H, Kidane AG, Burriesci G, Tavakoli M, Seifalian AM. Polymeric heart valves: new materials, emerging hopes.Trends Biotechnol 2009;27(6): 359-67

[22] Grauss RW, Hazekamp MG, Oppenhuizen F, van Munsteren CJ, Gittenberger-de Groot AC, De Ruiter MC. Histological evaluation of decellularised porcine aortic

valves: matrix changes due to different decellularisation methods. Eur J Cardiothorac Surg 2005;27(4): 566-71

[23] Rieder E, Kasimir MT, Silberhumer G, Seebacher G, Wolner E, Simon P, Weigel G. Decellularization protocols of porcine heart valves differ importantly in efficiency of cell removal and susceptibility of the matrix to recellularization with human vascular cells. J Thorac Cardiovasc Surg 2004;127(2): 399-405

[24] Bertipaglia B, Ortolani F, Petrelli L, Gerosa G, Spina M, Pauletto P, Casarotto D, Marchini M, Sartore S. Cell characterization of porcine aortic valve and decellularized leaflets repopulated with aortic valve interstitial cells: the VESALIO Project (Vitalitate Exornatum Succedaneum Aorticum Labore Ingenioso Obtenibitur). Ann Thorac Surg 2003;75: 1274–1282

[25] Iop L, Renier V, Naso F, Piccoli M, Bonetti A, Gandaglia A, Pozzobon M, Paolin A, Ortolani F, Marchini M, Spina M, De Coppi P, Sartore S, Gerosa G. The influence of heart valve leaflet matrix characteristics on the interaction between human mesenchymal stem cells and decellularized scaffolds. Biomaterials 2009;30(25): 4104-16

[26] L, Gandaglia A, Bonetti A, Marchini M, Spina M, Basso C, Thiene G, Gerosa G. *In vivo* Spontaneous Tissue Regeneration Of Allogeneic Decellularized Aortic Valves. Conference Proceedings *5th Biennial Meeting of the Society for Heart Valve Disease (Joint meeting with Heart Valve Society of America)* – Berlin, Germany, 27-30 June 2009

[27] Gallo M, Naso F, Poser H, Rossi A, Franci P, Bianco R, Micciolo M, Zanella F, Cucchini U, Aresu L, Buratto E, Busetto R, Spina M, Gandaglia A, Gerosa G. Physiological performance of a detergent decellularized heart valve implanted for 15 months in Vietnamese pigs: surgical procedure, follow-up, and explant inspection. Artif Organs 2012;36(6): E138-50

[28] Dohmen PM, Lembcke A, Holinski S, Kivelitz D, Braun JP, Pruss A, Konertz W. Mid-term clinical results using a tissue-engineered pulmonary valve to reconstruct the right ventricular outflow tract during the Ross procedure. Ann Thorac Surg 2007;84(3): 729-36

[29] Yang M, Chen CZ, Wang XN, Zhu YB, Gu YJ. Favourable effects of the detergent and enzyme extraction method for preparing decellularized bovinepericardium scaffold for tissue engineered heart valves.J Biomed Mater Res B Appl Biomater 2009;91(1): 354-61

[30] Cigliano A, Gandaglia A, Lepedda AJ, Zinellu E, Naso F, Gastaldello A, Aguiari P, De Muro P, Gerosa G, Spina M, Formato M. Fine structure of glycosaminoglycans from fresh and decellularized porcine cardiac valves and pericardium.Biochem Res Int 2012;2012: 979351

[31] Kuschert GS, Coulin F, Power CA, Proudfoot AE, Hubbard RE, Hoogewerf AJ, Wells TN. Glycosaminoglycans interact selectively with chemokines and modulate receptor binding and cellular responses.Biochemistry 1999;38(39): 12959-68

[32] Badylak SF, Freytes DO, Gilbert TW. Extracellular matrix as a biological scaffold material: Structure and function. Acta Biomater2009;5(1): 1-13

[33] Naso F, Gandaglia A, Formato M, Cigliano A, Lepedda AJ, Gerosa G, Spina M. Differential distribution of structural components and hydration in aortic and pulmonary heart valve conduits: Impact of detergent-based cell removal. Acta Biomater 2010;6(12): 4675-88

[34] Lau WL, Festing MH, Giachelli CM. Phosphate and vascular calcification: Emerging role of the sodium-dependent phosphate co-transporter PiT-1.Thromb Haemost 2010;104(3): 464-70

[35] Cebotari S, Tudorache I, Jaekel T, Hilfiker A, Dorfman S, Ternes W, Haverich A, Lichtenberg A. Detergent decellularization of heart valves for tissue engineering: toxicological effects of residual detergents on human endothelial cells.Artif Organs 2010;34(3): 206-10

[36] Bayrak A, Tyralla M, Ladhoff J, Schleicher M, Stock UA, Volk HD, Seifert M. Human immune responses to porcine xenogeneic matrices and their extracellular matrix constituents in vitro.Biomaterials 2010;31(14): 3793-803

[37] Schnell AM, Hoerstrup SP, Zund G, Kolb S, Sodian R, Visjager JF, Grunenfelder J, Suter A, Turina M. Optimal cell source for cardiovascular tissue engineering: venous vs. aortic human myofibroblasts. Thorac Cardiovasc Surg 2001;49(4): 221-5

[38] Zhu L, Williams WG, Bellhouse B, Pugh S, Rabinovitch M. Effective endothelialization of polyurethane surfaces. Response to shear stress and platelet adhesion. ASAIO Trans 1990;36(4): 811-6

[39] Bengtsson LA, Phillips R, Haegerstrand AN. In vitro endothelialization of photooxidatively stabilized xenogeneic pericardium. Ann Thorac Surg 1995;60(2 Suppl): S365-8

[40] Kim WG, Park JK, Park YN, Hwang CM, Jo YH, Min BG, Yoon CJ, Lee TY. Tissue-engineered heart valve leaflets: an effective method for seeding autologous cells on scaffolds.Int J Artif Organs 2000;23(9): 624-8

[41] Shinoka T, Shum-Tim D, Ma PX, Tanel RE, Langer R, Vacanti JP, Mayer JE Jr. Tissue-engineered heart valve leaflets: does cell origin affect outcome?Circulation 1997;96(9 Suppl): II-102-7

[42] Hoffman-Kim D, Maish MS, Krueger PM, Lukoff H, Bert A, Hong T, Hopkins RA. Comparison of three myofibroblast cell sources for the tissue engineering of cardiac valves.Tissue Eng 2005;11(1-2): 288-301

[43] Appleton AJ, Appleton CT, Boughner DR, Rogers KA. Vascular smooth muscle cells as a valvular interstitial cell surrogate in heart valve tissue engineering. Tissue Eng Part A 2009;15(12): 3889-97

[44] Hoerstrup SP, Kadner A, Melnitchouk S, Trojan A, Eid K, Tracy J, Sodian R, Visjager JF, Kolb SA, Grunenfelder J, Zund G, Turina MI. Tissue engineering of functional trileaflet heart valves from human marrow stromal cells. Circulation 2002;106(12 Suppl 1): I143-50

[45] Schmidt D, Achermann J, Odermatt B, Breymann C, Mol A, Genoni M, Zund G, Hoerstrup SP. Prenatally fabricated autologous human living heart valves based on amniotic fluid derived progenitor cells as single cell source. Circulation 2007;116(11 Suppl): I64-70

[46] Castrechini NM, Murthi P, Gude NM, Erwich JJ, Gronthos S, Zannettino A, Brennecke SP, Kalionis B. Mesenchymal stem cells in human placental chorionic villi reside in a vascular Niche. Placenta 2010;31(3): 203-12

[47] Iop L, Chiavegato A, Callegari A, Bollini S, Piccoli M, Pozzobon M, Rossi CA, Calamelli S, Chiavegato D, Gerosa G, De Coppi P and Sartore S. Different cardiovascular potential of adult and fetal-type mesenchymal stem cells in a rat model of heart cryoinjury. *Cell Transplantation* 2008;17: 679-694

[48] Schmidt D, Achermann J, Odermatt B, Genoni M, Zund G, Hoerstrup SP. Cryopreserved amniotic fluid-derived cells: a lifelong autologous fetal stem cell source for heart valve tissue engineering. J Heart Valve Dis 2008;17(4): 446–55

[49] Schmidt D, Mol A, Breymann C, Achermann J, Odermatt B, Gössi M, et al. Living autologous heart valves engineered from human prenatally harvested progenitors. Circulation 2006;114(1 Suppl): I125–31

[50] Sodian R, Schaefermeier P, Abegg-Zips S, Kuebler WM, Shakibaei M, Daebritz S, et al. Use of human umbilical cord blood-derived progenitor cells for tissue-engineered heart valves. Ann Thorac Surg 2010;89(3): 819–28

[51] Schmidt D, Mol A, Odermatt B, Neuenschwander S, Breymann C, Gössi M et al. Engineering of biologically active living heart valve leaflets using human umbilical cord-derived progenitor cells. Tissue Eng 2006;12(11): 3223–32

[52] Haniffa MA, Wang XN, Holtick U, Rae M, Isaacs JD, Dickinson AM, Hilkens CM, Collin MP. Adult human fibroblasts are potent immunoregulatory cells and functionally equivalent to mesenchymal stem cells. J Immunol 2007 1;179(3): 1595-604

[53] Batten P, Sarathchandra P, Antoniw JW, Tay SS, Lowdell MW, Taylor PM, et al. Human mesenchymal stem cells induce T cell anergy and downregulate T cell allo-responses via the TH2 pathway: relevance to tissue engineering human heart valves. Tissue Eng 2006;12: 2263–73

[54] Colazzo F, Sarathchandra P, Smolenski RT, Chester AH, Tseng YT, Czernuszka JT, Yacoub MH, Taylor PM. Extracellular matrix production by adipose-derived stem cells: implications for heart valve tissue engineering.Biomaterials 2011;32(1): 119-27

[55] Vaculik C, Schuster C, Bauer W, Iram N, Pfisterer K, Kramer G, Reinisch A, Strunk D, Elbe-Bürger A. Human dermis harbors distinct mesenchymal stromal cell subsets.J Invest Dermatol 2012;132(3 Pt 1): 563-74

[56] Pittenger MF, Mackay AM, Beck S, Jaiswal RK, Douglas R, Mosca JD, et al. Multilineage potential of adult human mesenchymal stem cells. Science 1999;284: 143–7

[57] Latif N, Sarathchandra P, Thomas PS, Antoniw J, Batten P, Chester AH, et al. Characterization of structural and signaling molecules by human valve interstitial cells and comparison to human mesenchymal stem cells. J Heart Valve Dis 2007; 16:56

[58] Della Rocca F, Sartore S, Guidolin D, Bertipaglia B, Gerosa G, Casarotto D, et al. Cell composition of the human pulmonary valve: a comparative study with the aortic valve – the VESALIO Project. Vitalitate Exornatum Succedaneum Aorticum Labore Ingenioso Obtenibitur. Ann Thorac Surg 2000;70: 1594–600

[59] Sutherland FW, Perry TE, Yu Y, Sherwood MC, Rabkin E, Masuda Y, et al. From stem cells to viable autologous semilunar heart valve. Circulation 2005; 111: 2783–91

[60] Bin F, Yinglong L, Nin X, Kai F, Laifeng S, Xiaodong Z. Construction of tissue engineered homograft bioprosthetic heart valves *in vitro*. ASAIO J 2006;52: 303–9

[61] Sales VL, Mettler BA, Engelmayr GC Jr, Aikawa E, Bischoff J, Martin DP, Exarhopoulos A, Moses MA, Schoen FJ, Sacks MS, Mayer JE Jr. Endothelial progenitor cells as a sole source for ex vivo seeding of tissue-engineered heart valves.Tissue Eng Part A 2010;16(1): 257-67

[62] Dvorin EL, Wylie-Sears J, Kaushal S, Martin DP, Bischoff J. Quantitative evaluation of endothelial progenitors and cardiac valve endothelial cells: proliferation and differentiation on poly-glycolic acid/poly-4-hydroxybutyrate scaffold in response to vascular endothelial growth factor and transforming growth factor beta1.Tissue Eng 2003;9(3): 487-93

[63] Fang NT, Xie SZ, Wang SM, Gao HY, Wu CG, Pan LF. Construction of tissue-engineered heart valves by using decellularized scaffolds and endothelial progenitor cells.Chin Med J (Engl) 2007;120(8): 696-702

[64] Hoerstrup SP, Sodian R, Sperling JS, Vacanti JP, Mayer JE. New pulsatile bioreactor for *in vitro* formation of tissue engineered heart valves. Tissue engineering 2000; 6: 75–79

[65] Ramaswamy S, Gottlieb D, Engelmayr GC Jr, Aikawa E, Schmidt DE, Gaitan-Leon DM, Sales VL, Mayer JE Jr, Sacks MS. The role of organ level conditioning on the promotion of engineered heart valve tissue development in-vitro using mesenchymal stem cells. Biomaterials 2010;31(6): 1114-25

[66] Wang L, Wilshaw SP, Korossis S, Fisher J, Jin Z, Ingham E. Factors influencing the oxygen consumption rate of aortic valve interstitial cells: application to tissue engineering. Tissue Eng Part C Methods 2009;15(3): 355-63

[67] Warnock JN, Konduri S, He Z, Yoganathan AP.Design of a sterile organ culture system for the ex vivo study of aortic heart valves. J Biomech Eng2005;127(5): 857-61

[68] Lichtenberg A, Tudorache I, Cebotari S, Suprunov M, Tudorache G, Goerler H, Park JK, Hilfiker-Kleiner D, Ringes-Lichtenberg S, Karck M, Brandes G, Hilfiker A, Haverich A. Preclinical testing of tissue-engineered heart valves re-endothelialized under simulated physiological conditions.Circulation2006;114(1 Suppl): I559-65

[69] Jockenhoevel S, Zund G, Hoerstrup SP, Schnell A, Turina M. Cardiovascular tissue engineering: a new laminar flow chamber for in vitro improvement of mechanical tissue properties.ASAIO J2002;48(1): 8-11

[70] Engelmayr GC Jr, Sales VL, Mayer JE Jr, Sacks MS. Cyclic flexure and laminar flow synergistically accelerate mesenchymal stem cell-mediated engineered tissue formation: Implications for engineered heart valve tissues.Biomaterials 2006;27(36): 6083-95

[71] Balachandran K, Alford PW, Wylie-Sears J, Goss JA, Grosberg A, Bischoff J, Aikawa E, Levine RA, Parker KK. Cyclic strain induces dual-mode endothelial-mesenchymal transformation of the cardiac valve.Proc Natl Acad Sci USA 2011;108(50): 19943-8

[72] Sierad LN, Simionescu A, Albers C, Chen J, Maivelett J, Tedder ME, Liao J, Simionescu DT. Design and Testing of a Pulsatile Conditioning System for Dynamic Endothelialization of Polyphenol-Stabilized Tissue Engineered Heart Valves.Cardiovasc Eng Technol 2010;1(2): 138-153

[73] Breuer CK, Shin'oka T, Tanel RE, Zund G, Mooney DJ, Ma PX, Miura T, Colan S, Langer R, Mayer JE, Vacanti JP.Tissue engineering lamb heart valve leaflets.Biotechnol Bioeng 1996;50(5): 562-7

[74] Zund G, Breuer CK, Shinoka T, Ma PX, Langer R, Mayer JE, Vacanti JP. The in vitro construction of a tissue engineered bioprosthetic heart valve.Eur J Cardiothorac Surg 1997;11(3): 493-7

[75] Sodian R, Hoerstrup SP, Sperling JS, Martin DP, Daebritz S, Mayer JE Jr, Vacanti JP. Evaluation of biodegradable, three-dimensional matrices for tissue engineering of heart valves.ASAIO J 2000;46(1): 107-10

[76] Sodian R, Hoerstrup SP, Sperling JS, Daebritz SH, Martin DP, Schoen FJ, Vacanti JP, Mayer JE Jr. Tissue engineering of heart valves: in vitro experiences.Ann Thorac Surg. 2000 Jul;70(1):140-4

[77] Kadner A, Hoerstrup SP, Tracy J, Breymann C, Maurus CF, Melnitchouk S, Kadner G, Zund G, Turina M. Human umbilical cord cells: a new cell source for cardiovascular tissue engineering.Ann Thorac Surg 2002;74(4): S1422-8

[78] Kadner A, Zund G, Maurus C, Breymann C, Yakarisik S, Kadner G, Turina M, Hoerstrup SP. Human umbilical cord cells for cardiovascular tissue engineering: a comparative study.Eur J Cardiothorac Surg 2004;25(4): 635-41

[79] Schmidt D, Breymann C, Weber A, Guenter CI, Neuenschwander S, Zund G, Turina M, Hoerstrup SP. Umbilical cord blood derived endothelial progenitor cells for tissue engineering of vascular grafts.Ann Thorac Surg 2004;78(6): 2094-8

[80] Sales VL, Engelmayr GC Jr, Johnson JA Jr, Gao J, Wang Y, Sacks MS, Mayer JE Jr. Protein precoating of elastomeric tissue-engineeringscaffolds increased cellularity, enhanced extracellular matrix protein production, and differentially regulated the phenotypes of circulating endothelial progenitor cells.Circulation 2007;116(11 Suppl): I55-63

[81] Bader A, Schilling T, Teebken OE, Brandes G, Herden T, Steinhoff G, Haverich A. Tissue engineering of heart valves--human endothelial cell seeding of detergent acellularized porcine valves. Eur J Cardiothorac Surg. 1998 Sep;14(3):279-84

[82] Cebotari S, Mertsching H, Kallenbach K, Kostin S, Repin O, Batrinac A, Kleczka C, Ciubotaru A, Haverich A. Construction of autologous human heart valves based on an acellular allograft matrix.Circulation 2002;106(12 Suppl 1): I63-I68

[83] Schenke-Layland K, Opitz F, Gross M, Döring C, Halbhuber KJ, Schirrmeister F, Wahlers T, Stock UA. Complete dynamic repopulation of decellularized heart valves by application of defined physical signals-an in vitro study.Cardiovasc Res 2003;60(3): 497-509

[84] Lichtenberg A, Tudorache I, Cebotari S, Ringes-Lichtenberg S, Sturz G, Hoeffler K, Hurscheler C, Brandes G, Hilfiker A, Haverich A. In vitro re-endothelialization of detergent decellularized heart valves under simulated physiological dynamic conditions.Biomaterials 2006;27(23): 4221-9

[85] Callegari A, Bollini S, Iop L, Chiavegato A, Torregrossa G, Pozzobon M, Gerosa G, De Coppi P, Elvassore N, Sartore S. Neovascularization induced by porous collagen scaffold implanted on intact and cryoinjured rat hearts. Biomaterials 2007;28(36): 5449-61

[86] Menon NG, Rodriguez ED, Byrnes CK, Girotto JA, Goldberg NH, Silverman RP. Revascularization of human acellular dermis in full-thickness abdominal wall reconstruction in the rabbit model. Ann Plast Surg 2003;50(5): 523-7

[87] Chue WL, Campbell GR, Caplice N, Muhammed A, Berry CL, Thomas AC, Bennett MB, Campbell JH. Dog peritoneal and pleural cavities as bioreactors to grow autologous vascular grafts. J Vasc Surg 2004;39(4): 859-67

[88] Kalfa D, Bel A, Chen-Tournoux A, Della Martina A, Rochereau P, Coz C, Bellamy V, Bensalah M, Vanneaux V, Lecourt S, Mousseaux E, Bruneval P, Larghero J, Menasché P. A polydioxanone electrospun valved patch to replace the right ventricular outflow tract in a growing lamb model.Biomaterials 2010;31(14): 4056-63

[89] Steinhoff G, Stock U, Karim N, Mertsching H, Timke A, Meliss RR, Pethig K, Haverich A, Bader A. Tissue engineering of pulmonary heart valves on allogenic acellular

matrix conduits: in vivo restoration of valve tissue.Circulation 2000;102(19 Suppl 3): III50-5

[90] Dohmen PM, Ozaki S, Yperman J, Flameng W, Konertz W. Lack of calcification of tissue engineered heart valves in juvenile sheep.Semin Thorac Cardiovasc Surg 2001;13(4 Suppl 1): 93-8

[91] Lutter G, Metzner A, Jahnke T, Bombien R, Boldt J, Iino K, Cremer J, Stock UA. Percutaneous tissue-engineered pulmonary valved stent implantation.Ann Thorac Surg 2010;89(1): 259-63

[92] Perri G, Polito A, Esposito C, Albanese SB, Francalanci P, Pongiglione G, Carotti A. Early and late failure of tissue-engineered pulmonary valve conduits used for right ventricular outflow tract reconstruction in patients with congenital heart disease. Eur J Cardiothorac Surg 2012;41(6): 1320-5

[93] Cebotari S, Lichtenberg A, Tudorache I, Hilfiker A, Mertsching H, Leyh R, Breymann T, Kallenbach K, Maniuc L, Batrinac A, Repin O, Maliga O, Ciubotaru A, Haverich A. Clinical application of tissue engineered human heart valves using autologous progenitor cells. Circulation 2006;114(1 Suppl): I132-7

[94] Dohmen PM, Lembcke A, Holinski S, Pruss A, Konertz W. Ten years of clinical results with a tissue-engineered pulmonary valve. Ann Thorac Surg 2011;92(4): 1308-14

[95] Weber B, Scherman J, Emmert MY, Gruenenfelder J, Verbeek R, Bracher M, Black M, Kortsmit J, Franz T, Schoenauer R, Baumgartner L, Brokopp C, Agarkova I, Wolint P, Zund G, Falk V, Zilla P, Hoerstrup SP. Injectable living marrow stromal cell-based autologous tissue engineered heart valves: first experiences with a one-step intervention in primates.Eur Heart J 2011;32(22): 2830-40

[96] Emmert MY, Weber B, Behr L, Frauenfelder T, Brokopp CE, Grünenfelder J, Falk V, Hoerstrup SP. Transapical aortic implantation of autologous marrow stromal cell-based tissue-engineered heart valves: first experiences in the systemic circulation.JACC Cardiovasc Interv 2011;4(7): 822-3

[97] Emmert MY, Weber B, Wolint P, Behr L, Sammut S, Frauenfelder T, Frese L, Scherman J, Brokopp CE, Templin C, Grünenfelder J, Zünd G, Falk V, Hoerstrup SP. Stem cell-based transcatheter aortic valve implantation: first experiences in a pre-clinical model.JACC Cardiovasc Interv 2012;5(8): 874-83

[98] Vincentelli A, Wautot F, Juthier F, Fouquet O, Corseaux D, Marechaux S, Le Tourneau T, Fabre O, Susen S, Van Belle E, Mouquet F, Decoene C, Prat A, Jude B. In vivo autologous recellularization of a tissue-engineered heart valve: are bone marrow mesenchymal stem cells the best candidates? J Thorac Cardiovasc Surg 2007;134(2): 424-32

[99] Dohmen PM, da Costa F, Yoshi S, Lopes SV, da Souza FP, Vilani R, Wouk AF, da Costa M, Konertz W. Histological evaluation of tissue-engineered heart valves im-

planted in the juvenile sheep model: is there a need for in-vitro seeding? J Heart Valve Dis 2006;15(6): 823-9

[100] Dohmen PM, da Costa F, Holinski S, Lopes SV, Yoshi S, Reichert LH, Villani R, Posner S, Konertz W. Is there a possibility for a glutaraldehyde-free porcine heart valve to grow? Eur Surg Res 2006;38(1): 54-61

[101] Affonso da Costa FD, Dohmen PM, Lopes SV, Lacerda G, Pohl F, Vilani R, Affonso Da Costa MB, Vieira ED, Yoschi S, Konertz W, Affonso da Costa I. Comparison of cryopreserved homografts and decellularized porcine heterografts implanted in sheep.Artif Organs 2004;28(4): 366-70

[102] Hopkins RA, Jones AL, Wolfinbarger L, Moore MA, Bert AA, Lofland GK. Decellularization reduces calcification while improving both durability and 1-year functional results of pulmonary homograft valves in juvenile sheep. J Thorac Cardiovasc Surg 2009;137(4):907-13, 913e1-4

[103] Baraki H, Tudorache I, Braun M, Höffler K, Görler A, Lichtenberg A, Bara C, Calistru A, Brandes G, Hewicker-Trautwein M, Hilfiker A, Haverich A, Cebotari S. Orthotopic replacement of the aortic valve with decellularized allograft in a sheep model.Biomaterials 2009;30(31): 6240-6

[104] Muratov R, Britikov D, Sachkov A, Akatov V, Soloviev V, Fadeeva I, Bockeria L. New approach to reduce allograft tissue immunogenicity. Experimental data. Interact Cardiovasc Thorac Surg 2010;10(3): 408-12

[105] Costa F, Dohmen P, Vieira E, Lopes SV, Colatusso C, Pereira EW, Matsuda CN, Cauduro S. Ross Operation with decellularized pulmonary allografts: medium-term results. Rev Bras Cir Cardiovasc 2007;22(4): 454-62

[106] CebotariS, Tudorache I, Ciubotaru A, Boethig D, Sarikouch S, Goerler A, Lichtenberg A, Cheptanaru E, Barnaciuc S, Cazacu A, Maliga O, Repin O, Maniuc L, Breymann T, Haverich A. Use of freshdecellularizedallografts for pulmonary valve replacement may reduce the reoperation rate in children and young adults: early report. Circulation 2011;124(11 Suppl): S115–23

[107] Brown JW, Elkins RC, Clarke DR, Tweddell JS, Huddleston CB, Doty JR, Fehrenbacher JW, Takkenberg JJ. Performance of the CryoValve SG human decellularized pulmonary valve in 342 patients relative to the conventional CryoValve at a mean follow-up of four years. J Thorac Cardiovasc Surg 2010;139(2): 339-48

[108] Burch PT, Kaza AK, Lambert LM, Holubkov R, Shaddy RE, Hawkins JA. Clinical performance of decellularized cryopreserved valved allografts compared with standard allografts in the right ventricular outflow tract. Ann Thorac Surg 2010;90(4): 1301-5

[109] Erdbrugger W, Konertz W, Dohmen PM, Posner S, Ellerbrok H, Brodde OE, Robenek H, Modersohn D, Pruss A, Holinski S, Stein-Konertz M, Pauli G. Decellularized xen-

ogeneic heart valves reveal remodeling and growth potential *in vivo*. Tissue Eng 2006;12(8): 2059-68

[110] Konertz W, Angeli E, Tarusinov G, Christ T, Kroll J, Dohmen PM, Krogmann O, Franzbach B, Pace Napoleone C, Gargiulo G. Right ventricular outflow tract reconstruction with decellularized porcine xenografts in patients with congenital heart disease. J Heart Valve Dis 2011;20(3): 341-7

[111] Bloch O, Golde P, Dohmen PM, Posner S, Konertz W, Erdbrügger W.Immune response in patients receiving a bioprosthetic heart valve: lack of response with decellularized valves. Tissue Eng Part A 2011;17(19-20): 2399-405

[112] Rüffer A, Purbojo A, Cicha I, Glöckler M, Potapov S, Dittrich S, Cesnjevar RA. Early failure of xenogenous de-cellularised pulmonary valve conduits--a word of caution! Eur J Cardiothorac Surg2010;38(1): 78-85

[113] Cicha I, Rüffer A, Cesnjevar R, Glöckler M, Agaimy A, Daniel WG, Garlichs CD, Dittrich S. Early obstruction of decellularized xenogenic valves in pediatric patients: involvement of inflammatory and fibroproliferative processes.Cardiovasc Pathol 2011;20(4): 222-31

[114] Simon P, Kasimir MT, Seebacher G, Weigel G, Ulrich R, Salzer U, Rieder E and Wolner E. Early failure of the tissue engineered porcine heart valve Synergraft™ in paediatric patients. Eur J Cardiothorac Surg 2003;23: 1002-6

[115] Sprangers B, Waer M, Billiau AD. Xenograft rejection-all that glitters is not Gal. Nephrol Dial Transplant 2006;21: 1486-8

[116] Terasaki PI, Cecka JM, Gjertson DW, Takemoto S, Cho YW, Yuge J. Risk rate and long-term kidney transplant survival. Clin Transpl 1996: 443-58

[117] Billingham ME, Cary NR, Hammond ME, Kemnitz J, Marboe C, McCallister HA, Snovar DC, Winters GL, Zerbe A. A working formulation for the standardization of nomenclature in the diagnosis of heart and lung rejection: Heart Rejection Study Group. The International Society for Heart Transplantation. J Heart Transplant 1990;9(6): 587-93

[118] Edge ASB, Gosse ME and Dinsmore J. Xenogeneic cell therapy: current progress and future developments in porcine cell transplantation. Cell Transplant 1998;7: 525-539

[119] Kobayashi T, Taniguchi S, Neethling FA, Rose A, Hancock WW, Ye Y, Niekrasz M , Kosanke S, Wright JL,White DJG and Cooper DKC. Delayed xenograft rejection of pig-to-baboon cardiac transplants after cobra venom factor therapy. Transplantation 1997; 64: 1255-1261

[120] Galili U, Clark MR, Shohet SB, Buehler J, Macher BA. Evolutionary relationship between the natural anti-Gal antibody and the Gal alpha 1-3Gal epitope in primates. Proc Natl Acad Sci USA 1987;84: 1369-1373

[121] Galili U, Shohet SB, Kobrin E, Stults CL, Macher BA. Man, apes, and Old World monkeys differ from other mammals in the expression of alpha-galactosyl epitopes on nucleated cells. J Biol Chem 1988;263(33): 17755-62

[122] Galili U, Rachmilewitz EA, Peleg A, Flechner I. A unique natural human IgG antibody with anti-alphagalactosyl specificity. J Exp Med 1984;160(5): 1519-31

[123] Galili U, Mandrell RE, Hamadeh RM, Shohet SB, Griffiss JM. Interaction between human natural anti-alphagalactosyl immunoglobulin G and bacteria of the human flora. Infect Immun 1988;56(7):1730

[124] Cooper DK, Good AH, Koren E, Oriol R, Malcolm AJ, Ippolito RM, Neethling FA, Ye Y, Romano E, Zuhdi N. Identification of alpha-galactosyl and other carbohydrate epitopes that are bound by human anti-pig antibodies: relevance to discordant xenografting in man. Transpl Immunol 1993;1(3): 198-205

[125] Koren E, Kujundzic M, Koscec M, Neethling FA, Richards SV, Ye Y, Zuhdi N, Cooper DK. Cytotoxic effects of human preformed anti-Gal IgG and complement on cultured pig cells. Transplant Proc 1994;26(3): 1336-9

[126] Alwayn IPJ, Basker M, Buhler L and Cooper DKC. The problem of anti-pig antibodies in pig-to-primate xenografting: current and novel methods of depletion and/or suppression of production of anti-pig antibodies. Xenotransplantation 1999; 6: 157-168

[127] Kozlowski T, Shimizu A, Lambrigts D, Yamada K, Fuchimoto Y, Glaser R, Monroy R, Xu Y, Awwad M, Colvin RB, Cosimi AB, Robson SC, Fishman J, Spitzer TR, Cooper DKC, Sachs DH. Porcine kidney and heart transplantations in baboons undergoing a tolerance induction regimen and antibody adsorption. Transplantation 1999;67: 18-30

[128] Schmoeckel M, Bhatti FN, Zaidi A, Cozzi E, Waterworth PD, Tolan MJ, Pino-Chavez G, Goddard M, Warner RG, Langford GA, Dunning JJ, Wallwork J, White DJ. Orthotopic heart transplantation in a transgenic pig-to-primate model. Transplantation 1998;65: 1570-7

[129] Minanov OP, Artrip JH, Szabolcs M, Kwiatkowski PA, Galili U, Itescu S, Michler RE. Triple immunosuppresion reduces mononuclear cell infiltration and prolongs graft life in pig-to-newborn baboon cardiac xenotransplantation. J Thorac Cardiovasc Surg 1998;115: 998-1006

[130] Lam TT, Paniagua R, Shivaram G, Schuurman HJ, Borie DC, Morris RE. Anti-non-Gal porcine endothelial cell antibodies in acute humoral xenograft rejection of hDAF-transgenic porcine hearts in cynomolgus monkeys. Xenotransplantation 2004;11: 531-535

[131] Costa C, Zhao L, Burton WV, Bondioli KR, Williams BL, Hoagland TA, Di Tullio PA, Ebert KM and Fodor WL. Expression of α1-2-fucosyltransferase in transgenic pigs

modifies the surface carbohydrate phenotype and confers resistance to human serum-mediated cytolysis. FASEB J 1999;6: 6-11

[132] Cozzi E, Yannoutsous N, Langford GA, Pino-Chavez G, Wallwork B and White DJG. Effect of transgenic expression of human decay-accelerating factor on the inhibition of hyperacute rejection of pig organs. In Xenotransplantation by Cooper DKC and Kemp E, pp. 665-682, Springer-Verlag, Berlin

[133] Kuwaki K, Tseng YL, Dor FJMF, et al. Heart transplantation in baboons using α1,3-galactosyltransferase gene-knockout pigs as donors: initial experience. Nat Med 2005;11: 29–31

[134] Kasimir MT, Rieder E, Seebacher G, Wolner E, Weigel G and Simon P. Presence and elimination of the xenoantigen Gal (α1-3) Gal in tissue-engineered heart valves. Tissue Engineering 2005;11: 1274-1280

[135] Naso F, Gandaglia A, Iop L, Spina M, Gerosa G. Alpha-Gal detectors in xenotransplantation research: a word of caution.Xenotransplantation 2012;19(4): 215-20

[136] Naso F, Gandaglia A, Iop L, Spina M, Gerosa G. First quantitative assay of alpha-Gal in soft tissues: presence and distribution of the epitope before and after cell removal from xenogeneic heart valves.Acta Biomater 2011;7(4): 1728-34

[137] Dijkman PE, Driessen-Mol A, Frese L, Hoerstrup SP, Baaijens FP. Decellularized homologous tissue-engineered heart valves as off-the-shelf alternatives to xeno- and homografts. Biomaterials 2012;33(18): 4545-54

[138] Krug EL, Markwald RR. Extracellular cardiac proteins activate chick endothelial transition to prevalvular mesenchyme. Prog Clin Biol Res1986;217B: 195-8

[139] de Lange FJ, Moorman AFM, Anderson H, Maenner J,. Soufan AT, de Gier-de Vries C, Schneider MD, Webb S, van den Hoff MJB, Christoffels VM. Lineage and Morphogenetic Analysis of the Cardiac Valves. Circ Res 2004;95; 645-654

[140] Snider P, Olaopa M, Firulli AB, Conway SJ. Cardiovascular Development and the Colonizing Cardiac Neural Crest Lineage. The Scientific World Journal 2007;7: 1090–1113

[141] Eisenberg LM, Markwald RR. Molecular Regulation of Atrioventricular Valvulo-septal Morphogenesis. Circulation Research 1995; 77:1-6

[142] von Wattenwyl R, Blumenthal B, Heilmann C, Golsong P, Poppe A, Beyersdorf F, Siepe M.Scaffold-based transplantation of vascular endothelial growth factor-overexpressing stem cells leads to neovascularization in ischemic myocardium but did not show a functional regenerative effect.ASAIO J 2012;58(3): 268-74

[143] Noiseux N, Gnecchi M, Lopez-Ilasaca M, Zhang L, Solomon SD, Deb A, Dzau VJ, Pratt RE. Mesenchymal stem cells overexpressing Akt dramatically repair infarcted

myocardium and improve cardiac function despite infrequent cellular fusion or differentiation.Mol Ther 2006;14(6): 840-50

[144] Takahashi K, Tanabe K, Ohnuki M, Narita M, Ichisaka T, Tomoda K, Yamanaka S.Induction of pluripotent stem cells from adult human fibroblasts by defined factors.Cell 2007;131(5): 861-72

[145] Jung CB, Moretti A, Mederos y Schnitzler M, Iop L, Storch U, Bellin M, Dorn T, Ruppenthal S, Pfeiffer S, Goedel A, Dirschinger RJ, Seyfarth M, Lam JT, Sinnecker D, Gudermann T, Lipp P, Laugwitz KL. Dantrolene rescues arrhythmogenic RYR2 defect in a patient-specific stem cell model of catecholaminergic polymorphic ventricular tachycardia.EMBO Mol Med 2012;4(3): 180-91

[146] Templin C, Zweigerdt R, Schwanke K, Olmer R, Ghadri JR, Emmert MY, Müller E, Küest SM, Cohrs S, Schibli R, Kronen P, Hilbe M, Reinisch A, Strunk D, Haverich A, Hoerstrup S, Lüscher TF, Kaufmann PA, Landmesser U, Martin U. Transplantation and tracking of human-induced pluripotent stem cells in a pig model of myocardial infarction: assessment of cell survival, engraftment, and distribution by hybrid single photon emission computed tomography/computed tomography of sodium iodide symporter transgene expression. Circulation 2012;126(4): 430-9

[147] Armstrong EJ and Bischoff J. Heart Valve Development: Endothelial Cell Signaling and Differentiation. Circ Res 2004;95; 459-470

[148] Combs MD and Yutzey KE. VEGF and RANKL Regulation of NFATc1 in Heart Valve Development. Circ Res 2009;105; 565-574

[149] de la Pompa JL. Notch Signaling in Cardiac Development and Disease. Pediatr Cardiol 2009;30: 643–650

[150] Rivera-Feliciano J, Tabin CJ. Bmp2 instructs cardiac progenitors to form the heart-valve-inducing field. Developmental Biology 2006;295:580–588

[151] MCCulley DJ, Kang J, Martin JF, Black BL. BMP4 is required in the anterior heart field and its derivatives for endocardial cushion remodeling, outflow tract septation, and semilunar valve development. Developmental Dynamics 2008;237: 3200–3209

[152] Lincoln J, Kist R, Scherer G, Yutzey KE. Sox9 is required for precursor cell expansion and extracellular matrix organization during mouse heart valve development. Developmental Biology 2007;305: 120–132

[153] Lie-Venema H, Eralp I, Markwald RR, van den Akker NM, Wijffels MC, Kolditz DP, van der Laarse A, Schalij MJ, Poelmann RE, Bogers AJ, Gittenberger-de Groot AC. Periostin expression by epicardium-derived cells is involved in the development of the atrioventricular valves and fibrous heart skeleton. Differentiation 2008;76(7): 809-19

[154] Norris RA, Potts JD, Yost MJ, Junor L, Brooks T, Tan H, Hoffman S, Hart MM,. Kern MJ, Damon B, Markwald RR, Goodwin RL. Periostin Promotes a Fibroblastic Lineage

Pathway in Atrioventricular Valve Progenitor Cells. Developmental Dynamics 2009;238: 1052–1063

[155] Scherz PJ, Huisken J, Sahai-Hernandez P, Stainier DYR. High-speed imaging of developing heart valves reveals interplay of morphogenesis and function. Development 2008;135: 1179-1187

[156] Ghosh AK, Nagpal V, Covington JW, Michaels MA, Vaughan DE. Molecular basis of cardiac endothelial-to-mesenchymaltransition (EndMT): differential expression of microRNAs during EndMT. Cell Signal 2012;24(5): 1031-6

[157] Hong H, Dong N, Shi J, Chen S, Guo C, Hu P, Qi H. Fabrication of a novel hybrid heart valve leaflet for tissue engineering: an in vitro study.Artif Organs2009;33(7): 554-8

[158] Paruchuri S, Yang JH, Aikawa E, Melero-Martin JM, Khan ZA, Loukogeorgakis S, Schoen FJ, Bischoff J. Human pulmonary valve progenitor cells exhibit endothelial/mesenchymal plasticity in response to vascular endothelial growth factor-A and transforming growth factor-beta2. Circ Res 2006;99(8): 861-9

[159] Chiu YN, Norris RA, Mahler G, Recknagel A, Butcher JT. Transforming growth factor β, bone morphogenetic protein, and vascular endothelial growth factor mediate phenotype maturation and tissue remodeling by embryonic valve progenitor cells: relevance for heart valve tissue engineering. Tissue Eng Part A 2010;16(11): 3375-83

[160] Sewell-Loftin MK, Chun YW, Khademhosseini A, Merryman WD. EMT-inducing biomaterials for heart valve engineering: taking cues from developmental biology.J Cardiovasc Transl Res 2011;4(5): 658-71

[161] Ramamurthi A, Vesely I. Evaluation of the matrix-synthesis potential of crosslinked hyaluronan gels for tissue engineering of aortic heart valves.Biomaterials2005;26(9): 999-1010

[162] Camci-Unal G, Nichol JW, Bae H, Tekin H, Bischoff J, Khademhosseini A. Hydrogel surfaces to promote attachment and spreading of endothelial progenitor cells.J Tissue Eng Regen Med 2012; doi: 10.1002/term.517

[163] Koens MJ, Faraj KA, Wismans RG, van der Vliet JA, Krasznai AG, Cuijpers VM, Jansen JA, Daamen WF, van Kuppevelt TH. Controlled fabrication of triple layered and molecularly defined collagen/elastin vascular grafts resembling the native blood vessel.Acta Biomater 2010;6(12): 4666-74

[164] Smith MD, Shearer MG, Srivastava S, Scott R, Courtney JM. Quantitative evaluation of the growth of established cell lines on the surface of collagen, collagen composite and reconstituted basement membrane.Urol Res 1992;20(4): 285-8

[165] Taite LJ, Yang P, Jun HW, West JL. Nitric oxide-releasing polyurethane-PEG copolymer containing the YIGSR peptide promotes endothelialization with decreased platelet adhesion.J Biomed Mater Res B Appl Biomater 2008;84(1): 108-16

[166] Andukuri A, Minor WP, Kushwaha M, Anderson JM, Jun HW. Effect of endothelium mimicking self-assembled nanomatrices on cell adhesion and spreading of human endothelial cells and smooth muscle cells.Nanomedicine 2010;6(2): 289-97

[167] Blindt R, Vogt F, Astafieva I, Fach C, Hristov M, Krott N, Seitz B, Kapurniotu A, Kwok C, Dewor M, Bosserhoff AK, Bernhagen J, Hanrath P, Hoffmann R, Weber C. A novel drug-eluting stent coated with an integrin-binding cyclic Arg-Gly-Asp peptide inhibits neointimal hyperplasia by recruiting endothelial progenitor cells.J Am Coll Cardiol2006;47(9): 1786-95

[168] einhart JG, Schense JC, Schima H, Gorlitzer M, Hubbell JA, Deutsch M, Zilla P. Enhanced endothelial cell retention on shear-stressed synthetic vascular grafts precoated with RGD-cross-linked fibrin.Tissue Eng2005;11(5-6): 887-95

[169] Andrieux A, Rabiet MJ, Chapel A, Concord E, Marguerie G. A highly conserved sequence of the Arg-Gly-Asp-binding domain of the integrin beta 3 subunit is sensitive to stimulation.J Biol Chem1991;266(22): 14202-7

[170] Hasegawa T, Okada K, Takano Y, Hiraishi Y, Okita Y. Autologous fibrin-coated small-caliber vascular prostheses improve antithrombogenicity by reducing immunologic response.J Thorac Cardiovasc Surg2007;133(5): 1268-76

[171] Flanagan TC, Cornelissen C, Koch S, Tschoeke B, Sachweh JS, Schmitz-Rode T, Jockenhoevel S. The in vitro development of autologous fibrin-based tissue-engineered heart valves through optimised dynamic conditioning.Biomaterials 2007;28(23): 3388-97

[172] Veleva AN, Heath DE, Cooper SL, Patterson C. Selective endothelial cell attachment to peptide-modified terpolymers.Biomaterials2008;29(27): 3656-61

[173] Rodas AC, Polak R, Hara PH, Lee EI, Pitombo RN, Higa OZ. Cytotoxicity and endothelial cell adhesion of lyophilized and irradiated bovine pericardium modified with silk fibroin and chitosan.Artif Organs 2011;35(5): 502-7

[174] Sarathchandra P, Smolenski RT, Yuen AH, Chester AH, Goldstein S, Heacox AE, Yacoub MH, Taylor PM. Impact of γ-Irradiation on Extracellular Matrix of Porcine Pulmonary Valves.J Surg Res 2012;176(2): 376-85

[175] Li S, Henry JJ. Nonthrombogenic approaches to cardiovascular bioengineering.Annu Rev Biomed Eng 2011;13: 451-75

[176] Hashi CK, Zhu Y, Yang GY, Young WL, Hsiao BS, Wang K, Chu B, Li S. Antithrombogenic property of bone marrow mesenchymal stem cells in nanofibrous vascular grafts. Proc Natl Acad Sci USA 2007;104(29): 11915-20

[177] Kito H, Matsuda T. Biocompatible coatings for luminal and outer surfaces of small-caliber artificial grafts.J Biomed Mater Res 1996;30(3): 321-30

[178] Gombotz WR, Wang GH, Horbett TA, Hoffman AS. Protein adsorption to poly(ethylene oxide) surfaces.J Biomed Mater Res 1991;25(12): 1547-62

[179] Jordan SW, Faucher KM, Caves JM, Apkarian RP, Rele SS, Sun XL, Hanson SR, Chaikof EL. Fabrication of a phospholipid membrane-mimetic film on the luminal surface of an ePTFE vascular graft. Biomaterials 2006;27(18): 3473-81

[180] Koo J, Galanakis D, Liu Y, Ramek A, Fields A, Ba X, Simon M, Rafailovich MH. Control of anti-thrombogenic properties: surface-induced self-assembly of fibrinogen fibers. Biomacromolecules 2012;13(5): 1259-68

[181] Smith DJ, Chakravarthy D, Pulfer S, Simmons ML, Hrabie JA, Citro ML, Saavedra JE, Davies KM, Hutsell TC, Mooradian DL, Hanson SR, Keefer LK. Nitric oxide-releasing polymers containing the [N(O)NO]- group.J Med Chem 1996;39(5): 1148-56

[182] Kolpakov V, Gordon D, Kulik TJ. Nitric oxide-generating compounds inhibit total protein and collagen synthesis in cultured vascular smooth muscle cells.Circ Res 1995;76(2): 305-9

[183] Yu J, Zhang Y, Zhang X, Rudic RD, Bauer PM, Altieri DC, Sessa WC. Endothelium derived nitric oxide synthase negatively regulates the PDGF-survivin pathway during flow-dependent vascular remodeling. PLoS One 2012;7(2): e31495

[184] Marks DS, Vita JA, Folts JD, Keaney JF Jr, Welch GN, Loscalzo J. Inhibition of neointimal proliferation in rabbits after vascular injury by a single treatment with a protein adduct of nitric oxide.J Clin Invest 1995;96(6): 2630-8

[185] Acharya G, Hopkins RA, Lee CH. Advanced polymeric matrix for valvular complications.J Biomed Mater Res A 2012;100(5): 1151-9

[186] De Scheerder I, Wang K, Wilczek K, Meuleman D, Van Amsterdam R, Vogel G, Piessens J, Van de Werf F. Experimental study of thrombogenicity and foreign body reaction induced by heparin-coated coronary stents.Circulation 1997;95(6): 1549-53

[187] Lahann J, Plüster W, Klee D, Gattner HG, Höcker H. Immobilization of the thrombin inhibitor r-hirudin conserving its biological activity.J Mater Sci Mater Med 2001;12(9): 807-10

[188] Hashi CK, Derugin N, Janairo RR, Lee R, Schultz D, Lotz J, Li S. Antithrombogenic modification of small-diameter microfibrous vascular grafts.Arterioscler Thromb Vasc Biol 2010;30(8): 1621-7

[189] Pastore CJ, Isner JM, Bacha PA, Kearney M, Pickering JG. Epidermal growth factor receptor-targeted cytotoxin inhibits neointimalhyperplasia in vivo. Results of local versus systemic administration.Circ Res 1995;77(3): 519-29

[190] Asahara T, Bauters C, Pastore C, Kearney M, Rossow S, Bunting S, Ferrara N, Symes JF, Isner JM. Local delivery of vascular endothelial growth factor accelerates reendo-

thelialization and attenuates intimal hyperplasia in balloon-injured rat carotid artery.Circulation 1995;91(11): 2793-801

[191] Leppänen O, Rutanen J, Hiltunen MO, Rissanen TT, Turunen MP, Sjöblom T, Brüggen J, Bäckström G, Carlsson M, Buchdunger E, Bergqvist D, Alitalo K, Heldin CH, Ostman A, Ylä-Herttuala S. Oral imatinib mesylate (STI571/gleevec) improves the efficacy of local intravascular vascular endothelial growth factor-C gene transfer in reducing neointimal growth in hypercholesterolemic rabbits.Circulation 2004;109(9): 1140-6

[192] Sirois MG, Simons M, Edelman ER. Antisense oligonucleotide inhibition of PDGFR-beta receptor subunit expression directs suppression of intimal thickening.Circulation 1997;95(3): 669-76

[193] Coleman KR, Braden GA, Willingham MC, Sane DC. Vitaxin, a humanized monoclonal antibody to the vitronectin receptor (alphavbeta3), reduces neointimalhyperplasia and total vessel area after balloon injury in hypercholesterolemic rabbits.Circ Res 1999;84(11): 1268-76

[194] Miniati DN, Hoyt EG, Feeley BT, Poston RS, Robbins RC.Circulation 2000;102(19 Suppl 3): III237-42

[195] Skelly CL, Curi MA, Meyerson SL, Woo DH, Hari D, Vosicky JE, Advani SJ, Mauceri HJ, Glagov S, Roizman B, Weichselbaum RR, Schwartz LB. Prevention of restenosis by a herpes simplex virus mutant capable of controlled long-term expression in vascular tissue in vivo.Gene Ther 2001;8(24): 1840-6

[196] Mallawaarachchi CM, Weissberg PL, Siow RC. Smad7 gene transfer attenuates adventitial cell migration and vascular remodeling after balloon injury.Arterioscler Thromb Vasc Biol2005;25(7): 1383-7

[197] Mallawaarachchi CM, Weissberg PL, Siow RC. Antagonism of platelet-derived growth factor by perivascular gene transfer attenuates adventitial cell migration after vascular injury: new tricks for old dogs?FASEB J2006;20(10): 1686–1688

[198] Garcia-Touchard A, Burke SE, Toner JL, Cromack K, Schwartz RS. Zotarolimus-eluting stents reduce experimental coronary artery neointimal hyperplasia after 4 weeks. Eur Heart J 2006;27(8): 988-93

[199] Chen YW, Smith ML, Sheets M, Ballaron S, Trevillyan JM, Burke SE, Rosenberg T, Henry C, Wagner R, Bauch J, Marsh K, Fey TA, Hsieh G, Gauvin D, Mollison KW, Carter GW, Djuric SW. Zotarolimus, a novel sirolimus analogue with potent antiproliferative activity on coronary smooth muscle cells and reduced potential for systemic immunosuppression.J Cardiovasc Pharmacol 2007;49(4): 228-35

[200] Zhao L, Ding T, Cyrus T, Cheng Y, Tian H, Ma M, Falotico R, Praticò D. Low-dose oral sirolimus reduces atherogenesis, vascular inflammation and modulates plaque composition in mice lacking the LDL receptor.Br J Pharmacol 2009;156(5): 774-85

[201] Patel JK, Kobashigawa JA. Everolimus for cardiac allograft vasculopathy--every patient, at any time?Transplantation. 2011 Jul 27;92(2):127-8

[202] Baek I, Bai CZ, Hwang J, Park J, Park JS, Kim DJ. Suppression of neointimalhyperplasia by sirolimus-eluting expanded polytetrafluoroethylene (ePTFE) haemodialysis grafts in comparison with paclitaxel-coated grafts.Nephrol Dial Transplant 2012;27(5): 1997-2004

[203] Thiene G, Valente M. Calcification of valve bioprosthesis: the cardiac surgeon's nightmare. Eur J Cardiothorac Surg 1994;8(9): 476-8

[204] Pettenazzo E, Deiwick M, Thiene G, Molin G, Glasmacher B, Martignago F, Bottio T, Reul H, Valente M. Dynamic *in vitro* calcification of bioprosthetic porcine valves: evidence of apatite crystallization. J Thorac Cardiovasc Surg 2001;121(3): 500-9

[205] Zhai W, Chang J, Lü X, Wang Z. Procyanidins-crosslinked heart valve matrix: anticalcification effect.J Biomed Mater Res B Appl Biomater 2009;90(2): 913-21

[206] Pettenazzo E, Valente M, Thiene G. Octanediol treatment of glutaraldehyde fixed bovine pericardium: evidence of anticalcification efficacy in the subcutaneous rat model.Eur J Cardiothorac Surg 2008;34(2): 418-22

[207] Lim HG, Kim SH, Choi SY, Kim YJ. Anticalcification effects of decellularization, solvent, and detoxification treatment for genipin and glutaraldehyde fixation of bovine pericardium.Eur J Cardiothorac Surg 2012;41(2): 383-90

[208] Connolly JM, Bakay MA, Alferiev IS, Gorman RC, Gorman JH 3rd, Kruth HS, Ashworth PE, Kutty JK, Schoen FJ, Bianco RW, Levy RJ. Triglycidyl amine crosslinking combined with ethanol inhibits bioprosthetic heart valve calcification.Ann Thorac Surg 2011;92(3): 858-65

[209] Sacks MS, Hamamoto H, Connolly JM, Gorman RC, Gorman JH 3rd, Levy RJ. In vivo biomechanical assessment of triglycidylamine crosslinked pericardium. Biomaterials 2007;28(35): 5390-8

[210] Koutsopoulos S, Kontogeorgou A, Dalas E, Petroheilos J. Calcification of porcine and human cardiac valves: testing of various inhibitors for antimineralization. J Mater Sci Mater Med 1998;9(7): 421-4

[211] da Costa FD, Costa AC, Prestes R, Domanski AC, Balbi EM, Ferreira AD, Lopes SV. The early and midterm function of decellularized aortic valve allografts.Ann Thorac Surg 2010;90(6): 1854-60

[212] Rodríguez M, Aguilera-Tejero E, Mendoza FJ, Guerrero F, López I. Effects of calcimimetics on extraskeletal calcifications in chronic kidney disease. Kidney Int Suppl 2008;(111): S50-4

[213] Jung S, Querfeld U, Müller D, Rudolph B, Peters H, Krämer S. Submaximal suppression of parathyroid hormone ameliorates calcitriol-induced aortic calcification and remodeling and myocardial fibrosis in uremic rats. J Hypertens 2012;30(11): 2182-91

[214] Alferiev I, Vyavahare N, Song C, Connolly J, Hinson JT, Lu Z, Tallapragada S, Bianco R, Levy R. Bisphosphonate derivatized polyurethanes resist calcification.Biomaterials 2001;22(19): 2683-93

[215] Ng KE, Joly P, Jayasinghe SN, Vernay B, Knight R, Barry SP, McComick J, Latchman D, Stephanou A. Bio-electrospraying primary cardiac cells: in vitro tissue creation and functional study.Biotechnol J 2011;6(1): 86-95

[216] Kaminski A, Klopsch C, Mark P, Yerebakan C, Donndorf P, Gäbel R, Eisert F, Hasken S, Kreitz S, Glass A, Jockenhövel S, Ma N, Kundt G, Liebold A, Steinhoff G. Autologous valve replacement-CD133+ stem cell-plus-fibrin composite-based sprayed cell seeding for intraoperative heart valvetissue engineering.Tissue Eng Part C Methods 2011;17(3): 299-309

[217] Lin Q, Ding X, Qiu F, Song X, Fu G, Ji J. In situ endothelialization of intravascular stents coated with an anti-CD34 antibody functionalized heparin-collagen multilayer.Biomaterials 2010;31(14): 4017-25

[218] Ye X, Zhao Q, Sun X, Li H. Enhancement of mesenchymal stem cell attachment to decellularized porcine aortic valve scaffold by in vitro coating with antibody against CD90: a preliminary study on antibody-modified tissue-engineered heart valve. Tissue Eng Part A 2009;15(1): 1-11

[219] Jordan JE, Williams JK, Lee SJ, Raghavan D, Atala A, Yoo JJ. Bioengineered self-seeding heart valves.J Thorac Cardiovasc Surg 2012;143(1): 201-8

[220] Hoffmann J, Paul A, Harwardt M, Groll J, Reeswinkel T, Klee D, Moeller M, Fischer H, Walker T, Greiner T, Ziemer G, Wendel HP. Immobilized DNA aptamers used as potent attractors for porcine endothelial precursor cells.J Biomed Mater Res A 2008;84(3): 614-21

[221] Schleicher M, Wendel HP, Fritze O, Stock UA. In vivo tissue engineering of heart valves: evolution of a novel concept.Regen Med 2009;4(4): 613-9

[222] Sun W, Darling A, Starly B, Nam J. Computer-aided tissue engineering: overview, scope and challenges. Biotechnol Appl Biochem 2004;39(Pt 1): 29-47

[223] Lalan S, Pomerantseva I, Vacanti JP. Tissue engineering and its potential impact on surgery.World J Surg 2001;25(11): 1458-66

[224] Norotte C, Marga FS, Niklason LE, Forgacs G. Scaffold-free vascular tissue engineering using bioprinting.Biomaterials 2009;30(30): 5910-7

[225] Masoumi N, Jean A, Zugates JT, Johnson KL, Engelmayr GC Jr. Laser microfabricated poly(glycerol sebacate) scaffolds for heart valve tissue engineering.J Biomed Mater Res A 2012. doi: 10.1002/jbm.a.34305

[226] Schmauss D, Schmitz C, Bigdeli AK, Weber S, Gerber N, Beiras-Fernandez A, Schwarz F, Becker C, Kupatt C, Sodian R. Three-dimensional printing of models for preoperative planning and simulation of transcatheter valve replacement. Ann Thorac Surg2012;93(2): e31-3

[227] Nakayama Y, Yamanami M, Yahata Y, Tajikawa T, Ohba K, Watanabe T, Kanda K, Yaku H. Preparation of a completely autologous trileaflet valve-shaped construct by in-body tissue architecture technology. J Biomed Mater Res B Appl Biomater 2009;91(2): 813-8

[228] Davies H. Catheter mounted valve for temporary relief of aortic insufficiency Lancet 1965;1: 250

[229] Bonhoeffer P, Boudjemline Y, Saliba Z, Merckx J, Aggoun Y, Bonnet D, Acar P, Le Bidois J, Sidi D, Kachaner J. Percutaneous replacement of pulmonary valve in a right-ventricle to pulmonary-artery prosthetic conduit with valve dysfunction.Lancet2000;356(9239): 1403-5

[230] Cribier A, Eltchaninoff H, Bash A, Borenstein N, Tron C, Bauer F, Derumeaux G, Anselme F, Laborde F, Leon MB. Percutaneous transcatheter implantation of an aortic valve prosthesis for calcific aortic stenosis: first human case description.Circulation2002;106(24): 3006-8

[231] Schmidt D, Dijkman PE, Driessen-Mol A, Stenger R, Mariani C, Puolakka A, Rissanen M, Deichmann T, Odermatt B, Weber B, Emmert MY, Zund G, Baaijens FP, Hoerstrup SP. Minimally-invasive implantation of living tissue engineered heart valves: a comprehensive approach from autologous vascular cells to stem cells.J Am Coll Cardiol2010;56(6): 510-20

[232] Schmidt D, Dijkman PE, Driessen-Mol A, Stenger R, Mariani C, Puolakka A, Rissanen M, Deichmann T, Odermatt B, Weber B, Emmert MY, Zund G, Baaijens FP, Hoerstrup SP. Minimally-invasive implantation of living tissue engineered heart valves: a comprehensive approach from autologous vascular cells to stem cells.J Am Coll Cardiol2010;56(6): 510-20

[233] Helmchen F, Denk W. Deep tissue two-photon microscopy. Helmchen F, Denk W. Nat Methods 2005;2(12): 932-40

[234] Schenke-Layland K, Riemann I, Opitz F, König K, Halbhuber KJ, Stock UA. Comparative study of cellular and extracellular matrix composition of native and tissue engineered heart valves.Matrix Biol 2004;23(2): 113-25

[235] Karamitsos TD, Myerson SG. The role of cardiovascular magnetic resonance in the evaluation of valve disease.Prog Cardiovasc Dis 2011;54(3): 276-86

[236] Dohmen PM, Lembcke A, Hotz H, Kivelitz D, Konertz WF. Ross operation with a tissue-engineeredheart valve.Ann Thorac Surg 2002;74(5):1438-42

[237] Ramaswamy S, Schornack PA, Smelko AG, Boronyak SM, Ivanova J, Mayer JE Jr, Sacks MS. Superparamagnetic iron oxide (SPIO) labeling efficiency and subsequent MRI tracking of native cell populations pertinent to pulmonary heart valve tissue engineering studies.NMR Biomed 2012;25(3): 410-7

[238] Aikawa E, Otto CM. Look more closely at the valve: imaging calcific aortic valve disease.Circulation2012;125(1): 9-11

[239] Liu L, Gardecki JA, Nadkarni SK, Toussaint JD, Yagi Y, Bouma BE, Tearney GJ. Imaging the subcellular structure of human coronary atherosclerosis using micro-opticalcoherencetomography.Nat Med 2011;17(8): 1010-4

[240] Ruggiero A, Thorek DL, Guenoun J, Krestin GP, Bernsen MR. Cell tracking in cardiac repair: what to image and how to image. Eur Radiol 2012;22(1): 189-204

[241] Ross DN. Homograft replacement of the aortic valve. Lancet 1962;2(7254): 487

[242] Jashari R, Tabaku M, Van Hoeck B, Cochéz C, Callant M, Vanderkelen A. Decontamination of heart valve and arterial allografts in the European Homograft Bank (EHB): comparison of two different antibiotic cocktails in low temperature conditions.Cell Tissue Bank 2007;8(4): 247-55

[243] Soo A, Healy DG, El-Bashier H, Shaw S, Wood AE. Quality control in homograft valve processing: when to screen for microbiological contamination?Cell Tissue Bank 2011;12(3): 185-90

[244] Jashari R, Goffin Y, Van Hoeck B, Vanderkelen A, du Verger A, Fan Y, Holovska V, Fagu A, Brahy O. Belgian and European experience with the European Homograft Bank (EHB) cryopreserved allograft valves.--assessment of a 20 year activity.Acta Chir Belg 2010;110(3): 280-90

[245] Wassenaar C, Bax WA, van Suylen RJ, Vuzevski VD, Bos E. Effects of cryopreservation on contractile properties of porcine isolated aortic valve leaflets and aortic wall.J Thorac Cardiovasc Surg 1997;113(1): 165-72

[246] Rendal Vázquez ME, Díaz Román TM, Rodríguez Cabarcos M, Zavanella Botta C, Domenech García N, González Cuesta M, Sánchez Dopico MJ, Pértega Díaz S, Andión Núñez C. Apoptosis in fresh and cryopreserved cardiac valves of pig samples.Cell Tissue Bank 2008;9(2): 101-7

[247] Gatto C, Dainese L, Buzzi M, Terzi A, Guarino A, Pagliaro PP, Polvani G, D'Amato Tothova J. Establishing a procedure for dimethyl sulfoxide removal from cardiovascular allografts: a quantitative study.Cell Tissue Bank 2012 Jul 27 [Epub ahead of print]

[248] Gerson CJ, Elkins RC, Goldstein S, Heacox AE. Structural integrity of collagen and elastin in SynerGraft® decellularized-cryopreserved human heart valves.Cryobiology. 2012 Feb;64(1):33-42

[249] Schenke-Layland K, Madershahian N, Riemann I, Starcher B, Halbhuber KJ, König K, Stock UA. Impact of cryopreservation on extracellular matrix structures of heart valve leaflets.Ann Thorac Surg 2006;81(3): 918-26

[250] Lisy M, Pennecke J, Brockbank KG, Fritze O, Schleicher M, Schenke-Layland K, Kaulitz R, Riemann I, Weber CN, Braun J, Mueller KE, Fend F, Scheunert T, Gruber AD, Albes JM, Huber AJ, Stock UA. The performance of ice-free cryopreserved heart valve allografts in an orthotopic pulmonary sheep model.Biomaterials 2010;31(20): 5306-11

[251] Rattazzi M, Iop L, Faggin E, Bertacco E, Zoppellaro G, Baesso I, Puato M, Torregrossa G, Fadini GP, Agostini C, Gerosa G, Sartore S, Pauletto P. Clones of interstitial cells from bovine aortic valve exhibit different calcifying potential when exposed to endotoxin and phosphate.Arterioscler Thromb Vasc Biol 2008;28(12): 2165-72

[252] Bertacco E, Millioni R, Arrigoni G, Faggin E, Iop L, Puato M, Pinna LA, Tessari P, Pauletto P, Rattazzi M. Proteomic analysis of clonal interstitial aortic valve cells acquiring a pro-calcific profile.J Proteome Res 2010;9(11): 5913-21

[253] New SE, Aikawa E. Cardiovascular calcification: an inflammatory disease.Circ J 2011;75(6): 1305-13

[254] Mathapati S, Verma RS, Cherian KM, Guhathakurta S.Inflammatory responses of tissue-engineered xenografts in a clinical scenario.Interact Cardiovasc Thorac Surg2011;12(3): 360-5

[255] Zhou J, Fritze O, Schleicher M, Wendel HP, Schenke-Layland K, Harasztosi C, Hu S, Stock UA. Impact of heart valve decellularization on 3-D ultrastructure, immunogenicity and thrombogenicity. Biomaterials 2010;31(9): 2549-54

[256] Arai S, Orton EC. Immunoblot detection of soluble protein antigens from sodium dodecyl sulphate- and sodium deoxycholate-treated candidate bioscaffold tissues. J Heart Valve Dis 2009;18(4): 439-43

[257] Barth PJ, KoÅNster H, Moosdorf R. CD34+ fibrocytes in normal mitral valves and myxomatous mitral valve degeneration. Pathol Res Pract 2005;201(4): 301-4

[258] Orkin SH. Diversification of haematopoietic stem cells to specific lineages. Nat Rev Genet 2000;1(1): 57-64

[259] Iop L, Basso C, Rizzo S, Piccoli M, Callegari M, Paolin A, De Coppi P, Thiene G, Sartore S, Gerosa G. Stem Cell Populations in Human Heart Valves: Identification, Isolation and Characterization in Valve Homografts and Surgical Specimens. Conference proceedings. World Conference on Regenerative Medicine– Leipzig, Germany, 29-31 October 2009

[260] Martinez FO, Sica A, Mantovani A, Locati M. Macrophage activation and polarization. Front Biosci 2008;13: 453-61

[261] Brown BN, Valentin JE, Stewart-Akers AM, McCabe GP, Badylak SF. Macrophage phenotype and remodeling outcomes in response to biologic scaffolds with and without a cellular component.Biomaterials 2009;30(8):1482-91

[262] Zheng C, Azcutia V, Aikawa E, Figueiredo JL, Croce K, Sonoki H, Sacks FM, Luscinskas FW, Aikawa M. Statins suppress apolipoprotein CIII-induced vascular endothelial cell activation and monocyte adhesion.Eur Heart J 2012 Aug 26 [Epub ahead of print]

[263] Monaghan M, Pandit A. RNA interference therapy via functionalized scaffolds. Adv Drug Deliv Rev 2011;63(4-5):197-208

Section 5

Bicuspid Aortic Valve

Chapter 10

Bicuspid Aortic Valve

George Tokmaji, Berto J. Bouma,
Dave R. Koolbergen and Bas A.J.M. de Mol

Additional information is available at the end of the chapter

http://dx.doi.org/10.5772/55325

1. Introduction

Bicuspid aortic valve (BAV) disease is one of the most frequent observed congenital heart abnormalities affecting 0.5-1.4% of the general population and has a 3:1 male predominance [1-4]. Although some genes have been described that found to be responsible for the abnormal valvulogenesis, little is known about BAV disease with respect to the genetic and embryological insight of calcification and why patients with BAV disease develop aortic valve calcification including severe aortic valve stenosis (AS) at an earlier age compared with degenerative tricuspid valve. BAV disease is also associated with several cardiovascular abnormalities including coarctation of the aorta (COA) and Turner Syndrome. While patients with BAV disease are often asymptomatic during the childhood, BAV disease is generally diagnosed in the adulthood using echocardiography when aortic stenosis with or without valve calcification, infective endocarditis, aortic regurgitation (AR), and proximal thoracic aortic dilatation are detected, often necessitating surgical intervention [5]. Patients with BAV disease require close observation before complications as heart failure and aortic dissection may occur. In this chapter, the contemporary knowledge regarding BAV disease will be discussed.

2. Anatomy and pathology

The anatomic features of BAV are characterized by smooth cusps margins and the fusion of two cusps of unequal size. These cusps often include a central raphé or false commissure which are usually in the centre of the larger cusp [Figure 2]. The main difference between a commissure and a raphé is that the commissure does not completely span into the cusp [6]. The raphé is to be considered as a hypoplastic commissure between two partially fused cusps. The most commonly seen variant of BAV is the fusion of the left and right coronary cusps (L-R BAV) also known as the latero-lateral cusps position which is seen in 70-86% of the BAV cases, whereas the fusion of the right and noncoronary cusps (R-N BAV; antero-posterior cusps position) are observed in 12-28% and the left and noncoronary cusps (L-N BAV) in 0.5-3% of the cases [7-11] [Figure 1]. R-N BAVs and asymmetrical sized cusps are relative risk factors that seem to accelerate the stenosis with 27 mm Hg per decade and are therefore more often associated with AS [12]. BAV with equal cusps and absence of raphé have also been reported [6, 7]. In some cases, the raphé can have a quite deep indentation, which could give a false echocardiographic image of a normal tricuspid aortic valve [13]. Calcium depositions are often confined to the raphé and the base of the cusps [7]. AS tend to develop in BAVs which contain no redundant cusp tissue whereas AR tend to develop in BAVs due to the different dimensions of the two cusps, valve prolapse or redundancy of one cusp [14-16]. Histological examination demonstrates that the raphé does not contain fibrous valve tissue but rather include elastin fibers [17]. BAV should also be distinguished from unicommisural valves that tend to calcify and degenerate even earlier in life. Unicommissural valves includes one commissure with normal height and two raphe's that are much lower height, while there is one large cusp, more or less moving like a bicuspid valve. Up to 90% of the individuals with normal tricuspid valve have right coronary artery dominance whereas 29% to 57% of the patients with BAV disease present with left coronary artery dominance. The average length of the left main stem for individuals with BAV and tricuspid valve is less than 5 mm (90% of the cases) and 10 mm in length, respectively. Recognition of these associations with BAV is mandatory due to the increased risk of perioperative myocardial infarction and a potential risk of insufficient myocardial preservation at the time of aortic valve replacement (AVR) [18, 19, 20]. L-R BAVs are often associated with right coronary artery taking its origin from the right sinus of Valsalva, while in the R-N BAVs, both coronary arteries derive from the anterior sinus [21]. The vast majority of the patients with COA present with a L-R BAV (66-90%) [9, 135, 136].

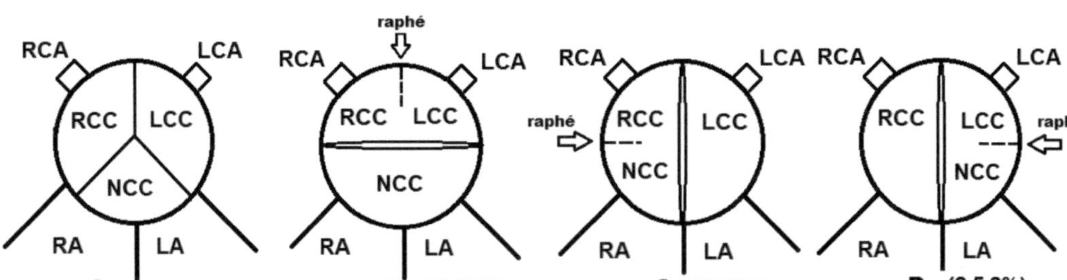

Figure 1. Schematic illustration of the anatomic variations of BAV. (A) normal tricuspid aortic valve. (B) Bicuspid aortic valve, fusion of the left and right coronary cusps. (C) Bicuspid aortic valve, fusion of the right and noncoronary cusps. (D) Bicuspid aortic valve, fusion of the left and noncoronary cusps.

http://dx.doi.org/10.5772/55325

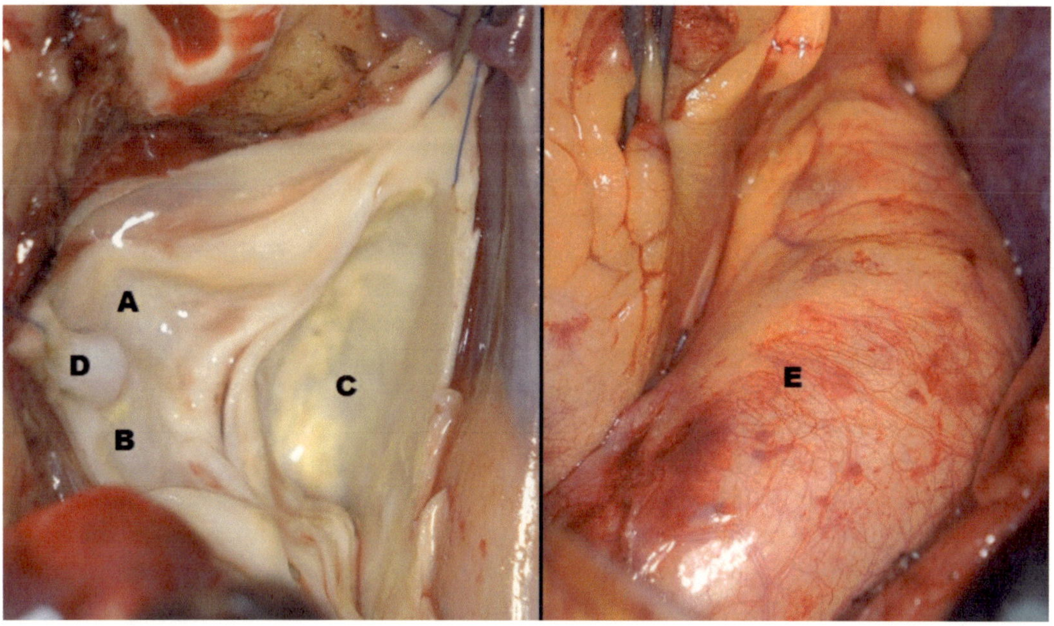

Figure 2. Macroscopic illustration of a bicuspid aortic valve with the fusion of the right and noncoronary cusps (left image) and a dilated ascending aorta (right image). A: Non coronary cusp, B: Right coronary cusp, C: Left coronary cusp, D: Raphé, E: Ascending aorta (dilated).

3. Morphologenesis

The embryogenesis of BAV is still not fully understood. It seems that both genetic predisposition and environmental factors, which could influence the valve morphogenesis, play an important role in the pathogenesis of BAV disease. Initially, the major factor in the formation of BAV is the fusion of the two cusps at the early foundation of the valvulogenesis [22]. The valve morphogenesis occurs in the early stage of foetal development. The heart is one of the first organs to develop through the specification and migration of the anterior lateral plate mesoderm cells which later forms the cardiac crescent [23]. At 3 weeks of gestation in humans, the cardiac progenitors migrate along the ventral midline where they fuse and form a linear heart tube. This beating heart tube is composed of an inner endocardial cell layer which is separated by the extracellular matrix (ECM). Cardiac looping occurs at 4 to 5 weeks of gestation which brings the atrial region of the linear tube into the posterior position of the common ventricles. This is followed by the increase of ECM production which causes the tissue to swell at several areas of the primitive heart, which leads to the formation of the endocardial cushions at the outflow tract (OFT) and atrioventricular (AV) canal. The inner endocardial cells transform into mesenchymal cells, also known as the epithelial-to-mesenchymal transformation (EMT). EMT initiates the formation of the aortic valve in the OFT. Afterwards, the cushions undergo massive cell proliferation, as a result growing towards each other with cushion fusion being the outcome. Subsequently, the endocardial cushions develop into thin protruding leaflets that are composed of endocardial cells and ECM which remodels the valves. This complex development is reliant on apoptosis, ECM remodeling and cell differentiation. The main contributors for the aortic valve in the OFT are the mesenchymal cells that reach the OFT cushions in association with the endocardial derived mesenchymal cells [24, 25]. Therefore, any disorder in the endocardial cushion development could lead to potential valve disorder including BAV. A disturbance in the neural crest migration which could lead to the fusion of the aortic valve cushions is thought to be a possible embryological explanation for the pathogenesis of BAV disease [22, 26-28]. Several aneurysms which originate from the neural crest including intracranial aneurysms, aortic aneurysms, and cervicocephalic aneurysm have also been observed in patients with BAV disease [29, 30]. Endothelial nitric oxide synthase is a vital protein for valve formation during embryogenesis. Knockout mice lacking this protein showed a high predisposition for BAV due to the fact that malformation in this protein could lead to disturbance of the intricate cell signals which are essential for valvulogenesis [31]. Moreover, it seems that L-R BAV and R-N BAV have different etiological attributes and genotypes. The pathogenesis of R-N BAV is most likely the result of morphogenetic defect which occurs before the OFT septation and is dependent on an aggravated nitric oxide–dependent epithelial-to-mesenchymal transformation. In contrast, L-R BAV is most probably the outcome from the anomalous septation of the proximal portion of the OFT which is caused by distorted activities of neural crest cells [32].

4. Genetics

Genetic burden also seem to contribute to the pathogenesis of BAV disease. It appears that BAV disease has a male-to-female ratio of roughly 3:1 [1-4]. Although some anatomical risk factors have been described, little is known about BAV disease with respect to the genetic insight of calcification process and why patients with BAV disease develop aortic valve calcification including stenosis at an earlier age compared with degenerative tricuspid valve. Chromosomal linkage with BAV disease has been discovered in chromosomal regions 5q, 13q and 18q [36]. Genetic mutations in the *NOTCH 1* gene, which is situated at chromosome 9q seems to be one of the major genetic contributors in the pathogenesis of BAV disease. *NOTCH 1* gene contributes to the pathogenesis of BAV disease through the pathological acceleration of aortic valvular calcium deposition by the increase of the osteogenesis due to the abnormalities in the signalling pathways [37]. Also, genetic mutations in the *ACTA2* gene which is located at chromosome 10q, is associated not only with BAV disease, but also with familial thoracic aortic aneurysms [38]. *ACTA2* gene encodes for the smooth muscle protein α-actin which is an important element of the contractile apparatus. Several familial clusters associated with BAV disease with an estimated prevalence of 24% of aortic valve disorder were found in relatives with more than one member with aortic valve disorder [33]. Additionally, an estimated BAV disease prevalence of up to 9% in first-degree family members of patients with BAV disease has been reported [34, 35]. Based on this known data, it is advisable for first-degree family members of BAV patients to receive an echocardiographic screening to exclude any potential congenital heart disease including thoracic aortic aneurysms [39, 67, 68].

5. Congenital associated cardiovascular malformations

Although the vast majority of BAV disease are isolated cases, patients with BAV could also present with additional congenital cardiovascular malformations [40-43]. BAV associated anomalies are illustrated in Table 1. Whereas most associated anomalies need treatment early in life, BAV often contributes to morbidity at an older age. COA and Turner Syndrome will be further discussed in this chapter.

5.1. Coarctation of the aorta

COA is a commonly seen congenital abnormality with an incidence of 50 of 100.000 births, whereby the aorta is narrowed in the region where the ductus arteriosus enters [figure 3]. COA can present itself as a simple or complex COA with simple COA referring to COA being an isolated defect and complex COA referring to a combination of COA with other cardiac defects. Congenital BAV is present in around 57% of the COA cases [44]. In the vast majority of the cases, COA in combination with BAV is observed with the fusion of left and right coronary cusps [9]. Patients with both BAV and COA have an increased risk for developing several aortic complications including aortic dissection, AS, AR, and aortic aneurysms [16, 44, 46, 49]. The overwhelming majority of BAV patients present with a L-R BAV (66-90%) [9, 135, 136].

Patients with both BAV and COA receive surgical intervention at a relative young age. Surgical options, mostly depending of the type of lesion include bypass of the coarctation, patch aortoplasty, aneurysm replacement, arch and descending aorta replacement, subclavian artery patch aortoplasty, tube graft replacement, ascending aorta–to– descending aorta bypass or 2-stage combined BAV surgery [69]. Endovascular balloon dilatation and stent placement are currently becoming successful novel interventional options to conventional open surgical treatment [70]. Around 11% to 14% of the patients require a reoperation somewhere in the adulthood [50]. A large cohort study showed that up to 41% of the patients who had a COA required a valve related re-operation [9]. Thus, long-term follow-up in (all) patients with COA including the evaluation of the function of the aortic valve, but also to trace re-coarctation and dilatation of the ascending aorta with routine MRI or echocardiographic evaluation is obligatory

5.2. Turner Syndrome

Turner Syndrome is a gonadal dysgenesis with complete or partial absence of one of the X chromosome. Cardiovascular defects are frequently observed in Turner Syndrome patients. Turner Syndrome is characterized as neck webbing, short stature, low hairline, and a shield-like chest. BAV disease is the most frequently seen cardiovascular abnormality in Turner Syndrome patients [51, 52]. In Turner Syndrome patients, cardiovascular abnormalities are often the primary cause of mortality including the increase risk of aortic dissection due to aortic root dilatation and therefore responsible for a much lower life expectancy in this subgroup of BAV disease [53, 54]. Due to the relative small body size, Turner Syndrome patients require an elective ascending aortic aneurysm replacement at a much smaller absolute size [54]. Moreover, it should be noted that the aortic size has to be properly indexed to the body surface area. Therefore, proper follow-up and evaluation of the cardiovascular lesions including imaging of the heart and the aorta for evidence of BAV disease or dilatation of the ascending aorta is mandatory. When imaging appears to be without any lesions and there are no additional risk factors for aortic dissection present, a repeated imaging should be conducted every 5 to 10 years or otherwise clinically indicated. In contrast, when abnormal imaging is present, regular imaging at smaller intervals should be made with echocardiography or CMRI [67].

• Coarctation of the Aorta	• Ascending Aortic Aneurysm
• Turner Syndrome	• Coronary Artery Anomalies
• Patent Ductus Arteriosus	• Sinus of Valsalva Aneurysm
• William's Syndrome	• Supravalvular Aortic Stenosis
• Ventricular Septal Defect	• Aortic Dissection
• Shone's Syndrome	

Table 1. Known cardiovascular abnormalities related to BAV disease.

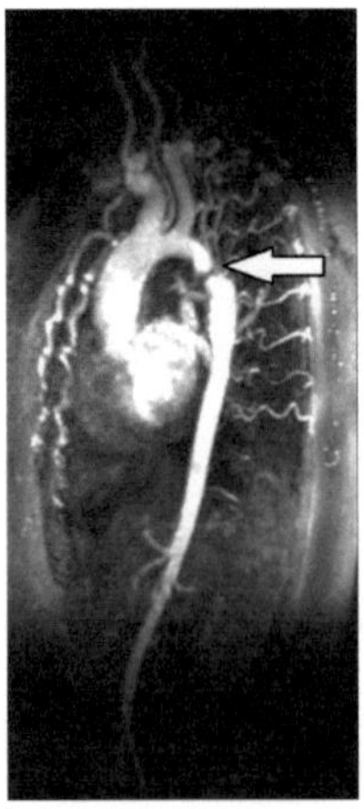

Figure 3. Sagittal plane cardiac magnetic resonance imaging illustrating coarctation of the aorta. Typical post ductal stenosis (arrow).

6. Diagnosis

6.1. Clinical examination

AS or AR can present themselves with significant symptoms in patients with BAV disease during activity, stress or rest including angina, shortness of breath, syncope or dizziness. In many cases, clinical examination reveals an ejection sound during auscultation at the apex. When AS is present, an ejection click can be often heard at the S1. The S2 is often simultaneously with P2 when AS is present. A diastolic murmur can often be heard when an AR is present. Heart failure of unknown cause could also be present during clinical examination. The ejection sound in BAV patients is most likely associated with anterior movement of the dome shaped BAV, and in rare cases heart failure could also be present during clinical examination in case of rapid deterioration [55]. AS, mitral valve prolapsed, AR, and COA are several associated pathological findings which have to be considered with BAV when a murmer is present.

6.2. Echocardiography

The current golden standards for diagnosing, surveilling and monitoring BAV disease are echocardiography and cardiac magnetic resonance imaging (CMRI) [39].

Both transthoracic echocardiography (TTE) and transesophageal echocardiography (TEE) can be used in the diagnosis of BAV disease. TTE has a sensitivity of 78% to 87% and a specificity of 91% to 96% for the diagnosis of BAV disease whereas TEE has a sensitivity and specificity of 87% and 96%, respectively [56, 57, 58]. However, up to 25% of TTE have non-diagnostic findings for aortic valve morphology due to severe valvular calcification [57].

The features of BAV on a TTE include systolic doming, an eccentric closure line in the parasternal long axis views, presence of a single commissural line in the diastolic phase with the occurrence of two cusps and the occurrence of two commisures in the parasternal short axis views [figure 4] [59, 60].

Moreover, both preoperative echocardiography and intraoperative TEE are essential for surgical preparation. When BAV disease is present, the degree of AS and AR should be determined with the help of Doppler analysis. After determining the severity of the AR, to ascertain the indication for surgery, especially TEE is needed to clarify the mechanisms that are responsible for AR. This is required to estimate the chance of successful repair and indispensible in surgical preparation. Moreover, any associated cardiovascular abnormalities or complications should be considered. Aortic diameters should therefore also be measured at several levels including valvular insertion, sinuses of Valsalva, sino-tubular junction and the ascending aorta. It should also be noted that in order to measure the severity of the AS by echocardiography- Doppler analysis, the aortic valve area and mean gradient should be applied rather than measuring only on peak systolic gradient, sequentially to prevent overestimation of the severity of the AS [39]. Also, aortic valve area should always be indexed to body surface area in order to correct for different habitus and body sizes, especially in Turner Syndrome patients [39, 54].

6.3. Cardiac magnetic resolution imaging

CMRI as a noninvasive diagnostic tool appears to have a high diagnostic sensitivity and specificity. CMRI showed a sensitivity of 100% and a specificity of 95% with steady state free-precession (SSFP) cine [61]. It seems that CMRI is more reliable than the standard TTE in diagnosing BAV [Figure 5]. When TTE is found to be non-diagnostic for aortic valve morphology, particularly in patients with severe AS, CMRI can be conducted as a complementary test [62].

When the diagnostic results of AR with the use of echocardiography is indefinite or at borderline, CMRI can be used to quantify the AR more accurately [39]. In addition, the valve can be visualized with any correlated lesion of the ascending aorta. This could be used for proper evaluation of the entire aortic and to prepare complex surgical interventions for both the aorta valve and the surrounding cardiovascular structures including the ascending aorta and the aortic root. Of importance, all patients with evidence of BAV should have the aortic root and ascending aorta inspected for indication of aortic dilatation with echocardiography or MRI [67].

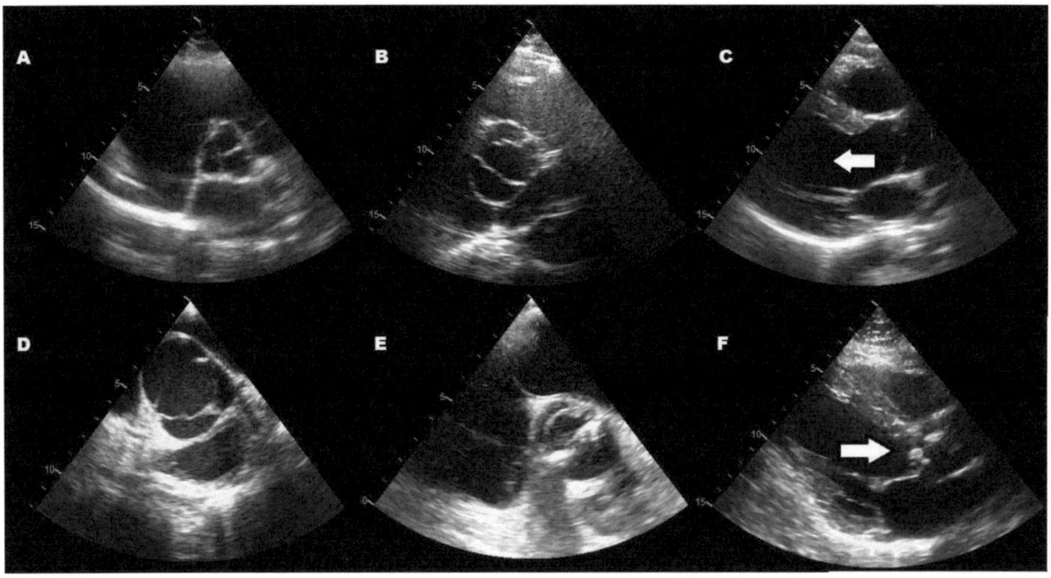

Figure 4. (A) Transthoracic echocardiography short axis view illustrating a normal tricuspid aortic valve. (B) Transthoracic echocardiography short axis view illustrating a bicuspid aortic valve with fusion of the left and right coronary cusps. (C) Transthoracic echocardiography long axis view illustrating a dilated ascending aorta (Arrow). (D) Transthoracic echocardiography short axis view illustrating a bicuspid aortic valve with fusion of the right and non coronary coronary cusps. (E) Transthoracic echocardiography short axis view illustrating a severe calcified bicuspid aortic valve with fusion of the right and non coronary coronary cusps. (F) Transthoracic echocardiography long axis view illustrating a severe calcified bicuspid aortic valve.

http://dx.doi.org/10.5772/55325

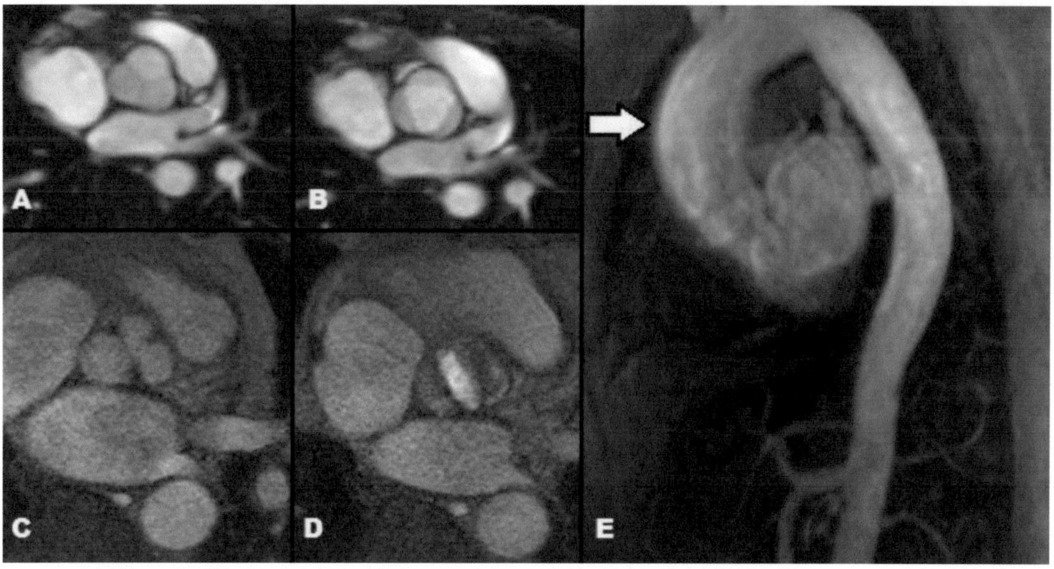

Figure 5. Panel (A, B) Cardiac magnetic resonance imaging in the axial plane illustrating a normal tricuspid valve in the diastolic (A) and systolic phase (B). (Panel C, D) Bicuspid aortic valve with fusion of the right coronary cusp and the non coronary cusp in the diastolic (C) and systolic (D) phase. (Panel E) Sagittal plane illustrating a dilatation of the ascending aorta (Arrow).

7. Complications associated with BAV

7.1. Aortic stenosis

Up to 50% of the adults who present with AS show evidence of BAV disease [71]. BAV degeneration is due to both fibrosis and calcification and is age related [16, 72, 73]. Additionally, the incidence of BAV related AS that is observed in patients with the age of under 60 years, 60 to 75 years, and more than 75 years are 59%, 40% and 32%, respectively [74].

Patients with BAV generally require AVR 5 years earlier compared with the patients who have an AS of the tricuspid valve [75]. Three-quarters of the patient with BAV who underwent AVR showed to have an isolated AS [7]. Both fibrosis and cusp calcifications occur in an accelerated pattern in BAV compared with tricuspid aortic valve [Figure 4, E &F] [76]. Moreover, several valve related factors seem to accelerate the calcification in BAV including larger sized cusp, presence of raphé and the overall BAV anatomy. It seems that sclerosis of the aortic valve starts in the second decade whereas calcification tends to develop around the fourth decade onwards with a 18 mmHg per decade increase of the average aortic valve gradient [75, 12]. Both R-N BAVs and asymmetrical sized cusps seem to contribute to the acceleration of the stenosis due to the progressive calcification and fibrosis with 27 mm Hg per decade [9, 45, 12]. It has to be noted that smoking and a poor lipid panel are both modifiable independent risk factors that could have a great impact on BAV degeneration [77]. In children, BAV with stenosis can sometimes be treated with balloon valvuloplasty whereas in other cases surgical commissurotomy is indicated [75, 78-80]. Severe fibrosis of the cusp tissue and calcified degeneration, which is found in the older population, make surgical repair difficult or impossible in most cases. AVR is therefore the primary surgical treatment of BAV with severe stenosis in adults.

7.2. Aortic regurgitation

AR most often involves patients with a young age and is less frequently seen than AS with prevalence ranging from 7% to 20% [15, 78, 81, 82]. AR can occur in the isolated form due to the prolapse of one of the cusps, but it could also occur due to and in combination with endocarditis, COA, and proximal aortic root dilatation [16, 25]. The presence of AR could have severe consequences for the patient's morbidity including the increased risk of heart failure, endocarditis and arrhythmia [80]. Aortic root dilatation is found in nearly half of the young adults with BAV disease, thus increasing the risk for AR [83]. In selected cases, patients with BAV disease and isolated AR can be a candidate for aortic valve repair [84].

7.3. Aortic dilatation and dissection

BAV disease is linked with dilatation of the proximal aortic root and ascending aorta and develops independently from stenotic or regurgitant aortic valvular lesions [91]. This process eventually leads to dissection or rupture of the aortic wall with potentially fatal consequences. Several molecular pathways have been discovered, possibly of genetic basis, which suggest that histopathologic modifications in the extracellular matrix of the dilated proximal aortic wall are a key pathogenesis of aortic dilatation in BAV patients. This includes the loss of smooth muscle cells, cystic medial necrosis and elastic fibre fragmentation [92, 93]. Furthermore, morphometric analysis of the aortic media showed deformities of the elastic lamellae and less elastic tissue in BAV patients in comparison with patients with tricuspid aortic valves [93, 94]. It appears that apoptosis is a key mechanism for the loss of the smooth muscle cells in the ascending aorta of BAV patients which can eventually lead to cardiovascular complications [95, 96, 97]. In addition, regarding the remodeling of the extracellular matrix, fibrillin-1 microfibrils were significantly reduced while the matrix metalloproteinase-2 and -9 activities were significantly increased in the aortic media of BAV patients. When fibrillin-1 deficiency is present, the release of enzymes, also known as matrix metalloproteinases, will increase and weaken the aortic wall by degrading elastic matrix components, thus resulting in aortic dilatation and degeneration [98, 99, 100].

Approximately 40% of the BAV cases develop proximal aortic root dilatation while an estimation of 6% lifetime risk is observed for aortic dissection [101].

Risk factors for developing an adverse aortic complications such as rupture or dissection in BAV patients include positive family history of aortic aneurism, dilatation of the sinotubular junction, the presence of AR, young age (<40 years), and aortic dilatation greater than 50 mm [101, 102]. Aortic dissection occurs most commonly in young adults with an asymptomatic medical history of BAV. A severe risk for aortic dissection is present when the aortic diameter surpasses 50 mm. [102]. When BAV is present in combination with aortic dilatation, the risk of aortic dissection is increased 9 fold compared with tricuspid valve cases [16]. Additionally, the area of the aortic dilation also varies among BAV patients. Some patients have a dilatation of the proximal ascending aorta dilation, while others have a dilation of the sinuses of Valsalva and yet other patients present with a dilatation of the transverse arch or a combination of these locations [103].

Aortic dilatation of the sinuses of Valsalva is often seen in patients with L-R BAV, whereas patients with R-N BAV present with the dilatation of the ascending aorta [10]. Of note, aortic dilatation and thoracic aortic aneurysm formation could also occur in BAV patients or related family members with the absence of significant valve pathology in the form of AS or AR [51, 68].

7.4. Infective endocarditis

Infective endocarditis is a condition high risk on mortality and morbidity which effects 10% to 30% of the BAV patients with actual risk assessment of 0.3% to 2% per patient-years in adults. Although these estimations are based on selected cases, the true incidence of BAV related infective endocarditis is most likely lower. [16, 85, 86]. Moreover, one-fourth of the infective endocarditis cases are a complication due to BAV. Infective endocarditis is frequently seen in young adults and adolescents rather than in elderly patients, particularly the male gender [16]. Almost three-quarters of the endocarditis related BAV cases are caused by *Viridans streptococci* and *Staphylococci* [87]. Poor dental hygiene, presence of a dialysis shunt and venous catheters are major independent risk factors for developing infective endocarditis due to the high risk of contamination [88]. Several complications due to infective endocarditis in BAV patient can occur including heart failure, the formation of myocardial or valvular abscess, and mortality within 6 month after hospital admission [89]. Antibiotic prophylaxis is nowadays no longer recommended for patients with BAV and with calcified aortic stenosis, except in BAV patients with a prior history of infective endocarditis, prosthetic heart valves, or prosthetic material used for heart valve repair [90].

8. Interventions

Surgical intervention is the key treatment option for patients with symptomatic BAV disease and the related aortic dilatation. Several factors are dependent on the surgical treatment management including the location and the severity of the aortic dilatation and the performance status of BAV.

8.1. Surgical indications for aortic valve repair/replacement

Surgical intervention for patients with BAV disease occurs at a relative earlier age than for degenerative tricuspid aortic valve disease [71]. In a study of 212 asymptomatic community residents, an average age for surgical intervention was reported for BAV disease versus degenerative tricuspid valve disease of 40± 20 years and 67 ± 16 years, respectively [85]. In Scheme 1, indications for surgical intervention in patients with BAV disease including AR, AS and/or proximal ascending aorta dilation are described. In adults with BAV disease, surgical intervention in the form of AVR is recommended when severe AS, chronic AR and left ventricle dysfunction (LV) with a LV ejection fraction (EF) of < 50% is present. Furthermore, adolescents and young adults with severe AR who have developing symptoms, persistent LV dysfunction with LV EF < 50%, or progressive LV dilatation, are also suitable candidates for AVR [39]. Several factors has to be kept in mind when choosing a patient tailored intervention namely, the risk for reoperation with bioprosthetic valves due to valve degeneration, and the necessity of lifelong anticoagulation with mechanical valve replacement. In athletic patients, bleeding risks due to chronic use of anticoagulation should be discussed, as well as the potential risk of teratogenic dangers of warfarine for women who desire pregnancy in the future. The discussion of the risk and benefits for both procedures is therefore mandatory.

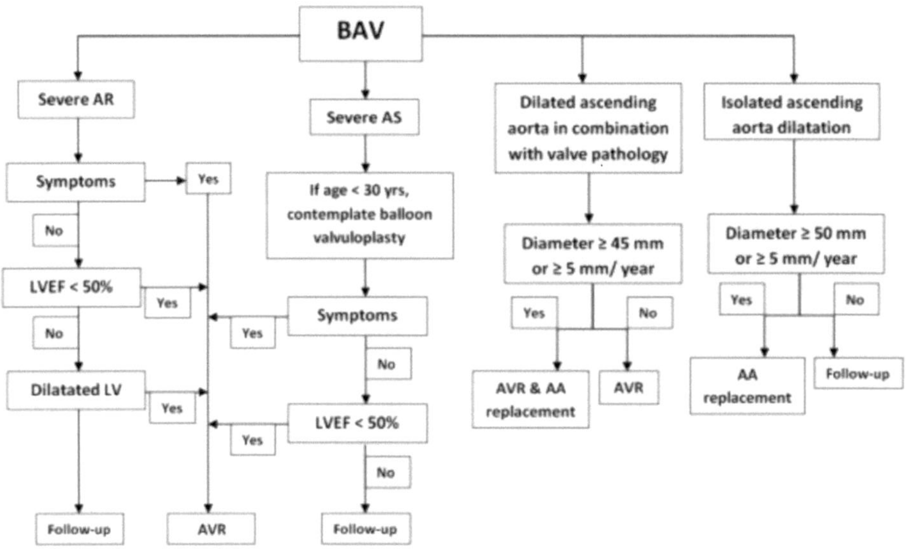

Scheme 1. Indication for cardiac surgical intervention in patients with bicuspid aortic valve disease including aortic regurgitation (AR), aortic stenosis (AS), and/or aortic dilatation. LVEF = left ventricle ejection fraction; LV dilatation = Left ventricle dilatation (End-systolic diameter > 55mm or end-diastolic diameter > 75 mm); Clinical symptoms include dyspnoea, angina, or syncope; Severe AS = jet velocity > 4 m/s, mean gradient. 40 mm Hg, valve area < 1 cm^2; severe AR = jet width < 65% of LOVT, vena contracta width > 0.6 cm, regurgitant volume > 60 mL, regurgitant fraction > 60%, regurgitant orifice area >0.3 cm^2. AVR = aortic valve replacement (Data derived from Bonow *et al.* [39]).

8.2. Surgical indications for ascending aorta dilation

As mentioned earlier, BAV disease is associated with aortic dilatation. BAV patients with the presence of AR or AS should receive surgical intervention of the ascending aorta when an aortic diameter of ≥ 45 mm is present. Conversely, BAV patients with absence of additional risk factors and co morbidities should receive surgical intervention at an aortic root or ascending aorta dilatation of ≥ 50 mm or a aortic dilatation expansion rate of ≥ 5 mm per year [39]. However, it seems that aortic size relative to body size could be a more superior novel technique to define high risk patients requiring surgical intervention [104]. Proper routine

http://dx.doi.org/10.5772/55325

evaluation of the aortic root and ascending aorta is therefore mandatory in patients with BAV with echocardiography or MRI to determine the potential presence of an aortic dilatation [67].

8.3. Pharmacological treatment options

Systematic high blood pressure is an independent risk factor for developing complications including aorta dissection in patients with stenotic BAV with aortic root dilatation. B-blocker therapy is therefore advisable for patients with BAV disease [39]. Moreover, osteogenic and proteolytic activities,which is a precursor to atherosclerotic and calcified degenerative AS, have been revealed in early aortic valve disease with the use of multimodality molecular imaging [115]. However, lipid lowering therapy didn't reduce calcific valve progression with respect to moderate to severe AS [116, 134]. Although, little evidence have acknowledged the beneficial use of statins in BAV disease, patients with BAV disease who have risk factors for atherosclerosis should receive statins with the purpose of reducing the degenerative risk in the aorta and potentially preventing atherosclerosis. Long-term vasodilator therapy is only recommended in BAV patients with AR if systematic hypertension is present [39]. Despite this, there is currently no concrete evidence suggesting that pharmacological treatments could alter the natural history or halt the development BAV calcifiation.

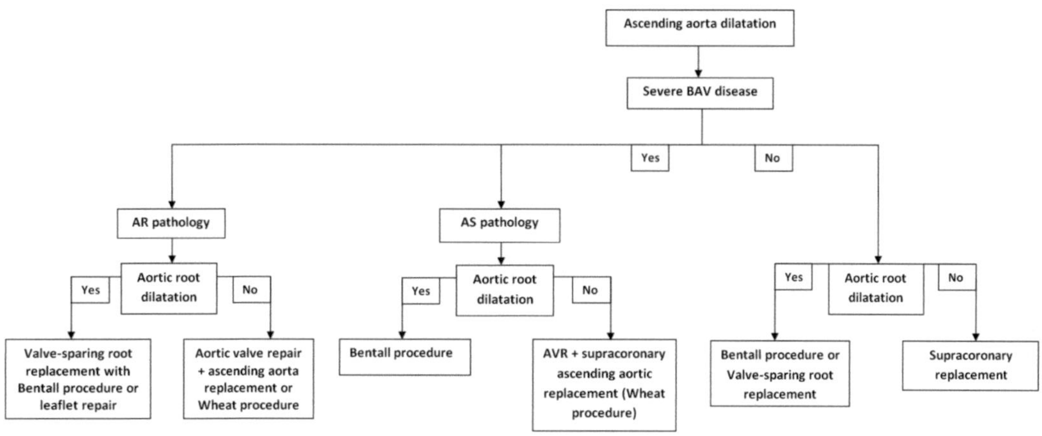

Scheme 2. Cardiac surgical options for aortic dilatation in patients with bicuspid aortic valve disease. AR = aortic regurgitation, AS = Aortic stenosis.

8.4. Surgical options

The surgical options are illustrated in Scheme 2 for BAV disease with aortic dilatation. When patients require an intervention of the aortic valve with an aortic diameter < 45 mm, the main surgical option is a bioprosthetic AVR, mechanical AVR, the Ross procedure which is contraindicated in older patients with BAV and onset of aortic dilatation, or aortic valve repair in selected cases of AR. In patients with > 45 mm ascending aorta root dilatation with significant aortic valve pathology, aortic root replacement therapy, (Bentall procedure) is the main surgical option.

8.5. Valve repair

Surgical repair can be considered when BAV disease is presented without any significant signs of calcification or valve thickening [105]. Several surgical repair options are available including raphé resection with or without leaflet placation, shortening or reinforcement of the free margin, augmentation of the pericardial patch cusp, aortic root repair, and subcommissural annuloplasty [105, 106]. Patients with BAV disease show evidence of sclerosis after the second decade and calcification associated with increasing stenosis at the fourth decade [12, 75]. This raises the question with respect to valve sparing replacement of a dilated aorta, especially in young patients. Although, it appears that the need for reoperation is greater in the surgical repair group for AR, this surgical option still remains attractive in both young adults with AR and women with BAV disease who want to become pregnant.

8.6. Ross procedure

The Ross procedure, also known as the pulmonary autograft, is a cardiac surgical procedure in which the pathological aortic valve is replaced with a patient's own pulmonary valve after which a pulmonary allograft is performed with a valve from a donor which is then used to substitute the patient's own pulmonary valve. Several benefits have been reported with the Ross procedure including the absence of anticoagulation, reduced endocarditis risk, and encouraging valve hemodynamic gradients [107]. However, major concerns have been raised including the most important concern regarding the durability of the autograft and allograft. In addition, another key concern is that histopathologic alterations of the pulmonary trunk may occur, after which the pulmonary trunk can show resemblances of the proximal aorta, thus increasing the risk for aortic aneurysms with a reoperation being the most likely end result [108]. The Ross procedure has no beneficial benefits over conventional AVR in adult patients with respect to hemodynamics or postoperative outcomes. Nevertheless, the Ross procedure offers adolescents, young adults and women with BAV disease who want to become pregnant, an adequate solution in the first decade after the operation. However, limitation with respect to the durability is evident by the end of the first postoperative decade, especially in younger patients [109]. Ross procedure in the setting of BAV disease still remains controversial and should only be performed in selected cases in specialized centres.

8.7. Bentall procedure

Due to the risk of aortic dilatation in patients with BAV disease, the majority of the surgeons evaluate the option of reinforcing or replace the ascending aorta with at the time of the valve surgery. The Bentall procedure is a widely used surgical procedure for patients with BAV and aortic root dilatation. This procedure includes the replacement of the aortic valve, aortic root and ascending aorta with the reimplantation of the coronary arteries [110]. Excellent long-term results have been observed with the Bentall procedure with respect to survival in patients with aortic valve disease and aorta dilatation [111]. This procedure is a suitable intervention in older

http://dx.doi.org/10.5772/55325

patients with severe BAV pathology with normal-sized sinuses and dilatation of the supra-coronary ascending aorta.

8.8. Yacoub and David procedure

Valve sparing aortic root replacement procedure may be an alternative to Bentall procedures in selected BAV patients such as young adults who present with aortic root lesion with normally functioning aortic valve including the absence of calcified aortic valves, multileaflet prolapsed and annular dilatation [112]. Two variations for this procedure have been described namely the remodeling (Yacoub) procedure and the re-implantation (David) procedure [113, 114]. The coronary artery ostia are removed as buttons in both procedures followed by reimplantation of a Dacron aortic graft with additional leaflet repair, if required. However, in the David procedure, the aortic root is mobilized to below the plane of the ventriculo-aortic junction followed by a Dacron graft replacement which is telescoped down outside the aortic root to provide a functional aortic annuloplasty. It seems that there is no significant difference between these two procedures in BAV patients. Valve sparing procedures are more surgically changeling than the traditional Bentall procedure and are only conducted in specialized aortic centres. When tubular ascending aorta dilatation is present with no root or valve pathology, supracoronary ascending aortic replacement is required in BAV patients. When valve pathology is present with this anatomical lesion, a Wheat procedure should be preformed. This procedure includes separate AVR or repair leaving the sinus segment intact. However, due to the fact that in most cases sclerosis of the aortic valve starts in the second decade and calcification begins to develop around the fourth decade, serious consideration have to be made with respect to valve-sparing replacement of a dilated aorta in young adults with normally functioning BAV [12, 75].

8.9. Balloon valvuloplasty

Due to the growth of adolescents during childhood, prosthetic valve insertion is unsatisfactory. Balloon valvuloplasty is therefore a successful treatment option because of the fact the aortic valve is not calcified at this age of the child and the fact that valvuloplasty disrupts the commissural fusion and reduces the obstruction when implemented. Balloon valvuloplasty is indicated in young adults and adolescents without significantly calcified BAV and no AR who experience symptoms with a peak-to-peak gradients of > 50 mm Hg. Also, asymptomatic adolescents who develop ST- or T wave changes with exercise or rest or demonstrate a peak-to-peak gradient of > 60 mm Hg should be considered candidates for balloon valvuloplasty. Additional indications for balloon valvuloplasty are asymptomatic adolescent or young adult who are interested in sport activities or becoming pregnant with a peak-to-peak gradient > 50 mm Hg. When severe AR is evident after balloon valvulplasty, AVR should be considered. Conversely, valvuloplasty is seldom performed in old adults due to often severe calcification of the aortic valve [39, 86]. However, balloon valvuloplasty should be considered as a bridge to surgery in adults with AS who have a high risk for AVR, who are hemodynamically unstable, or when AVR is not possible to perform due to secondary co morbidities. Excellent mid-term results have been observed after balloon valvuloplasty at experienced centres [117-119].

8.10. Transcatheter aortic valve implantation

Transcatheter aortic valve implantation (TAVI) is a novel minimally invasive technique indicated for patients who are contraindicated for cardiac surgery due to associated comorbilities or who have a high risk of perioperative mortality. TAVI is an alternative treatment for patients with valve disease in which a valve replacement is introduced through the femoral artery via a small incision or in some cases, an incision into the chest after which the catheter is inserted into the left ventricular apex, also known as the transapical approach. Other methods include subclavian in which the catheter is inserted beneath the collar bone and direct aortic incision in which the catheter is inserted directly into the aorta via a minimally invasive incision in the chest [120]. Due to the asymmetric anatomy which is observed with BAV disease, the TAVI device could potentially be affected to a noncircular expansion, thus creating an elevated risk of paravalvular leak [121]. Due to this major concern, BAV is considered a contraindication with respect to TAVI. BAV have been overall excluded in all the major TAVI trials in which little clinical experience is now known with regard to TAVI in BAV cases. However, several centres showed acceptable results in selected BAV patients with AS [121-123]. A high risk of suboptimal device seating has been observed in BAV patients with asymmetric valvular anatomy, AR, and bulky leaflets. Whether novel valve designs could improve TAVI performance in the BAV group, still remains uncertain.

9. Surveillance

All patients with BAV disease whether AS, AR, operated or not, should receive lifelong serial follow-up depending on symptoms and degree of the functional disorder. Moreover, serial follow-up with imaging assessment with respect to the cardiac and aortic anatomy including valve function, LV function, diameter of both ascending aorta, sinotublular junction, sinuses of Valsvalva and the annulus should be performed in BAV patients regardless the severity of the pathology. TTE is a reliable diagnostic tool to monitor the aortic valve and ascending aorta. However, it should be noted that it is difficult to obtain adequate imaging with the TTE regarding the mid and distal ascending aorta and arch, especially in BAV patients with large body index, in which MRI or CT scan should be used.

The occurrence of imaging should depend on the size of the aortic root at the initial assessment. If the aortic root is < 40 mm with no clinical symptom alternations, the ascending aorta should be reimaged every 2 years. Whereas, if the aortic root is ≥ 40 mm, it is should be reimaged annually or even more often if progression of the aortic root dilatation is present or whenever a change in clinical symptoms and/or findings occur with echocardiography or MRI [39]. Also of importance, first degree family members of patients with BAV disease should receive echocardiographic screening due to the increased risk of cardiovascular abnormalities [39].

http://dx.doi.org/10.5772/55325

10. Sport participation

The vast majority of young adults with BAV disease are asymptomatic. Little is known regarding the risks of aortic dissection and sudden cardiac death in young adults with BAV who participate in athletic activity. Also, the severity of the valve pathology and aortic root dilatation in this subgroup of BAV patients influence the clinical decision making with respect to strategy and recommendations for sport activity.

No restrictions are necessary with respect to BAV patients with an athletic lifestyle who present with a mild AS. However, asymptomatic BAV patients with moderate AS can only conduct low-intensity athletic competitive activities. Exercise stress testing is mandatory for BAV patients with moderate AS to detect any additional risk factors including unusual blood pressure during exercise, onset of symptoms during exercise or pathological arrhythmias, which could eventually alter the clinical strategy and recommendations. In addition, BAV patients with symptomatic moderate or severe AS should receive immediate surgical intervention and should therefore not participate in any form of competitive sport activities upon surgery [124].

BAV patients with mild enlargement of the left ventricular end-diastolic dimension and mild to moderate AR have no restriction in participating in all forms of athletic activity. Also in this case, an exercise stress testing should be performed to estimate the risk. Patients with BAV disease who have a definite LV enlargement of ≥ 60 mm, pulmonary hypertension, or any degree of LV systolic dysfunction at rest should avoid any form of competitive sport activities [124]. BAV patients who underwent an AVR should avoid any form of contact sport.

Also, BAV patients with severe AR and left ventricular end-diastolic diameter > 65 mm should avoid any form of competitive sport activities. This also includes BAV patients with mild-to moderate AR associated with positive symptoms for valve disease [124]. Young adults with uncalcified AS with a peak-to-peak gradient > 50 mm Hg should who play competitive sports are candidates for aortic balloon valvuloplasty [39]. The recommendation for sport activity for BAV patients with respect to dilatation of the proximal aortic root depends on the level of severity the aortic dilatation. BAV patients with an aortic root diameter of 40 to 45 mm should only perform low to moderate intensity sport activity and preferably avoid any form of contact sport. Moreover, BAV patients with an aortic root diameter of > 45 mm are allowed to conduct low-intensity sport activity due to due to the potential risk of aortic root dissection [125].

11. Pregnancy

Although, the vast majority of pregnancies with congenital AS go through labour uncomplicated, some pregnancies with severe AS have a higher risk rate of morbidity, although the mortality rates still remains rare [126, 127].

Severe AS is not well tolerated in pregnant women and is associated with high peripartum complications [75]. Around one-third of the pregnant women with maternal congenital AS showed clinical complications with a significant rate of abortion [128]. Of note, it is recommended that women with AS who are considering becoming pregnant receive prepregnancy counselling [39].

Nevertheless, mild-to-moderate AS is well tolerated by pregnant women and show no complications with respect to labour compared to pregnant women with severe AS who had a deterioration rate of 10% [126].

Asymptomatic severe AR is well endured by pregnant women unlike severe AS [129]. A possible explanation for this phenomenon is because of pregnancy related physiologic changes which presents with an afterload decrease and heart rate increase with a shortening of the diastole, thus reducing the level of AR.

Of note, several recommendations has to be considered in pregnant women with severe BAV pathology with symptoms including pre-pregnancy counselling, foetal echocardiography during the second trimester to investigate whether cardiac defects is present in the foetus, and close cardiac follow-up in the form of echocardiography to monitor changes in symptoms and further valve deterioration [39]. Several side effects have been reported when cardiac surgery requiring cardiopulmonary bypass is used including the potential risk of fetal distress, fetal wastage and growth retardation [130, 131]. Therefore, it should be noted that women with a high risk for complications during pregnancy should abstain from pregnancy until the valve pathology is properly surgically treated [124]. Moreover, parents should receive proper clinical counselling with respect to the genetic predisposition and the risk of congenital cardiac defect in their children [132].

Encouraging results have been observed with the balloon valvuloplasty during pregnancy including successful completion of the pregnancy [133]. However, concerns have been raised regarding symptomatic AR after balloon valvuloplasty which is also a burden for pregnant patients. Therefore, balloon valvuloplasty should be considered as a bridge to surgery in pregnant women with severe AS. When an unplanned pregnancy occurs in women with severe aortic pathology with symptoms, physical restriction with close cardiac follow-up are obligated. Furthermore, vasodilatation and volume depletion medicine should be avoided at all time. Due to the compression of the inferior vena cava by the gravid uterus, it is recommended that the delivery should be performed in the left lateral decubitus position.

12. Conclusion

BAV disease is a frequently seen congenital cardiac defect, complicated with proximal thoracic aortic aneurysm and associated with other cardiovascular malformations including Turner Syndrome and COA. Although little is known about the pathogenesis of BAV dis-

http://dx.doi.org/10.5772/55325

ease, it seems that BAV disease is linked with both genetic predisposition and defects in the early valvulogenesis. Further investigation is required with respect to the basic genetic and embryological defects associated with BAV disease and the proximal aortic dilatation including the cellular mechanisms and signalling pathways. This will give us more understanding regarding the background of the degeneration and calcification of the bicuspid valve, and the development of aortic aneurysm. This could offer new pharmacological targets to prevent calcification, degeneration and aortic dilatation.

The dilatation of the proximal thoracic aorta may lead to complications including ascending aortic aneurysm and dissection. Early detection, vigilant patient assessment and frequent follow-up by imaging including echocardiography, CT and CMRI can potentially persevere both long-term survival and quality of life in patients affected by BAV disease.

Several interventional options are available for patients with BAV disease and aortic dilatation. Balloon valvuloplasty is indicated in young adults and adolescents without significantly BAV calcification. Surgical repair (Yacoub and David procedure) should be considered when BAV disease is presented without any significant signs of calcification or valve thickening. In contrast, when calcified BAV disease is present, AVR, Bentall procedure or Ross procedure is necessary. Although in some cases these procedures are performed in valves without calcification. TAVI is relatively contraindicated due to the asymmetric anatomy which is observed patients with BAV disease. The TAVI device could potentially be affected to a noncircular expansion with the risk of paravalvular leak. BAV patients were excluded in the major TAVI studies. Future research should focus on novel valve designs.

Despite the fact that limited data exist with respect to prophylactic interventions, BAV disease associated aortic dilatation with absence of additional risk factors and co morbidities is indicated when the diameter is ≥ 50 mm or an aortic dilatation expansion rate of ≥ 5 mm per year. In patients with BAV disease with additional risk factors, such as COA, Turner Syndrome and a family history of aortic dissection, replacement should be considered when a diameter of ≥ 45 mm is present. Patients with symptoms of BAV disease due to AR or AS, or asymptomatic LV dysfunction all require surgery. If the ascending aorta exceeds 45 mm, the root should be replaced as well. Valve sparing aortic root replacement procedure is recommended in young patients who present with aortic root lesion with normally functioning aortic valve including the absence of calcified aortic valves, multileaflet prolapsed and annular dilatation. Future studies are mandatory, not only to predict the optimal timing for AVR when symptoms occur, but also to investigate whether prophylactic intervention of the ascending aorta at the time of AVR is necessary. Also, additional studies are required to determine the risks factors for aortic dissection and the optimal diameter at which replacement of the ascending aorta should be performed in patients with BAV disease. Future studies should also focus on sudden cardiac death in young adults with BAV disease who participate in athletic activity.

Author details

George Tokmaji[1], Berto J. Bouma[2], Dave R. Koolbergen[1,3] and Bas A.J.M. de Mol[1]

1 Department of Cardiothoracic Surgery, Academic Medical Center, Amsterdam, The Netherlands

2 Department of Cardiology, Academic Medical Center, Amsterdam, The Netherlands

3 Department of Cardiothoracic Surgery, Leiden University Medical Center, Leiden, The Netherlands

References

[1] Tadros TM, Klein MD, Shapira OM. Ascending aortic dilatation associated with bicuspid aortic valve. Pathophysiology, molecular biology, and clinical implications. Circulation 2009;119:880-890.

[2] Nistri S, Basso C, Marzari C, et al. Frequency of bicuspid aortic valve in young male conscripts by echocardiogram. Am J Cardiol. 2005;96:718–21.

[3] Tutar E, Ekici F, Atalay S, et al. The prevalence of bicuspid aortic valve in newborns by echocardiographic screening. Am Heart J. 2005;150:513–5.

[4] Basso C, Boschello M, Perrone C, et al. An echocardiographic survey of primary school children for bicuspid aortic valve. Am J Cardiol. 2004;93:661–3.

[5] Yener N, Oktar GL, Erer D, Yardimci MM, Yener A. Bicuspid aortic valve. Ann Thorac Cardiovasc Surg 2002;8:264–7.

[6] Roberts WC. The congenitally bicuspid aortic valve. A study of 85 autopsy cases. Am J Cardiol. 1970;26 (1):72–83.

[7] Sabet HY, Edwards WD, Tazelaar HD, Daly RC. Congenitally bicuspid aortic valves: a surgical pathology study of 542 cases (1991 through 1996) and a literature review of 2,715 additional cases. Mayo Clin Proc. 1999;74(1):14–26.

[8] Sievers HH, Schmidtke C. A classification system for the bicuspid aortic valve from 304 surgical specimens. J Thorac Cardiovasc Surg. 2007;133(5):1226–33.

[9] Fernandes SM, Sanders SP, Khairy P, Jenkins KJ, Gauvreau K, Lang P, et al. Morphology of bicuspid aortic valve in children and adolescents. J Am Coll Cardiol. 2004;44(8):1648–51.

[10] Schaefer BM, Lewin MB, Stout KK, Gill E, Prueitt A, Byers PH, et al. The bicuspid aortic valve: an integrated phenotypic classification of leaflet morphology and aortic root shape. Heart. 2008;94(12):1634–8.

[11] Russo CF, Cannata A, LanfranconiM, Vitali E, Garatti A, Bonacina E. Is aortic wall degeneration related to bicuspid aortic valve anatomy in patients with valvular disease? J Thorac Cardiovasc Surg. 2008;136(4):937–42.

[12] Beppu S, Suzuki S, Matsuda H, et al. Rapidity of progression of aortic stenosis in patients with congenital bicuspid aortic valve. Am J Cardiol 1993;71:322–7.

[13] Mancuso D, Basso C, Cardaioli P, Thiene G. Clefted bicuspid aortic valve. Cardiovasc Pathol 2002; 11:217–220.

[14] Peacock TB. Valvular disease of the heart. London: Churchill, 1865:2–33.

[15] Olson LJ, Subramanian R, Edwards WD. Surgical pathology of pure aortic insufficiency: a study of 225 cases. Mayo Clin Proc 1984;59:835–41.

[16] Ward C. Clinical significance of the bicuspid aortic valve. Heart 2000; 83:81–85.

[17] Johnson AD, Detwiler JH, Higgins CB. Left coronary artery anatomy in patients with bicuspid aortic valves. Br Heart J. 1978;40(5):489–93.

[18] Hutchins GM, Nazarian IH, Bulkley BH. Association of left dominant coronary arterial system with congenital bicuspid aortic valve. Am J Cardiol. 1978;42:57–9.

[19] Higgins CB,Wexler L. Reversal of dominance of the coronary arterial system in isolated aortic stenosis and bicuspid aortic valve. Circulation 1975;52:292–6.

[20] Murphy ES, Rosch J, Rahimtoola S. The frequency and significance of coronary arterial dominance in isolated aortic stenosis. Am J Cardiol 1977;39:505–9.

[21] Roberts WC. The structure of the aortic valve in clinically isolated aortic stenosis. An autopsy of 162 patients over 15 years of age. Circulation 1970; 42:91–97.

[22] Sans-Coma V, Fernandez B, Duran AC, Thiene G, Arque JM, Munoz- Chapuli R, Cardo M. Fusion of valve cushions as a key factor in the formation of congenital bicuspid aortic valves in Syrian hamsters. Anat Rec 1996; 244:490–498.

[23] R. Abu-Issa and M. L. Kirby, "Heart field: frommesodermto heart tube," Annual Review of Cell and Developmental Biology, vol. 23, pp. 45–68, 2007.

[24] R. R.Markwald, T. P. Fitzharris, and F. J.Manasek, "Structural development of endocardial cushions," American Journal of Anatomy, vol. 148, no. 1, pp. 85–119, 1977.

[25] A. D. Person, S. E. Klewer, and R. B. Runyan, "Cell biology of cardiac cushion development," International Review of Cytology, vol. 243, pp. 287–335, 2005.

[26] Duran AC, Frescura V, Sans-Coma V, et al. Bicuspid aortic valves in hearts with other congenital heart disease. J Heart Valve Dis 1995;4:581-90.

[27] Fernández B, Fernandez MC, Durán AC, et al. Anatomy and formation of congenital bicuspid and quadricuspid pulmonary valves in Syrian hamsters. Anat Rec 1998;250:70-9.

[28] Kappetein AP, Gittenberger-de Groot AC, Zwinderman AH, et al. The neural crest as a possible pathogenetic factor in coarctation of the aorta and bicuspid aortic valve. J Thorac Cardiovasc Surg 1991;102:830-6.

[29] Schievink WI, Mokri B. Familial aorto-cervicocephalic arterial dissections and congenitally bicuspid aortic valve. Stroke 1995;26: 1935– 40.

[30] Schievink WI, Mokri B, Piepgras DG, Gittenberger-de Groot AC. Intracranial aneurysms and cervicocephalic arterial dissections associated with congenital heart disease. Neurosurgery 1996;39:685–9, discussion 689–90.

[31] Lee TC, Zhao YD, Courtman DW, Stewart DJ. Abnormal aortic valve development in mice lacking endothelial nitric oxide synthase. Circulation 2000;101:2345– 8.

[32] Fernández B, Durán AC, Fernández-Gallego T, Fernández MC, Such M, Arqué JM, Sans-Coma V. Bicuspid aortic valves with different spatial orientations of the leaflets are distinct etiological entities. J Am Coll Cardiol. 2009 Dec 8;54(24):2312-8.

[33] Glick BN, Roberts WC. Congenitally bicuspid aortic valve in multiple family members. Am J Cardiol. 1994 Feb 15;73(5):400-4.

[34] Cripe L, Andelfinger G, Martin J, et al. Bicuspid aortic valve is heritable. J Am Coll Cardiol. 2004;44:138–43.

[35] Huntington K, Hunter AG, Chan KL. A prospective study to assess the frequency of familial clustering of congenital bicuspid aortic valve. J Am Coll Cardiol. 1997;30:1809–12.

[36] Martin LJ, Ramachandran V, Cripe LH, et al. Evidence in favor of linkage to human chromosomal regions 18q, 5q and 13q for bicuspid aortic valve and associated cardiovascular malformations. Hum Genet. 2007;121:275–84.

[37] Garg V, Muth AN, Ransom JF, et al. Mutations in NOTCH 1 cause aortic valve disease. Nature. 2005;437:270–4.

[38] Guo DC, Pannu H, Tran-Fadulu V, et al. Mutations in smooth muscle alpha-actin (ACTA2) lead to thoracic aortic aneurysms and dissections. Nat Genet. 2007;39:1488–93.

[39] Warnes CA, Williams RG, Bashore TM, et al. ACC/AHA 2008 guidelines for the management of adults with congenital heart disease: a report of the American College of Cardiology/American Heart Association Task Force on Practice Guidelines (Writing Committee to Develop Guidelines on the Management of Adults With Congenital Heart Disease). J Am Coll Cardiol 2008;52:e1–121.

http://dx.doi.org/10.5772/55325

[40] Bolling SF, Iannettoni MD, Dick M. Shone's anomaly: operative results and late outcome. Ann Thorac Surg 1990;49:887-93.

[41] Oppenheimer-Dekker A, Gittenberger-de Groot AC, Bartelings MM. Abnormal architecture of the ventricles in hearts with an overriding aortic valve and a perimembranous ventricular septal defect. Int J Cardiol 1985;9:341-55.

[42] Neumayer U, Stone S, Somerville J. Small ventricular septal defects in the adult. Eur Heart J 1998;9:1573-82.

[43] Sugayama SM, Moises RL, Wagenfur J, Ikari NM, Abe KT, Leone C, et al. Williams-Beuren syndrome: cardiovascular abnormalities in 20 patients diagnosed with fluorescence in situ hybridization. Arq Bras Cardiol. 2003;81(5):462–73.

[44] Oliver JM, Gallego P, Gonzalez A, et al. Risk factors for aortic complications in adults with coarctation of the aorta. J Am Coll Cardiol 2004;44:1641-7.

[45] Kuboki K. Clinicopathologic study of congenital bicuspid aortic valve in the aged. Cardio 2000; 35:287–296.

[46] Abbott ME. Coarctation of the aorta of adult type; statistical study and historical retrospect of 200 recorded cases with autopsy; of stenosis or obliteration of descending arch in subjects above age of two years. Am Heart J 1928;3:574.

[47] Luijendijk P, Franken RJ, Vriend JW, Zwinderman AH, Vliegen HW, Winter MM, Groenink M, Bouma BJ, Mulder BJ. Increased risk for ascending aortic dilatation in patients with complex compared to simple aortic coarctation. Int J Cardiol. 2012 Feb 25

[48] Attenhofer Jost CH, Schaff HV, Connolly HM, et al. Spectrum of reoperations after

[49] air of aortic coarctation: importance of an individualized approach because of

[50] xistent cardiovascular disease. Mayo Clin Proc 2002;77:646-53.

[51] Roos-Hesselink JW, Scholzel BE, Heijdra RJ, et al. Aortic valve and aortic arch pathology after coarctation repair. Heart 2003;89:1074-7.

[52] Miller MJ, Geffner ME, Lippe BM, et al. Echocardiography reveals a high incidence of bicuspid aortic valve in Turner syndrome. J Pediatr 1983;102:47-50.

[53] Price WH, Clayton JF, Collyer S, et al. Mortality ratios, life expectancy, and causes of death in patients Turner's syndrome. J Epidem Comm Health 1986;40:97-102.

[54] Matura LA, Ho VB, Rosing D, et al. Aortic dilation and dissection in Turner syndrome. Circulation 2007;116:1e7.

[55] Perloff, JK. The Clinical Recognition of Congenital Heart Disease, 4th ed. Philadelphia, PA: W.B. Saunders, 1994.

[56] Espinal M, Fuisz AR, Nanda NC, Aaluri SR, Mukhtar O, Sekar PC. Sensitivity and specificity of transeophgeal echocardiography for determination of aortic valve morphology. A Heart J. 2000;139 (6):1071-6.

[57] Brandenburg Jr RO, Tajik AJ, Edwards WD, Reeder GS, Shub C, Seward JB. Accuracy of 2-dimensional echocardiographic diagnosis of congenitally bicuspid aortic valve: echocardiographic-anatomic correlation in 115 patients. Am J Cardiol. 1983;51(9): 1469–73.

[58] Espinal M, Fuisz AR, Nanda NC, Aaluri SR, Mukhtar O, Sekar PC. Sensitivity and specificity of transesophageal echocardiography for determination of aortic valve morphology. Am Heart J. 2000;139 (6):1071–6.

[59] Fowles RE, Martin RP, Abrams JM, et al. Two dimensional echocardiographic features of bicuspid aortic valve. Chest 1979;75:434-40.

[60] Nanda NC, Gramiak R. Echocardiographic recognition of the congenital bicuspid aortic valve. Circulation 1974;49:870-5.

[61] Gleeson TG,Mwangi I, Horgan SJ,Cradock A, Fitzpatrick P, Murray JG. Steady-state free-precession (SSFP) cine MRI in distinguishing normal and bicuspid aortic valves. J Magn Reson Imaging. 2008;28(4):873–8.

[62] Malaisrie SC, Carr J, Mikati I, Rigolin V, Yip BK, Lapin B, McCarthy PM. Cardiac magnetic resonance imaging is more diagnostic than 2-dimensional echocardiography in determining the presence of bicuspid aortic valve. J Thorac Cardiovasc Surg. 2012 Aug;144(2):370-6.

[63] McElhinney DB, Lock JE, Keane JF, et al. Left heart growth, function, and reintervention after balloon aortic valvuloplasty for neonatal aortic stenosis. Circulation 2005; 111:451.

[64] Maskatia SA, Ing FF, Justino H, et al. Twenty-five year experience with balloon aortic valvuloplasty for congenital aortic stenosis. Am J Cardiol 2011; 108:1024.

[65] Rehnström P, Malm T, Jögi P, Fernlund E, Winberg P, Johansson J, Johansson S. Outcome of surgical commissurotomy for aortic valve stenosis in early infancy. Ann Thorac Surg. 2007 Aug;84(2):594-8.

[66] Alexiou C, Langley SM, Dalrymple-Hay MJ, Salmon AP, Keeton BR, Haw MP, Monro JL. Open commissurotomy for critical isolated aortic stenosis in neonates. Ann Thorac Surg. 2001 Feb;71(2):489-93.

[67] Hiratzka LF, Bakris GL, Beckman JA, et al. 2010 ACCF/AHA/AATS/ACR/ASA/SCA/SCAI/SIR/STS/SVM Guidelines for the diagnosis and management of patients with thoracic aortic disease. A Report of the American College of Cardiology Foundation/American Heart Association Task Force on Practice Guidelines, American Association for Thoracic Surgery, American College of Radiology,American Stroke Association, Society of Cardiovascular Anesthesiologists, Society for Cardiovascular

Angiography and Interventions, Society of Interventional Radiology, Society of Thoracic Surgeons,and Society for Vascular Medicine. J Am Coll Cardiol. 2010 Apr 6;55(14):e27-e129.

[68] Loscalzo ML, Goh DL, Loeys B, et al. Familial thoracic aortic dilation and bicommissural aortic valve: a prospective analysis of natural history and inheritance. Am J Med Genet A. 2007;143A:1960–7.

[69] Svensson LG, Crawford ES. Cardiovascular and Vascular Disease of the Aorta. Philadelphia, PA: WB Saunders Co; 1997.

[70] Kutty S, Greenberg RK, Fletcher S, et al. Endovascular stent grafts for large thoracic aneurysms after coarctation repair. Ann Thorac Surg. 2008;85:1332– 8.

[71] Roberts WC, Ko JM. Frequency by decades of unicuspid, bicuspid, and tricuspid aortic valves in adults having isolated aortic valve replacement for aortic stenosis, with or without associated aortic regurgitation. Circulation 2005; 111:920–925.

[72] Wallby L, Janerot-Sjoberg B, Steffensen T, et al. T lymphocyte infiltration in nonrheumatic aortic stenosis: a comparative descriptive study between tricuspid and bicuspid aortic valves. Heart 2002;88:348-51.

[73] Subramanian R, Olson LJ, Edwards WD. Surgical pathology of pure aortic stenosis: a study of 374 Cases.Mayo Clin Proc 1984;59:683–90.

[74] Pomerance A. Pathogenesis of aortic stenosis and its relation to age. Br Heart J 1972;34:569–74.

[75] Mautner GC, Mautner SL, Cannon RD, et al. Clinical factors useful in predicting aortic valve structure in patients >40 years of age with isolated valvular aortic stenosis. Am J Cardiol 1993;73:194–8.

[76] Wallaby L, Janerot-Sjoberg B, Steffensen T, Broqvist M. T-lymphocyte infiltration in non-rheumatic aortic stenosis: a comparative descriptive study between tricuspid and bicuspid aortic valves. Heart 2002; 88:348–351.

[77] Chan KL, Ghani M, Woodend K, Burwash IG. Case-controlled study to assess risk factors for aortic stenosis in congenitally bicuspid aortic valve. Am J Cardiol 2001; 88:690–693.

[78] Pachulski RT, Chan KL. Progression of aortic valve dysfunction in 51 adult patients with congenital bicuspid aortic valve: assessment and follow-up by Doppler echocardiography. Br Heart J 1993; 69:237–240.

[79] Yotsumoto G, Moriyama Y, Toyohira H, Shimokawa S, Iguro Y, Watanabe S, et al. Congenital bicuspid aortic valve: analysis of 63 surgical cases. J Heart Valve Dis 1998; 7:500–503.

[80] Fedak PWM, Verma S, Tirone ED, Leask RL, Weisel RD, Butany J. Clinical and pathophysiological implications of a bicuspid aortic valve. Circulation 2002; 106:900–904.

[81] Roberts WC, Morrow AG, McIntosh CL, Jones M, Epstein SE. Congenitally bicuspid aortic valve causing severe, pure aortic regurgitation without superimposed infective endocarditis. Analysis of 13 patients requiring aortic valve replacement. Am J Cardiol. 1981;47(2):206–9.

[82] Lewin MB, Otto CM. The bicuspid aortic valve: adverse outcomes from infancy to old age. Circulation. 2005;111(7):832–4.

[83] Nistri S, Sorbo MD, Marin M, et al. Aortic root dilatation in young men with normally functioning bicuspid aortic valves. Heart 1999;82:19–22.

[84] Cosgrove DM, Valvuloplasty for aortic insufficiency. J Thorac Cardiovasc Surg 1991, 102, 571–576.

[85] Michelena HI, Desjardins VA, Avierinos JF, et al. Natural history of asymptomatic patients with normally functioning or minimally dysfunctional bicuspid aortic valve in the community. Circulation 2008; 117:2776–84.

[86] Tzemos N, Therrien J, Yip J, et al. Outcomes in adults with bicuspid aortic valves. JAMA 2008;300:1317–25.

[87] Thiene G, Basso C Pathology and pathogenesis of infective endocarditis in native heart valves. Cardiovasc Pathol 2006, 15, 256–263.

[88] Habib G, Hoen B, Tornos P, et al. Guidelines on the prevention, diagnosis, and treatment of infective endocarditis (new version 2009): the Task Force on the Prevention, Diagnosis, and Treatment of Infective Endocarditis of the European Society of Cardiology (ESC). Endorsed by the European Society of Clinical Microbiology and Infectious Diseases (ESCMID) and the International Society of Chemotherapy (ISC) for Infection and Cancer. Eur Heart J. 2009 Oct;30(19):2369-413.

[89] Lamas GC, Eykyn SJ. Bicuspid aortic valve—a silent danger: analysis of 50 cases of infective endocarditis. Clin Infect Dis 2000;30:336-41.

[90] Nishimura RA, Carabello BA, Faxon DP et al. ACC/AHA 2008 guideline update on valvular heart disease: focused update on infective endocarditis: a report of the American College of Cardiology/American Heart Association Task Force on Practice Guidelines: endorsed by the Society of Cardiovascular Anesthesiologists, Society for Cardiovascular Angiography and Interventions, and Society of Thoracic Surgeons. Circulation. 2008 Aug 19;118(8):887-96.

[91] Keane MG, Wiegers SE, Plappert T et al. (2000) Bicuspid aortic valves are associated with aortic dilatation out of proportion to coexistent valvular lesions. Circulation, 102, III35–III39.

[92] Niwa K, Perloff JK, Bhuta SM, Laks H, Drinkwater DC, Child JS, Miner PD. Structural abnormalities of great arterial walls in congenital heart disease. Light and electron microscopic analyses. Circulation 2001; 103:393– 400.

[93] Parai JL, Masters RG, Walley VM, Stinson WA, Veinot JP. Aortic medial changes associated with bicuspid aortic valve: myth or reality? Can J Cardiol 1999; 15:1233–1238.

[94] Bauer M, Pasic M, Meyer R. Morphometric analysis of aortic media in patients with bicuspid and tricuspid aortic valve. Ann Thorac Surg 2002; 74:58–62.

[95] Bonderman D, Gharehbaghi-Schnell E, Wollenek G, Maurer G, Baumgartner H, Lang IM. Mechanisms underlying aortic dilatation in congenital aortic valve malformation. Circulation 1999; 99:2138–2143.

[96] Schmid FX, Bielenberg K, Schneider A, Haussler A, Keyser A, Birnbaum D. Ascending aortic aneurysm associated with bicuspid and tricuspid aortic valve: involvement and clinical relevance of smooth muscle cell apoptosis and expression of cell death-initiating proteins. Eur J Cardiothorac Surg 2003; 23:537–543.

[97] Nataatmadja M, West M, West J, Summers K, Walker P, Nagata M, Watanabe T. Abnormal extracellular matrix protein transport associated with increased apoptosis of vascular smooth muscle cells in Marfan syndrome and bicuspid aortic valve thoracic aortic aneurysm. Circulation 2003; 108 (suppl II):329–334.

[98] Fedak PW, de Sa MP, Verma S, Nili N, Kazemian P, Butany J, et al. Vascular matrix remodeling in patients with bicuspid aortic valve malformations: implications for aortic dilatation. J Thorac Cardiovasc Surg 2003; 126:797–806.

[99] Boyum J, Fellinger EK, Schmoker JD, Trombley L, McPartland K, Ittleman FP, Howard AB. Matrix metalloproteinase activity in thoracic aortic aneurysms associated with bicuspid and tricuspid aortic valves. J Thorac Cardiovasc Surg 2004; 127:686–691.

[100] Koullias GJ, Korkolis DP, Ravichandran P, Psyrri A, Hatzaras I, Elefteriades JA. Tissue microarray detection of matrix metalloproteinases, in diseased tricuspid and bicuspid aortic valves with or without pathology of the ascending aorta. Eur J Cardiothorac Surg 2004; 26:1098–1103.

[101] El-Hamamsy I, Yacoub MH. A measured approach to managing the aortic root in patients with bicuspid aortic valve disease. Curr Cardiol Rep. 2009;11 (2):94–100.

[102] Roberts CS, Roberts WC (1991) Dissection of the aorta associated with congenital malformation of the aortic valve. J Am Coll Cardiol, 17, 712–716.

[103] Fazel SS, Mallidi HR, Lee RS, Sheehan MP, Liang D, Fleischman D, Herfkens R, Mitchell RS, Miller DC: The aortopathy of bicuspid aortic valve disease has distinctive patterns and usually involves the transverse aortic arch. J Thorac Cardiovasc Surg 2008, 135 (4):901–907, 907 e901-902.

[104] Davies RR, Gallo A, Coady MA, Tellides G, Botta DM, Burke B, Coe MP, Kopf GS, Elefteriades JA. Novel measurement of relative aortic size predicts rupture of thoracic aortic aneurysms. Ann Thorac Surg. 2006 Jan;81(1):169-77.

[105] Borger MA, David TE. Management of the valve and ascending aorta in adults with bicuspid aortic valve disease. Semin Thorac Cardiovasc Surg. 2005;17(2):143–7.

[106] El Khoury G, Vanoverschelde JL, Glineur D, Pierard F, Verhelst RR, Rubay J, et al. Repair of bicuspid aortic valves in patients with aortic regurgitation. Circulation. 2006;114(1 Suppl):I610–1616.

[107] Cameron DE, Vricella LA. What is the proper place of the Ross procedure in our modern armamentarium? Curr Cardiol Rep. 2007;9(2):93–8.

[108] de Sa M, Moshkovitz Y, Butany J, David TE. Histologic abnormalities of the ascending aorta and pulmonary trunk in patients with bicuspid aortic valve disease: clinical relevance to the ross procedure. J Thorac Cardiovasc Surg. 1999;118(4):588–94.

[109] Takkenberg JJ, Klieverik LM, Schoof PH, van Suylen RJ, van Herwerden LA, Zondervan PE, Roos-Hesselink JW, Eijkemans MJ, Yacoub MH, Bogers AJ. The Ross procedure: a systematic review and meta-analysis. Circulation. 2009 Jan 20;119(2):222-8.

[110] Bentall H, De Bono A. A technique for complete replacement of the ascending aorta. Thorax. 1968;23 (4):338–9.

[111] Etz CD, Bischoff MS, Bodian C, et al. The Bentall procedure: is it the gold standard? A series of 597 consecutive cases. Ann Thorac Cardiovasc Surg. 2010;140:S64–71.

[112] Schmitto JD, Mokashi SA, Chen FY, Chen EP. Aortic valve-sparing operations: state of the art. Curr Opin Cardiol. 2010 Mar;25(2):102-6.

[113] David TE, Feindel CM. An aortic valve-sparing operation for patients with aortic incompetence and aneurysm of the ascending aorta. J Thorac Cardiovasc Surg 1992; 103:617–621.

[114] Sarsam MA, Yacoub M. Remodeling of the aortic valve annulus. J Thorac Cardiovasc Surg 1993; 105:435–438.

[115] Aikawa E, Nahrendorf M, Sosnovik D, et al. Multimodality molecular imaging identifies proteolytic and osteogenic activities in early aortic valve disease. Circulation. 2007;115:377– 86.

[116] Cowell SJ, Newby DE, Prescott RJ, et al. A randomized trial of intensive lipid-lowering therapy in calcific aortic stenosis. N Engl J Med. 2005 Jun 9;352(23):2389-97

[117] Moore P, Egito E, Mowrey H, Perry SB, Lock JE, Keane JF. Midterm results of balloon dilation of congenital aortic stenosis: predictors of success. J Am Coll Cardiol 1996;27:1257– 63.

[118] McCrindle BW, for the Valvuloplasty and Angioplasty of Congenital Anomalies (VACA) Registry Investigators. Independent predictors of immediate results of percutaneous balloon aortic valvotomy in children. Am J Cardiol 1996;77:286 –93.

[119] Rosenfeld HM, Landzberg MJ, Perry SB, Colan SD, Keane JF, Lock JE. Balloon aortic valvuloplasty in the young adult with congenital aortic stenosis. Am J Cardiol 1994;73:1112–7.

[120] Holmes DR Jr, Mack MJ, Kaul S, et al. 2012 ACCF/AATS/SCAI/STS expert consensus document on transcatheter aortic valve replacement. J Am Coll Cardiol. 2012 Mar 27;59(13):1200-54.

[121] Wijesinghe N, Ye J, Rodes-Cabau J, et al. Transcatheter aortic valve implantation in patients with bicuspid aortic valve stenosis. J Am Coll Cardiol Intv. 2010;3:1122–5.

[122] Delgado V, Tops LF, Schuijf JD, et al. Successful deployment of a transcatheter aortic valve in bicuspid aortic stenosis: role of imaging with multislice computed tomography. Circ Cardiovasc Imaging. 2009;2: e12–3.

[123] Chiam PT, Chao VT, Tan SY, et al. Percutaneous transcatheter heart valve implantation in a bicuspid aortic valve. J Am Coll Cardiol Intv. 2010;3:559–61.

[124] Bonow RO, Carabello BA, Kanu C, et al. ACC/AHA 2006 guidelines for the management of patients with valvular heart disease: a report of the American College of Cardiology/American Heart Association Task Force on Practice Guidelines (Writing Committee to Revise the 1998 Guidelines for the Management of Patients With Valvular Heart Disease). J Am Coll Cardiol 2006;48:e1–148.

[125] Bonow RO, Cheitlin MD, Crawford MH, Douglas PS. Task Force 3: valvular heart disease. J Am Coll Cardiol. 2005;45(8):1334–40.

[126] Silversides C, Colman JM, Sermer M, et al. Early and intermediate-term outcomes of pregnancy with congenital aortic stenosis. Am J Cardiol 2003;91:1386-9.

[127] Hameed A, Karaalp IS, Tummala PP, et al. The effect of valvular heart disease on maternal and fetal outcome of pregnancy. J Am Coll Cardiol. 2001;37:893–9.

[128] Lao TT, Sermer M, Magee L, et al. Congenital aortic stenosis. Am J Obstet Gynecol 1993;169:540-5.

[129] Elkayam U, Bitar F. Valvular heart disease and pregnancy part I: native valves. J Am Coll Cardiol. 2005 Jul 19;46(2):223-30.

[130] Sullivan HJ. Valvular heart surgery during pregnancy. Surg Clin North Am 1995;75:59-75.

[131] Goldstein I, Jakobi P, Gutterman E, et al. Umbilical artery flow velocity during maternal cardiopulmonary bypass. Ann Thorac Surg 1995;60:1116-8.

[132] Brickner ME. Valvar aortic stenosis. In: Gatzoulis MA, Webb GD, Daubeney PE, editors. Diagnosis and Management of Adult Congenital Heart Disease. Philadelphia, PA: Churchill Livingstone, 2003.

[133] Banning AP, Pearson JF, Hall RJ. Role of balloon dilatation of the aortic valve in pregnant patients with severe aortic stenosis. Br Heart J 1993;70:544-5.

[134] Teo KK, Corsi DJ, Tam JW, Dumesnil JG, Chan KL Lipid lowering on progression of mild to moderate aortic stenosis: meta-analysis of the randomized placebo-controlled clinical trials on 2344 patients. Can J Cardiol. 2011 Nov-Dec;27(6):800-8.

[135] Ciotti GR, Vlahos AP, Silverman NH. Morphology and function of the bicuspid aortic valve with and without coarctation of the aorta in the young. Am J Cardiol. 2006 Oct 15;98(8):1096-102.

[136] Wendell DC, Samyn MM, Cava JR et al. Including aortic valve morphology in computational fluid dynamics simulations: Initial findings and application to aortic coarctation. Med Eng Phys. 2012 Aug 20.

Chapter 11

The Bicuspid Aortic Valve

Mehmet Demir

Additional information is available at the end of the chapter

http://dx.doi.org/10.5772/52567

1. Introduction

Bicuspid aortic valve (BAV) represents the most common cardiac congenital malformation in the adult age, with strong male predominance. It may occur in isolation, or in association with other congenital heart diseases. The BAV is seen in 1% to 2% of the population and may be complicated by aortic stenosis or aortic insufficiency and infective endocarditis. It may be associated with abnormalities of the aortic wall such as coarctation of the aorta, aortic dissection, and aortic aneurysm. Most patients with a BAV develop some complications during life [1,2].

Congenital coronary anomalies, coronary atherosclerosis, and calcification have been described in association with BAV[3].

BAV has been identified at a prevalence of 4.6 cas-es per 1000 live births. The prevalence of BAV according to sex has been found to be 7.1 cases per 1000 among male neonates, and 1.9 per 1000 among female neonates.

The congenitally BAV may function normally throughout life, may develop progressive calcification and stenosis or may develop regurgitation with or without infection. Aortic root dilatation is common in BAV, even when the valve is haemodynamically normal, and consequently aortic dissection usually occurs in previously asymptomatic patients [4,5].

Aortic stenosis and regurgitation, infective endocarditis and aortic dissection are the most common complications. Left coronary artery dominance is more common in patients with a BAV (29-56.8%) and in 90% of cases, the left main coronary artery is less than 5 mm in length [6-8]. The ignorance of these associations may cause an inadequate myocardial preservation and an increased risk of myocardial infarction[9,10].

Accordingly, associated congenital cardiovascular anomalies have been reported in as many as 25% of patients. Patent ductus arteriosus and ventricular septal defect are the most frequent heart defects associated with BAVdisease [11].

1.1. Embryology and pathogenesis

The definitive fetal cardiac structure is evident from the second week of gestation, whereas separation of the heart into four chambers is completed during the sixth and seventh weeks of gestation resulting in separated systemic and pulmonary circulation[12]. The process of aortic valve morphogenesis begins from the cardiac cushions located in the ventricular outflow tract of the primary heart tube. In the outflow tract, the truncal cushion swellings contribute to form three leaflet valves of the aorta and pulmonary artery.The initial endocardial cushions, which will contribute to all four cardiac valves, are formed by the thickening of the extracellular matrix in the region of the atrioventricular and outflow tract.This process is initiated by the secretion of extracellular matrix proteins such as fibronectin and transferrin across the cardiac jelly to the adjacent endocardium. The endocardium then secretes transforming growth factor beta family members, which act synergistically with bone morphogenetic protein-2 secreted by the myocardium, to increase mesenchyme formation and proliferation, which results in the growth of the endothelial cushions. The myocardial cells then invade the margins of the cellular endothelial cushions [13].

The semilunar valves form the division of the truncus arteriosus into two separate channels which form the aortic and pulmonary trunks..The channels are created by the fusion of two truncal ridges across the lumen. In each channel a third swelling occurs opposite the first two which will form the 3rd leaflet. In the normal aortic valve the left and right leaflets of the adult valve are formed from the respective swellings while the posterior leaflet is formed from a swelling in the aortic trunk.

The pathogenesis of BAV is not yet fully understood. There is certainly a genetic component, especially given the association of BAV with other congenital abnormalities. However, fusion of the right and left valve cushions at the beginning ofvalvulogenesis appears to be a key factor in BAV formation [14].

A previous study suggested that BAV is a consequence of the anomalous behavior of cells derived from the neural crest because BAV often is associated with congenital aortic arch malformations and other neural crest-derived systems [15]. Other studies suggest that extracellular matrix proteins may affect the initiation of cell differentiation during valvulogenesis, while a molecular abnormality in this process may lead to the formation of abnormal cusps [16,17]. Some researchers suggest that a molecular abnormality in the extracellular matrix may lead to abnormal valvulogenesis, becouse matrix proteins help direct cell differentiation and cusp formation during valvulogenesis [16-18]. This could also explain why BAVis often linked to other cardiovascular anomalies.

These abnormalities cause the fusion of two cusps and lead to one larger cusp; therefore, the BAV usually includes two unequally sized cusps, the presence of a central raphe, and smooth cusp margin. A previous studies showed that raphal position was between the right and left cusp in 86% of cases [19]. An anomalous origin of coronary arteries depends on the

http://dx.doi.org/10.5772/52567

spatial orientation of the two cusps. When the orientation of the cusps is anteroposterior, the coronary arteries originate from the anterior sinus or if cusps laterlateral oriented the right coronary artery originate from the common trunk and right Valsava's sinus [20].

A recent study has demonstrated that BAVs with fused right and noncoronary leaflets and those with fused right and left leaflets are different etiological entities. BAVs with fused right and noncoronary leaflets result from a morphogenetic defect that occurs before cardiac outflow tract septation on the basis of an exacerbated nitric oxide-dependent epithelialto-mesenchymal transformation. On the other hand, BAVs with fused right and left leaflets result from anomalous septation of the proximal portion of the cardiac outflow tract, caused by dysfunctional neural crest cells [21].

The pulmonary valve can also be bicuspid, although this is much rarer and is most commonly associated with congenital heart disease such as Tetralogy of Fallot. There have been less than 10 cases reported in the literature of an isolated bicuspid pulmonary valve [22].

Deficient fibrillin-1 content in the vasculature of BAV patients may trigger matrix metalloproteinase production, thereby leading to matrix disruption and dilation. It has been noted that the fibrillin-1 content was remarkably reduced in the aorta of BAV patients, compared with that of patients with a tricuspid aortic valve. Aortic elasticity measurements of BAV patients suggest that diminished aortic elasticity is at least part of its causation [23-25].

1.2. Anatomy

The bicuspid valve is composed of two leaflets, of which one is usually larger (due to fusion of two cusps leading to one larger cusp), and unequal cusp size the presence of a central raphe (usually in the center of the larger of the two cusps). The raphe or fibrous ridge is the site of congenital fusion of the two components of the conjoined cusps and does not contain valve tissue (Figure 1) Three morphologies are identified: type 1, fusion of right coronary cusp and left coronary cusp; type 2, fusion of right coronary cusp and noncoronary cusp; and type 3, fusion of left coronary cusp and noncoronary cusp. The most common is type 1 (70% to 85%), followed by type 2 (10% to 30%) and most rare type 3 (1%) [13,19,26] (Figure 2).

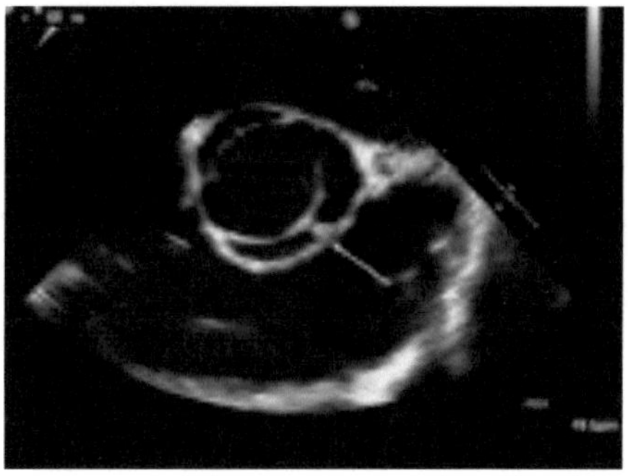

Figure 1. Transesophageal short-axis view of a BAV. There is fusion of the right and left cusps. The arrow points to the raphe.

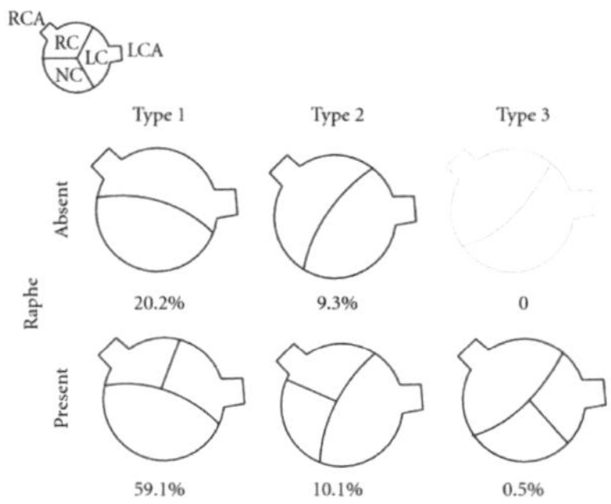

Figure 2. The classification and incidence of BAVs.

The site of cusp fusion can have e ▪ ects on the prognosis of BAV [27], with the suggestion that type 1 BAVs are more likely to stenose as adults while type 2 valves will have complications at a younger age. The fused valve leaflet in BAV is actually smaller in area. Valvular incompetence is usually caused by the redundancy of one cusp, since the two cusps usually have different dimensions [28]

The coronary anatomy can be abnormal. Most patients with BAV disease have a left dominant coronary circulation [29]. This left coronary can arise from the pulmonary artery. The left main can also be up to 50% shorter than in normal in up to 90% of cases. This is an important consideration for any aortic valve surgery. The commonest abnormality associated with BAV is dilatation of the thoracic aorta, also known as aortopathy. This is thought not only to be due to the altered flow in the aorta, but also due to cellular structural abnormalities including decreased fibrillin, causing smooth muscle cell detachment, and cell death [30].

The other abnormality found in conjunction with BAV disease is coarctation of the aorta. [22,31]. The presence of coarctation and a poor result from repair can lead to more rapid failure of the valve or aortic dissection.

1.3. Genetics

BAV is an inheritable disorder, with a family recurrence rate of approximately 35% [33]. Recent clinical studies have reported a 9% prevalence of BAV in first-degree relatives of patients with BAV which was the estimated population prevalance of 1-2% [33-35].

BAV is likely due to mutations in different genes with dissimilar patterns of inheritance [33].

The first genetic cause of BAV is Anderson syndrome, which is reported to be a result of mutations in the potassium channel gene KCNJ2 (chromosome 17q24.3)], whereas it clinically presents as ventricular arrhythmias, periodic paralysis, and scoliosis [36]. Another mutations in a gene called NOTCH1(gene map locus 9q34.3), a transmembrane receptor that has a role in determining cell outcome in organogenesis, were noted in two families with BAV [37]. Regions 18q, 5q, and 13q are reported to contain genes responsible for BAV and/or associated cardiovascular malformations [38,39]. The region 10q contains the ACTA2 gene, which encodes for smooth muscle alpha-actin (ACTA2), and mutation in this gene can result in thoracic aneurysm and, in some instances, BAV [40]. Also the ubiquitin fusion degradation 1–like gene UFD1L (chromosome 22q11.2) expressed in the outflow tract during embryogenesis is down-regulated in BAV tissue when compared with trileaflet valve tissue [41]. The UFD1L gene encodesa component of a multi-enzyme complex involved in the degradation of ubiquitin fusion proteins, and is highly expressed during embryogenesis in certain tissues. It seems to play a key role in the development of ectoderm-derived structures, including neural crest cells.Downregulation of the UFD1L gene, hypothetically resulting from an anomalous behavior of neural crest cells, may lead to reduced degradation activities, and may finally lead to fusion of valve cushions, a key factor in the development of congenital BAV[42]. Recent American College of Cardiology (ACC)/American Heart Association (AHA) adult congenital heart disease guidelines suggest echocardiographic screening for BAV and aortopathy in first-degree relatives of patients with BAV [43,44].

Although these valves are more common in males than females by a factor of 2:1 in the general population, the prevalance was equal in males and females in families having more than one affected individual [45,46].

2. Diagnosis

Clinical findings are usually limited to auscultation with most patients having an ejection systolic murmur heard loudest at the apex [47]. The S1 usually is normal but sometimes may be associated with ejection click. The S2 is soft, and when aortic stenosis is present, S2 occurs simultaneously with P2. In aortic stenosis, an ejection systolic murmur is heard in the left second intercostal space but may also be transmitted to the carotid arteries. If aortic incompetence is present, a diastolic murmur of aortic regurgitation may be heard.

The electrocardiogram is usually normal; and ECG changes are not specific in patients with BAV: left ventricular hypertrophy, atrial enlargement, and arrhythmias may be present.

The mainstay of diagnosis is echocardiography (transthoracic or transoesophageal) which can provide a definitive diagnosis in the majority of patients [92% sensitivity and 96% specificity) [48,49]. Transesophageal echocardiography (TEE) is also very important for evaluating the aortic valve and thoracic aorta, whereas the sensitivity and specifity of multiplane technique for assessing aortic valve morphology is high [13].

The parasternal short axis view allows for direct visualization of the valve cusps. In this view the normal triangular opening shape is lost, becoming more "fish mouth-"like in appearance, more similar to the mitral valve. This is especially pronounced in systole, as in diastole the raphe can appear similar to a commissure of the third cusp. Differentiating severe bicuspid aortic stenosis from severe other aortic stenosis can also be difficult. In order to establish the diagnosis, the valve must be visualized in systole in the short-axis view. In the long-axis view, the valve often has an eccentric closure line and there is doming of the leaflets. If there is uncertainty in diagnosis, a TEE can improve visualization of the leaflets [50].

For BAV associated with stenosis, mean gradient and maximal flow velocity should be measured, but when regurgitation is present, the effective regurgitant area and Doppler jet size should be evaluated. For asymptomatic patients with aortic stenosis, echocardiography is recommended for evaluating disease progression. In asymptomatic patients, TTE recommended: every year for severe aortic stenosis, ever 1-2 years for moderate aortic stenosis and every 3-5 years for mild aortic stenosis [51].

In patients with poor acustic window, cardiac magnetic resonance (MRI) and multidetector computed tomography are useful for measuring the aortic valve area and is an alternative method to echocardiography in selected cases. MRI especially will enable views of the valve to be obtained without interference from calcification. It also allows for excellent assessment of the aorta. A recent study of 123 patients with confirmed BAV found that 10% of the patients were misidentified as having a tricuspid valve using transthoracic echo and 28% had a nondiagnostic study, in comparison to 4% being misidentified as having a tricuspid valve by MRI and 2% having a non-diagnostic study [52].

The current guidelines suggest that cardiac magnetic resonance imaging or cardiac computed tomography is reasonable in patients with BAVs when aortic root dilatation is detected by echocardiography to further quantify severity of dilatation and involvement of theascending aorta (Clas IIa; Level of Evidence: B)[53].

3. Clinic

The clinical presentation of patients with BAV can vary from severe valve disease in infancy to asymptomatic valve disease in old age. It may be associated with abnormalities of the aortic wall such as coarctation of the aorta, aortic dissection, and aortic aneurysm. Most patients with a BAV develop some complications during life [1,2].

Congenital coronary anomalies, coronary atherosclerosis, and calcification have been described in association with BAV[3].

The congenitally BAV may function normally throughout life, may develop progressive calcification and stenosis or may develop regurgitation with or without infection. Aortic root dilatation is common in BAV, even when the valve is haemodynamically normal, and consequently aortic dissection usually occurs in previously asymptomatic patients [4,5].

Sudden death may occur as a result of obstruction of the left ventricular outflow tract by a congenital BAV [54]. BAV are in most cases remain undetected until infection or calcification supervenes [55].

Aortic stenosis and regurgitation, infective endocarditis and aortic dissection are the most common complications. Left coronary artery dominance is more common in patients with a BAV (29-56.8%) and in 90% of cases, the left main coronary artery is less than 5 mm in length [7,8]. The ignorance of these associations may cause an inadequate myocardial preservation and an increased risk of myocardial infarction[9,10].

Symptoms associated with aortic stenosis are angina pectoris, syncope, and congestive heart failure. The most common complication of aortic stenosis is congestive heart failure symptomatically presented with dyspnea, which is a result of combined diastolic and systolic dysfunction [56]. Angina pectoris occurs in patients with severe aortic stenosis and in those who do not have coronary artery disease; it may be a result of ventricular hypertrophy.

Syncope is another common symptom in patients with BAV. Syncope reflects the cerebral hypoperfusion caused by the inability to increase stroke volume during physical activity.

The clinical presentation in patients with BAV and presence of other cardiac congenital defects depends from structural complexity of the heart. In patients with interventricular septal defects, the clinical presentation depends on the size of the defect area and the grade of aortic stenosis. If the interventricular defect is small, the patient may be asymptomatic, but when the interventricular defect is large, cardiac output will decrease and Eisenmenger syndrome will develop.

Two large recent series reported that clinical course of unoperated patients with BAV depends on age, stenosis, and aortic incompetence. The severe aortic stenosis, and severe aortic incompetence in older patients increases the risk of primary cardiac events including cardiac death. Both these studies suggest that intervention on the basis of early symptoms or incipient cardiac dysfunction may decreases the mortality of patients with BAV [57,58].

The natural history of BAV has been evaluated several cohort studies. It is known to be variable and of course somewhat dependent on associated abnormalities. It can range from severe aortic stenosis in childhood to asymptomatic disease until old age. There have indeed been incidental findings of a minimally calcified BAV in patients in their 70s.More commonly however [in around 75% of patients] there is progressive fibrocalcific stenosis of the valve eventually requiring surgery. This usually leads to presentation in middle age only around 2% of children have clinically significant BAV disease [59].

The prevalence of fibrosis, cystic medial necrosis, elastic fragmentation, and inflammation has been shown to be significantly higher in patients with fusion of the left coronary and right coronary cusps. fusion of the left coronary and right coronary cusps was associated with a larger aortic root diameter and a smaller aortic arch,than was fusion of the right coronary and non-coronary cusps. Another study demonstraed that fusion of the right coronary and non-coronary cusps correlated with the more rapid growth of ascending aortic diameter in the pediatric population [60-63].

There have been a couple of studies looking at long-term followup of patients with unoperated BAV. A cohort of 212 asymptomatic patients with BAV were found to have the same 20-year survival rate as the normal population but an increased frequency of cardiac events including aortic valve surgery, ascending aorta surgery and any other cardiovascular surgery. Predictive factors for cardiovascular events were found to be age ≥50 years and valve degeneration at diagnosis while baseline ascending aorta ≥40 mm independently predicted surgery for aorta dilatation. Another study [64] 642 patients were followed up for a mean of 9 years, again with a 10-year survival rate similar to the normal population [96%]. One or more primary cardiac events occurred in 25% including cardiac death in 3, intervention on aortic valve or ascending aorta in 22%, aortic dissection or aneurysm in 2%, and congestive heart failure requiring hospital admission in 2%. Independent predictors of primary cardiac events were age older than 30 years, moderate or severe aortic stenosis, and moderate or severe aortic regurgitation [50].

In the another study [61].the incidence of aortic dissection was found to be 1.5% in all patients regardless of the progression of BAV; however this increased markedly in patients aged 50 or older at baseline to 17.4% and even more in those found to have aneurysm formation at baseline to [44.9%]. 25-year rate for aortic surgery was 25% and there was a significant burden of progression of disease to cause aortic dissection with 49 of the 384 patients without baseline aneurysms developing them during followup [22].

Although the clinical presentation of patients with BAV can vary from severe valve disease in infancy to asymptomatic valve or thoracic aortic disease in old age, symptomstypically develop in adulthood. The clinical manifestations relate to the function of the aortic valve,the aortopathy/dissection, and acquired complications such as endocarditis. However in childhood, BAV disease is commonly asymptomatic [61]

Estimates of late cardiac events were approximately 25% at a mean age of 44 years in the study from Toronto and 40% at a mean age of 52 years in the Olmsted County study [62,63]. In the Olmsted County series, 27% of adults with BAV and no significant valve disease at baseline required cardiovascular surgery within 20 years of follow-up. Twenty-two percent of the patients in the Toronto cohort required intervention within 9 years of follow-up. In both studies, age was an important determinant of outcomes supporting the notion held by many that eventually most patients with BAV would require some form of intervention.

3.1. Aortic stenosis

A common complication of BAV disease is aortic stenosis. BAV is recognized as a frequent cause of aortic stenosis in adults. Aortic stenosis has been found in 72% of adults with BAV. In 388 patients with severe aortic valve disease alone, BAVs were found in 45% of the patients with aortic stenosis and 24% of the patients with aortic regurgitation. In 110 patients with severe combined aortic and mitral valve disease, BAVs were found in only 12% [64].

Among the 600 patients analyzed, 213 (36%) had pure aortic stenosis, 265 (44%) had pure aortic regurgitation and 122 (20%) had combined stenosis and regurgitation. BAVs represented 18%, as the third most important cause of aortic disorder following degenerative and rheumatic changes, followed by infective endocarditis (5%) [65].

The main symptoms are exertional dyspnea, syncope, and chest pain. These patients should be evaluated and managed similarly to patients with tricuspid aortic valve stenosis.

In the Joint Study of the Natural History of Congenital Heart Defects, one-third of the children in the cohort had increases in catheterization gradients during the 4- to 8-year follow-up period. In the follow-up study, children with baseline peak left ventricular to aortic gradients >50 mm Hg were at risk for serious cardiac events at a rate of 1.2% per year. In theUnited Kingdom cohort.20% of children with mild aortic stenosis at baselinehad mild disease after 30 years of follow-up. Age was the primary determinant of valvular disease progression [50,66].

In adults, with BAV, stenosis occurs by similar methods to the process in patients with tricuspid aortic valves. It is felt to be due to calcification, endothelial dysfunction, inflammation, lipoprotein deposition, and ossification of the aortic side of the valve leaflets. There has been a suggestion that leaflet orientation may be a predictive factor in the rate of valve stenosis. The folding and creasing of the valves and the turbulent flow are felt to contribute to development of fibrosis and calcification [59].more rapid progression in aortic valve gradients occurred in patients with anteroposteriorly located cusps[60]. However, not all studies have found this association, and the 2 large studies in adults have not identified leaflet orientation as a risk factor for late adverse events. Olmsted County study identified a composite index of valve degeneration, which incorporated valve thickening, calcification, and mobility, that was an independent predictor of long-term cardiac events in a population of adults with no baseline valve dysfunction. The predictive role of both morphology and function in adults with BAV parallels that observed in series examining older adults with aortic stenosis mostly of acquired basis [50,62,63].

3.2. Aortic incompetence

Primary aortic regurgitation without infective endocarditis was uncommon, and 32% had an apparently normally functioning aortic valve [67].

One cohort of 118 BAV patients found that of 70 patients without aortic stenosis, 28 (40% had moderate to severe aortic regurgitation. The mechanisms of aortic incompetence in children are usually due to prolapsing cusps, myxoid degeneration, postvalve surgery and after balloon valvuloplasty or endocarditis, while as the patients age dilatation of the ascending aorta can lead to a functionally regurgitant valve[68,69]. With age, aortic incompetence may also develop secondary to dilation of the ascending aorta. In the Olmstead study of asymptomatic adults, 47% had some degree of aortic incompetence at baseline; however, interventions for severe aortic incompetence were relatively uncommon, occurring in only 3% of the cohort during follow-up. In the Toronto study 21% of the population had moderate or severe aortic incompetence at baseline; however, only 6% had an intervention for symptomatic aortic incompetence or progressive left ventricular dysfunction [62,63].

3.3. Aortopathy/aortic dissection

BAV patients tend to develop vascular abnormalities of the aorta, such as dilation, coarctation and dissection. Aortic dilation in BAV patients is thought to be caused by intrinsic aortic disease that is characterized by cystic medial necrosis and disruption of the extracellular matrix due to fibrillin deficiency. BAV is often associated with dilatation of the aortic root and the ascending aorta. This is otherwise known as aortopathy. This can lead to aneurysm and dissection. The dilatation has been reported during childhood, and it has also been suggested that increased aortic size at baseline is predictive for earlier dilatation and worse outcomes. Aortic size is larger generally in patients with BAV compared to those with normal valves. The most likely risk factor for progression is felt to be age. Aortic root size itself is related to valve morphology and the presence of significant disease [22,6]; however, a recent study did suggest that while most patients with BAV and ascending aortic aneurysm had severe valve dysfunction, there was a small proportion of patients (5%) who did have aneurysm formation without any aortic valve dysfunction [50].

In the ascending aorta as well as the pulmonary trunk, the severity of cystic medial necrosis, elastic fragmentation and changes in the smooth muscle cell orientation have been found to be significantly more severe in patients with bicuspid valves than in those with tricuspid valves.

Factors leading to aortic dissection four years after the Bentall operation have been considered to be an impact of congenital BAV or proximal anastomosis of venous grafts, or both [70].

Studies have suggested that patients with BAV have an intrinsic defect in the aortic wall that results in aortic disease, regardless of aortic valve function. BAV was associated with significantly less intimal change, and less fragmentation and loss of elastic tissue, compared with patients with a tricuspid aortic valve. Type I and III collagens were significantly decreased in dilated aortas of BAV patients, compared with controls, particularly at the convexity. Expression of messenger RNA [ribonucleic acid] for collagens was lower than normal only in the regurgitant subgroup. Fewer smooth muscle cells and greater severity of elastic fiber fragmentation were observed at the convexity than at the concavity [71-73].

Among 119 cases of fatal dissecting aneurysm of the aorta, 11 cases of congenital BAV (9%) were observed. Among the latter, three had coarctation of the aorta and one had Turner's syndrome without coarctation. In each case, cystic medial necrosis of the aorta was present. Hypertension was either established or inferred from cardiac weight in 73% of the cases. The high incidence among subjects with dissecting aneurysm suggested a causative relationship between BAV and aortic dissecting aneurysm [74].

Many theories have been postulated for the mechanism of BAV aortopathy. For a long time there has been felt to be a genetic component; however there is increasing evidence for a haemodynamic mechanism. It is felt that it is due to defects in the aortic media, such as elastin fragmentation, loss of smooth muscle cells, and an increase in collagen [6,22]. Systemic features have also been noted in BAV patients which may predispose to aneurysm formation including systemic endothelial dysfunction and higher plasma levels of matrix metalloproteinases [75].

Pathological examination of surgical specimens from the aortic wall of patients with aortic dissection associated with BAV showed cystic medial necrosis or mucoid degeneration [76].

Matrix metalloproteinases (endogenous enzymes that degrade matrix components) have been implicated in atherosclerotic aortic aneurysm formation and appear to be elevated in the aorta of patients with BAVs [77].

The histological findings of BAV are nonspecific, and had been described by several authors in patients with Marfan syndrome [78-80]. The histopathological appearance of thoracic aortic aneurysm in Marfan and BAV is similar, and includes evidence of vascular smooth

http://dx.doi.org/10.5772/52567

muscle cell (VSMC) apoptosis and extracellular matrix degeneration in the absence of a significant inflammatory response [81].

Abnormalities in the ascending aorta of the patients with BAV, specifically premature medial layer VSMC apoptosis, have been described, explaining the higherthan-expected prevalance of aortic dissection in these patients [82].

Also recently studies show less elastic tissue in the aortas of BAV patients [83,84].

In patient with BAV there are fibrillin, fibronectin, and tenascin abnormality. Additionally Bonderman et al suggested that a primary role for VMSC apoptosis in the development of aneurysm these patients [85].

The FBN1 gene encodes fibrillin-1, a large glycoprotein that is secreted from cells and deposited in the extracellular matrix in structures called microfibrils. Microfibrils are found at the periphery of elastic fibers, including the elastic fibers in the medial layer of the ascending aorta, and in tissues not associated with elastic fibers.

The histopathological appearance of thoracic aortic aneurysm in Marfan and BAV is similar, and includes evidence of VSMC apoptosis and extracellular matrix degeneration in the absence of a significant inflammatory response. Abnormalities in the ascending aorta of the patients with BAV, specifically premature medial layer smooth muscle cell apoptosis, have been described, explaining the higherthan-expected prevalance of aortic dissection in these patients [82,83].

Aortic root dilation has been documented in childhood, suggesting that this process begins early in life. Furthermore, children with BAV have greater increases in aortic dimensions than do children with trileaflet valves. In both children and adults, progressive dilation of the aorta is more common in patients with larger aortas at baseline. In BAV disease, the aortic annulus, sinus, and proximal ascending aorta are larger than those found in adults with trileaflet valves [50].

In the Olmsted County study, the prevalence of ascending aorta dilation (>40 mm) was 15% and in the subset of patients with repeat measurements, the prevalence increased to 39% at study completion. Dilation of the ascending aorta was an independent risk factor for ascending aorta surgery. Although there are a number of risk factors associated with dilation of the ascending aorta including increased systolic blood pressure, male sex, and significant valve disease, the most important variable is likely age [50,63,64]. Aortic root size is shown to be related to valve morphology and the presence of significant valve disease. In the Toronto series, the prevalence of dissection was 0.1% per patient-year of follow-up, and in the Olmsted County study, there were no cases of dissection. Despite the low rates of dissection, the increased-prevalence of BAV disease relative to Marfan syndrome make dissections due to BAV equal to or more common than dissections due to Marfan syndrome [86]. Dissection in BAV, when it occurs, typically involves the ascending aorta, but involvement of the descending aorta has been reported in older patients. Although dissection is more common in patients with dilated aortas, there are reports of dissection in normal-sized aortic roots and after valve replacement. Risk factors for dissection have included aortic size, aortic stiffness, male sex, family history, and the presence of other lesions such as coarctation of the aorta or Turner syndrome [50].

3.4. Endocarditis

Endocarditis is more common in BAV. The estimated incidence is 0.16% per year in unoperated children and adolescents [87]. In adults the case series by Michelena give an incidence of 2% per year [56].

Outcomes in BAV patients with infective endocarditis tend to be worse than in those with normal valves. A recent study of 310 patients with infective endocarditis found that the 50 patients with BAV were younger at presentation and had a higher incidence of aortic perivalvular abscess. In-hospital mortality and 5-year survival were also comparable to patients with normal valves [22].

Most patients are unaware of their condition until the onset of infective endocarditis

Patients with BAV endocarditis are young, and there is strong male predominance. Staphylococci and viridans streptococci account for nearly three-quarters of the cases affecting BAVs. Endocarditis can lead to severe acute aortic incompetence, heart failure and it is poorly tolerated [88].

Endocarditis risk was estimated to range between 2% or 0.3%/year. Because the risk of endocarditis is felt to be low, the ACC/AHA practice guidelines no longer suggest bacterial endocarditis prophylaxis in patients with straightforward BAV disease, except in patients with a prior history ofendocarditis [50,89].

3.5. Coronary artery disorders

Some reports have also suggested that the involvement of coronary arteries, including congenital coronary artery anomalies, coronary artery fistulas, spontaneous coronary artery dissection, immediate bifurcation and a shorter length of the left main coronary artery [6,13]. The incidence of left dominance in BAVs has been found to be unusually high (24.4-56.8%), compared with the incidence in tricuspid valves [9.5%]. Patients with BAVs have higher incidence of immediate bifurcation of the left main coronary artery, and higher incidence of left main coronary length less than 10 mm. The mean length of the left main coronary artery is significantly shorter in BAV patients [90].

Anomalous origins of the right 20,21 and left 22 coronary arteries, association with annuloaortic ectasia, and anomalous origins of the left circumflex coronary artery 23 and single left coronary artery,24 have been noted in patients with BAVs. Spontaneous coronary artery dissection may occur in BAV patients [91]

There have also been some case reports describing patients with BAVdisease associated with coronary heart disease [92] and even with acute myocardial infarction[10].

Also Recently studies[93]Yuan et al. suggested that the prevalence rate of angiographic coronary heart disease was higher among the patients with BAVdisease.

3.6. Congenıtal heart defects

Patent ductus arteriosus and ventricular septal defect are the most frequent congenital heart defects associated with BAV. Patent ductus arteriosus is usually present in pediatric patients with BAV and may be associated with hand anomalies. BAV is reported to be present in up to 30 % of adult patients with small ventricular septal defects. However, BAV may also be associated with large ventricular septal defects and poor clinical outcome. There is significantly higher incidence of aortic arch obstruction (51.1%). The frequency of BAV in specimens with complete transposition of great arteries has been found to be 1% [13,50].

Hypoplastic left heart syndrome, complete atrioventricular canal defect, Ebstein's anomaly, partial or total anomalous pulmonary venous return, tetralogy of Fallot, double-outlet right ventricle, septal left ventricular diverticulum,Williams syndrome,Down syndrome and annuloaortic ectasia are occasionally associated with BAV. Shone's complex, which is defined by four cardiovascular defects including supravalvular mitral membrane, valvular mitral stenosis with a parachute mitral valve, subaortic stenosis and aortic coarctation, is a rare entity and forms another association in BAV cases [94].

It has been reported that BAV is presented in > 50 % of patients with coarctation of the aorta [COA]. Patients with COA and BAV are reported to have more severe disease associated with aortic stenosis, aortic regurgitation, and aortic aneurysm. The risk of dissection of the aorta and death is greater when COA and BAV are comorbid.

Turner syndrome characterized by a defect in or the absence of one X chromosome. Except for gonadal dysgenesis, cardiovascular defects are commonly present in this group of patients. Clinical research on patients with Turner Syndrome reports that BAV is present in 30% of cases, that over 95% of BAV s result from fusion of the right and left coronary leaflets, and that aortic ascending diameters are significantly greater in this group of patients [13].

3.7. Thromboembolism

Thrombus formation in a native BAV is a rare complicaton. Pathological studies have indicated that post-inflammatory changes ocur in the resected BAV, which is prone to develop thrombosis on the valve surface or in the calcification area [95].

Microthrombus formation and valve thickening with incompetence could result in embolization, and subsequent cerebrovascular events [96].

Embolization from calcific BAVs may lead to stroke and myocardial infarction. Conservative management with anticoagulation, to treat associated post-stagnation thrombosis, or aortic valve replacement as the treatment, is debatable [97].

4. Management

4.1. Medical

Medical therapies are to try and alleviate symptoms and slow progression. It is generally felt that blood pressure should be aggressively controlled to try and slow the progression of aortopathy [51].

High blood pressure should be aggressively treated in patients with BAV disease. In Marfan-associated aortopathy, treatment with beta-blockers to slow the rate of progression is the standard of care at many centers, although debate exists about their effectiveness [50,101]. The ACC/AHA guidelines for the management of adult congenital heart disease and guidelines for the management of patients with valvular heart disease suggest that it is reasonable to use beta-blockers in this population [Class IIa recommendation] [53]. There are emerging data in animal models and in 1 small study in humans supporting the use of angiotensin II receptor blockers to decreased aortic root dilation in Marfan syndrome [50]. Whether these agents will have a role in BAV aortopathy has not yet been demonstrated. Also long-term vasodilator therapy in BAV disease with aortic regurgitation is only recommended if there is concomitant systemic hypertension [47]. The relationship between risk factors for atherosclerosis and the development and progression of degenerative aortic valve disease has been well studied [99]. However, the role of treatment with cholesterol-lowering agents is unresolved. The use of lipid lowering agents specifically in young patients with BAV has not been studied, and the current ACC/AHA guidelines for the management of patients with valvular heart disease do not endorse the use of statins to slow the degenerative process in this population [51]. Concomitant conditions and risk factors should be treated as in the normal population.

4.2. Surgical

Indications for valve surgery in patients with BAV are similar to those with tricuspid aortic valve disease or degenerative aortic valve disease [100].

The 2006 AHA/ACC guidelines also suggest concomitant replacement of the ascending aorta if it is greater than 45 mm in diameter [51]. Estimated 15-year freedom from complications was 86% in patients with an aortic diameter less than 40 mm, dropping down to 81% in those with diameter 40–44 and 43% in patients with a diameter 45 mm or greater.

When rheumatic disease is excluded, a significant portion of adults undergoing surgery for aortic valve disease will have a congenitally malformed valve. During childhood, insertion of a prosthetic valve is suboptimal because of the continuing growth of the child. Fortunately, at this stage, the aortic valve is usually not calcified and valvuloplasty can successfully disrupt the commissural fusion and relieve obstruction. Valvuloplasty is the interventional strategy of choice in children and in some young adults with BAV and aortic stenosis. Symptomatic aortic stenosis is an indication for intervention, similar to standard indications for trileaflet valve disease. However, in the pediatric setting, indications include children with peak-topeak gradients >50 mm Hg who develop symptom at rest or with exercise. An additional indication includes asymptomatic children with peak-to-peak gradients >60 mm Hg. In adulthood, aortic valve replacement is the most common intervention for either aortic valve stenosis or incompetence, and valvuloplasty is rarely performed [50,51,62].

BAV disease involves younger patients and involves both the valves and the ascendan aorta; therefore, surgical decision making is more complicated. Approximately 30% of adults undergoing aortic valve replacement will also need aortic root surgery[63]. The guideline suggest that a cutoff of 5.0 cm be used for intervention or 4.5 cm if the surgery is otherwise being performed for valve indications. In addition, suggest that changes in root size more than 0.5 cm/year are an indication for root replacement [53].

Recently published Guidelines [53] for the diagnosis and management of patients with thoracic aortic disease recommendations for BAV are summarized below:

CLASS I

1. First-degree relatives of patients with a BAV, premature onset of thoracic aortic disease with minimal risk factors, and/or a familial form of thoracic aortic aneurysm and dissection should be evaluated for the presence of a BAV and asymptomatic thoracic aortic disease. (Level of Evidence: C)

2. All patients with a BAV should have both the aortic root and ascending thoracic aorta evaluated for evidence of aortic dilatation (Level of Evidence: B)

3. Should undergo elective operation at smaller diameters (4.0 to 5.0 cm)to avoid acute dissection or rupture. ()Level of Evidence: C)

4. Patients with a growth rate of more than 0.5 cm/year in an aorta that is less than 5.5 cm in diameter should be considered for operation. (Level of Evidence: C)

5. Patients undergoing aortic valve repair or replacement and who have an ascending aorta or aortic root of greater than 4.5 cm should be considered for concomitant repair of the aortic root or replacement of the ascending aorta. (Level of Evidence: C)

6. Elective aortic replacement is reasonable for patients with BAV when the ratio of maximal ascending or aortic root area ($\pi r2$) in cm2 divided by the patient's height in meters exceeds 10 (CLASS IIa, Level of Evidence: C).

In regard to valve surgery, there is controversy regarding the use of the Ross procedure and the use of valve repairs in this population. Abnormalities of the media are seen in both the aorta and the pulmonary artery in BAV disease. Intrinsic abnormalities in the wall of the pulmonary artery [neoaorta] may contribute to progressive neoaortic root dilation and/or aortic regurgitation when the pulmonary root is placed in the systemic position [101].

When to surgically treat asymptomatic patients with BAV remains controversial. The risk of sudden death in asymptomatic adult patients with severe aortic stenosis is reported to be less than 1% per year, however, current practice guidelines recommended aortic valve replacement in patients with reduced left ventricular systolic function (EF < 50%) without oth er explanation even when they are asymptomatic [51].

For high-risk patients to undergo conventional novel methods including aortic balloon valvulotomy or transfemoral valve implantation may be helpful. A patient considered inoperable should be treated orally with angiotensin converting enzyme (ACE) inhibitors, diuretics, and digitalis. In patients with depressed LV associated with pulmonary congestion and atrial fibrillation, diuretics and digitalis may be used with the understanding that in some cases intensive hemodynamic monitoring is needed. Patients with aortic root dilatation > 4.0cm who are not candidate for surgical treatment should be given β-adrenergic blocking agents [51].

4.3. Pregnancy

During pregnancy there are changes in hemodynamics as well as changes in the aortic media, and therefore, women with BAV and significant aortic stenosis and/or dilated aortic roots are at risk for complications during pregnancy.

In rare instances, women will develop progressive symptoms during pregnancy and require either valvuloplasty or valve surgery. Both interventions can be performed during pregnancy, but are associated with both maternal and fetal risks and should be performed only when necessary.

Although pregnancy can be successfully completed in most instances, aortic surgery may be required early after pregnancy in some women with severe aortic stenosis. Pregnancy itself seems to accelerate the need for surgery postpartum in women with moderate or severe aortic stenosis, perhaps by affecting the ability of the left ventricle to adapt to the fixed outflow obstruction. It is therefore important that women be counseled about both the risk of pregnancy and the potential for late complications [102,103].

Additionally, guidelines suggest that women with BAV and significant aortopathy (ascending aorta diameter >4.5 cm)"should be counseled against the high risk of pregnancy" [43].

4.4. Exercise

There are little data available to support recommendations regarding exercise in subjects with BAV. In children with congenital severe aortic stenosis, for instance, sudden death can occur during exercise [121]. The Task Force on Exercise in Patients with Heart Disease recommends that athletes with severe aortic stenosis or severe aortic incompetence with left ventricular dilation [left ventricular dimensions >65 mm] should not participate in competitive athletics. Athletes with or without aortic valve disease who have dilated aortic roots (>45 mm) are advised to only participate in low-intensity competitive sports. No restrictions exist for those with BAV with no significant valve dysfunction or aortic root/ascending aorta dilation(>40 mm) [50,104,105].

5. Conclusions

Consequently aortic stenosis and regurgitation, infective endocarditis and aortic dissection are the most common complications of BAV additionaly this process continues after valve replacement. The person with BAV requires continuous surveillance to treat associated lesions and prevent complications. Arterial hypertension should be meticulously controlled. Smoking should be discouraged and control of hypercholesterolaemia considered, in view of the impact of these factors on the development of aortic stenosis. Aortic root dilatation is common in BAV, even when the valve is haemodynamically normal, and consequently aortic dissection usually occurs in previously asymptomatic patients. Beta-blockers and statins are the possibilities for medical treatment, and aortic valve repair/replacement and ascending aorta replacement are indicated for patients with a severely diseased aortic valve and aorta. All patients should therefore be regularly reviewed to identify progressive root dilatation [6,94].

Author details

Mehmet Demir

Bursa Yüksek İhtisas Education and Research Hospital, Cardiology Department, Bursa, Turkey

References

[1] Braverman AC, Güven H, Beardslee MA, et al.The bicuspid aortic valve. Curr Probl Cardiol 2005;30:470-522.

[2] Yener N, Oktar GL, Erer D, et al. Bicuspid aortic valve. Ann Thorac Cardiovasc Surg. 2002 Oct;8[5]:264-7.

[3] Ward C. Clinical significance of the bicuspid aortic valve. Heart 2000; 83: 81–5.

[4] Tadros TM, Klein MD, Shapira OM. Ascending aortic dilatation associated with bicuspid aortic valve: pathophysiology, molecular biology, and clinical implications Circulation. 2009 17;119[6]:880-90.

[5] Pachulski RT, Weinberg AL, Chan KL. Aortic aneurysm in patients with functionally normal or minimally stenotic bicuspid aortic valve. Am J Cardiol 1991; 67:781–2.

[6] Demir M. Current Approach to Bicuspid Aortic Valve: Review. Global Advanced Research Journal of Medicine and Medical Sciences. 2012: 1[5]; 105-107.

[7] Hutchins GM, Nazarian IH, Bulkley BH. Association of left dominant coronary arterial system with congenital bicuspid aortic valve. Am J Cardiol 1978; 42: 57–9.

[8] Higgins CB, Wexler L. Reversal of dominance of the coronary arterial system in isolated aortic stenosis and bicuspid aortic valve. Circulation 1975; 52: 292 6.

[9] Presbitero P, Demarie D, Villani M, et al. Long term results [15-30 years] of surgical repair of aortic coarctation. Br Heart J 1987; 57: 462–7.

[10] Demir M. Acute myocardial infarction in a young patient with bicuspid aortic valve. Turk Kardiyol Dern Ars. 2009 Oct;37[7]:490-2.

[11] Suzuki T, Nagai R, Kurihara H, et al. Stenotic BAVassociated with a ventricular septal defect in an adult presenting with congestive heart failure: a rare observation. European Heart Journal. 1994;15:402-403.

[12] Rabkin-Aikawa E, Farber M, Aikawa M,et al. Dynamic and reversible changes of interstitial cell phenotype during remodeling of cardiac valves. The Journal of heart valve disease 2004; 13:841-847.

[13] Blerim Berisha, Xhevdet Krasniqi,Dardan Kocinaj, Ejup Pllana and Masar Gashi Bicuspid Aortic Valve.In: Ying-Fu Chen and Chwan-Yau Luo. (ed) Aortic valve. Rijeka: InTech; 2011.

[14] Sans-Coma V, Fernández B, Durán AC, et al. Fusion of valve cushions as a key factor in the formation of congenital bicuspid aortic valves in Syrian hamsters. Anat Rec. 1996;244[4]:490-8.

[15] Kappetein AP, Gittenberger-de Groot AC, Zwinderman AH, et al. The neural crest as a possible pathogenetic factor incoarctation of the aorta and bicuspid aortic valve. The Journal of Thoracic and Cardiovascular Surgery 1991; 102[6]:830-836.

[16] Eisenberg LM, Markwald RR. Molecular regulation of atrioventricular valvuloseptal morphogenesis. Circulation Research, 1995; 77[1]: 1-6.

[17] Fedak PW, Verma S, DavidTE,et al. Clinical and pathophysiological implications of a bicuspid aortic valve. Circulation 2002;106:900-4.

[18] Hinton RB, Jr, Lincoln J, Deutsch GH, et al. Extracellular matrix remodeling and organization in developing and diseased aortic valves. Circulation Research 2006; 98[11]:1431-1438.

[19] Sabet HY, Edwards WD, Tazelaar HD, et al. Congenitally bicuspid aortic valves: a surgical pathology study of 542 cases [1991 through 1996] and a literatüre review of 2715 additional cases. Mayo Clinic Proceedings 1996;74[1]:14–26.

[20] Schang SJ, Pepine CJ, Bemiller CR, et al. Anomalous coronary artery origin and bicuspid aortic valve. Vasc Surg 1975; 9: 67–72.

[21] Fernández B, Durán AC, Fernández-Gallego T, et al. Bicuspid aortic valves with different spatial orientations of the leaflets are distinct etiological entities. J Am Coll Cardiol.2009;54[24]:2312-8.

[22] Ify Mordi, Nikolaos Tzemos. BAVDisease: A Comprehensive Review. Cardiology Research and Practice 2012];

[23] Leme MP, David TE, Butany J, et al. Molecular evaluation of the great vessels of patients with BAVdisease. Rev Bras Cir Cardiovasc. 2003;18[2]:148-56.

[24] Sá MPL, Bastos ES, Murad H. Valva aórtica bicúspide: fundamentos teóricos e clínicos para substituição simultânea da aorta ascendente [Bicuspid aortic valve: theoretical and clinical aspects of concomitant ascending aorta replacement]. Rev Bras Cir Cardiovasc.2009;24[2]:218-24.

[25] Yap SC, Nemes A, Meijboom FJ, et al. Abnormal aortic elastic properties in adults with congenital valvular aortic stenosis. Int J Cardiol. 2008;128:336–41.

[26] Fernandes SM, Sanders SP, Khairy P, et al. Morphology of BAVin children and adolescent. Journal of the American College of Cardiology 2004;44[8]:1648-1651.

[27] T. J. Calloway, L. J. Martin, X. Zhang, et al. "Risk factors for aortic valve disease inbicuspid aortic valve: a family-based study," American Journal of Medical Genetics 2011;155[5]:1015–1020.

[28] De Mozzi P, Longo UG, Galanti G, et al. Bicuspid aortic valve: a literature review and its impact on sport activity. British Medical Bulletin 2008;85:63-85.

[29] W. C. Roberts. The congenitally bicuspid aortic valve. A study of 85 autopsy cases. The American Journal of Cardiology 1970;26[1]:72–83.

[30] E. S. Murphy, J Rosch, S. H. Rahimtoola. Frequency and significance of coronary arterial dominance in isolated aortic stenosis. American Journal of Cardiology 1977;39[4]: 505–509.

[31] B. Stewart, R. Ahmed, C. M. Travill,et al. Coarctation of the aorta life and health 20–44 yers after surgery repair. British Heart Journal 1993;69[1]:65–70.

[32] Larson EW, Edwards WD. Risk factors for aortic dissection: a necropsy study of 161 cases. Am J Cardiol 1984;53:849–55.

[33] Cripe L, Andelfinger G, Martin J, Shooner K, Benson DW. BAVis heritable. J Am Coll Cardiol 2004;44:138–43.

[34] Huntington K, Hunter AG, Chan KL. A prospective study to assess the frequency of familial clustering of congenital bicuspid aortic valve. J Am Coll Cardiol 1997;30:1809-12.

[35] Glick BN, Roberts WC. Congenitally BAVin multiple family members. Am J Cardiol 1994;73:400–4.

[36] Andelfinger G, Tapper AR, Welch RC, et al. KCNJ2 mutation results in Andersen syndrome with sex-specific cardiac and skeletal muscle phenotypes. American Journal of Human Genetics 2002;71[3]:663-668.

[37] Garg V, Muth AN, Ransom JF, et al. Mutations in NOTCH1 cause aortic valve disease. Nature 2005;437:270–4.

[38] Mohamed SA, Aherrahrou Z, Liptau H, et al. Novel missense mutations [p.T596M and p.P1797H] in NOTCH1 in patients with bicuspid aortic valve. Biochem Biophys Res Commun 2006;345:1460–5.

[39] Martin LJ, Ramachandran V, Cripe LH, et al. Evidence in favor of linkage to human chromosomal regions 18q, 5q and 13q for BAVand associated cardiovascular malformations. Hum Genet 2007;121:275–84.

[40] Guo DC, Pannu H, Tran-Fadulu V, et al. Mutations in smooth muscle alpha-actin [ACTA2] lead to thoracic aortic aneurysms and dissections. Nat Genet 2007;39:1488–93.

[41] Mohamed SA, Hanke T, Schlueter C, et al.Ubiquitin fusion degradation 1-like gene dysregulation in bicuspid aortic valve. The Journal of thoracic and cardiovascular surgery 2005;130:1531-36.

[42] Yamagishi C, Hierck BP, Gittenberger-De Groot AC, et al. Functional attenuation of UFD1l, a 22q11.2 deletion syndrome candidate gene, leads to cardiac outflow septation defects in chicken embryos. Pediatric Research 2003;53:546-553.

[43] Warnes CA, Williams RG, Bashore TM, et al. ACC/AHA 2008 guidelines for the management of adults with congenital heart disease: a report of the American College of Cardiology/American Heart Association Task Force on Practice Guidelines [Writing Committee to Develop Guidelines on the Management of Adults With Congenital Heart Disease]. J Am Coll Cardiol 2008;52:e1–121.

[44] Novaro GM, Griffin BP. Congenital BAVand rate of ascending aortic dilatation. Am J Cardiol 2004;93:525–6.

[45] Emanuel R, Withers R, O'Brien K, et al. Congenitally bicuspid aortic valves: clinicogenetic study of 41 families. Br Heart J 1978; 40: 1402-7.

[46] Clementi M, Notari L, Borghi A, et al. Familial congenital bicuspid aortic valve: a disorder of uncertain inheritance. Am J Med Genet 1996; 62: 336-8.

[47] P. Mills, G. Leech, M. Davies, et al. The natural history of a non-stenotic bicuspid aortic valve. British Heart Journal 1978;40:951-957.

[48] K. L. Chan, W. A. Stinson, J. P. Veinot. Reliability of transthoracic echocardiography in the assessment of aortic valve morphology: pathological correlation in 178 patients. Canadian Journal of Cardiology 1999;15:48-52.

[49] R. Tanaka, K. Yoshioka, H. Niinuma,et al. Diagnostic value of cardiac CT in the evaluation of bicuspid aortic stenosis: comparison with echocardiography and operative findings. American Journal of Roentgenology 2010;195:895-899.

[50] Samuel C. Siu, Candice K. Silversides.BAVDisease. J Am Coll. Cardiol 2010;55;2789-2800.

[51] Bonow RO, Carabello BA, Kanu C, et al. ACC/AHA 2006 guidelines for the management of patients with valvular heart disease: a report of the American College of Cardiology/American Heart Association Task Force on Practice Guidelines [Writing Committee to Revise the 1998 Guidelines for the Management of Patients With Valvular Heart Disease]. J Am Coll Cardiol 2006;48:e1–148.

[52] S. C. Malaisrie, J. Carr, I. Mikati et al. Cardiac magnetic resonance imaging is more diagnostic than 2-dimensional echocardiography in determining the presence of bicuspid aortic valve. The Journal of Thoracic and Cardiovascular Surgery.

[53] Hiratzka LF, Bakris GL, Beckman JA, et al. 2010 ACCF/AHA/AATS/ACR/ASA/SCA/SCAI/SIR/STS/SVM Guidelines for the diagnosis and management of patients with thoracic aortic disease. A Report of the American College of Cardiology Foundation/

American Heart Association Task Force on Practice Guidelines, American Association for Thoracic Surgery, American College of Radiology,American Stroke Association, Society of Cardiovascular Anesthesiologists, Society for Cardiovascular Angiography and Interventions, Society of Interventional Radiology, Society of Thoracic Surgeons,and Society for Vascular Medicine. J Am Coll Cardiol. 2010 6;55[14]:e27-e129

[54] Karayel F, Ozaslan A, Turan AA, et al. Sudden death in infancy due to bicuspid aortic valve. J Forensic Sci. 2006;51[5]:1147-50.

[55] Lamas CC, Eykyn SJ. Bicuspid aortic valve–A silent danger: analysis of 50 cases of infective endocarditis.Clin Infect Dis 2000; 30: 336–41.

[56] Michelena HI, Desjardins VA, Avierinos JF, et al. Natural history of asymptomatic patients with normally functioning or minimally dysfunctional BAVin the community. Circulation 2008; 117:2776-84.

[57] J. J. Fenoglio Jr, H. A. McAllister, C. M. DeCastro. Congenital BAVafter age 20. Am J Cardiol 1977;39:164–169.

[58] Schaefer BM, Lewin MB, Stout KK, et al. The bicuspid aortic valve: an integrated phenotypic classification of leaflet morphology and aortic root shape. Heart 2008;94:1634-1638.

[59] Hoffman JI. Congenital heart disease: incidence and inheritance. Pediatr Clin North Am 1990;37:25-43.

[60] H. I. Michelena, V. A. Desjardins, J. F. Avierinos et al. Natural history of asymptomatic patients with normally functioning or minimally dysfunctional BAVin the community. Circulation 2008;117:2776-2784.

[61] H. I. Michelina, A. D. Khanna, D. Mahoney et al. Incidence of aortic complications in patients with bicuspid aortic valves.The Journal of the American Medical Association. 2011;306:1104–1112.

[62] Tzemos N, Therrien J, Yip J, et al. Outcomes in adults with bicuspid aortic valves. JAMA 2008;300:1317–25.

[63] Michelena HI, Desjardins VA, Avierinos JF, et al. Natural history of asymptomatic patients with normally functioning or minimally dysfunctional BAVin the community. Circulation 2008;117:2776–84.

[64] Turina J, Turina M, Krayenbühl HP. [Significance of the BAVin the incidence of aortic valve defects in adults]. Schweiz Med Wochenschr. 1986;116[44]:1518-23.

[65] Matsumura T, Ohtaki E, Misu K, et al. Etiology of aortic valve disease and recent changes in Japan: a study of 600 valve replacement cases. Int J Cardiol. 2002;86[2-3]: 217-23.

[66] Wallby L, Janerot-Sjoberg B, Steffensen T, et al. T lymphocyte infiltration in non-rheumatic aortic stenosis: a comparative descriptive study between tricuspid and bicuspid aortic valves. Heart 2002;88:348–51.

[67] Fenoglio JJ Jr, McAllister HA Jr, DeCastro CM, et al. Congenital BAVafter age 20. Am J Cardiol. 1977;39[2]:164-9.

[68] Roman MJ, Devereux RB, Niles NW, et al. Aortic root dilatation as a cause of isolated, severe aortic regurgitation. Prevalence, clinical and echocardiographic patterns, and relation to left ventricular hypertrophy and function. Ann Intern Med 1987;106:800-7.

[69] Roberts WC, Morrow AG, McIntosh CL,et al. Congenitally BAVcausing severe, pure aortic regurgitation without superimposed infective endocarditis. Analysis of 13 patients requiring aortic valve replacement. Am J Cardiol 1981;47:206-9.

[70] Morishita A, Shimakura T, Nonoyama M, et al. Ascending aorta dissection associated with bicuspid aortic valve. Considerations 4 years after combined coronary artery bypass grafting and mitral valve replacement. Jpn J Thorac Cardiovasc Surg. 2001;49[6]:368-72.

[71] Hahn RT, Roman MJ, Mogtader AH, et al. Association of aortic dilation with regurgitant, stenotic and functionally normal bicuspid aortic valves. J Am Coll Cardiol. 1992;19[2]:283-8.

[72] Collins MJ, Dev V, Strauss BH, Fedak PW, Butany J. Variation in the histopathological features of patients with ascending aortic aneurysms: a study of 111 surgically excised cases. J Clin Pathol. 2008;61[4]:519-23.

[73] Cotrufo M, Della Corte A, De Santo LS, et al. Different patterns of extracellular matrix protein expression in the convexity and the concavity of the dilated aorta with bicuspid aortic valve:preliminary results. J Thorac Cardiovasc Surg. 2005;130:504-11.

[74] Edwards WD, Leaf DS, Edwards JE. Dissecting aortic aneurysm associated with congenital bicuspid aortic valve. Circulation. 1978;57[5]:1022-5.

[75] N. Tzemos, E. Lyseggen, C. Silversides et al. Endothelial function, carotid-femoral sti ▪ ness, and plasma matrix metalloproteinase-2 in men with BAVand dilated aorta," Journal of the American College of Cardiology 2010;55:660-668.

[76] Ando M, Okita Y, Matsukawa R, et al. Surgery for aortic dissection associated with congenital bicuspid aortic valve. Jpn J Thorac Cardiovasc Surg. 1998;46[11]:1069-73.

[77] Fedak PW, de Sá MP, Verma S, et al. Vascular matrix remodeling in patients with BAVmalformations: implications for aortic dilatation. J Thorac Cardiovasc Surg. 2003;126[3]:797-806.

[78] McKusick VA. Association of congenital BAVand erdheim's cystic medial necrosis. Lancet.1972;1[7758]:1026-7.

[79] Keane MG, Wiegers SE, Plappert T, Pochettino A, Bavaria JE, Sutton MG. Bicuspid aortic valves are associated with aortic dilatation out of proportion to coexistent valvular lesions.Circulation. 2000;102[19 Suppl 3]:III35-9.

[80] Sá M, Moshkovitz Y, Butany J, David TE. Histologic abnormalities of the ascending aorta and pulmonary trunk in patients with BAVdisease: clinical relevance to the Ross procedure. J Thorac Cardiovasc Surg.1999;118[4]:588-94.

[81] Schmid FX, Bielenberg K, Holmer S, et al. Structural and biomolecular changes in aorta and pulmonary trunk of patients with aortic aneurysm and valve disease: implications for the Ross procedure. Eur J Cardiothorac Surg. 2004;25[5]:748-53.

[82] Nistri S, Sorbo MD, Basso C, Thiene G. Bicuspid aortic valve: abnormal aortic elastic properties. J Heart Valve Dis. 2002 May;11[3]:369-73.

[83] Parai JL, Masters RG, Walley VM, Stinson WA, Veinot JP. Aortic medial changes associated with bicuspid aortic valve: myth or reality? Can J Cardiol 1999; 15:1233–8.

[84] De Backer JF, Devos D, Segers P, Matthys D, Francois K, Gillebert TC et al.Primary impairment of left ventricular function in Marfan syndrome. Int J Cardiol 2006;112:353–8.

[85] Bonderman D, Gharehbaghi-Schnell E, Wollenek G, et al. Mechanisms underlying aortic dilatation in congenital aortic valve malformation. Circulation.1999;99:2138 2143.

[86] Pape LA, Tsai TT, Isselbacher EM, et al., on behalf of International Registry of Acute Aortic Dissection [IRAD] Investigators. Aortic diameter >5.5 cm is not a good predictor of type A aortic dissection: observations from the International Registry of Acute Aortic Dissection [IRAD]. Circulation 2007;116:1120–7.

[87] W. M. Gersony, C. J. Hayes, D. J. Driscoll et al., "Bacterial endocarditis in patients with aortic stenosis, pulmonary stenosis, or ventricular septal defect," Circulation, vol. 87, no.2, pp. I121–I126, 1993.

[88] Lamas CC, Eykyn SJ. Bicuspid aortic valve--A silent danger: analysis of 50 cases of infective endocarditis. Clin Infect Dis. 2000;30[2]:336-41.

[89] Nishimura RA, Carabello BA, Faxon DP, et al. ACC/AHA 2008 guideline update on valvular heart disease: focused update on infective endocarditis: a report of the American College of Cardiology/American Heart Association Task Force on Practice Guidelines.J Am Coll Cardiol 2008;52:676–85.

[90] Johnson AD, Detwiler JH, Higgins CB. Left coronary artery anatomy in patients with bicuspid aortic valves. Br Heart J. 1978;40[5]:489-93.

[91] Labombarda F, Legallois D, Sabatier R. Spontaneous coronary artery dissection and bicuspid aortic valve. Arch Cardiovasc Dis. 2009;102[12]:857-8.

[92] Yokoyama S, Ashida T, SugiyamaT, et al. An autopsied case with a BAVwho had progressive angina pectoris and heart failure during follow-up of 27 years. Nippon Ronen Igakkai Zasshi 2002;39:444-447.

[93] Yuan SM, Jing H, Lavee J.The BAVand its relation to aortic dilation. Clinics [Sao Paulo] 2010;65:497-505.

[94] Shi-Min Yuan, Hua Jing. The BAVand related disorders. Sao Paulo Med J. 2010; 128[5]:296-301.

[95] Chuangsuwanich T, Warnnissorn M, Leksrisakul P, et al. Pathology and etiology of 110 consecutively removed aortic valves. J Med Assoc Thai. 2004;87[8]:921-34.

[96] Pleet AB, Massey EW, Vengrow ME. TIA, stroke, and the bicuspid aortic valve. Neurology.1981;31[12]:1540-2.

[97] Mahajan N, Khetarpal V, Afonso L. Stroke secondary to calcific bicuspid aortic valve: Case report and literature review. J Cardiol. 2009;54[1]:158-61.

[98] Shores J, Berger KR, Murphy EA, et al. Progression of aortic dilatation and the benefit of long-term beta-adrenergic blockade in Marfan's syndrome. N Engl J Med 1994;330:1335–41.

[99] Stewart BF, Siscovick D, Lind BK, et al. Clinical factors associated with calcific aortic valve disease. Cardiovascular Health Study. J Am Coll Cardiol 1997;29:630–4.

[100] H. M. Rosenfeld, M. J. Landzberg, S. B. Perry, et al. Balloon aortic valvuloplasty in the young adult with congenital aortic stenosis. Am J Cardiol 1994;73:1112-1117.

[101] David TE, Omran A, Ivanov J, et al. Dilation of the pulmonary autograft after the Ross procedure. J Thorac Cardiovasc Surg 2000;119:210–20.

[102] Silversides CK, Colman JM, Sermer M, et al.Early and intermediate-term outcomes of pregnancy with congenital aortic stenosis. Am J Cardiol 2003;91:1386-9.

[103] Tzemos N, Silversides CK, Colman JM, et al. Late cardiac outcomes after pregnancy in women with congenital aortic stenosis. Am Heart J 2009;157:474–80.

[104] Lambert EC, Menon VA, Wagner HR, Vlad P. Sudden unexpected death from cardiovascular disease in children. A cooperative international study. Am J Cardiol 1974;34:89-96.

[105] Graham TP Jr, Driscoll DJ, Gersony WM, et al.Task Force 2: congenital heart disease. J Am Coll Cardiol 2005;45:1326-33.

Section 6

Current Treatment Approaches

Chapter 12

Surgical Valve Replacement (Bioprosthetic vs. Mechanical)

Stamenko Šušak, Lazar Velicki, Dušan Popović and Ivana Burazor

Additional information is available at the end of the chapter

http://dx.doi.org/10.5772/53687

1. Introduction

The aortic valve separates the left ventricular outflow tract from the aorta. It is a tricuspid valve consisting of three semilunar cusps and the aortic valve annulus. The aortic valve annulus is a collagenous structure lying at the level of the junction of the aortic valve and the ventricular septum, which is the nadir of the aortic valve complex. This area is also referred to as the aortic ring and serves to provide structural support to the aortic valve complex. The annulus is shaped like a crown and extends to the level of the aortic sinuses. It attaches to the aortic media distally and the membranous and muscular ventricular septum proximally and anteriorly. There are 3 aortic valve cusps, each half-moon shaped or semilunar in appearance. A small dilatation of the proximal aorta is associated with each cusp; collectively, these are referred to as the sinuses of Valsalva or aortic sinuses, named after the Italian anatomist Antonio Valsalva. Their association with the respective coronary ostia identifies them: left, right, and posterior (or noncoronary).[1]

Aortic stenosis (AS) is one of the most common diseases of the aortic valve. The most common causes of AS are degenerative calcification, bicuspid aortic valve and rheumatic etiology. Age – related degenerative calcific AS is currently the most common cause of AS in adults and most frequent reason for aortic valve replacement (AVR).[2] That atherosclerosis is a cause of AS is derived primarily from five pieces of evidence: 1) that patients with familial homozygous hyperlipidemia usually develop calcific deposits on the aortic aspects of their aortic valve cusps at a very young age, usually by the teenage years (These individuals have serum total cholesterol levels >800 mg/dl from the time of birth.); 2) that progression of AS can be slowed by lowering total and low-density lipoprotein cholesterol levels by statins; 3) that patients >65 years of age with AS involving a three-cuspid aortic valve (unassociated with mitral valve disease) usually have extensive atherosclerosis involving the major epicardial coronary arteries and usually other systemic arterial systems; 4) that serum total cholesterol levels and concomitant coronary bypass grafting tend to be higher in patients with AS involving three-cuspid aortic valves than in patients of similar age and sex without AS or with congenitally bicuspid aortic valves; and 5) that histologic study of three-cuspid stenotic aortic valve demonstrates features similar to those in atherosclerotic plaques.[2] Rare causes of aortic stenosis include obstructive, infective endocarditis, Paget's disease, renal failure, drug induced, familial hypercholesterolemia, systemic lupus erythematosus, irradiation, and ochronosis.[3] As the valves stenosis, valvular abnormality produces turbulent flow, which traumatizes the leaflets and eventually leads to progressive cell proliferation, extracellular matrix production, and calcification of the valve. It is degenerative process that leads to proliferative and inflammatory changes that leading to calcification of the aortic valve. Progressive calcification leads to immobilization of the cusps.[3]

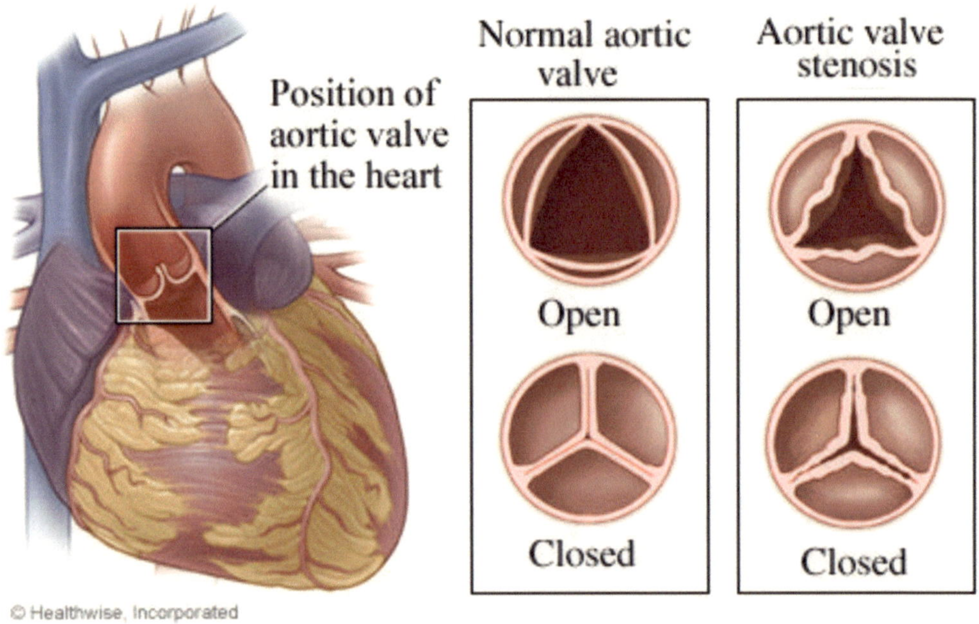

Figure 1. Normal aortic valve and stenotic aortic valve

The pathophysiology of valvular aortic stenosis is one of progressive obstruction and the resultant compensatory changes. With increasing left ventricular outflow tract obstruction, there is pressure hypertrophy of the left ventricle. Left ventricular cavity size and systolic function is initially maintained, as the increase in left ventricular wall thickness acts as a compensatory mechanism to normalize wall stress. The development of pressure hypertrophy is initially a beneficial adaptation. However, this hypertrophy may result in reduced coronary flow reserve and oxygen supply–demand mismatch. These hypertrophied hearts are also more sensitive to diffuse subendocardial ischemic injury, which may result in both systolic and diastolic dysfunction. As the obstruction progresses to a critical level, the high afterload "overwhelms" the left ventricle and systolic function begins to decrease. With continued severe afterload excess, myocyte degeneration and fibrosis occurs and produces irreversible left ventricular systolic dysfunction. In these patients, both the high afterload and the intrinsic myocardial disease significantly increase wall stress and a vicious cycle of deterioration in ventricular function ensues.[3]

The evaluation of aortic stenosis is based upon the history, the physical examination, and a comprehensive echocardiography. For most patients, two-dimensional echocardiography readily identifies the calcified stenotic aortic valve, and Doppler echocardiography reliably estimates the severity of aortic stenosis in the majority of patients. Many patients with aortic stenosis will remain asymptomatic for decades. The diagnosis of aortic stenosis is usually made in the asymptomatic patient on the basis of a systolic murmur on auscultation and confirmed by echocardiography. Symptoms, when they occur, usually consist of one or more of the classic triad of exertional dyspnea, angina, and syncope. Following symptom onset, there is a high mortality rate with an average survival of 2–3 years. The development of symptoms therefore is a critical point in the natural history of patients with aortic stenosis. Sudden death rarely is the initial manifestation of severe aortic stenosis, occurring at a rate of less than 1% per year in asymptomatic patients.[3] Two-dimensional and Doppler echocardiography is the imaging modality of choice for the diagnosis and quantification of aortic stenosis. Short-axis images from two-dimensional echocardiography demonstrate the number of aortic cusps and the degree of cusp fusion or restricted cusp opening in valvular aortic stenosis. Two dimensional echocardiography is also useful for determining the status of the left ventricle and the degree of hypertrophy. Left atrial enlargement indicates concomitant diastolic dysfunction. The normal area of the adult aortic valve is 3.0 to 4.0 cm^2. Reduction of the normal area usually does not produce symptoms until the valve reaches one-fourth of its normal dimension.[4] The graduation of AS is given in Table 1.

Severity	Aortic jet velocity (m per second)	Mean gradient (mm Hg)	Aortic valve area (cm^2)
Normal	< 2.5	-	3 to 4
Mild	2.5 to 2.9	< 25	1.5 to 2
Moderate	3 to 4	25 to 40	1 to 1.5
Severe	> 4	> 40	< 1

Table 1. Classifications of Aortic Stenosis Severity[4]

There is no effective medical therapy for AS. AVR is the only effective treatment for severe aortic stenosis in adults. Following AVR for AS, one can expect resolution of symptoms, left ventricular hypertrophy (LVH) regression, and improved left ventricular (LV) systolic function secondary to reduced afterload. Importantly, postoperative survival is similar to age-matched controls after AVR for AS when performed prior to the development of LV dysfunction or congestive heart failure (CHF). Similarly, incomplete regression of LVH after AVR has been associated with adverse outcomes such as reduced long-term survival. Contrary to the immediate improvement in systolic performance, diastolic dysfunction may persist for several more years after AVR. In fact, Gjertsson et al. recently evaluated diastolic dysfunction in AS and found that the proportion of patients with moderate-to-severe diastolic dysfunction actually increased with time after AVR despite normalization of LV mass and appropriate adjustments for senile diastolic dysfunction. Finally, AVR is associated with improved quality of life scores, particularly among the elderly, and has been found to be similar to age-matched individuals without heart disease. [3,5,6]

The American College of Cardiology (ACC) and the American Heart Association (ACH) have jointly developed guidelines in which they published indications for AVR:

a. Definite indications:

- Patients who have severe AS and presented with one or more of its classical symptoms (angina, syncope, heart failure, etc.)
- Patients who have severe AS and required coronary artery bypass surgery, surgery on the aorta or other heart valves
- Patients who have severe AS and left ventricle systolic dysfunction (ejection fraction less than 50 %)

b. Possible indications:

- Patients who have moderate AS and required coronary artery bypass surgery, surgery on the aorta or other heart valves
- Asymptomatic patients with severe AS with abnormal exercise test, or an increase in transaortic gradient during exercise, or left ventricle systolic dysfunction (ejection fraction less than 50 %), or left ventricular dilatation, or significantly elevated left ventricular diastolic pressure. [7]

The European Society of Cardiology (ESC) has also developed guidelines in which they published indications for AVR (Table 2).[8] They strongly recommended early AVR in all symptomatic patients with severe AS.

Management of asymptomatic patients requires careful weighing of benefits against risks. Early elective surgery at these patients can only be recommended in selected patients, at low operative risk. This could be the case in:

- The rare asymptomatic patients with depressed LV function not due to another cause
- Those with echocardiographic predictors of poor outcome suggested by the combination of a markedly calcified valve with a rapid increase in peak aortic velocity of ≥ 0.3 m/s per year
- If the exercise test is abnormal, particularly if it shows symptom development, which is a strong indication for surgery in physically active patients.

http://dx.doi.org/10.5772/53687

- However, on the other hand, breathlessness on exercise may be difficult to interpret in patients with only low physical activity, particularly the elderly, making decisionmaking more difficult. There is no strict age limit for performance of exercise testing and it is reasonable to propose it in patients > 70 years old who are still highly active.[8]

Patients with severe AS and any symptoms	**IB**
Patients with severe AS undergoing coronary artery bypass surgery, surgery of the ascending aorta, or on another valve	IC
Asymptomatic patients with severe AS and systolic LV dysfunction (LVEF < 50%) unless due to other cause	IC
Asymptomatic patients with severe AS and abnormal exercise test showing symptoms on exercise	IC
Asymptomatic patients with severe AS and abnormal exercise test showing fall in blood pressure below baseline	IIaC
Patients with moderate AS undergoing coronary artery bypass surgery, surgery of the ascending aorta or another valve	IIaC
Asymptomatic patients with severe AS and moderate-to-severe valve calcification, and a rate of peak velocity progression ≥ 0.3 m/s per year	IIaC
AS with low gradient (< 40 mmHg) and LV dysfunction with contractile reserve	IIaC
Asymptomatic patients with severe AS and abnormal exercise test showing complex ventricular arrhythmias	IIbC
Asymptomatic patients with severe AS and excessive LV hypertrophy (≥ 15 mm) unless this is due to hypertension	IIbC
AS with low gradient (< 40 mmHg) and LV dysfunction without contractile reserve	IIbC

Table 2. Indications for AVR in AS

In last 50 years, the varieties of prostheses that have become available for use are numerous. An ideal aortic prosthesis would be simple to implant, widely available, possess long-term durability, would have no intrinsic thrombogenicity, would not have a predilection foe endocarditis and would have no residual transvalvular pressure gradient. Such a valve does not currently exist. Currently available options include mechanical valves, stented biological valves, stentless biological valves, allograft valves and pulmonary autograft valves. Commonly in us are mechanical and biological prostheses.[9] When selecting between mechanical and biologic heart valves, the surgeon and patient must balance the risks and benefits of each choice.

2. Mechanical prostheses

Charles Hufnagel in 1952. Used aortic valve ball and cage prosthesis heterotopically in the descending aorta to treat aortic insufficiency. The first aortic valve replacement with an intra cardiac mechanical prosthesis, which led to long terms survivors, was performed in 1960. Mechanical valves are classified according to their structure as caged-ball, single-tilting-disk or bileaflet-tilting-disk valves. The Starr-Edwards caged-ball valve has been available since the 1960's and comprises a silastic ball, which rests on the sewing ring when closed and moves forward into the cage when the valve opens. The single-disk valves, for example, the Bjork-Shiley prosthesis and the Medtronic-Hall prosthesis, contain a disk that tilts between two struts of the orifice housing. The most popular of the mechanical valves at present are the bileaflet valves, of which the St. Jude Medical valve and the Carbomedics valve are widely implanted. Both these devices are implanted within the aortic annulus. The two semi-circular leaflets of the bileaflet valve are connected to the housing by a butterfly hinge mechanism and swing apart during opening of the valve creating three outflow tracts, one central and two peripheral respectively. In contrast to the configuration of the latter, the Carbomedics Top Hat (Sulzer Carbomedics, Austin, TX) bileaflet aortic valve that was introduced in 1993 has a unique supra-annular design with all its components incorporated within the aortic sinuses.[10,11]

Mechanical valves are made from carbon, Teflon, Dacron, titanium and polyester and are very durable. The current designs for the aortic and mitral positions include ball-and-cage valves, single tilting disc prostheses, and bileaflet prostheses. Bileaflet mechanical valves are the standard in current practice, with the St. Jude Medical (St. Jude Medical, Inc., St. Paul, MN) prosthesis the modern prototype, having been first implanted in 1977. Most of these valves are constructed using carbon strengthened with silicon carbide additives. Other examples of bileaflet mechanical valves include those manufactured by CarboMedics (Austin, TX); Advancing the Standard Medical (ATS, Minneapolis, MN); Medtronic, Inc. (Minneapolis, MN); and Medical Carbon Research Institute, LLC (MCRI, Austin, TX). [10,11,12] The On-XR mechanical valve (MCRI) was introduced in Europe in 1996 and differs from other bileaflet mechanical valves in that it is made from pure pyrolytic carbon. The PROACT (Prospective Randomized On-X R Valve Anticoagulation Trial) study is an FDA-approved multicenter trial, sponsored by MCRI, currently enrolling patients to determine whether or not defined patient groups receiving AVR (low versus high risk for TE events) with the On-X R _ valve may be safely maintained on lower doses of warfarin or, for patients in the lowrisk aortic valve arm, on antiplatelet drugs (aspirin plus clopidogrel) alone compared with standard anticoagulation regimens. No single mechanical valve has shown superior patient outcomes, and all demonstrate extremely low rates of structural valve deterioration, the major advantage of mechanical valves.[3]

http://dx.doi.org/10.5772/53687

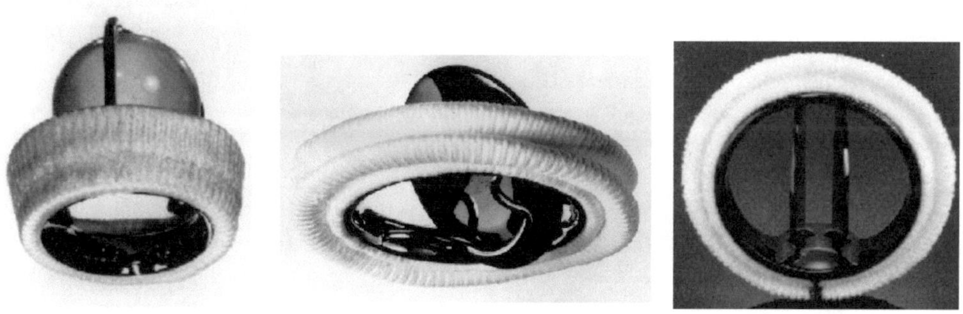

Figure 2. Mechanical valves: a) Starr-Edwards cage-ball valve, b) Bjork-Shiley mono-leaflet valve and c) St. Jude Medical bileaflet valve

3. Biological prosthesis

The biological prostheses include a wide variety of devices. Included within this broad category are the bioprostheses, a term which is used for valves with non-viable tissue of biological origin. The bioprostheses include the heterografts, composed of porcine (actual valves of a pig) or bovine tissue (pericardium of a cow) and the allografts, which are preserved human aortic valves. The initial bioprostheses were mounted on stents to which the leaflets and sewing ring were attached but subsequently stentless valves, which are sewn in free hand, have been developed.[13] Stented bioprosthetic valves, which incorporate a semi-rigid external support structure for the valve leaflets, represent the majority of tissue valves implanted in clinical practice. The external support provides accurate valve mounting, improving ease of implantation. Two types of stented bioprosthetic valves are currently available in the United States: porcine aortic valves, which incorporate chemically stabilized porcine valve leaflets mounted on a stented structure or frame, and bovine pericardial valves. The leaflets of the latter valve type are constructed from bovine pericardium and subsequently mounted on a stented frame. Available porcine valves include the Medtronic Mosaic valve (Medtronic Inc., Minneapolis, MN), the St. Jude Medical Biocor and Biocor Supra valves (St. Jude Medical, Inc., St. Paul, MN), and the Carbomedics Mitroflow valve (Carbomedics, Inc., Austin, TX). Bovine pericardial valves include the Carpentier–Edwards (C–E) Perimount (Edward Lifesciences, Irvine, CA) and the CE Perimount Magna valves as well as the Sorin Soprano (Sorin Group, Saluggia, Italy) valves. At present, based on the best available data, no one bioprosthetic valve appears superior with regard to patient outcomes and none requires systemic anticoagulation with warfarin, which is their major advantage. Their major disadvantage is the incidence of structural valve deterioration and subsequent need for reoperation, although the lifespan of the latest generation of tissue valves is unknown. Recent evidence also suggests that stentless biological valves may have better coronary flow reserve compared to stented valves. Additionally, compared with stented bovine pericardial valves, stentless valves have been associated with increased transvalvular EOA and decreased pressure gradients during extended follow-up. However, as seen in other studies, LV mass regression after stentless valve implantation was not different from stented aortic bioprostheses.[3,14]

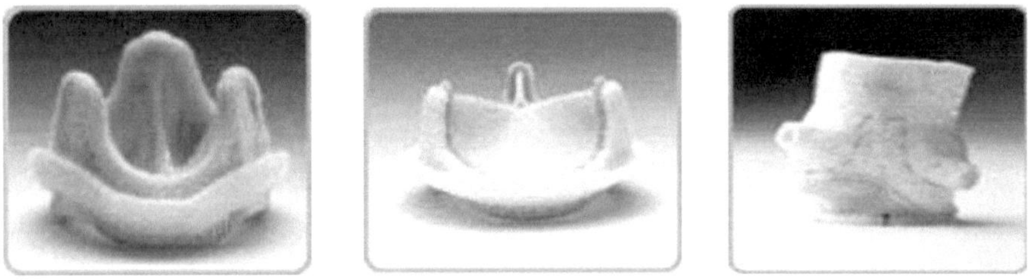

(a) (b) (c)

Figure 3. Biological prosthesis: a) stented porcine bioprosthesis, b) pericardial bovine bioprosthesis and c) stentless porcine bioprosthesis

4. Outcomes after aortic valve replacement

The Ad Hoc Liaison Committee for Standardizing Definitions of Prosthetic Heart Valve Morbidity of the American Association of Thoracic Surgery and the Society of Thoracic Surgeons published guidelines during years, which are now widely used in reporting outcomes after valve surgery. They presented a list of developing specific valve-related events during patients remaining lifetime. These valve-related events are:

1. Structural valvular deterioration
2. Nonstructural dysfunction
3. Valve thrombosis
4. Embolism
5. Valvular endocarditis and
6. Bleeding events.[7, 15]

Structural valvular deterioration - Any change in function or deterioration (a decrease of one New York Heart Association functional class or more) of an operated valve due to an intrinsic abnormality, which causes stenosis or regurgitation. Changes intrinsic to the valve include wear, fracture, poppet escape, calcification, leaflet tear stent creep and suture line disruption of the components of the operated valve. The definition excludes changes due to infection or thrombosis. *Mechanical prostheses* are extremely resistant to material fatigue or structural valve deterioration. This is characteristic of mechanical valves whether they are aortic or mitral valves.[16] Because of the long-term durability of mechanical prostheses a valve replacement rate is less than 2% over 25 years. The most common reasons for reimplantation are pre- and postoperative endocarditis, paravalvular leak and valve thrombosis.[17] *Bioprosthetic valves* are not as durable, have a shorter lifespan and are more susceptible to calcification than human and mechanical valves.[13] Bioprostheses have a significantly higher rate of reoperation due to structural valve deterioration. In large series, freedom from reoperation is > 90% at 10 years, but < 70 % at 15 years.[17,18,19] There is an important predisposition for premature bioprosthetic structural valve deterioration in younger patients, especially those under the age of 40 years.[17]

Nonstructural dysfunction - Any abnormality that is not intrinsic to the valve per se, which causes stenosis or regurgitation. Examples for this include entrapment of pannus, tissue or suture; paravalvular leak; inappropriate sizing or positioning; residual leak and clinically important hemolytic anemia. This definition also excludes changes due to infection and thrombosis. Subvalvular pannus formation is rare with *mechanical bileaflet valves.*[20] Panus overgrowth and prosthetic structural degeneration interfering with normal valve opening and closure may cause hemolysis severe enough for reoperation. Paravalvular leak is an operative complication and it is related to operative technique and to endocarditis.[21]

Valve thrombosis – Any thrombus, in the absence of infection, which is attached to or near an operated valve that occludes part of the blood flow path or that interferes with function of the valve. The incidence of prosthesis thrombosis is < 0.2 % per year and it occurs more often in *mechanical prostheses.*[22] It is most commonly due to inadequate anticoagulation or noncompliance. Freedom from valve thrombosis at 20 years is > 97 %.[23,24]

Embolism – Any embolic event that occurs, in the absence of infection, after the immediate peri-operative period. This could be either a neurologic or peripheral embolic event. A neurologic event includes any new, temporary or permanent focal or global neurologic deficit. A peripheral embolic event is due to an embolus that produces symptoms from obstruction of a peripheral (non-cerebral) artery. The incidence of thromboembolic events between bioprostheses and mechanical prostheses are the same.[25] This is a continuous risk factor that is present through the life of patients with *mechanical valve prosthesis,* so they must maintain therapeutic anticoagulant levels. The embolic risk is highest in the first few months, before the ring and valve components have fully endothelialized.[26] Acceptable thromboembolic rates range between 0.8 and 2.3 % per patient-year.[21,22,25] 50 % of these events are neurologic, 40 % are transient and 10 % are peripheral.[21]

Valvular endocarditis – Any infection involving an operated valve diagnosed by customary clinical criteria. It is rare case with prophylactic antibiotics. Around 60 % of events occur early and are associated with staphylococci. The mortality for this event is high. Freedom from endocarditis with mechanical prosthesis is 97 to 98 % at 20 to 25 years. A number of studies have reported a higher incidence of valvular endocarditis after *mechanical valve* replacement in comparison with the biologic valve replacement during the initial few months after implantation. *Bioprostheses* are less susceptible to early infection, which is often restricted to the leaflets, making cure with antibiotics more likely but increasing the chances of late failure due to degeneration of the cusps.[27,28,29]

Bleeding event – Formerly classified as anti-coagulant hemorrhage, a bleeding event is an episode of major internal or external bleeding that causes death, hospitalization, and permanent injury or requires transfusion. This definition applies to all patients, irrespective of anticoagulation status. *Mechanical valves* are durability but anticoagulation is key of long-term success. International Normalized Ratio (INR) is the standard to which anticoagulation levels should be targeted. Level of INR should be individual for each person. Complications occur during fluctuations in the INR and less during steady-state levels, be they high or low.[30,31] When levels of INR increase, bleeding episodes become more common, and when levels of INR decrease thromboembolic episodes become more common. Some studies showed that around 40 % of the bleeding episodes occurred in the first year after surgery, when levels of INR are more likely to fluctuate. Many studies suggested that in the early postoperative period slowly raise the level of INR to therapeutic levels is needed, to prevent bleeding events. [21,32,33] According to ACC and ACH after mechanical AVR, the goal of antithrombotic therapy is usually to achieve an INR of 2.5 to 3.5 for the first 3 months after surgery and 2.0 to 3.0 beyond that time. At that level of anticoagulation, the risk of significant hemorrhage appears to be 1% to 2% per year.[7] Low-dose aspirin is also indicated in addition to warfarin to result in a lower incidence of thromboembolic event, with a low possibility for bleeding.[34] Older patients are at higher risk for thromboembolic event because of the greater number of risk factors that accumulate with aging.[30] Anticoagulation-related hemorrhage (ARH) is the most common valve-related event. More often it will occur during fluctuations in INR, which happens most often early after valve replacement.[21,22] The most common places for ARH are gastrointestinal tract and central nervous system.[21] Acceptable ARH rates range from 1.0 to 2.5% per patient-year in long term reports.[21,22,25,35] It is very dangerous complication, because mortality more often occurs in relation to bleeding events than in relation to thromboembolic events.[21]

Operative mortality – Operative mortality is defined as all-cause mortality within 30 days of operation. According to the Society of Thoracic Surgeons mortality for isolated AVR is 4.3% and for AVR with concomitant coronary artery disease is 8%.[36] Many factors have been associated with an increased risk of operative mortality in isolated AVR. Some of these risk factors are age, female gender, diabetes, renal failure, and emergency status, previous operation, advanced preoperative NYHA class, lower cardiac index, concomitant coronary artery bypass grafting and longer aortic crossclamp and cardiopulmonary bypass time respectively.[37] In the absence of major comorbidities and preserved ejection fraction, isolated AVR can be performed with an expected mortality of less than 2%.[38]

Several studies have evaluated independent risk factors for operative mortality after AVR. Five variables predictive of increased mortality risk after AVR are common to each of these analyses: preoperative renal failure, urgency of AVR, preoperative heart failure, presence of CAD or recent MI, and redo cardiac operation. Other factors independently associated with operative mortality from the individual studies include preoperative atrial fibrillation, active endocarditis, preoperative stroke, advanced age, lower body surface area, multiple valve procedures, and hypertension. [39, 40]

http://dx.doi.org/10.5772/53687

5. Factors affecting long-term outcome after AVR

- Demographic
  - Older age
  - Male sex
- Clinical
  - Higher pre-operative NYHA functional class
  - Pre-operative atrial fibrillation and non-sinus rhythm
  - Pure aortic regurgitation
  - Hypertension
  - Diabetes mellitus
  - Renal failure
- Surgery-related
  - Longer cardiopulmonary bypass time
- Morphological
  - Previous myocardial infarction
  - Left ventricular structure and functional abnormality
  - Previous aortic valve surgery
  - Coronary artery disease (CAD)

Older patients have a lot of comorbiditis and they are at higher risk for valve-related events. Atrial fibrillation is one of the risk factor for thromboembolism, because of that INR levels must be higher (INR 2.5 to 3.5) than regular.[30,34] The majority of patients undergoing AVR have other cardiac lesions, most commonly CAD, and more complex pathology has been associated with increased risk. Combined myocardial revascularization and AVR increases cross-clamp time and has the potential to increase perioperative myocardial infarction and early postoperative mortality compared with patients undergoing isolated AVR.[7] In addition to severity of CAD and AS, the multivariate factors for late postoperative mortality include low ejection fraction, severity of LV dysfunction, age greater than 70 years (especially in women), and presence of NYHA functional class IV symptoms.[36]

6. Patient selection

Propter selection of patients for valve replacement can bring us excellent long-term results, long-term survival and low incidence of valve-related complications.

In some studies of patients followed over longer time frames, freedom from all valve-related events and freedom from reoperation were improved in patients with mechanical valve prostheses as compared to patients with biological prostheses. [9,16,25] Key of long-term success of mechanical valve prostheses is anticoagulation. Patients that are inconsistent, noncompliant or incapable of managing medications are not good candidates for long-term chronic anticoagulation.[39,41] Also patients with higher levels of education and those from geographic areas with a good medical infrastructure have better compliance with necessary medications and anticoagulant monitoring.[31]

Many centers used bioprosthetic valves for patients who are older than 70 year, based on data by Akins.[42] In patients younger than 60 years of age, the best solution would be implantation of mechanical valves, based on prosthesis durability and they have low-risk for valve-related events.[21] In decade between 60 and 70 years of age, other factors have to be taken into account.[7] According to some studies, patients over 65 years at the time of surgery should receive a biologic valve. Patients under the age of 60 should have a mechanical prosthesis to minimize the risk of structural failure requiring repeat AVR in an octogenarian. Patients between 60 and 65 represent the group in whom there is still considerable debate regarding prosthesis selection. Those patients who have comorbidities such as severe CAD may be less likely to outlive their prosthesis and should receive a biologic valve. A detailed discussion of these risks and benefits of prosthesis selection should occur with all patients and their families prior to entering the operating room. [3,7,22,24,25,37,38]

In the early follow-up period, anticoagulation – related hemorrhage is the most common unwanted event for mechanical valve prostheses. Over the first 10 years of follow-up there is a higher incidence of valve-related events in patients with mechanical prostheses as opposed to those with biologic valves.[32] However, in the next 10 to 20 years after AVR, the incidence of valve failure and valve-related complications are much higher at biologic prostheses than those with mechanical valve prostheses. Some series showed that the time to biologic valve failure was only 7.6 years.[43] This failure rate will increase over time. However, freedom from valve-related events is more strongly influenced by pre-existing comorbidities than the presence of mechanical prostheses.[21], [22, 25, 31]

The elderly patient with severe aortic stenosis poses a therapeutic challenge. In considering elderly patients for aortic valve replacement, important factors include the presence of symptoms, physiologic age, patient expectations, anticipated future activities, and comorbidity. The operation itself carries a higher risk than in younger patients. Extensive calcification of the aorta and annulus as well as fragile tissue presents significant technical difficulties for the surgeon. In addition, particularly in women, the aortic root and annulus may be small and require concomitant enlargement to accommodate the valve prosthesis. Furthermore, protruding arch atheroma occurs in one-fifth of patients > 65 years of age and significantly increases the risk of stroke and mortality during cardiac surgery. Major postoperative complications, nevertheless, remain high, with the incidence of permanent stroke between 4 and 6%. Rehabilitation can also be a problem, as elderly patients take longer to recover from surgery. Survival has clearly improved in these elderly patients with severe symptomatic aortic stenosis who undergo aortic valve replacement. Survival is 80–85% at 1 year and 60–

http://dx.doi.org/10.5772/53687

70% at 5 years, which is similar to an age- and sex-matched population without aortic valve disease. Most patients report improved functional capacity and quality of life, with more than 90% of patients feeling better after surgery.[3]

A major deterrent to mechanical valve replacement in the younger patient is the impact of long-term anticoagulation. Mechanical valves are, however, more ideal for younger patients due to their excellent durability characteristics. Most importantly, younger patients (i.e., patients under the age of 50 years) are a low-risk subset for valve related events. These individuals have very few risk factors for TE, and thus anticoagulation can be run at the lower end of the therapeutic target range, decreasing the incidence of anticoagulant-related hemorrhage without altering the incidence of TE. In fact, many infants and children have been managed with only aspirin with quite good long term results. While this is not recommended in patients older than infancy, it is a feasible alternative. A recent study in patients under 50 years of age followed 254 patients for up to 20 years and found an exceedingly low rate of valve related events, an exceptional long-term overall survival of nearly 88%, and event-free survival probability of 92% at 19 years.[3,44,45]

Patients with an absolute requirement for long-term anticoagulation such as atrial fibrillation, previous thromboembolic events, hypercoagulable state, severe LVD, another mechanical heart valve in place, or intracardiac thrombus, should receive a mechanical valve regardless of age. Patients in whom anticoagulation with warfarin is contraindicated, such as women of child-bearing age wishing to become pregnant, patients with other bleeding disorders, or those who refuse anticoagulation should receive a bioprosthesis. There is growing interest in using mechanical prostheses in women of child-bearing age and providing anticoagulation with subcutaneous low-molecular weight heparin injections. Patients with end-stage renal failure were previously believed to have significantly elevated risk for early bioprosthetic structural valve deterioration. However, increased anticoagulation- related complications are also more likely in this group, and the current ACC/AHA guidelines do not recommend routine use of mechanical prostheses in these patients.[3,7,8,9,10]

The decision between bioprosthetic and mechanical valve should be made by the patient with educated input regarding the pros and cons of each option from the patient's physicians. Today surgeons implant bioprosthetic valves in younger patients who wish to avoid anticoagulation due to lifestyle concerns (e.g. young, active individual, desire to become pregnant, etc.), although surgeons generally will guide patients toward a mechanical option at the time of redo-AVR if their life expectancy exceeds 10–15 years at that time.[3]

7. Operative technique

Aortic valve replacement is most frequently done through a median sternotomy, meaning the incision is made by cutting through the sternum. Once the pericardium has been opened, the patient is put on a cardiopulmonary bypass machine. This machine takes over the task of breathing for the patient and pumping their blood around while the surgeon replaces the heart valve.

Once the patient is on bypass, a cut is made in the aorta and a crossclamp applied. The surgeon then removes the patient`s diseased aortic valve and a mechanical or biological valve is put in its place. Once the valve is in place and aorta has been closed, the patient is taken off the heart-lung machine. Transesophageal echocardiogram can be used to verify that the new valve is functioning property. Pacing wires are usually put in place, so that the heart can be manually paced should any complications arise after surgery. Drainage tubes are also inserted to drain fluids from the chest and pericardium following surgery. These are usually removed within 36-48 hours while the pacing wires are generally left in place until right before the patient is discharged from the hospital.

8. Patient-prosthesis mismatch

Prosthesis-patient mismatch (PPM) is that a smaller than expected effective orifice area (IEOA) in relation to the patient's body surface area (BSA) will result in higher transvalvar gradients. It is condition that occurs when the valve area of a prosthetic valve is less than the area of that patient's normal valve.[46] Several authors suggest that prosthesis-patient mismatch occurs at an IEOA of 0.85 cm^2/m^2.[46,47] Transvalvular gradients begin to rise substantially at IEOAs below this value, and these elevated gradients potentially cause increased left ventricular work that prevents adequate regression of left ventricular hypertrophy. Several factors including age, body mass index (BMI), and pre-operative status of left ventricular function may potentially influence the effect of PPM on post-operative outcomes.[46] PPM is associated with a significant reduction in cardiac index during the postoperative course. The incidence of congestive heart failure was significantly higher in patients with PPM.[48] Several studies reported that early mortality is significantly increased in patients with PPM.[47, 48, 49, 50]

The projected indexed EOA should be systematically calculated at the time of the operation to estimate the risk of PPM. PPM can be avoided by using a simple strategy at the time of operation. Pibarot suggested that surgeon first calculate the patient's BSA from his or her weight and height. Than multiply BSA by 0.85 cm^2/m^2, the result being the minimum EOA that the prosthesis to be implanted should have to avoid PPM, and than choose the prosthesis and the reference values for the different types and sizes of prosthesis.[46, 47]

Due to concerns over PPM, stentless bioprosthetic valves, which generally have a larger EOA sizefor- size compared with mechanical or stented bioprosthetic valves, have been increasingly utilized for AVR. In initial evaluation, stentless valves had better hemodynamics and improved survival rates relative to stented biological or mechanical valves and were more durable than stented biological valves. Stentless valves may be preferred in patients with a small aortic root, and arguments have been made that wider utilization of stentless valves may minimize PPM. Stentless valves also appear to have better hemodynamic profiles than stented valves during exercise testing. Technical reasons for not implanting stentless valves include extensive aortic root calcification, coronary ostia opposed by 180, presence of the two coronary ostia in close proximity, or unusual disproportion between the sinotubular junction and the aortic annulus. Whereas stented valves allow

http://dx.doi.org/10.5772/53687

perfect valve mounting within the aortic annulus, thus reducing the risk of implanting an incompetent valve, postoperative AR and limited durability remain a concern with the free-hand stentless valve insertion technique. This issue may be circumvented with full aortic root replacement using a stentless porcine root.[3.49,50]

Author details

Stamenko Šušak[1*], Lazar Velicki[1], Dušan Popović[1] and Ivana Burazor[2]

*Address all correspondence to: drsusak@gmail.com

1 Institute of Cardiovascular Diseases Vojvodina, Sremska Kamenica, Serbia

2 Clinical Centers, Nis, Serbia

References

[1] Malouf, J. F, Edwards, W. D, Tajik, A. J, & Seward, J. Functional anatomy of the heart. In: Fuster V, O'Rourke RA, Walsh RA, Poole-Wilson P, eds. Hurst's The Heart. 12th ed. New York, NY: McGraw-Hill Companies, Inc; (2008).

[2] Otto, C. M, Lind, B. K, Kitzman, D. W, et al. Association of aortic valve sclerosis with cardiovascular mortality and morbidity in the elderly. N Eng J Med (1999).

[3] Andrew WangThomas S. Bashore. Valvular Heart Disease. Humana Press, a part of Springer Science Business Media, LLC (2009).

[4] Gjertsson, P, Caidahl, K, Farasati, M, et al. Preopeartive moderate to severe diastolic dysfunction: A novel Doppler echocardiographic long-term prognosis factor in patients with severe aortic stenosis. J Thorac Cardiovasc Surg (2005).

[5] Connolly, H. M, Oh, J. K, Orszulak, T. A, et al. Aortic valve replacement for aortic stenosis with severe left ventricular dysfunction: prognostic indicators. Circulation (1997)., 95, 2395-400.

[6] Gjertsson, P, Caidahl, K, & Bech-hanssen, O. Left ventricular diastolic dysfunction late after aortic valve replacement in patients with aortic stenosis. Am J Cardiol (2005)., 96, 722-7.

[7] Bonow, R. O, Carabello, B. A, & Chatterjee, K. de Leon AC Jr, Faxon DP, Freed MD, Gaasch WH, Lytle BW, Nishimura RA, O'Gara PT, O'Rourke RA, Otto CM, Shah PM, Shanewise JS. ACC/AHA 2006 guidelines for the management of patients with valvular heart disease: a report of the American College of Cardiology/American Heart Association Task Force on Practice Guidelines (Writing Committee to Develop

Guidelines for the Management of Patients With Valvular Heart Disease). Circulation. (2006). ee231. DOI:CIRCULATIONAHA.106.176857, 84.

[8] The European Society of Cardiology Guidelines on the management of valvular heart disease European Heart Journal (2007.

[9] Gott, V. L. Alejo DE: Mechanical heart valves: 50 years of evolution. Ann Thorac Surg (2003). S2230

[10] Bloomfield, P. Choice of heart valve prosthesis. Heart. (2002). , 87, 583-9.

[11] Dewall, R. A, Qasim, N, & Carr, L. Evolution of Mechanical Heart valves. Ann Thorac Surg. (2000). , 69, 1612-21.

[12] Bonow, R. O, Carabello, B. A, Chatterjee, K. C, De Leon, J. R, Faxon, A. C, Freed, D. P, Shah, M. D, & Acc, P. M. AHA 2006 guidelines for the management of patients with valvular heart disease. Journal of the American College of Cardiology, 48(3), 1-148.doi:10.1016/j.jacc.2006.05.021

[13] YangThang, "Mechanical Versus Bioprosthetic Valve Replacement in Valvular Heart Disease: A Systematic Review" ((2011). School of Physician Assistant Studies. Paper 240.http://commons.pacificu.edu/pa/240

[14] Tsialtas, D, Bolognesi, R, Beghi, C, et al. Stented versus stentless bioprostheses in aortic valve stenosis: effect on left ventricular remodeling. Heart Surg Forum (2007). E, 205-10.

[15] Golubovic, M, Mihajlovic, B, Kovacevic, P, Cemerlic-adjic, N, Pavlovic, K, Velicki, L, & Susak, S. Postoperativne neletalne komplikacije posle operacije na otvorenom srcu. Vojnosanitetski pregled (2012). , 69(1), 27-31.

[16] Stamenko, S. Susak. Mitralna regurgitacija- kardiohirurski aspekti dijagnostike i terapije. Mediterran Publishing, Biblioteka Academica, knjiga 15, Novi Sad (2010).

[17] Emery, R. W, Arom, K. V, Krogh, C. C, et al. Reoperative valve replacement with the St.Jude Medical valve prosthesis: long-term follow up. J Am Coll Cardiol (2004). A

[18] Desai, N. D, Merin, O, Cohen, G. N, et al. Long-term results of aortic valve replacement with the St.Jude Toronto stentless porcine valve. Ann Thorac Surg (2004).

[19] Grunkemeier, G. L, Jamieson, W. R, & Miller, D. C. Starr A: Actuarial versus actual risk of porcine structural valve deterioration. J Thorac Cardiovasc Surg (1994).

[20] Vongpatanasin, W, & Hills, L. D. Lange RA: Prosthetic heart valve. N Eng J Med (1996).

[21] Emery, R. W, Krogh, C. C, Arom, D. V, et al. The ST. Jude Medical cardiac valve prosthesis: A year experience with single valve replacement. Ann Thorac Surg (2005). , 25.

[22] Ikonomidis, J. S, Kratz, J. M, Crumbley, A. J, et al. Twenty-year experience with the St.Jude Medical mechanical valve prosthesis. J Thorac Cardiovasc Surg (2003).

[23] Lengyel, M. Vandor L: The role of thrombolysis in the management of left-sided prosthetic valve thrombosis: a study of 85 cases diagnosed by transesophageal echocardiography. J Heart Valve Dis (2001).

[24] Durrleman, N, Pellerin, M, Bouchard, D, et al. Prosthetic valve thrombosis: twenty-year experience at the Montreal Heart Institute. J Thorac Cardiovasc Surg (2004).

[25] Khan, S. S, Trento, A, Derobertis, M, et al. Twenty-year comparison of tissue and mechanical valve replacement. J Thorac Cardiovasc Surg (2001).

[26] Heras, M, Chesebro, J. H, Fuster, V, et al. High risk of thromboemboli early after bioprosthetic cardiac valve replacement. J Am Coll Cardiol (1995).

[27] Mahesh, B, Angelini, G, Caputo, M, Jin, X. Y, & Bryan, A. (2005). Prosthetic valve endocarditis. Ann. Thorac. Surg., 0003-4975, 80(3), 1151-1158.

[28] Velicki, L, Susak, S, Cemerlic-adjic, N, & Redzek, A. Aortic valve endocarditis, Chapter in: Ying-Fu Chen and Chwan-Yau Luo- Aortic valve, InTech Publishing (2011).

[29] Velicki, L, Susak, S, & Srdanovic, I. Kovacevic M; Infective endocarditis of native aortic valve: destruction of leaflet with an aorto-cavitary fistula to the right ventricle, Chirurgia (2010)., 23(6), 261-266.

[30] Koertke, H, Minami, K, Boethig, D, et al. INR self-management permits lower anticoagulation levels after mechanical heart valve replacement. Circulation (2003). Suppl II):II-75.

[31] Butchart, E. G, Ionescu, A, Payne, N, et al. A new scoring system to determine thromboembolic risk after heart valve replacement. Circulation (2003). Suppl II):II-68.

[32] Kumar, D, & Elefteriades, J. Ezekowitz MD: Anticoagulation in patients with prosthetic heart valves. Cardiac Surg Today (2004).

[33] Koo, S, Kucher, N, Nguyen, P. L, et al. The effect of excessive anticoagulation on mortality and morbidity in hospitalized patients with anticoagulant-related major hemorrhage. Arch Intern Med (2004).

[34] Massel, D. Little SH: Risk and benefits of adding antiplatelet therapy to warfarin among patients with prosthetic heart valves: a metaanalysis. J Am Coll Cardiol (2001).

[35] Lund, O, Nielsen, S. L, Arildsen, H, et al. Standard aortic St. Jude valve at 18 years: performance, profile and determinants of outcome. Ann Thorac Surg (2000).

[36] Society of Thoracic Surgeons National Cardiac Surgery DatabaseAvailable at: http://www.sts.org/documents/pdf/STS-ExecutiveSummaryFall2005.pdf. November (2005).

[37] Edwards, F. H, Peterson, E. D, Coombs, L. P, et al. Prediction of operative mortality after valve replacement surgery. J Am Coll Cardiol (2001).

[38] David TE: Surgery of the aortic valve. (1999). *Curr Probl Surg.*

[39] Rankin, J. S, Hammill, B. G, Ferguson, T. B, et al. Determinants of operative mortality in valvular heart surgery. J Thorac Cardiovasc Surg (2006). , 131, 547-57.

[40] Kuduvalli, M, Grayson, A. D, Au, J, et al. A multi-centre additive and logistic risk model for in-hospital mortality following aortic valve replacement. Eur J Cardiothorac Surg (2007). , 31, 607-13.

[41] Butchart, E. G, Payne, N, Li, H, et al. Better anticoagulation control improves survival after valve replacement. J Thorac Cardiovasc Surg (2002).

[42] Akins, C. W, Buckley, M. J, Daggett, W. M, et al. Risk of reoperative valve replacement for failed mitral and aortic bioprostheses. Ann Thorac Surg (1998).

[43] Potter, D. D, & Sundt, T. M. rd, Zehr KJ, et al: Operative risk of reoperative aortic valve replacement. J Thorac Cardiovasc Surg (2005).

[44] Cabalka, A. K, & Emery, R. W. Petersen RJ: Long-term follow-up of the St. Jude Medical prosthesis in pediatric patients. Ann Thorac Surg (1995). S618

[45] Emery, R. W, Erickson, C. A, Arom, K. V, et al. Replacement of the aortic valve in patients under 50 years old with the St. Jude Medical prosthesis. Ann Thorac Surg (2003).

[46] Dumesnil, J. G. Pibarot P: Prosthesis-patient mismatch and clinical outcomes: the evidence continues to accumulate. J Thorac Cardiovasc Surg (2006).

[47] Pibarot, P, & Dumesnil, J. G. Prosthesis-patient mismatch: definition, clinical impact, and prevention. Heart. (2006). , 92, 1022-9.

[48] Milano, A D, De Carlo, M, Mecozzi, G, et al. Clinical outcome in patients with 19-mm and 21-mm St. Jude aortic prostheses: comparison at long-term follow-up, Ann Thorac Surg (2002). , 7337-43.

[49] Rao, V, Jamieson, W, & Ivanov, E. J. et al Prosthesis-patient mismatch affects survival following aortic valve replacement. Circulation (2000). IIIIII9.III9, 5.

[50] Blais, C, Dumesnil, J G, Baillot, R, et al. Impact of prosthesis-patient mismatch on short-term mortality after aortic valve replacement. Circulation (2003). , 108983-988.

Chapter 13

Current Treatment Options in Aortic Stenosis

Fahrettin Oz, Fatih Tufan, Ahmet Ekmekci,
Omer A. Sayın and Huseyin Oflaz

Additional information is available at the end of the chapter

http://dx.doi.org/10.5772/54355

1. Introduction

There is a trend towards a worldwide aging in the last decades and diseases which are common in the elderly people would take important place in clinical practice. Although patients with aortic stenosis (AS) usually remain asymptomatic for a long time, once the classic triad of angina, syncope, and exertional dyspnea develop, the prognosis becomes dramatically worse. Accurate diagnosis and efficient treatment are getting more important as aortic valve replacement is the treatment of choice for severe AS.

We present a detailed description of the different therapeutic procedures that are being developed and increasingly used as an alternative to standard surgical treatment. However special surgical techniques as low-profile mechanical prosthesis, biological prosthesis (both stented and stentless), homograft and Ross technique (pulmonary autograft in aortic position and homograft in pulmonary position) will also be discussed in this chapter. We would also like to mention special considerations about treatment in special groups such as elderly.

2. Medical treatment

The standard therapy for symptomatic patients with severe aortic stenosis (AS) due to any cause is replacement of the valve. Since the prognosis dramatically worsens once the symptoms of AS develop, this is a late stage for an effective medical treatment. Patient education regarding the disease course and typical symptoms is an important priority. Current management of patients with AS comprises monitoring disease progression. Unfortunately, in patients with AS medical therapy may not prolong life nor improve progression and has limited utility in alleviating symptoms. Severe AS is adversely affected by changes in preload and afterload. In patients with severe AS, drugs that reduce preload or afterload should be used with caution because any medical treatment option used in these patients may worsen the patients' conditions. Meanwhile, there is a growing body of evidence about TAVI which is currently used mainly in patients with multi-morbidity and high surgical risk. In patients with rheumatic valve disease, rheumatic fever prophylaxis is strongly recommended to prevent repetitive valve scarring [1]. It has been hypothesized that some of the risk factors and pathophysiologic mechanisms in atherosclerosis play an important role in the development of calcific AS. Therefore theoretically, anti-inflammatory and anti-proliferative agents might slow or prevent disease progression. Because patients with severe AS are mostly older adults, some important and common issues like kidney insufficiency (KI), autonomic dysfunction, conduction disturbances, propensity to falls, and osteoporosis should always be kept in mind in the medical management of these patients.

2.1. Hypertension

Hypertension is not uncommon in patients with AS and approximately 40 percent of patients have hypertension [2]. In patients with concomitant hypertension and AS, left ventricular afterload is elevated as result of the "double-load" of increased systemic vascular resistance and valve stenosis [3]. For this reason reducing afterload may improve the degree of valvular opening and stroke volume. Therefore treatment of hypertension is recommended in patients with asymptomatic AS by many clinicians. There are a few studies assessing the safety of anti-hypertensive treatment in patients with AS [4]. Angiotensin converting enzyme (ACE) inhibitors seem to be well tolerated both in patients with mild-to-moderate and severe AS [5, 6]. Recently, ACE inhibitors and angiotensin receptor blockers (ARBs) were reported to be associated with improved survival and reduced cardiovascular (CV) events [7]. On the other hand, the recently published Simvastatin and Ezetimibe in Aortic Stenosis (SEAS) study reported an increased risk of CV events associated with antihypertensive treatment. However, this study was not a dedicated study on HT in AS and the only type of anti-hypertensive drug group associated with increased CV events was alpha-blockers [4]. This finding is in accordance with the results of Antihypertensive and Lipid-Lowering Treatment to Prevent Heart Attack Trial [8]. Blood pressure lowering agents should be initiated at low doses and gradually titrated with frequent monitoring, especially in older patients with increased risk of falls and osteoporotic fractures. Especially older patients given alpha blockers or diuretics should be informed about orthostatic hypotension to avoid falls.

2.2. Coronary artery disease

Coronary artery disease (CAD) is rather common in patients with AS and evaluation regarding conventional atherosclerotic risk factors is recommended in these patients. Tobacco use should be discouraged. The current US Preventive Services Task Force recommends usage of low dose aspirin for primary prevention when CV risk outweighs the risk of gastrointestinal hemorrhage in men between 45-79 years and when the risk of ischemic stroke outweighs the risk of gastrointestinal hemorrhage in women between 55-79 years [9]. It is also stated that the current evidence is insufficient to assess the balance of benefits and harms of aspirin in patients 80 years or older [9]. A recently published article reported the outcomes of percutaneous coronary intervention (PCI) in patients with concomitant severe AS and CAD [10]. In this well-matched trial, 30-day mortality after PCI was similar in patients with and without severe AS. In this study AS patients with low EF (≤30) and high Society of Thoracic Surgeons score (≥10) were associated with significantly increased 30-day mortality after PCI. Patients with mild AS should not be restricted from physical activity. Patients with severe AS should avoid competitive or vigorous activities that involve high dynamic and static muscular demands, although other forms of exercise are safe. Exercise may also improve functional capacity and may prevent skeletal muscle mass loss (i.e. sarcopenia).

2.3. Atrial fibrillation

Valvular heart disease, particularly left-sided valvular lesions precipitate the development of atrial fibrillation (AF). Although it has been less well studied in AS compared to mitral valve disorders, AF often complicates uncorrected aortic valve disorders [11]. In the recently published SEAS study, baseline or prior was present in approximately 9% of patients with mild-to-moderate AS [12]. The study excluded the patients with baseline and prior AF and sought the effect of simvastatin plus ezetimibe on new-onset AF. During an average of 4.3±0.8 years of follow up, 6% of the patients developed AF and the rate was similar between the simvastatin plus ezetimibe and placebo groups. In this study, increased age and left ventricular mass index were independent predictors of new onset AF. New-onset AF was associated with two-fold higher risk of AF related outcomes and four-fold higher risk of nonfatal nonhemorrhagic stroke. In a previously asymptomatic patient, new onset AF may cause overt heart failure symptoms due to the noncompliant left ventricle which is associated with a relative shift of left ventricular filling to the later part of diastole with a greater dependence upon atrial contraction. Similar treatment approaches for AF in patients with AS can be used as in patients without AS. Heart rate control is important to enable an adequate diastolic filling time. Although guidelines generally recommend rate control over rhythm control in patients with AS, there is a trend towards preference of rhythm control with the benefits of early rhythm control and options of left atrial catheter ablation and new anti-arrhythmic drugs [13, 14]. Within the current ECS guidelines on AF, severe AS is stated as a contraindication for verkalant usage [14]. It is also important to screen for coronary disease in patients with AS before the initiation of class Ic anti-arrhythmic drugs for rhythm control for AF [11]. Significant ventricular hypertrophy or dysfunction increases the risk of proarrhythmia associated with class Ic and most class III anti-arrhythmic drugs. In such patients amidodarone is the preferred agent [11]. However, when medications for heart rate control such as beta blockers and non-dihydropridine calcium channel blockers are used, their potential to depress LV systolic function and cause clinical deterioration should be kept in mind. Specific considerations about drug choices to control heart-rate are depicted in the following specific drug classes section. Specific considerations about warfarin treatment are depicted in the following specific drug classes section.

2.4. Heart failure

In patients with severe AS, aortic valve replacement (AVR) is indicated when symptomatic heart failure develops. Even when severe AS is present, transvalvular pressure gradients may not be found high because of left ventricular systolic dysfunction. Reduced EF is associated with worse clinical outcome. A recent study compared the outcomes of severe AS patients with an EF of ≤30 or >30 who was followed with medical treatment or underwent TAVI [15]. While an EF of ≤30 was associated with worse prognosis in the medically treatment group, TAVI was associated with an improvement in EF and functional class and patients who underwent TAVI had better prognoses irrespective of their baseline EF. When patients with mild or moderate AS have HF, there is generally other causes of HF like coronary heart disease and medical therapy of HF is preferable to AVR. Vasodilator therapy and beta blockers may be started with careful dose titration and closely monitoring. Volume status of patients should also be determined and followed up carefully [3, 16].

Invasive hemodynamic monitoring in the intensive care unit should be considered for decompensated patients with severe AS [3]. Nitroprusside rapidly and markedly improves cardiac function in patients with decompensated HF due to severe left ventricular systolic dysfunction and severe AS. It provides a safe and effective bridge to AVR or oral vasodilator therapy in these critically ill patients [17].

Phosphodiesterase type 5 inhibition had beneficial effects on pressure overload in preclinical models and a preliminary study of oral sildenafil in 20 patients with severe symptomatic AS showed that it was associated a reduction in systemic and pulmonary vascular resistance and pulmonary artery and wedge pressures [18]. Although sildenafil was also resulted in 11% decrease in mean systemic arterial pressure, it was not associated with any episodes of symptomatic hypotension.

2.5. Metabolic syndrome

Metabolic syndrome (MS) is a worldwide problem with increased risk of CV events. The results of Multi-Ethnic Study of Atherosclerosis (MESA) and another recent prospective trial suggest that MS is independently associated with progression of AS, particularly in younger individuals [19, 20]. Although these findings need to be confirmed in larger studies, studies assessing the effects of lifestyle modification and reduction of insulin resistance on the incidence and progression rate of AS could be of value.

2.6. Malnutrition

Malnutrition is a common and important health problem in the older adults and being underweight is associated with a worse prognosis than being overweight in this population [21]. Association of malnutrition and heart valve disorders is rarely reported in the literature. Otto et al reported increased long-term mortality independently associated with cachexia in 674 elderly patients who underwent balloon aortic valvuloplasty for AS [22]. Another observational study showed association of heart valve calcification with malnutrition in patients on hemodialysis [23]. In this study evaluation of malnutrition was done only with albumin level which is not specific for malnutrition. Wang et al demonstrated the correlation of fetuin-A, which has recently been identified as an important circulating inhibitor of calcification, with the presence and degree of malnutrition in patients on peritoneal dialysis [24].

There is also data indicating undernutrition is associated with worse outcomes after cardiac valve surgery. In a retrospective study, impact of BMI and albumin levels on morbidity and mortality after cardiac surgery was assessed in 5168 patients undergoing coronary artery bypass or valve operations [25]. Preoperative low albumin (<2.5 g/dl) and low BMI (<20 kg/m2) were independently associated with increased postoperative mortality. Tepsuwan et al. assessed the impact of cardiac cachexia retrospectively in 353 patients who underwent cardiac valve surgery [26]. The study population was relatively young and mitral stenosis and mitral regurgitation were the most frequent valve disorders. They found significant association between cachexia and worse New York Heart Association functional class and worse postoperative outcomes. Thourani et al investigated the impact of body mass index (BMI) on outcomes after cardiac valve surgery in 4247 patients [27]. Most of the procedures were isolated AVR (47.2%). They showed increased in-hospital and all-cause long-term mortality in patients with a BMI of less than 25 compared to patients with a BMI of 25-35 or higher than 35. In this study, no laboratory or clinical data about nutritional status was reported.

Patients with AS may suffer from dietary restriction due to reduced physical capacity and depressive mood. When concomitant mesenteric vessel atherosclerosis is present, abdominal angina may cause avoidance from eating. All these factors may render these patients susceptible to infectious diseases, osteoporosis, skeletal muscle loss (i.e. sarcopenia) and fall related fractures. Unfortunately, there is no study evaluating the role of nutritional intervention, which may potentially improve muscle and bone mass, muscle functions, and functional capacity, on clinical outcomes in patients with AS.

2.7. Depression

Later-life depression (LLD) is associated with disability and poor outcomes [28]. Among various chronic medical conditions, cardiac disease and arthritis are the most commonly ones associated with depression [29]. Underlying medical problems may affect the prognosis of depression and depression may decrease compliance to medical treatment thus delay recovery from medical illnesses [28]. The importance of screening for depression in patients with heart disease is well established, but identifying patients with depression may be difficult. Organic somatic symptoms possibly unrelated to mood may increase the score on depression scales and patients with depression may deny and do not report their depressive symptoms [28]. Furthermore, there are many shared symptoms of heart disease and depression like insomnia, fatigue, shortness of breath, weight loss, palpitations, and exercise intolerance. Vascular depression is associated with late onset, treatment-resistant symptoms, vascular disease, vascular risk factors, and extensive cerebrovascular lesions [28]. Although there is no specific data about the association of vascular depression and AS in the elderly, atherosclerosis has pivotal role in the pathogenesis of both.

Beta blocker treatment, which is being used commonly in patients with heart disease, may potentially precipitate depression. Although there is conflicting data about the association of beta blockers and depression, and individual susceptibility to depression may be important, patients with risk factors for depression should be followed up in terms of development of depression [30]. Lipophilic beta blockers like propranolol, timolol, pindolol, metoprolol, carvedilol and nebivolol are more strongly associated with depression than hydrophilic beta blockers like atenolol, nadolol, practolol and sotalol [30]. When there are strong indications like CAD and CHF for beta blocker treatment are present, depression should not be considered as an absolute contraindication. SSRI are among the most commonly used medications in the treatment of depression. There is some data that indicate use of SSRI in patients with CAD and depression may improve CV outcomes [31]. Because treatment with SSRI may reduce platelet functions as severe AS do, bleeding complications of surgical procedures may be increased in patients with severe AS under SSRI treatment. Sodium levels should be monitored in older patients under SSRI treatment, especially if concomitant diuretic use is present because both of them may be associated with hyponatremia.

2.8. Perioperative medical treatment

Careful manipulation of hemodynamics in the perioperative period is crucial in patients with AS [32]. Maintaining sinus rhythm, a relatively slow heart rate, and adequate preload and afterload are important goals to minimize the perioperative CV risk [32]. Ideal heart rate is between 60 and 70 beats per minute and bradicardia should be avoided. Careful assessment of hydration status and providing adequate hydration is also important to maintain preload which these patients are dependent upon. Careful monitoring of the arterial blood and central venous pressures is also important. Hypotension should be controlled with pure α agonists because they do not cause tachycardia. Routine antibiotic prophylaxis is not recommended unless the patient has a previous history of infective endocarditis [33]. Severe AS may be associated with markedly reduced platelet functions. One recent double-blind placebo controlled trial investigated effects of infusion of desmopressin (0.3 μg/kg) on platelet functions and postoperative blood loss [34]. The authors recommend assessing of platelet functions in the preoperative period in patients with severe AS and usage of desmopressin to avoid increased blood loss in patients with reduced platelet functions.

Delirium is rather common after cardiac valve surgery and is independently associated with increased risk of short and long term morbidity and mortality [35, 36]. Hyperactive delirium is easily recognized because of agitation, hallucinations and delusions. Routine assessment of attention and orientation is crucial to detect hypoactive delirium because it is easily and frequently overlooked. Providing adequate volume status, following up of renal functions and electrolyte levels, controlling postoperative pain and rational selection of medications may reduce the risk of delirium. Many drugs like anticholinergics, antihistaminics, narcotics and central acting drugs may precipitate delirium. Maldonado et al. investigated the effects of postoperative sedation on the development of delirium in patients undergoing cardiac valve surgery [35]. In this open label study, dexmedetomidine was associated with a significantly decreased rate of delirium with compared to propofol and midazolam (rates of delirium 3%, 50% and 50% respectively).

2.9. Perioperative medical treatment for non-cardiac surgery

Beta blocker treatment is recommended in patients with CAD or more than one of the cardiac risk factors which are listed in Table 1 [37]. However, the multicenter POISE trial showed an increased rate of death associated with perioperative beta blocker treatment despite a significant reduction in the primary composite endpoint of CV death, nonfatal MI or nonfatal cardiac arrest [38]. This trial resulted in the following recommendation in the current guidelines: "Routine administration of high-dose beta blockers in the absence of dose titration is not useful and may be harmful to patients not currently taking beta blockers who are undergoing noncardiac surgery" [37]. Titration of beta blockers to heart rate and blood pressure is recommended if the patient will undergo high- or intermediate-risk surgery [37]. Like it is recommended for many drug classes, starting beta blockers in low doses and careful titration is important in elderly patients who are at increased risk for bradycardia and hypotension. The role of beta blockers in intermediate- and low-risk patients is not well known. Optimal type, dose, timing, duration, and titration of beta blockers are also lacking [37]. Withdrawal of beta blockers in the preoperative period may be associated with adverse events and should not be performed unless necessary. Metformin and renin-angiotensin-aldosterone system (RAS) blockers increase the risk of postoperative lactic acidosis and KI respectively and it is recommended to stop them before the surgery.

History of ischemic heart disease
History of compensated or prior heart failure
History of cerebrovascular disease
Diabetes Mellitus
Renal insufficiency (defined as a preoperative serum creatinine of greater than 2 mg/dL)

Table 1. Clinical risk factors for perioperative cardiovascular complications

2.10. Specific drug classes

2.10.1. Statins

It has been considered that the valve lesion in calcific AS might share similar pathogenetic mechanisms with atherosclerosis and progression may be related to known atherosclerotic risk factors [39]. Statins are now well established in the primary and secondary prevention of CAD. Several studies have suggested that statins may cause regression of CAD and reduce the calcific volume of coronary plaques [40]. In accordance with this finding, presence and progression of aortic valve calcification are reported to be increased in patients with a serum LDL cholesterol >130 mg/dL [41].

While some earlier studies indicate that statin therapy is associated with a slower rate of hemodynamic progression of AS [42-45], some more recent trials have inconsistent results of different statin preparations on the progression of AS [46-49]. SALTIRE (Scottish aortic stenosis and lipid lowering therapy, impact on regression) trial was the first double blind randomized controlled trial of lipid lowering treatment in patients with calcific AS. This trial of 155 adults with calcific AS showed that, although atorvastatin 80 mg daily, more than halved serum LDL cholesterol concentrations, there was no difference in the rate of increase in aortic jet velocity or of progression of aortic valve calcification as measured by Doppler echocardiography or helical computed tomography [46]. The prospective open-label RAAVE study (The Rosuvastatin Affecting Aortic Valve Endothelium) comprised of 121 consecutive patients with moderate to severe AS. Treatment with rosuvastatin 20 mg was given when LDL-cholesterol was greater than 130 mg/dL and no statin therapy was given when LDL-cholesterol was less than 130 mg/dL. Patients treated with rosuvastatin had significantly attenuated rates of deterioration in mean aortic valve area and aortic jet velocity compared to patients who did not receive rosuvastatin [47]. The prospective and placebo controlled SEAS trial sought the effect of statins on calcific AS. In this study, 1873 adults (mean age 68) with mild-to-moderate AS were enrolled and randomly assigned to treatment with simvastatin plus ezetimibe or placebo [48]. At median follow-up of 52 months there were no differences in the peak aortic jet velocity or valve area noted between the 2 groups. There was also no difference in CV death, aortic valve replacement, non-fatal myocardial infarction, hospitalized unstable angina pectoris, and heart failure due to progression of AS, coronary artery bypass grafting, percutaneous coronary interventions, or non-hemorrhagic stroke. Although there were fewer ischemic events in the treatment group, this difference was only due to a lower rate of coronary bypass grafting at the time of aortic valve surgery so the clinical relevance of this finding is unclear. SEAS study results show that the effect of statin therapy on disease process does not provide convincing evidence [48]. The investigators of SEAS study recently reported the results of simvastatin plus ezetimibe on new-onset AF in 1421 patients with asymptomatic mild-to-moderate AS [6]. The rate of new-onset AF was similar in the simvastatin plus ezetimibe group compared to placebo group. Aortic Stenosis Progression Observation (ASTRONOMER) is the most recently published trial regarding effect of statins on AS. This double-blind prospective trial randomized 269 younger asymptomatic patients with mild to-moderate AS with no indications for lipid-lowering agents to rosuvastatin 40 mg daily (134 patients) or placebo (135 patients). Unlike earlier trials in which bicuspid aortic valve was rare, a bicuspid valve was present in nearly half of the subjects in this study. After a mean follow-up of 3.5 years, there were no significant differences in the transaortic gradient or aortic valve area in the rosuvastatin group compared to placebo [49].

At present, if atherosclerotic vascular disease or other indications do not coexist, statin therapy solely for AS cannot be recommended. It should be noted that effect of therapy has not been evaluated in earlier stages of the disease.

2.10.2. Angiotensin converting enzyme inhibitors

Although expression of angiotensin II has not been shown the in normal valves, sclerotic aortic valve tissues demonstrably express angiotensin II and angiotensin converting enzyme (ACE). Therefore it may contribute to valve inflammation, calcification, and disease progression [50]. It has been shown that ACE inhibitors suppress ventricular fibrosis and inhibit angiotensin II

http://dx.doi.org/10.5772/54355

type 1 receptor in the cardiomyocytes and therefore decrease systolic and diastolic dysfunction in patients with left ventricular hypertrophy and AS [51]. For these reasons ACE inhibitors may have a role in the management of patients with AS. Two preliminary observational studies examined the effect of ACE inhibitors in patients with AS in preventing further changes in the valve leaflets. Rosenhek et al showed that hemodynamic progression of AS did not occur in 211 patients with moderate AS after at least 6 months of treatment with the ACE inhibitors. Furthermore, the presence of hypertension did not appear to influence the outcome [44]. Another retrospective study by Obrien et al of 123 patients evaluated the aortic valve calcium score by electron beam computed tomographic scans. The study showed that ACE inhibitor treatment was associated with a 71% reduction in the progression of aortic valve calcification in 123 patients with AS [52]. At the present, there are no published randomized prospective studies using ACE inhibitors to delay the progression of calcific AS. Some potential targets for therapy in AS such as the pathways involved in inflammation and tissue calcification have not yet been studied. ACE inhibitors have beneficial effects on ventricular systolic and diastolic functions and are well tolerated, increase exercise capacity, and reduce dyspnea in symptomatic patients with mild to moderate AS [6]. ACE inhibitors may provide symptomatic relief when patients with severe AS who are not good candidates for surgery develop symptoms of left heart failure. It should also be kept in mind that ACE inhibitors may increase the transvalvular gradient by reducing afterload or preload and cause sudden clinical deterioration in patients with severe AS. In older adults, ACE inhibitors should be initiated at low doses and gradually increased to avoid hypotension and fall related fractures. Because elderly patients with severe AS generally have extensive atherosclerosis, before initiation of ACE inhibitors bilateral renal artery stenosis should be considered and investigated if suspected.

2.10.3. Angiotensin receptor blockers

Angiotensin receptor blockers have similar hemodynamic effects like ACE inhibitors. A recently published observational study indicates that both ACE inhibitors and ARBs are associated with lower mortality and CV events in patients with AS [7]. However, prospective and controlled studies are needed to test this finding. Although similar precautions as in ACE inhibitors should be considered when starting and maintaining ARBs, they have some benefits like less incidence of cough. Because compelling evidence does not exist for neither ACE inhibitors nor ARBs for these patients, when RAS blockage is planned ACE inhibitors may be selected in the first step and switching to ARBs may be considered if adverse effects like chronic cough develop.

2.10.4. Beta blockers

Beta blockers are a not part of routine medical treatment. Because beta blockers may aggravate the symptoms of HF, patients with symptoms and signs of HF are not good candidates for this treatment option. Beta blockers may be used in AS patients with angina pectoris or AF with rapid ventricular response. Because older adults are at increased risk for hypotension, bradycardia, conduction disturbances and diabetes, a close follow-up should be performed when patients with AS are given beta blocker treatment.

2.10.5. Diuretics

Diuretics are not indicated in patients without signs of congestion because of their potential for reducing preload, which may lead to fall in cardiac output and exacerbation in symptoms of HF. Therefore, diuretics are not first-line treatment options in hypertensive patients with severe AS without findings of congestion. Diuretics may improve symptoms of HF by reducing left ventricular end-diastolic pressure in patients with lung congestion, ascites or edema. Older patients may not excrete free water effectively, and they may more easily develop hyponatremia after diuretic treatment [53]. Thiazide diuretics cause hyponatremia more frequently than loop diuretics [54]. These older patients also have increased tendency to diuretic induced hyponatremia, because concomitant use of other medications like selective serotonin reuptake inhibitors (SSRI), which precipitate hyponatremia, is common. Because of disruption of normal circadian rhythm of antidiuretic hormone, nocturia is frequently seen in elderly patients and may be bothersome and increase the risk of falls when evening or night doses of diuretics are used [55]. Administration of diuretics in earlier hours of the day may be safer. Patients with urgency incontinence may need urinary anti-cholinergics under diuretic treatment to avoid urgency induced falls and significant physical exertion. Diuretics also lead to orthostatic hypotension by inducing volume depletion. Because falls are more frequent and are associated with great morbidity and mortality in these older patients, monitoring of blood pressure at home and avoidance of hypotension is crucial.

2.10.6. Nitrates

Nitrates may be used in symptomatic treatment of angina pectoris in patients with severe AS. They should be initiated at low doses and gradually increased to avoid sudden hypotension. Concomitant use of phosphodiesterase inhibitors for erectile dysfunction should be avoided to prevent substantial hypotension.

2.10.7. Digoxin

Digoxin has a narrow therapeutic index and the risk of adverse events associated with it may be more common in older patients [56]. Digoxin levels may be increased in older patients with impaired kidney functions. Because creatinine levels may be normal or minimally increased in older adults with impaired kidney functions when significant loss of muscle mass (i.e. sarcopenia) is present. It is recommended in the recent ACC/AHA guideline that an initial dose of 0.125 mg daily or every other day is chosen if the patient is older than 70 years old, has impaired kidney function, or has a low lean body mass [57]. Digoxin above 0.125 mg/d is also listed among the potentially inappropriate medications (PIMs) list in the recent Beers criteria [58]. Because digoxin concentrations above 1 ng/ml are not associated with better clinical outcomes and may adversely increase morbidity and mortality, a target digoxin concentration of 0.5-1 ng/ml is recommended despite conventional therapeutic serum concentration is defined as 0.8-2 ng/ml [56, 57]. When there is concomitant hypokalemia, hypomagnesemia or hypothyroidism, digoxin toxicity may occur in lower concentrations [57]. Older patients under digoxin treatment may develop adverse effects like anorexia, nausea, vomiting, confusion, visual problems, and rhythm and conduction disturbances more commonly [56]. Clarithro-

http://dx.doi.org/10.5772/54355

mycin, erythromycin, amiodarone, itraconazole, cyclosporine, verapamil, and quinidine can increase serum digoxin concentrations [57]. Digoxin should not be used in patients with severe AS and sinus rhythm. Digoxin may be used to reduce the ventricular rate in patients with AF and a rapid ventricular rate especially when hemodynamic deterioration is present. When these harms are taken into consideration, should be used with caution as an adjunctive agent for heart rate control. Alternatively, beta blockers, which are associated with improved survival in patients with HF and may effectively control heart rate alone, may be used as first line agents in these patients. However, when hypotension and significant HF signs are present, digoxin may be a better agent for symptomatic treatment.

2.10.8. Calcium channel blockers

Although published data regarding anti-hypertensive drugs in patients with AS is limited, calcium channel blockers like amlodipine do not appear to depress LV function and may be safe to use in patients with AS. Non-dihydropridine agents like diltiazem and verapamil may influence left ventricular systolic functions and may cause clinical deterioration.

2.10.9. Alpha blockers

Peripheral alpha blocker use may possibly lead to hypotension or syncope, decreased coronary perfusion due to reduced afterload and should generally be avoided. Alpha blockers are listed among the PIMs in the recent Beers criteria and routine use for the treatment of hypertension is not recommended [58]. Alpha blockers are also listed among the PIMs in patients with a history of syncope [58].

2.10.10. Warfarin

Warfarin treatment is generally recommended in patients with AS and AF to decrease the incidence of stroke and systemic arterial embolism. Assessing the risk of embolism associated with AF and bleeding associated with warfarin treatment should be carefully performed. It is very important to educate the patient and his/her relatives about the benefits and risks of warfarin treatment and the details of follow-up. Integration of the patients' relatives in the treatment plan is crucial especially in older adults with significant cognitive problems. A meta-analysis which was published in 2007 indicated that aspirin was associated with a 22% reduction in the rate of stroke, while warfarin was associated with 64% reduction [59]. Because warfarin is associated with a significantly lower risk of stroke than aspirin, simply prescribing aspirin without discussing the benefits and risks of warfarin treatment with the patients and their relatives would be therapeutic nihilism. Although there are newer anticoagulant medications like dabigatran which do not require therapeutic monitoring, we need more data especially in the older individuals in order to prescribe them instead of warfarin. For instance, dabigatran is associated with greater risk of bleeding than with warfarin in patients $\geq$ 75 years and efficacy and safety is not known in patients with a creatinine clearance below 30 ml/min [58].

Warfarin is also the drug of choice in patients with AVR with mechanical prostheses. To date there is no alternative for warfarin for these patients and a higher international normalized ratio (2.5-3.5) is targeted. This translates into increased risk of bleeding associated with warfarin especially in the older patients. These patients may also have other bleeding risk factors like concurrent anti-platelet, SSRI or ginkgo biloba use and platelet dysfunction associated with KI or significant AS. Whether warfarin treatment is appropriate for the patient, may even determine if AVR might be performed and if a mechanical prosthesis might be used. Patients, in whom warfarin treatment is planned, should also be carefully assessed about the risk of falls which may lead to significant bleeding, most importantly to intracranial hemorrhage. If warfarin is started, ensuring precautions by educating the patients and their relatives to avoid falls is also crucial.

3. Transcathater aortic valve implantation

Surgical AVR is currently the gold-standard treatment for patients with severe symptomatic AS. Without surgery, the prognosis is extremely poor, with a 3-year survival rate of <30%.However, in the huge Euro Heart multinational registry in Europe, 33% of symptomatic patients over the age of 65 years were not referred for surgery [60]. The reasons for not planning surgery were not always the co morbidities. David Bach's series showed the same issue and 33% of symptomatic patients were not referred for surgery, some of whom had a low Euro Score risk [61]. Balloon aortic valvuloplasty, which was described in the 1980s, was the first alternative to surgical therapy [62]. Despite high rates of initial procedural success, restenosis is frequently encountered in the long term. The procedure has generally been abandoned in adult patients except as a palliative procedure often prior to surgical AVR [63]. Trans-catheter aortic valve implantation (TAVI) was first described by Andersen et al in 1992 [64]. They implanted an expandable aortic valve by a catheter technique in a closed chest pig model. The first attempt to use TAVI in man was in 2002 by Cribier et al [65]. A percutaneous bioprosthesis was successfully implanted within the diseased native aortic valve through an antegrade trans-septal approach. In more recent years, the technology has developed very rapidly and, to date, more than 40,000 transcathater valves have been implanted worldwide. The results of several large multicenter registries and randomized Placement of Aortic Transcathater Valves (PARTNER) trial, TAVI is now the standard of care for extremely high risk or 'inoperable ' patients and is a valid alternative to surgery for selected high-risk but ' operable ' patients with symptomatic AS [66-68].

Patients might be considered candidates for TAVI if they fulfill the following criteria: symptomatic severe AS, a life expectancy of >1year, contraindications for surgery, high risk for surgery (clinical judgment plus Euro Score (logistic) >20%; STS Score>10%), and/or porcelain aorta, history of thoracic irradiation, severe thoracic deformity, patent coronary bypass, cachexia, recurrent pulmonary emboli, right ventricular insufficiency and cirrhosis.

Contraindications for TAVI are as follows: an aortic annulus of <18 mm or >27 mm, bicuspid valves or unicuspid or noncalcified valve, severe aortic regurgitation or mitral regurgitation, estimated life expectancy < 12 months, evidence of an acute myocardial infarction within one month, MRI confirmed CVA within six months, ejection fraction < 20 %, heavy calcification in front of LM, presence of LV thrombus and need for CABG

Risk Estimation: Accurate estimation of the risk of SAVR performed by an experienced cardiothoracic surgeon and cardiologist is vital to appropriate evaluation of potential candidates for TAVI. Some risk score algorithms like Ambler score, logistic EuroSCORE and Society of Thoracic Surgeons Predicted Risk of Mortality (STS-PROM) are widely used to identify patients at high risk for cardiac surgery. Ambler score was dedicated to predict in-hospital mortality after heart valve surgery [69]. EuroSCORE integrates increased age, female gender, chronic pulmonary disease, extracardiac arteriopathy, neurological dysfunction, previous cardiac surgery, increased serum creatinine, active endocarditis, critical perioperative state, unstable angina, LV dysfunction, recent MI, and pulmonary hypertension as patient and cardiac related factors and some operation related factors like emergency, other than isolated CABG, surgery on thoracic aorta, and postinfarct septal rupture. An online calculator is available in their official website (http://www.euroscore.org/). Logistic EuroSCORE appears to overestimate mortality risk in patients undergoing high-risk aortic valve replacement. The STS-PROM risk scoring which is more complicated integrates age, gender, race, weight, creatinine level, various chronic cardiac and non-cardiac diseases, previous cardiovascular interventions, perioperative cardiac status, hemodynamic status, and operative risk factors. This scoring estimates the rates of postoperative morbidity, mortality, permanent stroke, prolonged ventilation, renal failure, and reoperation. It is updated regularly and calculation can be performed only via the online calculator (http://www.sts.org/). However the STS-PROM model may provide more accurate risk stratification than other scores, more appropriate scoring systems are not currently available. In clinical practice, it seems reasonable that high –risk patients should be evaluated using clinical judgment and a combination of several scores [70, 71].

4. Overview of procedure

4.1. Approaches used for TAVI

Stented valves placed either transapically or percutaneously are garnering much attention. In the percutaneous approach, the valve is deployed either antegradely via the transseptal route,or retrogradely across the native aortic valve.

Transfemoral Approach: The transfemoral approach is simper and quick to access the aortic valve. This route is the first choice of approach in the vast majority of centers performing TAVI procedures. Although surgical cutdown was the technique used for the transfemoral approach at the beginning of the TAVI experience, most centers are now using a fully percutaneous technique. The aortic valve is corossed and a stiff wire is placed in the LV with a large loop. Within these procedures, firstly balloon aortic valvotomy is undertaken and a stented bioprosthesis is then deployed over a balloon intothe aortic annulus. Inflation of the balloon anchors the valve in place in the annulus,effectively achieving AVR. Some specific contraindications for transfemoral approach are; narrow peripheral arteries (diameter < 8-9 mm), severe tortuousity or calcification, history of aorto-femoral by pass, aneurysm of abdominal aorta with thrombosis, and severe atheroma of the arch.

Transapical approach: Transapical approach necessitates a thoracotomy but the valve is deployed into the beating heart and extracorporeal circulation is not performed. This approach is particularly suited to patients with severe peripheral artery disease and heavily calcified ascending aorta and arch. The transapical approach includes the following other benefit: no stored tension in the delivery system, more reliable device control and feedback and no size limitations. The main disadvanteges are the need for thoracotomy; a greater degree of myocardial injury and the potentially life threating bleeding complications associated with the surgical repair.

Subclavian Approach: A subclavian approach allows patient with unfavorable iliofemoral artery anatomy or extensive disease to be treated with TAVI. A surgical cutdown is needed to isolate the subclavian artery. However no specific complications for subclavian access reported, any injury of the subclavian artery would translate into a major intrathoracic bleeding that might be difficult control.

Transaortic approach: In 2009 and 2010, transaortic approach with direct access to the ascending aorta though an anterior minithorocatomy has been advocated. Altough requiring sternotomy, avoidance of LV apical injury and avoidance of the use of large cathaters are potential advantages of this novel approach.

4.2. TAVI systems and placement

Currently two valve systems are approved for TAVI: the balloon expandable Edwards valve-the first generation Cribier-Edwards, second generation Edwards SAPİEN, and the third generation Edwards SAPIEN XT versions and the self expandable CoreValve (Medtronic CV) system.

The EdwardsSAPİEN System consists of a trileaflet pericardial bovine valve mounted in a stainless steel,and it is available in three sizes: 23 mm, 26 mm and 29 mm for transfemoral, transapical and subclavian approaches [Fig1]. The third generation SAPİEN XT calve is available in 20 mm, 23 mm, and 29 mm sizes and is introduced via an 18 F sheath.

The CoreValve ReValving System consist of three porcine pericardial leaflets mounted in a self expandable nitinol frame housed within a percutaneus delivery catheter. This system is available two sizes, 26 mm and 29 mm. The valve is introduced via an 18 F sheath [Fig 2].

Balloon aortic valvuloplasty is systematically performed before valve implantation to facilitate passage of the prosthesis through the stenotic native valve. Although, Grube at al. have suggested direct implantation of the CoreValve system with no prior balloon valvuloplasty [72]. The balloon expandable valve is positioned using fluoroscopy and echocardiography, and ventricular burst pacing is used at balloon inflation to decrease transvalvular flow and avoid expulsion of the system toward the aorta. The self-expandable valve is deployed without burst pacing, by the retracting the outer sheath of the delivery catheter.

http://dx.doi.org/10.5772/54355

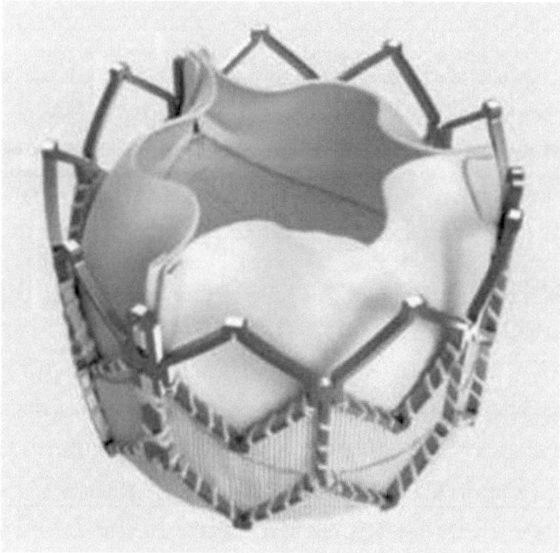

Figure 1. The EDWARS SAPİEN system

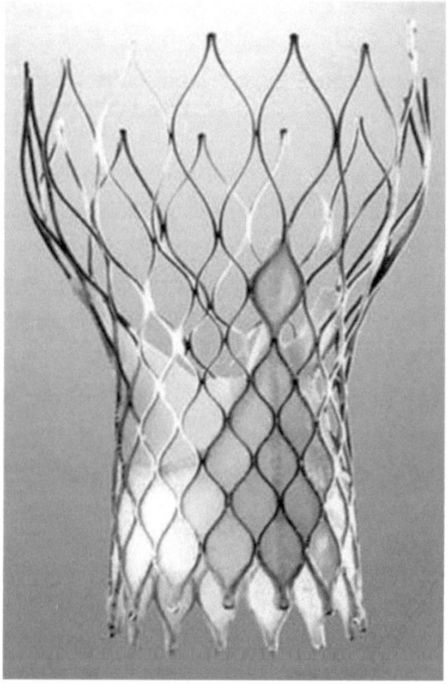

Figure 2. The CoreValve ReValving System

5. Outcomes

Overall, the procedural success rate was >90% in all studies. Valve embolization or conversion to open heart surgery occurred in ~1% of the patients (0.3–3.0% for valve embolization; 0.5–2.3% for conversion to open heart surgery) [73].

5.1. Mortality

In the multicenter registries and series, mortality was systematically <10% in patients treated using the transfemoral approach and ranged from 11.3% to 16.9% in patients treated using the transapical approach, probably owing to the higher risk profile of the patients treated via the latter route [73-74].At 1-year follow-up, the survival rates were ~80% (75–85%) for the transfemoral approach and ~70% (63–78%) for the transapical approach.

As the first of two parallel trials was completed, the results of PARTNER IB showed that TF TAVI was superior to standard therapy in patients not deemed candidates for surgery [73]. The primary endpoint of all-cause mortality was markedly reduced by 46% (P, 0.001). Recently reported 2-year outcomes showed continued encouraging results. At 2 years, the primary endpoint of all-cause mortality was reduced from 67.6% in the standard treatment arm to 43.3% in the TAVI arm (P, 0.001). The PARTNER cohort IA compared TAVI with SAVR and met its non-inferiority endpoint: the all-cause 1-year mortality in the TAVI group was non-inferior to the SAVR group (24.2 vs. 26.8%;P: 0.44; P: 0.001 for non-inferiority) [74]. Some concerns were raised with regard to neurologic events that were somewhat higher with TAVI than SAVR at 30 days (5.5 vs. 2.4%; P: 0.04) and 1 year (8.3 vs. 4.3%; P: 0.04). Although the recently published 2-year results showed that stroke rates were similar for TAVI and SAVR during 1 and 2 years with a hazard ratio of 1.22 (95% CI 0.67–2.23, P: 0.52), the issue of stroke warrants further investigation and should not be underestimated The rate of the composite of all-cause death and stroke was encouragingly nearly identical after TAVI (37.1%) and SAVR (36.4%) at 2 years (P: 0.85)[73-74]

Predictors of mortality — Risk factors for early and late mortality were identified in a study of 663 patients undergoing TAVR with CoreValve. Intraprocedural mortality was 0.9 percent. Mortality was 5.4 percent at 30 days and 15 percent at one year. Independent predictors of mortality at 30 days included certain procedural complications (conversion to open heart surgery, cardiac tamponade, major vascular or access site complications) as well as baseline characteristics (left ventricular ejection fraction <40 percent, prior balloon valvuloplasty, and diabetes mellitus). Independent predictors of mortality between 30 days and one year included prior stroke, postprocedural paravalvular leak ≥2+, prior acute pulmonary edema, and chronic kidney disease.

Indeed, in the past few years, 1-year survival rates from some registries have been reported to be ≥80%, and we can expect better survival rates at the 2-year and 3-year follow-ups in the coming years. Importantly, no structural failures of the transcatheter valves have been seen in studies with a follow-up of more than 1 year [73-74].

In addition to baseline and procedural factors, the learning-curve phenomenon and the improvements in valve prosthesis and delivery catheters have also been associated with a substantial improvement in the results obtained with TAVI.

5.2. Symptom improvement

Three-year follow-up data have been published and are consistent with lasting improvement in cardiac symptoms [72]. While 86% of patients were in NYHA class III or IV at baseline, 93%

of surviving patients were in NYHA class I/II at 3-year follow-up. Similarly, the PARTNER trial showed that patients treated with TAVI compared with patients treated with standard medical therapy have better symptom control at 1 year. Indeed, the 1-year rate of NYHA class III or IV was 25.2% for the TAVI group compared with 58.0% for the standard medical therapy group (P, 0.001).

6. Complications

Stroke: The occurrence of stroke is one of the most –fearing complication of TAVI. The most frequent etiology of procedural stroke is likely to be atheroembolism from the ascending aorta or the aortic arh. Other several factors include manipulation of a wire, positioning of device, performance of the balloon aortic valvuloplasty, air embolism, dissection of the arc vessels and inadequate blood flow to brain during rapid pacing. Reported 30 day stroke rate was 3.5 (ranging from 1.2% to 6.7%) [76]. Additionaly Kahlert et al observed that using diffusion-weighed MRI has underlined this issue, demonstrating multiple embolic cerebral lesion in all patients after TAVI. Although most of these lesions were clinically silent, silent cerebral infarcts are associated with subtle cognitive change. Efforts have been directed towards prevention of stroke. Procedural anticoagulation to reach a target activated clotting time over 250 s is suggested. Empiric dual antiplatelet therapy is recommended for 3 to 6 months followed by long-term daily low dose aspirin. Additionally less traumatic valve delivery system and embolic protection devices (Embrella embolic deflector system) currently under devolepment might lower the risk of stroke. However some authors have suggested that stroke risk might be lower with transapical access, this has not been a universal finding.

Vascular Complication: Common vascular complication arterial dissection, closure device failure, arterial stenosis, haematoma in the accsess site. Artery avulsion, vessel perforation, annulus rupture represent more severe complications which are fatal if not rapidly treated. In the SOURCE registry, 10.6 % of patients had major vascular complication and major vascular complications were less frequent in the transapical approach (2.4 %) [73-74]. Small vessel diameter, severe atherosclerosis, bulky calcification, and tortusosity are the main determinats of vascular complications. In the future delivery catheter and sheath size will likely decrease which should be associated with reductions in the risk of vascular injury. Additionally, for patients with unsuitable access, alternatives include apical, axillar/subclavian or transaortic approaches, or treatment of iliofemoral lesion with stents or grafts.

Coronary obstruction and myocardial infarction: Coronary ostia obstruction (especially of the left main coronary artery) might occur if an obstructive portion of the valve frame or the sealing cuff is placed directly over a coronary ostium however this is very rare but potentially fatal event [77]. Some cases may require immediate coronary angioplasty or coronary artery bypass graft operation. TAVI has been associated with a variable rate of myocardial infarction, ranging from 0% to 16.3% [73-74] Myocardial infarction could be explained by myocardial tissue compression, hypotension due to rapid pacing, atheroembolism and mechanic complication such as coronary ostia obstruction. Additionally myocardial infarction was associated with an increased cardiac mortality at midterm follow up

Heart Block: High grade atrioventricular block and consecutive pacemaker implantation are frequent (especially in CoreValve) complications following TAVI. CoreValve implantation is associated with a need for permanent pacemaker in 20 % of patients compared with in 5 % of patients implanted with the balloon expandable valves [78]. Potential risk factors include aggressive over sizing, low implantation of the prosthesis, small annulus diameter, using CoreValve and the presence of preexisting infranodal block such as RBBB [79, 80].

Cardiogenic Schock and low cardiac output: This complication may be induced by ischemia, rapid pacing, volume depletion, anesthesia and interruption in cardiac output during valve implantation. Vasopresor agents and intraaortic balloon support to maintain adequate perfusion pressure are often helpful. Rarely elective femoral cardiopulmonary bypass is an option for patients at hemodynamic instability.

Paravalvuler Regurgitation: However paravalvuler aortic regurgitation is common, occurring in about 85 %, Grade > 2 + regurgitation is found in 7-24 % [72,73].Trivial, mild and even moderate degrees of regurgitation seem well tolerated, although grade > 2+ regurgitation associated with increased short and long term mortality [81]. Causes of paravalvular regurgitation include a heavily calcified annulus,large annulus size, an undersized prosthesis, device failure and inadequate balloon aortic valvuloplasty. Redilatation or implantation of a second, overlapping transcathater valve can often correct the problem.

Acute Kidney Injury: Angiographic contrast injection, hypotension, atheroembolism, periprocedural blood transfusion might contribute to acute renal failure. The incidence of acute kidney injury after TAVI has been reported with incidence of 8 %. Additionally need for hemodialysis has ranged from 1.4% to 15.7 %, respectively [82]. Predictors of acute kidney injury include hypertension, decrease baseline renal function, previous myocardial infarction, high logistic EuroSCORE and chronic obstructive pulmonary disease [83].

Other Complication: Other significant and very rare complications include aortic rupture, aortic dissection, periaortic hematoma, ventricular or aortic embolization of valve, structural valve failure, cardiac tamponade and acute mitral regurgitation due to mitral valve apparatus damage [73-74].

Valve-in-valve — A valve-in-valve procedure involves catheter-based valve implantation inside an already implanted bioprosthetic valve. This approach may provide an alternative to replacement of a degenerated surgically-implanted valve, or a means of salvaging suboptimal implantation of a catheter-based valve during the initial implantation procedure.

Conclusion: Despite continual technical advancement of TAVI devices and procedures, the combined mortality and morbidity is still high in the range of 5-10%, especially when we are facing a group of high surgical risk patients. In addition TAVR offered no survival benefit compared to standard therapy in patients with an STS score of > 15 % because of high degree of comorbid conditions in these patients. In the future when it is a safer and more reliable procedure and further refinement of the device (i.e. smaller size delivery systems and multiple valve size options) is done, utilization of the procedure in patients with lower surgical risk may be possible.

7. Surgery

In 1912, Theodore Tuffier was the first to attempt opening AS using his finger. Russel Brock and then Bailey used dilatators for stenotic aortic valves. Today more than 1000 patients have aortic valve surgery per year and surgery for AS is more common than it is for aortic insufficiency [84]. Aortic valve surgery has been improved with the developments of new technologies in cardiopulmonary bypass techniques and valve industry. Approximately 2% to 5% of elderly individuals aged 75 years present with signs of severe AS and they are scheduled for elective AVR. AVR is the treatment of choice for patients with severe degenerative AS, offering both symptomatic relief and a potential for improved long term survival [85].

It's obvious that AVR is indicated in all symptomatic patients and asymptomatic patients with severe AS undergoing open heart surgery. The surgery should immediately be programmed if the patient becomes symptomatic. Despite LV dysfunction, the risk of aortic valve replacement for AS was satisfactory and related to meanaortic gradient and additional coronary artery disease, and long-term survival was related to also coronary disease and cardiac output [86].

5-year survival for adults after aortic valve replacement is 80-90%. The results of the conventional surgery for octogenarians are also satisfactory and 5% to 10% of mortality is noted for isolated AVR (2). On the other hand, elderly patients stay longer in the hospitals and intensive care units during the postoperative period [87]. United Kingdom heart valve registry observed 1100 elderly patients (56% women) who underwent AVR that the 30-day mortality was 6.6% [88]. The actuarial survival was 89% at 1 year, 79% at 3 years, 69% at 5 years, and 46% at 8 years. The mortality is rising up to 10% per year for the patient becoming symptomatic. The indications for AVR in patients with AS according to the current ACC/AHA guidelines are listed in Table 2 [89]. Although the surgery for the asymptomatic patients is preferred due to sudden death, surgery for asymptomatic octogenarians is controversial. The complex cardiac procedures have high risks for elderly patients.

The mortality rate of valve surgery and risk of sudden death without surgery have to be carefully considered. Postoperatively symptoms diminish and quality of life is improved in the majority of patients ≥75 years who had undergone aortic valve surgery, but long term survival was not affected [90].

AVR usually performed under general anesthesia using conventional techniques of open heart surgery with median sternotomy. Minimally invasive surgery has continued to be an evolving concept after the first publication of Cosgrove in 1996 [91] Minimally invasive procedures are associated with acceptable mortality and morbidity rates even in high risk patients. 30-day in-hospital mortality was 0.8% for 1,103 minimally invasive aortic valve procedures [92].

The major advantages of minimally access surgeries are improved cosmesis with reduced insicion size, decreased surgical trauma, less pain, better respiratory function and early return to work [92].

These procedures can be performed through different approaches. These are upper mini sternotomy, transverse sternotomy and right parasternal or anterolateral mini thoracotomy,

Class I
AVR is indicated for symptomatic patients with severeAS.* *(Level of Evidence: B)*
AVR is indicated for patientswith severe AS* undergoing coronaryartery bypass graft surgery(CABG). *(Level of Evidence: C)*
AVR is indicated for patientswith severe AS* undergoing surgeryon the aorta or other heartvalves. *(Level of Evidence: C)*
AVR is recommended for patientswith severe AS* and LV systolicdysfunction (ejection fractionless than 0.50). *(Level of Evidence: C)*
Class IIa
AVR is reasonable for patients with moderate AS*undergoingCABG or surgery on the aorta or other heart valves(see Section3.7 on combined multiple valve disease and Section10.4 on AVRin patients undergoing CABG). *(Level of Evidence: B)*
Class IIb
AVR may be considered for asymptomatic patientswith severeAS* and abnormal response to exercise (e.g., developmentofsymptoms or asymptomatic hypotension). *(Level of Evidence: C)*
AVR may be considered for adults with severe asymptomaticAS* if there is a high likelihood of rapid progression (age,calcification, and CAD) or if surgery might be delayed at thetime of symptom onset. *(Level of Evidence: C)*
AVR may beconsidered in patients undergoing CABG who havemild AS* whenthere is evidence, such as moderate to severevalve calcification,that progression may be rapid. *(Level of Evidence: C)*
AVRmay be considered for asymptomatic patients with extremelysevereAS (aortic valve area less than 0.6 cm^2, mean gradientgreaterthan 60 mm Hg, and jet velocity greater than 5.0 m persecond)when the patient's expected operative mortalityis 1.0%or less. *(Level of Evidence: C)*
Class III
AVR is not useful for the prevention of sudden deathin asymptomaticpatients with AS who have none of the findingslisted underthe class IIa/IIb recommendations. *(Level of Evidence: B)*

Table 2. Indications for Aortic Valve Replacement.

using port access technique or not. Although mini sternotomy is the most common approach, the outcomes after right anterior thoracotomy have satisfactory results [93]. The arterial cannulation sites are either aorta or femoral artery. The venous cannulation sites are right atrium, femoral vein or percutanous supeior vena cava with femoral vein. The incisions differ from 5 to 10 cm and small incisions may provide low infection rates [94]. This procedure has advantages such as less 1 surgical trauma, decreased pain and faster recovery. It reduces blood transfusions and shortens the length of hospital and ICU stay [95]. It is a safe operation and results lower incidence of atelectasis inthe cardiac ICU [96]. Port access aortic surgery also allows patients to be extubated earlier [97]. Avoidance of full sternotomy for patients prompts a comfortable postoperative period. Although the number of the aortic valve procedures increase worldwide, the ideal valve choice is still a debate. There are several options for valves. These are mechanical valve prosthesis, stented and stentless bioprosthetic valves, aortic homograft and pulmonary autograft. The use of these valves differs from patient to patient due to comorbidities and anticoagulant needs. The bioprosthetic valves are good alternatives for elderly patients and women who want to be pregnant because long term anticoagulation use is not required. The other situation for the patients undergoing AVR is the injurious effects of Cardiopulmonary bypass to the life organs. This results as a systemic inflammatory response and this may affect the post-operative course of the patients. Paroxysmal or chronic AF is a risk factor for mortality in patients with severe AS and a LVEF <35% undergoing AVR. Of 83 elderly patients with severe AS and an LVEF <35%, 29 (35%) had paroxysmal or chronic AF [86]. The perioperative mortality was 24% in the group with AF versus 5,5% in the group without AF.

The Ross procedure is another surgical technique for aortic valve replacement. This is more commonly used in pediatric cases but also good alternative for especially young adult patients and women want have child. In this operation the patient's own pulmonary valve and main pulmonary artery are used as an autograft and they are implanted to the aortic position, with reimplantation of coronary arteries.

The primary indication for the Ross procedure is to provide a permanent valve replacement among younger patients who will grow potentially. Other possible indications include complex left ventricular outflow obstructive disease, native or prosthetic valve endocarditis, and adult aortic insufficiency with a dilated aortic annulus [98].

One of the most commonly seen complications of Ross procedure is autograft regurgitation and sinus or ascending aortic dilatation, which can usually be corrected with a valve-sparing root replacement. In a study 212 patients underwent Ross aortic valve replacement; 51% were older than 19 years old. There were just 2 early deaths. At 15 years, freedom from autograft sinus or ascending aortic dilatation was 79%, autograft dysfunction, 91%. And actuarial survival was 98% [99].

Recent years aortic valve repair also become popular when valve morphology is amenable to repair. But this is a limited procedure among patients who have aortic regurgitation (AR) without aortic stenosis. Aortic valve repair is commonly indicated commonly in patients with a dilated aortic annulus without any degeneration of the leaflets [100]

Author details

Fahrettin Oz[1], Fatih Tufan[2], Ahmet Ekmekci[3], Omer A. Sayın[4] and Huseyin Oflaz[1]

1 Istanbul University, Istanbul School of Medicine, Department of Cardiology, Turkey

2 Istanbul University, Istanbul School of Medicine, Department of Internal Medicine, Division of Geriatrics, Turkey

3 Istanbul University, Istanbul School of Medicine, Department of Internal Medicine, Turkey

4 Istanbul University, Istanbul School of Medicine, Department of Cardiovascular Surgery, Turkey

References

[1] Gerber MA, Baltimore RS, Eaton CB, Gewitz M, Rowley AH, Shulman ST, Taubert KA. Prevention of rheumatic fever and diagnosis and treatment of acute Streptococcal pharyngitis: a scientific statement from the American Heart Association Rheumatic Fever, Endocarditis, and Kawasaki Disease Committee of the Council on Cardiovascular Disease in the Young, the Interdisciplinary Council on Functional Genomics and Translational Biology, and the Interdisciplinary Council on Quality of Care and Outcomes Research: endorsed by the American Academy of Pediatrics. Circulation. 2009;119(11):1541-51.

[2] Antonini-Canterin F, Huang G, Cervesato E, Faggiano P, Pavan D, Piazza R, Nicolosi GL. Symptomatic aortic stenosis: does systemic hypertension play an additional role? Hypertension. 2003;41(6):1268-72.

[3] Zile MR, Gaasch WH. Heart failure in aortic stenosis - improving diagnosis and treatment. N Engl J Med. 2003;348(18):1735-6.

[4] Rieck ÅE, Cramariuc D, Boman K, Gohlke-Bärwolf C, Staal EM, Lønnebakken MT, Rossebø AB, Gerdts E. Hypertension in aortic stenosis: implications for left ventricular structure and cardiovascular events. Hypertension. 2012;60(1):90-7.

[5] O'Brien KD, Zhao XQ, Shavelle DM, Caulfield MT, Letterer RA, Kapadia SR, Probstfield JL, Otto CM. Hemodynamic effects of the angiotensin-converting enzyme inhibitor, ramipril, in patients with mild to moderate aortic stenosis and preserved left ventricular function. J Investig Med. 2004;52(3):185–191.

[6] Chockalingam A, Venkatesan S, Subramaniam T, Jagannathan V, Elangovan S, Alagesan R, Gnanavelu G, Dorairajan S, Krishna BP, Chockalingam V. Safety and efficacy of angiotensin-converting enzyme inhibitors in symptomatic severe aortic stenosis: Symptomatic Cardiac Obstruction-Pilot Study of Enalapril in Aortic Stenosis (SCOPE-AS). Am Heart J. 2004;147(4):E19.

[7] Nadir MA, Wei L, Elder DH, Libianto R, Lim TK, Pauriah M, Pringle SD, Doney AD, Choy AM, Struthers AD, Lang CC. Impact of renin-angiotensin system blockade therapy on outcome in aortic stenosis. J Am Coll Cardiol. 2011;58(6):570–576.

[8] ALLHAT Collaborative Research Group. Major cardiovascular events in hypertensive patients randomized to doxazosin vs chlorthalidone: the Antihypertensive and Lipid-Lowering Treatment to Prevent Heart Attack Trial (ALLHAT). JAMA. 2000;283(15):1967–1975.

[9] U.S. Preventive Services Task Force. The Guide to Clinical Preventive Services 2010 - 2011: Recommendations of the U.S. Preventive Services Task Force. Rockville (MD): Agency for Healthcare Research and Quality (US); 2010 Aug.

[10] Goel SS, Agarwal S, Tuzcu EM, Ellis SG, Svensson LG, Zaman T, Bajaj N, Joseph L, Patel NS, Aksoy O, Stewart WJ, Griffin BP, Kapadia SR. Percutaneous coronary inter-

vention in patients with severe aortic stenosis: implications for transcatheter aortic valve replacement. Circulation. 2012 Feb 28;125(8):1005-13.

[11] Darby AE, Dimarco JP. Management of atrial fibrillation in patients with structural heart disease. Circulation. 2012;125(7):945-57.

[12] Bang CN, Greve AM, Boman K, Egstrup K, Gohlke-Baerwolf C, Køber L, Nienaber CA, Ray S, Rossebø AB, Wachtell K. Effect of lipid lowering on new-onset atrial fibrillation in patients with asymptomatic aortic stenosis: the Simvastatin and Ezetimibe in Aortic Stenosis (SEAS) study. Am Heart J. 2012;163(4):690-6.

[13] Camm AJ, Savelieva I. Atrial fibrillation: the rate versus rhythm management controversy. J R Coll Physicians Edinb. 2012;42 Suppl 18:23-34.

[14] Authors/Task Force Members, Camm AJ, Lip GY, De Caterina R, Savelieva I, Atar D, Hohnloser SH, Hindricks G, Kirchhof P; ESC Committee for Practice Guidelines (CPG), Bax JJ, Baumgartner H, Ceconi C, Dean V, Deaton C, Fagard R, Funck-Brentano C, Hasdai D, Hoes A, Kirchhof P, Knuuti J, Kolh P, McDonagh T, Moulin C, Popescu BA, Reiner Z, Sechtem U, Sirnes PA, Tendera M, Torbicki A, Vahanian A, Windecker S; Document Reviewers, Vardas P, Al-Attar N, Alfieri O, Angelini A, Blömstrom-Lundqvist C, Colonna P, De Sutter J, Ernst S, Goette A, Gorenek B, Hatala R, Heidbüchel H, Heldal M, Kristensen SD, Kolh P, Le Heuzey JY, Mavrakis H, Mont L, Filardi PP, Ponikowski P, Prendergast B, Rutten FH, Schotten U, Van Gelder IC, Verheugt FW. 2012 focused update of the ESC Guidelines for the management of atrial fibrillation: An update of the 2010 ESC Guidelines for the management of atrial fibrillation * Developed with the special contribution of the European Heart Rhythm Association. Europace. 2012 Aug 24. [Epub ahead of print] No abstract available.

[15] Pilgrim T, Wenaweser P, Meuli F, Huber C, Stortecky S, Seiler C, Zbinden S, Meier B, Carrel T, Windecker S. Clinical outcome of high-risk patients with severe aortic stenosis and reduced left ventricular ejection fraction undergoing medical treatment or TAVI. PLoS One. 2011;6(11):e27556.

[16] Chockalingam A, Venkatesan S, Subramaniam T, Jagannathan V, Elangovan S, Alagesan R, Gnanavelu G, Dorairajan S, Krishna BP, Chockalingam V; Symptomatic Cardiac Obstruction-Pilot Study of Enalapril in Aortic Stenosis. Safety and efficacy of angiotensin-converting enzyme inhibitors in symptomatic severe aortic stenosis: Symptomatic Cardiac Obstruction Pilot Study of Enalapril in Aortic Stenosis (SCOPE-AS). Am Heart J. 2004;147(4):E19.

[17] Khot UN, Novaro GM, Popović ZB, Mills RM, Thomas JD, Tuzcu EM, Hammer D, Nissen SE, Francis GS. Nitroprusside in critically ill patients with left ventricular dysfunction and aortic stenosis. N Engl J Med. 2003;348(18):1756-63.

[18] Lindman BR, Zajarias A, Madrazo JA, Shah J, Gage BF, Novak E, Johnson SN, Chakinala MM, Hohn TA, Saghir M, Mann DL. Effects of phosphodiesterase type 5 inhibi-

tion on systemic and pulmonary hemodynamics and ventricular function in patients with severe symptomatic aortic stenosis. Circulation. 2012;125(19):2353-62.

[19] Katz R, Budoff MJ, Takasu J, Shavelle DM, Bertoni A, Blumenthal RS, Ouyang P, Wong ND, O'Brien KD. Relationship of metabolic syndrome with incident aortic valve calcium and aortic valve calcium progression: the Multi-Ethnic Study of Atherosclerosis (MESA). Diabetes. 2009;58(4):813-9

[20] Capoulade R, Clavel MA, Dumesnil JG, Chan KL, Teo KK, Tam JW, Côté N, Mathieu P, Després JP, Pibarot P; ASTRONOMER Investigators. Impact of metabolic syndrome on progression of aortic stenosis: influence of age and statin therapy. J Am Coll Cardiol. 2012;60(3):216-23.

[21] Berrington de Gonzalez A, Hartge P, Cerhan JR, Flint AJ, Hannan L, MacInnis RJ, Moore SC, Tobias GS, Anton-Culver H, Freeman LB, Beeson WL, Clipp SL, English DR, Folsom AR, Freedman DM, Giles G, Hakansson N, Henderson KD, Hoffman-Bolton J, Hoppin JA, Koenig KL, Lee IM, Linet MS, Park Y, Pocobelli G, Schatzkin A, Sesso HD, Weiderpass E, Willcox BJ, Wolk A, Zeleniuch-Jacquotte A, Willett WC, Thun MJ. Body-mass index and mortality among 1.46 million white adults. N Engl J Med. 2010;363(23):2211-9.

[22] Otto CM, Mickel MC, Kennedy JW, Alderman EL, Bashore TM, Block PC, Brinker JA, Diver D, Ferguson J, Holmes DR Jr, Lambrew CT, McKay CR, Palacios IF, Powers ER, Rahimtoola SH, Weiner BH, Davis KB. Three-year outcome after balloon aortic valvuloplasty. Insights into prognosis of valvular aortic stenosis. Circulation. 1994;89(2):642-50.

[23] Ikee R, Honda K, Oka M, Maesato K, Mano T, Moriya H, Ohtake T, Kobayashi S. Association of heart valve calcification with malnutrition-inflammation complex syndrome, beta-microglobulin, and carotid intima media thickness in patients on hemodialysis. Ther Apher Dial. 2008;12(6):464-8.

[24] Wang AY, Woo J, Lam CW, Wang M, Chan IH, Gao P, Lui SF, Li PK, Sanderson JE. Associations of serum fetuin-A with malnutrition, inflammation, atherosclerosis and valvular calcification syndrome and outcome in peritoneal dialysis patients. Nephrol Dial Transplant. 2005;20(8):1676-85.

[25] Engelman DT, Adams DH, Byrne JG, Aranki SF, Collins JJ Jr, Couper GS, Allred EN, Cohn LH, Rizzo RJ. Impact of body mass index and albumin on morbidity and mortality after cardiac surgery. J Thorac Cardiovasc Surg. 1999;118(5):866-73.

[26] Tepsuwan T, Schuarattanapong S, Woragidpoonpol S, Kulthawong S, Chaiyasri A, Nawarawong W. Incidence and impact of cardiac cachexia in valvular surgery. Asian Cardiovasc Thorac Ann. 2009;17(6):617-21.

[27] Thourani VH, Keeling WB, Kilgo PD, Puskas JD, Lattouf OM, Chen EP, Guyton RA. The impact of body mass index on morbidity and short- and long-term mortality in cardiac valvular surgery. J Thorac Cardiovasc Surg. 2011;142(5):1052-61.

[28] Maixner SM, Struble L, Blazek M, Kales HC. Later-life depression and heart failure. Heart Fail Clin. 2011;7(1):47-58.

[29] Bisschop MI, Kriegsman DM, Deeg DJ, Beekman AT, van Tilburg W. The longitudinal relation between chronic diseases and depression in older persons in the community: the Longitudinal Aging Study Amsterdam. J Clin Epidemiol. 2004;57(2): 187-94.

[30] Verbeek DE, van Riezen J, de Boer RA, van Melle JP, de Jonge P. A review on the putative association between beta-blockers and depression. Heart Fail Clin. 2011;7(1): 89-99.

[31] Kimmel SE, Schelleman H, Berlin JA, Oslin DW, Weinstein RB, Kinman JL, Sauer WH, Lewis JD. The effect of selective serotonin re-uptake inhibitors on the risk of myocardial infarction in a cohort of patients with depression. Br J Clin Pharmacol. 2011;72(3):514-7.

[32] Frogel J, Galusca D. Anesthetic considerations for patients with advanced valvular heart disease undergoing noncardiac surgery. Anesthesiol Clin. 2010;28(1):67-85.

[33] Nishimura RA, Carabello BA, Faxon DP, Freed MD, Lytle BW, O'Gara PT, O'Rourke RA, Shah PM. ACC/AHA 2008 Guideline update on valvular heart disease: focused update on infective endocarditis: a report of the American College of Cardiology/ American Heart Association Task Force on Practice Guidelines endorsed by the Society of Cardiovascular Anesthesiologists, Society for Cardiovascular Angiography and Interventions, and Society of Thoracic Surgeons. J Am Coll Cardiol. 2008;52(8): 676-85.

[34] Steinlechner B, Zeidler P, Base E, Birkenberg B, Ankersmit HJ, Spannagl M, Quehenberger P, Hiesmayr M, Jilma B. Patients with severe aortic valve stenosis and impaired platelet function benefit from preoperative desmopressin infusion. Ann Thorac Surg. 2011;91(5):1420-6.

[35] Maldonado JR, Wysong A, van der Starre PJ, Block T, Miller C, Reitz BA. Dexmedetomidine and the reduction of postoperative delirium after cardiac surgery. Psychosomatics. 2009;50(3):206-17.

[36] Giltay EJ, Huijskes RV, Kho KH, Blansjaar BA, Rosseel PM. Psychotic symptoms in patients undergoing coronary artery bypass grafting and heart valve operation. Eur J Cardiothorac Surg. 2006;30(1):140-7.

[37] Fleisher LA, Beckman JA, Brown KA, Calkins H, Chaikof EL, Fleischmann KE, Freeman WK, Froehlich JB, Kasper EK, Kersten JR, Riegel B, Robb JF. 2009 ACCF/AHA focused update on perioperative beta blockade incorporated into the ACC/AHA 2007 guidelines on perioperative cardiovascular evaluation and care for noncardiac surgery: a report of the American college of cardiology foundation/American heart association task force on practice guidelines. Circulation. 2009;120(21):e169-276.

[38] POISE Study Group, Devereaux PJ, Yang H, Yusuf S, Guyatt G, Leslie K, Villar JC, Xavier D, Chrolavicius S, Greenspan L, Pogue J, Pais P, Liu L, Xu S, Málaga G, Avezum A, Chan M, Montori VM, Jacka M, Choi P. Effects of extended-release metoprolol succinate in patients undergoing non-cardiac surgery (POISE trial): a randomised controlled trial. Lancet. 2008;371(9627):1839-47.

[39] Agmon Y, Khandheria BK, Meissner I, Sicks JR, O'Fallon WM, Wiebers DO, Whisnant JP, Seward JB, Tajik AJ. Aortic valve sclerosis and aortic atherosclerosis: different manifestations of the same disease? Insights from a population-based study. J Am Coll Cardiol. 2001;38(3):827-34.

[40] Callister TQ, Raggi P, Cooil B, Lippolis NJ, Russo DJ. Effect of HMG-CoA reductase inhibitors on coronary artery disease as assessed by electron-beam computed tomography. N Engl J Med. 1998;339(27):1972-8.

[41] Pohle K, Mäffert R, Ropers D, Moshage W, Stilianakis N, Daniel WG, Achenbach S. Progression of aortic valve calcification: association with coronary atherosclerosis and cardiovascular risk factors. Circulation. 2001;104(16):1927-32.

[42] Novaro GM, Tiong IY, Pearce GL, Lauer MS, Sprecher DL, Griffin BP.Effect of hydroxymethylglutaryl coenzyme a reductase inhibitors on the progression of calcific aortic stenosis. Circulation. 2001;104(18):2205-9.

[43] Bellamy MF, Pellikka PA, Klarich KW, Tajik AJ, Enriquez-Sarano M. Association of cholesterol levels, hydroxymethylglutaryl coenzyme-A reductase inhibitor treatment, and progression of aortic stenosis in the community. J Am Coll Cardiol 2002; 40:1723-30.

[44] Rosenhek R, Rader F, Loho N, Gabriel H, Heger M, Klaar U, Schemper M, Binder T, Maurer G, Baumgartner H. Statins but not angiotensin-converting enzyme inhibitors delay progression of aortic stenosis. Circulation 2004; 110:1291-5.

[45] Aronow WS, Ahn C, Kronzon I, Goldman ME. Association of coronary risk factors and use of statins with progression of mild valvular aortic stenosis in older persons. Am J Cardiol 2001; 88:693-5.

[46] Cowell SJ, Newby DE, Prescott RJ, Bloomfield P, Reid J, Northridge DB, Boon NA; Scottish Aortic Stenosis and Lipid Lowering Trial, Impact on Regression (SALTIRE) Investigators. A randomized trial of intensive lipid-lowering therapy in calcific aortic stenosis. N Engl J Med 2005; 352:2389-97.

[47] Moura LM, Ramos SF, Zamorano JL, Barros IM, Azevedo LF, Rocha-Gonçalves F, Rajamannan NM. Rosuvastatin affecting aortic valve endothelium to slow the progression of aortic stenosis. J Am Coll Cardiol 2007; 49:554-61.

[48] Rossebø AB, Pedersen TR, Boman K, Brudi P, Chambers JB, Egstrup K, Gerdts E, Gohlke-Bärwolf C, Holme I, Kesäniemi YA, Malbecq W, Nienaber CA, Ray S,

Skjaerpe T, Wachtell K, Willenheimer R; SEAS Investigators. Intensive lipid lowering with simvastatin and ezetimibe in aortic stenosis. N Engl J Med. 2008;359(13):1343-56.

[49] Chan KL, Teo K, Dumesnil JG, Ni A, Tam J; ASTRONOMER Investigators. Effect of Lipid lowering with rosuvastatin on progression of aortic stenosis: results of the aortic stenosis progression observation: measuring effects of rosuvastatin (ASTRONOMER) trial. Circulation. 2010;121(2):306-14.

[50] Helske S, Lindstedt KA, Laine M, Mäyränpää M, Werkkala K, Lommi J, Turto H, Kupari M, Kovanen PT. Induction of local angiotensin II-producing systems in stenotic aortic valves. J Am Coll Cardiol 2004;44:1859–66.

[51] Routledge HC, Townend JN. ACE inhibition in aortic stenosis: dangerous medicine or golden opportunity? J Hum Hypertens. 2001;15(10):659-67.

[52] O'Brien KD, Probstfield JL, Caulfield MT, Nasir K, Takasu J, Shavelle DM, Wu AH, Zhao XQ, Budoff MJ. Angiotensin-converting enzyme inhibitors and change in aortic valve calcium. Arch Intern Med. 2005;165(8):858-62.

[53] Clark BA, Shannon RP, Rosa RM, Epstein FH. Increased susceptibility to thiazide-induced hyponatremia in the elderly. J Am Soc Nephrol. 1994;5(4):1106-11.

[54] Hwang KS, Kim GH. Thiazide-induced hyponatremia. Electrolyte Blood Press. 2010;8(1):51-7.

[55] Moon DG, Jin MH, Lee JG, Kim JJ, Kim MG, Cha DR. Antidiuretic hormone in elderly male patients with severe nocturia: a circadian study. BJU Int. 2004;94(4):571-5.

[56] Cheng JW, Nayar M. A review of heart failure management in the elderly population. Am J Geriatr Pharmacother. 2009;7(5):233-49.

[57] Hunt SA, Abraham WT, Chin MH, Feldman AM, Francis GS, Ganiats TG, Jessup M, Konstam MA, Mancini DM, Michl K, Oates JA, Rahko PS, Silver MA, Stevenson LW, Yancy CW. 2009 focused update incorporated into the ACC/AHA 2005 Guidelines for the Diagnosis and Management of Heart Failure in Adults: a report of the American College of Cardiology Foundation/American Heart Association Task Force on Practice Guidelines: developed in collaboration with the International Society for Heart and Lung Transplantation. Circulation. 2009;119(14):e391-479. Epub 2009 Mar 26. Review. No abstract available. Erratum in: Circulation. 2010 Mar 30;121(12):e258.

[58] American Geriatrics Society 2012 Beers Criteria Update Expert Panel. American Geriatrics Society updated Beers Criteria for potentially inappropriate medication use in older adults. J Am Geriatr Soc. 2012;60(4):616-31.

[59] Hart RG, Pearce LA, Aguilar MI. Meta-analysis: antithrombotic therapy to prevent stroke in patients who have nonvalvular atrial fibrillation. Ann Intern Med. 2007;146(12):857-67.

[60] Iung, B; Baron, G; Butchart, E.G; Delahaye, F; Gohlke-Bärwolf, C; Levang, O.W; Tornos, P;Vanoverschelde, J.L; Vermeer F, Boersma, E; Ravaud P; Vahanian, A. A pro-

spective survey of patients with valvular heart disease in Europe: The Euro Heart Survey on valvular heart disease. Eur Heart J. 2003; 24: 1231 – 1243.

[61] Bach D.S, Nina, C, Deeb G.M. Unoperated Patients With Severe Aortic Stenosis. J Am Coll Cardiol. 2007;50: 2018-2019.

[62] Cribier A, Savin T, Saoudi N, Rocha P, Berland J, Letac B. Percutaneous transluminal valvuloplasty of acquired aortic-stenosis in elderly patients alternative to valve-replacement. Lancet. 1980;1: 63–7.

[63] Eltchaninoff H, Cribier A, Tron, C; Anselme F, Koning R, Soyer R, Letac B. Balloon aortic valvuloplasty in elderly patients at high-risk for surgery, or inoperable-immediate and mid-term results. Balloon aortic valvuloplasty in elderly patients at high-risk for surgery, or inoperable-immediate and mid-term results. Eur Heart J. 1992;16: 1079–84.

[64] Andersen H.R, Knudsen L.L, Hasenkam J.M. Transluminal implantation of artificial heart valves. Description of a new expandable aortic valve and initial results with implantation by catheter technique in closed chest pigs. Eur Heart J. 1992; 13: 704-708.

[65] Cribier A, Eltchaninoff H, Bash A, Borenstein N, Tron C, Bauer F, Derumeaux G, Anselme F, Laborde F, Leon M.B. Percutaneous transcatheter implantation of an aortic valve prosthesis for calcific aortic stenosis: first human case description. Circulation. 2002;106:3006–8.

[66] Buellesfeld L, Gerckens U, Schuler G, Bonan R, Kovac J, Serruys PW, Labinaz M,den Heijer P, Mullen M, Tymchak W, Windecker S, Mueller R, Grube E. 2-year follow-up of patients undergoing transcatheter aortic valve implantation using a self-expanding valve prosthesis. J Am Coll Cardiol 2011;57:1650–1657.

[67] Cribier A, Eltchaninoff H, Tron C, Bauer F, Agatiello C, Nercolini D, Tapiero S,Litzler PY, Bessou JP, Babaliaros V. Treatment of calcific aortic stenosis with the percutaneous heart valve: mid-term follow-up from the initial feasibility studies: the French experience. J Am Coll Cardiol 2006;47:1214–1223.

[68] D'Onofrio A, Rubino P, Fusari M, Salvador L, Musumeci F, Rinaldi M, Vitali EO, Glauber M, Di Bartolomeo R, Alfieri OR, Polesel E, Aiello M, Casabona R, Livi U, Grossi C, Cassese M, Pappalardo A, Gherli T, Stefanelli G, Faggian GG, Gerosa G. Clinical and hemodynamic outcomes of 'all-comers' undergoing transapical aortic valve implantation: results from the Italian Registry of Trans-Apical Aortic Valve Implantation (I-TA). J Thorac Cardiovasc Surg 2011;142:768–775

[69] Ambler G, Omar R.Z, Royston P, Kinsman R, Keogh B.E, Taylor K.M. Generic, simple risk stratification model for heart valve surgery. Circulation. 2005;112:224-31

[70] Vahanian A, Otto CM. Risk stratification of patients with aortic stenosis. Eur Heart J, 2010; 31: 416–423

[71] Piazza N, Wenaweser P, van Gameren M et al. Relationship between the logistic EuroSCORE and the Society of Thoracic Surgeons Predicted Risk of Mortality score in patients implanted with the CoreValve ReValving System: A Bern-Rotterdam Study. Am Heart J, 2010; 159: 323–329.

[72] Eberhard Grube, Christoph Naber, Alexandre Abizaid, Eduardo Sousa, Oscar Mendiz, Pedro Lemos, Roberto Kalil Filho, Jose Mangione, Lutz Buellesfeld. Feasibility of transcatheter aortic valve implantation without pre-dilation: a pilot study. JACC Cardiovasc. Intervent. 2011; 4:751–757

[73] Leon MB, Smith CR, Mack M, Miller DC, Moses JW, Svensson LG, Tuzcu EM, Webb JG, Fontana GP, Makkar RR, Brown DL, Block PC, Guyton RA, Pichard AD, Bavaria JE, Herrmann HC, Douglas PS, Petersen JL, Akin JJ, Anderson WN, Wang D, Pocock S; PARTNER Trial Investigators. Transcathater aortic valve implantation for aortic stenosis in patients who cannot undergo surgery. N. Engl. J. Med. 2010;363: 1597–607

[74] Smith CR, Leon MB, Mack MJ, Miller DC, Moses JW, Svensson LG, Tuzcu EM, Webb JG, Fontana GP, Makkar RR, Williams M, Dewey T, Kapadia S, Babaliaros V, Thourani VH, Corso P, Pichard AD, Bavaria JE, Herrmann HC, Akin JJ, Anderson WN, Wang D, Pocock SJ; PARTNER Trial Investigators. Transcatheter versus Surgical Aortic-Valve Replacement in High-Risk Patients. N. Engl. J. Med. 2011; 364: 2187–2198

[75] Godino C, Maisano F, Montorfano M, Latib A, Chieffo A, Michev I, Al-Lamee R, Bande M, Mussardo M, Arioli F, Ielasi A, Cioni M, Taramasso M, Arendar I, Grimaldi A, Spagnolo P, Zangrillo A, La Canna G, Alfieri O, Colombo A. Outcomes after transcatheter aortic valve implantation with both Edwards-SAPIEN and CoreValve devices in a single center: the Milan experience. JACC Cardiovasc Interv 2010;3:1110–1121.

[76] Rodés-Cabau J, Webb JG, Cheung A, Ye J, Dumont E, Feindel CM, Osten M, Natarajan MK, Velianou JL, Martucci G, DeVarennes B, Chisholm R, Peterson MD, Lichtenstein SV, Nietlispach F, Doyle D, DeLarochellière R, Teoh K, Chu V, Dancea A, Lachapelle K, Cheema A, Latter D, Horlick E. Transcatheter aortic valve implantation for the treatment of severe symptomatic aortic stenosis in patients at very high or prohibitive surgical risk. Acute and late outcomes of the multicenter Canadian experience. J. Am. Coll. Cardiol.2010; 55: 1080–1090.

[77] Webb JG, Chandavimol M, Thompson CR, Ricci DR, Carere RG, Munt BI, Buller CE, Pasupati S, Lichtenstein S. Percutaneous aortic valve implantation retrograde from the femoral artery. Circulation. 2006; 113: 842–850

[78] Ge´ne´reux P, Head SJ, Van Mieghem NM, Kodali S, Kirtane AJ, Xu K, Smith CR, Serruys PW, Kappetein AP, Leon MB. Clinical outcomes after transcatheter aortic valve replacement using Valve Academic Research Consortium definitions: a weighted meta-analysis of 3519 patients from 16 studies. J Am Coll Cardiol 2012; 59:2317–2326

[79] Piazza N, Onuma Y, Jesserun E, Kint PP, Maugenest AM, Anderson RH, de Jaegere PP, Serruys PW. Early and persistent intraventricular conduction abnormalities and requirements for pacemaking after percutaneous replacement of the aortic valve. JACC Cardiovasc Interv 2008;1:310–316.

[80] Godin M, Eltchaninoff H, Furuta A, Tron C, Anselme F, Bejar K, Sanchez-Giron C, Bauer F, Litzler PY, Bessou JP, Cribier A. Frequency of conduction disturbances after transcatheter implantation of an Edwards Sapien aortic valve prosthesis. Am J Cardiol. 2010;106:707–712.

[81] Gurvitch R, Wood DA, Tay EL, Leipsic J, Ye J, Lichtenstein SV, Thompson CR,Carere RG, Wijesinghe N, Nietlispach F, Boone RH, Lauck S, Cheung A, Webb JG. Transcatheter aortic valve implantation: durability of clinical and hemodynamic outcomes beyond 3 years in a large patient cohort. Circulation. 2010;122: 1319–1327.

[82] Barbour, J.R. & Ikonımidis, J.S. Aortic Valve Replacement, In: Johns Hopkins Manual of Cardiothoracic Surgery, Yuh, DD; Vricella, L.A. & Baumgartner W.A. 561-606. Mc Graw-Hill Companies, ISBN-13:978-0-07-141652-8, United States of America)

[83] Heinze, H; Sier, H; Schäfer, U, Heringlake, M. Percutaneous aortic valve replacement: overview and suggestions for anesthestic management. J Clin Anesth, 2010; 22:373-8.

[84] Connolly HM, Oh JK, Orszulak TA, Osborn SL, Roger VL, Hodge DO, Bailey KR, Seward JB, Tajik AJ.Aortic valve replacement for aortic stenosis with severe left ventricular dysfunction. Prognosticindicators. Circulation. 1997; 20:2395-400.

[85] Maganti K, Rigolin V.H, Sarano M.E, Bonow O.R. Valvular Heart Disease: Diagnosis and Management. Mayo Clin Proc. 2010; 85(5): 483–500

[86] Avery, G.J; Ley, S.J; Hill, J.D; Hershon, J.J, Dick S.E. Cardiac surgery in the octogenarian: evaluation of risk, cost, and outcome. Ann Thorac Surg. 2001;71:591-6.

[87] Aronow, W.S. Valvular aortic stenosis in the elderly. Cardiol Rev. 2007;15:.217-25.

[88] Taylor KM, Gray SA, Livingstone S, Brannan JJ. The United Kingdom Heart Valve Registry. J Heart Valve Dis. 1992;1(2):152-9

[89] Bonow, R.O; Carabello, B.A; Chatterjee, K; de Leon, A.C. Jr.; Faxon, D.P; Freed, M.D; Gaasch W.H, Lytle B.W, Nishimura R.A, O'Gara P.T, O'Rourke R.A, Otto C.M, Shah P.M, Shanewise J.S, Smith S.C. Jr; Jacobs, A.K; Adams, C.D; Anderson J.L; Antman, E.M, Fuster, V; Halperin, J.L; Hiratzka, L.F; Hunt, S.A; Lytle, B.W; Nishimura, R; Page, R.L, Riegel B. ACC/AHA 2006 practice guidelines for the management of patients with valvular heart disease: Executive Summary. A Report of the American College of Cardiology/ American Heart Association Task Force on Practice Guidelines (Writing Committee to Revise the 1998 Guidelines for the Management of Patients With Valvular Heart Disease). Developed in collaboration with the Society of Cardiovascular Anesthesiologists. Endorsed by the Society for Cardiovascular An-

giography and Interventions and the Society of Thoracic Surgeons. J Am Coll Cardiol. 2006; 48:1-148

[90] Petersen R.S & Poulsen A. (2010). Quality of life after aortic valve-replacement in patients > or = 75 years. Ugeskr Laeger, Vol.172, No.5, (February, 2010), pp.355-9

[91] Minimally invasive cardiac surgery Daniel J. Goldstein, Mehmet C. Oz. 21 Minimally invasive aortic valve surgery 293-307

[92] Svensson LG. Minimally invasive surgery with a partial sternotomy "J" approach. Semin Thorac Cardiovasc Surg. 2007;19(4):299-303.

[93] GlauberM, MiceliA, BevilacquaS, FarnetiPA.Minimally invasive aortic valve replacement via right anterior minithoracotomy:Early outcomes and midterm follow-up. J Thorac Cardiovasc Surg. 2011;142(6):1577-9.

[94] Olin C.L, Péterffy A. Minimal access aortic valve surgery. Eur J Cardiothorac Surg. 1999; 15:39-43.

[95] Korach A, Shemin R.J, Hunter C.T, Bao Y, Shapira O.M. Minimally invasive versus conventional aortic valve replacement: a 10-year experience. J Cardiovasc Surg. 2010;51: 417-21.

[96] Foghsgaard S, Gazi D, Bach K, Hansen H, Schmidt T.A, Kjaergard H.K. Minimally invasive aortic valve replacement reduces atelectasis in cardiac intensive care. Acute Cardiac Care. 2009;11: 169-72.

[97] Wheatley G.H, Prince S.L, Herbert M.A, Ryan W.H. Port-access aortic valve surgery: a technique in evolution. Heart Surg Forum. 2004;7:628-31

[98] Morita K, Kurosawa H. Indications for and clinical outcome of the Ross procedure: a review]. Nihon Geka Gakkai Zasshi. 2001;102(4):330-6.

[99] Brown JW, Ruzmetov M, Shahriari A, Rodefeld MD, Mahomed Y, Turrentine MW.Midterm results of Ross aortic valve replacement: a single-institution experience. Ann Thorac Surg. 2009 ;88(2):601-7.

[100] Fattouch K, Murana G, Castrovinci S, Nasso G, Mossuto C, Corrado E, Ruvolo G, Speziale G. Outcomes of aortic valve repair according to valve morphology and surgical techniques. Interact Cardiovasc Thorac Surg. 2012;15(4):644-50

Chapter 14

Stentless Bioprostheses for Aortic Valve Replacement in Calcific Aortic Stenosis

Kaan Kirali

Additional information is available at the end of the chapter

http://dx.doi.org/10.5772/55373

1. Introduction

The classic case of aortic stenosis is a healthy middle-aged patient with/without symptoms, but in practical life, patients with severe calcific aortic valve come with several and severe comorbidities such as advanced age, coronary artery disease, atherosclerotic aorta, significant left ventricular dysfunction. Aortic valve replacement (AVR) is the only options in these patients, and it requires patient-by-patient analysis of clinical, echocardiograhic, and hemodynamic data with associated pathologies. The curative treatment of calcific aortic valve stenosis is the replacement of the aortic valve with a prosthetic valve, and selection of a perfect prosthetic valve is the main goal to get a successful treatment. But, there is no any perfect heart valve prosthesis which may mimic the characteristics of the normal native aortic valve: excellent hemodynamics, life-long durability, thromboresistance, and excellent implantability. That means that native valve disease will be traded for prosthetic valve disease and the outcome of AVR is affected by the type of prosthetic valve. Mechanical valves are non-limited durable, but have a substantial risk of hematologic complications (thromboemboli, thrombotic obstruction, hemorrhage related life-long anticoagulation therapy) with/without hemolysis potential. In contract, bioprosthetic valves have a low risk of thromboembolism without anticoagulation, but their durability is limited by calcific or noncalcific tissue deterioration. Biological prostheses, especially homografts, are often believed to be the substitute of choice in AVR, but the limited availability of homografts prevents their more broadly usage. To overcome this problem and all possible complications of mechanical valves, xenogenic biological prostheses have been developed. The design of bioprosthetic valves purports to mimic the anatomy of the native aortic valve and their flow characteristics are better than mechanical valves, whereas stentless bioprostheses have hemodynamic performance similar to the healthy native aortic valve. Although stented bioprostheses can be implanted easier, they decrease the effective orifice area due to the rigid stent and result turbulent flow through the valve. Stented valves also increase stress at the attachment of the stent which cause earlier primary tissue failure. Stentless biologic valves have been introduced into clinical practice to solve all these problems and to reproduce the anatomy and function of the native aortic valve, but their clinical use has still not exceeded the number of stented aortic bioprostheses because of more demanding technique of implantation. To gain more widespread clinical use and general recommendation of stentless bioprostheses, their advantages and simple implantation techniques must be popularized.

It is believed that the aortic root is probably the best stent for the native or prosthetic aortic valve. The anatomy and function of the aortic root may dampen the mechanical stress to which the leaflets are subjected during diastole. The ideal stentless prosthesis should have no synthetic materials, preserve the aortic root dynamics, restore flexibility and distensibility of the native valve annulus after decalcification, and have minimal xenograft aortic wall, short implantation time, and excellent hemodynamic performance to facilitate the recovery of left ventricular function.

1.1. Historical background

Homografts were the first biological prostheses used in clinical practice to treat aortic valve stenosis in early 1960s, and they were the first stentless valves, too [1,2]. The authors used the aortic root of the patient to secure the homograft aortic valve in the subcoronary position. The most complicated implantation technique and the restricted availability of homografts prevented their widespread usage. First stentless pig and calf xenografts were used in limited patients, but the valves were abandoned because of poor tissue fixation [3]. Stented bioprostheses were considered as the gold standard for several years, but abnormal stress on the leaflets was believed to decrease durability. To overcome this problem with a rigid stent on the aortic position, stentless bioprostheses were re-introduced in the middle of 80's [4], whereas new designed stentless xenografts were proposed and popularized in daily use at the beginning of 1990s [5]. The main problem (early failure of bioprostheses) was solved with new bioengineering improvement (antimineralization, zero-pressure fixation) [6]. The other problem was partial dehiscence when the heterograft contained muscular bar resulting paravalvular leakage in the area corresponding to the muscular bar, and this problem was abolished with a fine Dacron cloth covered the outside wall of the stentless porcine aortic valve along its inflow [7]. Recognizing the range of aortic root variability and disease of the root itself, the concept of stentless valve replacement was expanded to replacement of the entire aortic root. Full root replacement with a bioprosthesis brought the challenges of homeostasis and coronary reimplantation. In spite of hemodynamic advantages proven for the root replacement technique, acceptance was slowed by risk/benefit ratio concerns. The whole aortic root could be prepared and implanted with modified root inclusion or subcoronary implant techniques.

Biological stentless valve can be prepared by pulmonary autograft, homograft, xenograft, autologous or xenogenic pericardium. Pulmonary autograft has limited durability beyond the first decade [8]. The same problem has been observed with homografts in the aortic position,

http://dx.doi.org/10.5772/55373

especially in younger patients, which are less durable than commercially available stentless bioprostheses and cannot be recommended as the ideal device [9]. The use of the patients own pericardium for constructing a heart valve prosthesis is biologically more appealing than the use of animal tissue or heterologous material. The feasibility of autologous pericardial stentless aortic valve was shown in an animal study [10]. The feasibility and durability of truly stentless autologous pericardial AVR sutured directly onto the aortic wall has been also performed in human recently [11]. Stentless porcine or pericardial xenogenic bioprostheses have been introduced to get better long-term durability and become a routine device when a stentless biologic valve is implanted.

There are a lot of stentless bioprostheses with/without the aortic root in the market, but some of them are not used widespread and implantation of a few xenografts is stopped (Table 1). The first modern (first generation) stentless valves were glutaraldehyde-fixed porcine prostheses with a fully scalloped shape or a complete aortic root (Figure 1). The most preferred approach was root replacement technique because subcoronary approach needed more suture line. The second generation of stentless valves improved the technical difficulties related to free-hand implantation with two rows of sutures for subcoronary implantation of porcine bioprostheses (Figure 2). The third generation of stentless prostheses are made by xenogenic pericardium, because the pericardial valve is free from the compromises of the porcine aortic root, it is flexible, and easy to implant either with an interrupted or running suture technique (Figure 3). There are different xenogenic pericardial valves (bovine or equine), and horse pericardium is thinner, however, stronger than the bovine pericardium and also much more pliable. The fourth generation of stentless valves are produced by a proprietary process and the unique conditioning technology paves the way for autologous repopularization of the valve in patients. The durability of current bioprosthetic heart valves is diminished by glutaraldehyde-associated leaflet calcification or by the host immune reaction. As a novel tissue engineering approach to improving replacement heart valve durability, a new acellular (nonglutaraldehyde-fixed) tissue heart valve for autologous recellularization is developed to limit xenograft antigenicity. As no glutaraldehyde is used in the whole process lack of calcification and also lack of toxicity, and the method delivers a very pliable valve with very low gradients. To use of autologous pericardium fixed with glutaraldehyde avoids any immune reaction between the host and the implanted heart valve and so minimizes tissue calcification and pannus formation. The last generation of stentless valves provides avoidance of suture lines during AVR: closed [transcatheter (transfemoral or transapical)] or open (transaortic = sutureless) techniques (Figure 4).

2. Hemodynamic recovery

Every effort should be made to avoid moderate prosthesis-patient mismatch during AVR. Stentless valves enable to select the largest bioprosthesis to the patient's annulus and provide better aortic root and valve behavior, larger effective orifice area (EOA), reduced transprosthetic gradient and greater left ventricular mass regression.

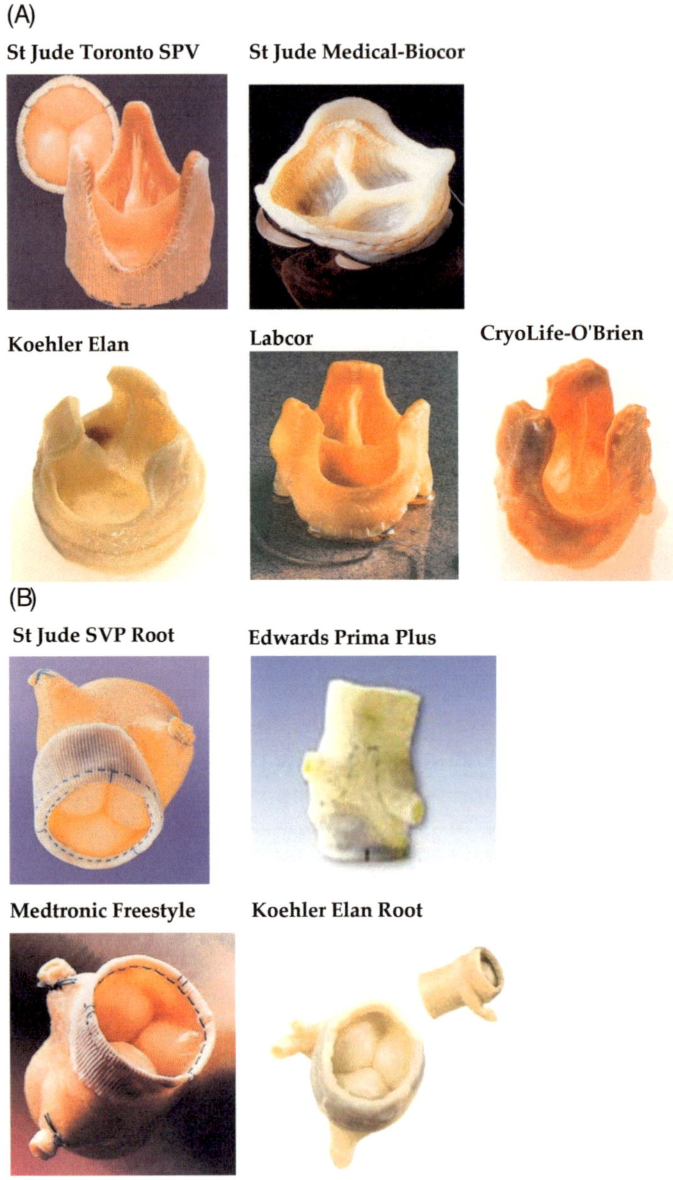

Figure 1. First generation bioprostheses (Porcine Stentless Xenografts) A) Scalloped stentless porcine bioprostheses B) Root stentless porcine bioprostheses.

To prevent early or late prosthetic failure, maintenance of the aortic root with physiological anatomy must be the primary goal during AVR with a stentless prosthesis. Any kind of bioprosthetic valve will deviate from native aortic valve in terms of leaflet dynamics. Stiffening of the aortic root either by glutaraldehyde or by stent degenerates the opening (wrinkles and blurry edges of leaflets) and closing (asynchronism) behavior of native aortic valve leaflets.

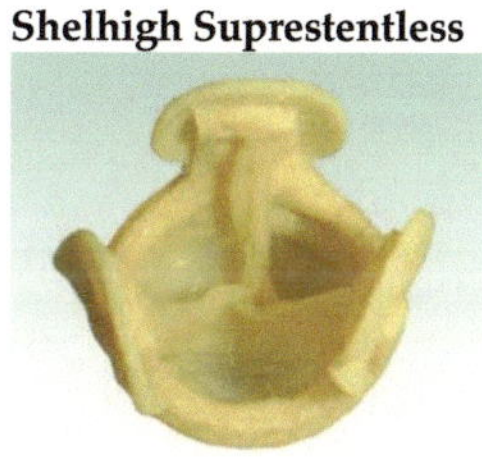

Figure 2. Second generation bioprostheses.

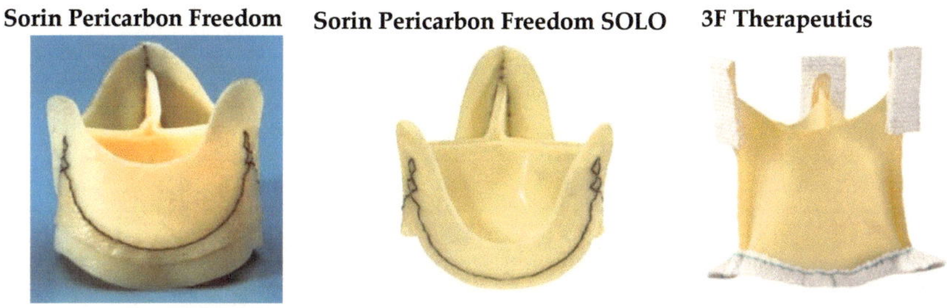

Figure 3. Third generation bioprostheses (Pericardial Stentless Xenografts)

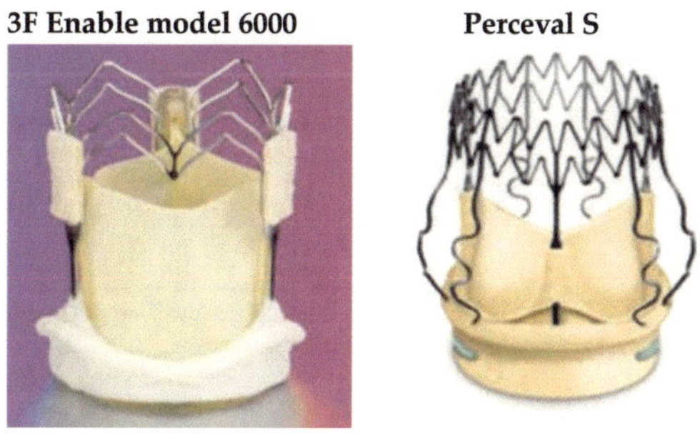

Figure 4. Sutureless Pericardial Stentless Xenografts

Stented valves fixe the native commissures and do not allow cyclic change of the commissural dimension as it normally occurs. This cyclic expansion of the commissural area serves reduction of stress on the leaflets, which is preserved by stentless bioprostheses. Second, the intrinsically obstructive nature of the stented bioprostheses increases pressure gradient and creates turbulent flow patterns, however, normal laminar flow patterns can be restored after AVR with stentless tissue valves. The opening and closing of the stentless biologic valve constitute a passive mechanism responding to pressure difference between the left ventricle and the aorta. Like the native aortic valve, a stress created by this difference heads toward the central coaptation area of the bioprosthesis during diastole. The negative pressure difference during diastole helps prosthetic valve to be closed. The valve opens rapidly at the beginning of ejection because of rising of pressure difference and persists to remain open as a tunnel

A. Autograft	
B. Homograft	
C. Xenografts	
I. First generation (Stentless Porcine Bioprosthesis)	
Dacron reinforced inflow tract	
Toronto SPV (stentless porcine valve)	St Jude Medical, Inc., St Paul, MN, USA
St Jude Medical-Biocor	St Jude, Belo Horizonte, MG, Brazil
CryoLife-O'Brien Model 3000	CryoLife International Inc, Atlanta, GA, USA
Toronto SPV Root	St Jude Medical, Inc., St Paul, MN, USA
Edwards Prima Plus	Edwards Lifesciences, Inc., Irvine, CA,USA
Medtronic Freestyle	Medtronic, Inc., Minneapolis, MN, USA
pericardial reinforced inflow tract	
Koehler Elan	Koehler, Bellshill, Scotland
Koehler Elan Root	
tri-composite design (three noncoronary leaflets)	
Labcor	Labcor, Inc., Belo Horizonte, MG, Brazil
II. Second generation (porcine with single suture line, No-react treatment)	
Shelhigh Suprestentless	Shelhigh, Inc, Millburn, NJ, USA
III. Third generation (Stentless Pericardial Bioprosthesis)	
porcine pericardium	
Sorin Pericarbon Freedom	Sorin Biomedica Cardio SpA, Saluggia, Italy
Sorin Pericarbon Freedom SOLO	
horse (equine) pericardium	
3F Therapeutics	3F Therapeutics, Inc., Lake Forest, CA, USA
IV. Fourth generation (non-gluteraldayhde fixed + decellularized)	
Matrix A	
V. Sutureless generation (Sutureless + Stentless Pericardial Bioprosthesis)	
3F Enable model 6000	3F Therapeutics, Inc., Lake Forest, CA, USA
Perceval S	Sorin Biomedica Cardio SpA, Saluggia, Italy
D. Autologous pericardium	

Table 1. Stentless Bioprostheses.

during systole, and the aortic root may also expanse at the late diastole to help opening of the leaflets (in native aortic valve, expansion of the aortic root is about 12% and that starts opening the leaflets to about 20%). At the end of systole, the backward blood flow into the sinuses of Valsalva (behind prosthetic leaflets) and initialization of pressure difference help prosthetic leaflets to revert to their original closed position. An in-vivo-study has showed that there is no difference in opening velocities among native, stented and subcoronary stentless valves in a porcine model [12]. However, the closing velocities are significantly higher in the pericardial valves. The bending deformation increases when implanting a glutaraldehyde-treated valve subcoronary. Porcine stentless valves display a distinct folding pattern during opening resulting in an altered stress distribution and also tend to fold during opening causing increased leaflet bending stress [13].

One of the key parameters for stentless xenograft performance is the EOA. In spite of the EOA is significantly higher in stentless bioprostheses it is also dependent on the design and the implantation technique of the prostheses. The EOA will increase especially during the first year and the transvalvular gradient drops dramatically in the first 3 to 6 months after surgery, but some further drop may be seen more later [14]. The reason may be remodeling of the left ventricular outflow tract, diminished aortic root edema, and slight dilatation of the aortic root. Transvalvular gradient is closely related to the EOA: the larger orifice area the lower is the transvalvular gradient. The second reason to increase transvalvular gradient is usage of a rigid stent. Avoidance of a stent enlarges inner diameter of prosthetic valve and eliminates intraluminal obstruction which increases the EOA. Several studies have shown transvalvular gradient across stentless valves is always lower than for their stented valves, especially mean and/or peek gradients [15-1617]. The third possible reason can be excessive tissue of a bioprosthesis: the lesser tissue implanted within the recipient aortic root the lesser obstruction. The full root prostheses reduce the intraluminar obstruction because nothing is implanted inside, and they have larger EOA than subcoronary prostheses. The main differences of stentless biologic tissue valves are the specific gravity of the leaflets which is not equal to that of blood like native human aortic leaflets and the specific thickness of the leaflets which is thinner in pericardial tissue valves. Both parameters cause transvalvular gradient during ejection which is lesser in fully pericardial stentless valves than porcine. The other reasons may be small aortic annulus and physically active patients. The change in gradients during exercise is interesting: when cardiac output increases it also increases the transvalvular flow and raises transprosthetic gradient, but these gradients under exercise are lower with stentless valves than stented bioprostheses, which provide better opening closing behavior [18].

Left ventricular output is maintained by the development of the left ventricular hypertrophy which results in a large pressure gradient across the stenotic valve. The left ventricle mass increases and becomes less compliant. Left ventricular hypertrophy and increased mass can be correlated with sudden death, congestive heart failure, and other cardiovascular events. Left ventricular hypertrophy will regress after AVR regardless of the type of prostheses, and an improved hemodynamic performance of prostheses should result in a faster regression, especially in patients with severe calcific aortic stenosis and left ventricular hypertrophy, because incomplete regression after AVR is related to poor long-term outcome [19]. This regression is related to EOA and transvalvular gradient constituted by the prosthetic valve. A significant improvement will occur in all type of valves in the first year, but this improvement is greater and faster with the stentless bioprostheses [20]. A lasting benefit beyond the first year is possible, especially in severely enlarged ventricles [21]. These improvements include mass regression, wall thickening, fractional shortening, and diastolic relaxation. Patients with small aortic annuli or with compromised left ventricular function (EF < 50%) might benefit more from stentless prostheses [22,23].

3. Structural and nonstructural durability

One of the foremost concern of any tissue valve is its long-term patency, because the limited durability represents the main disadvantage of these devices. Tissue valve degeneration causing stenosis or regurgitation is the primer indication for reoperation.

Durability of any kind of stentless bioprosthesis can be affected adversely by internal (structural) or external (nonstructural) factors.

Structural valve deterioration (SVD) is a primary tissue failure after biological valve implantation. A major cause of SVD is cusp tear with consequent aortic regurgitation where urgent or emergent reoperation is necessary due to congestive heart failure and hemolytic anemia. The other major reason is prosthetic valve sclerosis and calcification which could permit an elective reoperation in stable condition. An in vivo animal study has shown that native aortic valves are significantly more distensible at the level of the sinotubular junction, commissures and ascending aorta when compared with all-valve prosthesis [24]. There is no any study to evaluate how the late scar with/without calcification tissue formation spread and effect this distensibility. We can argue that annular calcification developed during follow-up acts similar in native and stentless valves and fixes the aortic annulus. The zero-pressure fixation and antimineralization techniques have improved durability of tissue valves. To avoid from well known limited durability of xenogenic bioprostheses owing to structural degeneration and calcification, the use of autologous pericardium may be an attractive alternative with several advantages: no immune reaction, minimum tissue calcification and pannus formation, excellent hemodynamics and dynamics of the aortic root, no complicated reoperation [11].

Nonstructural valve deterioration (NSVD) is independent on the xenograft's tissue. In spite of leaflets of xenografts work very well, stentless bioprosthesis shows incompetence. There are several reasons causing prosthetic stenosis or regurgitation (Table 2).

Technical inadequacy during stentless valve implantation cause hemodynamic problems like regurgitation, turbulent flow, uncoaptation or stretching of leaflets which aggregate tissue degeneration. Any increase in mechanical stress causing by surgical implantation techniques has a negative impact on durability. Description of all implantation techniques with their tips is not adequate to avoid iatrogenic valve degeneration, all details of these techniques should be well known. The best way to avoid mechanical stress may be to use the full root replacement technique, but most surgeon do not like to replace the aortic root without any pathology

A. Endocarditis
B. Technically implantation errors
C. Aortic root enlargement
I. Sinotubular junction dilatation
II. Sinus of Valsalva aneurysm (± rupture)
III. Aortic dissection
IV. Left ventricular dilatation
D. Partial dehiscence after preserved non-coronary sinus
E. Insufficiently decalcification
I. Poor decalcification (intra-operatively)
II. Suture rupture or loosening (post-operatively)
III. Calcification on the native aorta (follow-up)
F. Subvalvular fibrous band
G. Hematologic problems (hemolysis, thrombocytopenia)

Table 2. Non-structural Deterioration (regurgitation or stenosis).

(dilatation, calcification) because of higher operative risk. Subcoronary implantation technique is more acceptable approach for isolated AVR with stentless bioprostheses. Technical errors relating to xenograft sizing and failure to achieve appropriate geometry of the xenograft within the aortic root are 2 major reasons for early valve failure. The learning curve associated with subcoronary implantation is the main reason for these technical errors. Suboptimal implantation resulting in distortion of the valve or bulking of valve tissue into the outflow tract may be involved in the evolution of higher gradients. Undersizing of xenograft results regurgitation due to handicapping leaflet coaptation, whereas oversizing may cause higher transvalvular gradient due to making leaflet opening difficult. The other error is to decide and apply the wrong implantation technique, especially in small or dilated aortic root, and subcoronary technique might be associated with higher gradient or regurgitation [25].

On the other hand, improvement of the long term patency of an aortic prosthetic valve is dependent on avoidance of paravalvular complications which can be very serious and cause reoperation. Paravalvular regurgitation is a dangerous long-term result of insufficient decalcification, which causes incompetence suturing or suture rupture during follow-up.

Partial dehiscence of the stentless xenograft indeed occurs and that it has a strong predilection for the preserved non-coronary sinus after modified subcoronary technique. Supposedly, proteolytic enzymes from captured blood cells in the dead space between native and donor aortas or the potential usefulness of biologic glues might prevent adequate fusion of the walls and healing of the anastomosis [26].

Subvalvular fibrous band is a rare complication resulting significant left ventricular outflow tract obstruction, which can be a derivative of the pannus discovered on the sewing ring of stented valves. The etiology is unknown, but it may result from thrombus formation or inflammation related to host factors. A chronic inflammatory infiltrate composed of lymphocytes and macrophages occurs in equine or porcine stentless valves, which suggests equal immunogenicity among different various biologic graft materials [27].

4.1. Aortic valve surgery

4.1.1. Cardiopulmonary bypass

Aortic valve surgery can be performed through a median full sternotomy or upper ministernotomy with conventional or minimal skin incision. The distal ascending aorta cannulation is usually the standard approach in most patients, but the arcus aorta or axiller artery can be also cannulated when the ascending aorta should be replaced [28]. A single dual-stage venous cannula is inserted through the right atrium appendage. After cardiopulmonary bypass is initiated the aorta is clamped and cardiac arrest is be achieved with antegrade isothermic blood cardioplegia administered into the aortic root. Myocardial protection is continued due to retrograde cardioplegic cannula during whole procedure, and retrograde cardioplegia is continuously infused whenever clear visulation of the aortic root is not required [29]. Rarely the retrograde cannula cannot be introduced safely into the coronary sinus, in this situation intermittent antegrade isothermic blood cardioplegia is performed using selective coronary ostial cannulation after transverse aortotomy incision. If both approaches are unsuccessful, bicaval cannulation is performed and the retrograde cannula is placed in the coronary sinus under direct vision. A vent cannula is inserted into the left atrium through the right upper pulmonary vein after cross clamp to prevent the left ventricle distention. Mild-moderate hypothermia (30-32°C) is achieved and continued during extracorporeal circulation, and rewarming of patients is started before the closure of the aortotomy.

4.1.2. Aortotomy

A small transverse aortotomy incision is made initially at least 15 to 20 mm above the origin of the right coronary ostium or the sinotubular junction. The calcific aortic valve and whole aortic root should be investigated under direct vision and decided which approach will be preferred. If the aortic root will not be replaced then the transverse aortotomy incision is extended on both sides until 3D view of the aortic root appears. That helps surgeons for excision of the severe calcific aortic valve, selection of an appropriate stentless bioprosthesis and insertion simple and/or continuous sutures easily and correctly. A transverse aortotomy is also required to image 3D shape of the aortic root which is the main condition for resuspention of the prosthetic commissures and to hold a stentless tissue valve in corrected position for prevention of the iatrogenic valve degeneration. An oblique or hockey-stick incision is preferred very seldom, but it could be useful in patients with small aortic root. If the aortic root is replaced it is excised completely and aortic root implantation technique is performed. Reoperation for severe calcific aortic stenosis is not rare in patients with previously coronary artery bypass surgery, and patent proximal anastomoses on the ascending aorta can be a serious problem during aortotomy. I have offered a simple aortotomy incision "Reverse U aortotomy" to save proximal anastomoses and if it is necessary to apply direct antegrade cardioplegia through proximal anastomoses [30].

4.1.3. Excision of the calcific aortic valve

Aortic valve stenosis appears with fusion of one or both commissures, thickening and retraction of the cusps, and restriction of effective orifice area. Calcific involvement of native aortic valve is the last step which can be widespread very aggressively: aortic annulus, mitral annulus, aortic root, coronary ostia. The typically pathologic findings of calcific aortic stenosis are discrete, focal lesions on the aortic side of the leaflets. The severe form is characterized by diffuse calcification of the aortic root and the deposits involve the sinuses of Valsalva and the ascending aorta (porcelain aorta). The calcification presents as a cauliflower-like mass within the leaflets and often extends deep into the annulus and surrounding tissues. All these contiguous anatomical structures can have adverse affects on the surgical techniques.

A surgically complete decalcification of the aortic annulus is an important point. The flexible continuity of the aortic annulus with sub- and supra-annular tissues is indispensable condition to get better durability and hemodynamics with stentless xenografts, and to avoid from a whole aortic root replacement technique, which hinders surgeons to perform AVR with a stentless xenograft. Surgeons must care 1) not to leave any calcific tissue around the aortic annulus, 2) not to allow fragments of calcium to fall into the left ventricle, 3) not to disrupt the annulus as possible, 4) not to detach the anterior mitral leaflet from the annulus (non-coronary sinus), 5) not to rupture subannular muscular septum (right coronary sinus), 6) not to perforate outside the heart (left coronary sinus).

The calcific aortic valve is excised and trimmed with a scissor leaving a 2-3 mm margin at the annulus if the annular margin of the leaflets are healthy. The frequent scenario is conversely that and extensive calcific involvement of the whole aortic annulus is observed very often. First of all, complete resection of the calcific aortic valve should be performed without any complication listed above. Excision of the calcific leaflets with a scissor is usually unsuccessful and dangerous because of breaking of calcification and falling calcium debris into the left ventricle. The best alternative to remove the diseased tissue is excision all of them with a lancet (number 15). A folded segment of sponge or tampon is not necessary to place in the left ventricle and it hinders to see the cavity and to remove any calcium particle. The easiest excision with the lancet is to perforate the healthy leaflet near the annulus in partial calcified aortic valve or to begin excision at the commissure between the non-coronary and right coronary leaflets in en-bloc calcific aortic valve. Cutting of the calcification is begun at the nearest end and the lancet incises the calcified valve from the healthy annular tissue. The sharp edge of the lancet should be headed toward the calcified valve, and cutting is performed just below of calcification. The whole calcified valve must be incised as en-block, without fragmentation. If calcification is very heavy or invaded into the annulus it can be cut with the scissor and then the residual calcifications will be gently crushed and removed with a rounger. After completion of the aortic valve excision, all residual diseased and/or calcified tissue or particles should be removed from around the annulus. Before sizing the prosthesis, the left ventricular cavity is flushed and irrigated with saline solution.

4.1.4. Sizing the stentless aortic bioprosthesis

The stented prostheses must fit snugly in the annulus, because a very loose or tight fit indicates inadequate effective orifice area (patient-prosthesis mismatch) or oversizing the prosthesis. For the truly measurement of a stented valve, the seizer should be inserted through the aortic annulus and the same (supra-annular) or one number smaller (intra-annular) stented prosthesis must be chosen.

Sizing a stentless bioprosthesis is different from stented valves. The most important phase is the choice of an appropriate stentless bioprosthesis, and measurement of the aortic annulus must be done with the seizer that corresponds to the specific bioprosthesis. The true seizer should be chosen to implant the appropriate tissue valve with the optimum size. If the prosthetic valve is too small, the inflow end obstructs the EOA which increases transvalvular gradient and the outflow end is stretched out with decreased leaflet coaptation which causes more regurgitation. On the other hand, oversizing to fit a larger sinotubular junction leads to buckling of the inflow end which can produce both relative stenosis and regurgitation as well as harmful turbulent flow. How the stentless valves sized and implanted will influence its function and durability in future. The larger surface area of the cusps allows greater coaptation area which reduces the risk of bioprosthesis regurgitation. This relatively larger bioprosthesis can simplify replacement, especially the running sutures for all sinuses. But, it is imperative to avoid over-sizing of stentless valves with the tubular structure achieved by three tabs on the commissures, and if sizing is uncertainty the smaller prosthesis should be implanted.

In normal aortic root, the diameter of the aortic annulus is 10-15% larger than those of the sinotubular junction and measurement of the aortic annulus is the correct way to choice an appropriate sized stentless valve. However, most patients with calcific aortic stenosis have an abnormal aortic root and the relationship between both diameters is usually altered. In this situation, the diameter of the sinotubular junction is more important because the three commissures of stentless valves are secured at approximately the level of the sinotubular junction if not the full-root replacement technique will be used.

A cylindrical silicon seizer is more practical to measure the true valve size when both the annulus and the sinotubular junction are measured. The rule is that the sinotubular junction should be dominate during measuring and if there is a major difference (> 3 mm) subcoronary implantation technique can be not used because the commissures of stentless valves are pulled outward and cause valvular insufficiency and an alternative technique (root replacement) or stented bioprosthesis must be used. Supra-annular sizing is the best measurement method to choice an appropriate stentless bioprosthesis, especially during single suture line technique. I prefer this more practical way and put the appropriate seizer into the aortic root in supra-annular position (not into the annulus) where I put continuous proximal suture line, so I can choice an acceptable size that is equal to the sinotubular junction size or one number larger stentless prosthesis can be chosen if the seizer fits aortic orifice tightly in patients with aortic root enlargement. Trans-annular measurement is adequate to get a fit stentless valve for subcoronary implantation in patients with normal aortic root, but preferring one size larger prosthesis is better if full-root replacement technique will be performed or a small aortic root is present. I never suggest to play some traction sutures at the commissures or in the nadir of the annulus to open the aortic orifice. It can be useful during the replacement of a stented valve, but it will be better to release the aortic root in its original shape during sizing stentless valves.

5. Implantation techniques

Stentless aortic biologic prostheses can be different in origin: autogenous, homogenous, heterogeneous. Procuring of aortic auto- or homograft is not easy, but production of xenografts is a sufficiently technical supply of the industry for the treatment of aortic valve diseases. All stentless biologic valves can be implanted using different techniques: the subcoronary method, the full root implantation technique, and the root inclusion alternative.

The subcoronary technique is the simplest method for implantation, and either a porcine root can be adapted intra-operatively or a prefabricated tissue valve can be utilized. The main advantages are to avoid the manipulation of coronary ostia and bleeding from suture lines. The disadvantages could be difficulties occurring in the small aortic annulus and calcified aortic root, and possibilities of valve insufficiency by changing the shape of the stentless valve in a diseased aortic root [31]. Subcoronary implantation technique can be performed in two methods: double suture lines (classic) or single suture line (simple) approach.

In classical subcoronary implantation technique, stentless valves are fixed into the host aortic root using double suture lines. The first suture line attaches the inflow site of the stentless bioprosthesis in the left ventricular outflow tract: annular suture line. The second suture line, which is constructed using 1 or 3 continuous sutures, connects the outflow site of the prosthesis with the aortic wall below the coronary ostia: supra-annular suture line. The first suture line consists usually of interrupted sutures, but to reduce cross-clamp and cardiopulmonary times a continuous suture can be preferred [32]. Because the conventional continuous inflow suture line can increase the postoperative heart block risk, an alternative subcoronary technique has been reported in which the inflow suture line is raised at the level of right-non-coronary commissure [33].

The single suture line technique is a simple, quick, safe and reliable method to replace the native aortic valve with a stentless valve. This approach is used for implantation of scalloped new generation tissue valves in supra-annular position and placement of the sutures below or through the annulus should be avoided. Running sutures avoid any prosthetic dead space between prosthetic valve and native aortic wall, and selecting a prosthesis a size larger than the host annulus minimizes the stress on the suture lines. These new generation pericardial valve can have manufactured scalloped design [34] or it can be prepared by trimming away all the extra tissue of the valve inflow side ond scalloping the outflow side [35]. If stentless prostheses are designed with a tubular structure, the tabs on the commissures should be attached to the aortic wall [36].

The total root technique requires reimplantation of coronary arteries using the button technique. The main advantages are normal physiological shape of the aortic root and choice of a larger valve in small aortic annulus, and both avoid any patient-prosthesis mismatch. The total root technique also prevents torsions of the commissures which avoiding postoperative prosthetic dysfunction. The main disadvantages are implantation difficulties, requirement of interposition a vascular tubular graft between xenograft and native ascending aorta, and xenograft aortic wall calcification making reoperation difficulty. The learning curve seems to be more pronounced when using the total root technique, whereas single suture line technique may be also performed by young surgeons without any problem. Surgeons decide on their experience and the patient's anatomy pre- and intra-operatively which approach with appropriate stentless bioprosthesis type they will use for AVR. Isolated AVR using the subcoronary technique is the best and easiest way in calcific aortic stenosis and using single suture line technique increases the success of implantation a stentless xenograft.

The direct suture of autologous pericardium to the aortic wall creating a new aortic valve does not need any supporting stent, sewing ring or cuff, allowing to rebuilt 3 symmetrical aortic cusps independent of the geometry of the native aortic valve. Harvesting a circular pericardium about 8-10 cm in diameter, treating with glutaraldehyde, sizing-cutting-shaping (a trefoil) with a specially designed instrument, and suturing the cut pericardium mounted on a tissue holder are the steps of this technique which does not take more time. The important goal is to reconstruct a newly geometrically symmetric valve and to ensure adequate coaptation with no prolapse. the suture technique is similar to the single suture line technique and running sutures are placed onto supra-annular aortic wall.

5.1. Subcoronary implantation technique

This approach is a simple method to implant a stentless bioprosthesis. In spite of the only handicap is the inexperience in this field, geometric thinking is the key point to perform a successful stentless AVR using this approach. A transverse aortotomy helps to image 3D shape of the aortic root which simplifies sizing and implanting a stentless valve. The proximal suture line is performed with the simple interrupted suture technique. This technique requires 18-24 sutures (4/0 Ticron or Polypropylene) which are placed in a circular plane coursing through the aortic annulus (annular suture line) and passed through the inflow end of the stentless valve (subannular suture line). All sutures are passed through the Dacron skirt of the bioprosthesis just below the lowest aspect of the cusps, but the sutures at the native commissures must be passed through the same level of prosthetic commissures to create a geometrical shape without any distortion. It is also important not to injury or perforate the prosthetic cusps when the needles are passed through the skirt of the stentless valve. If the aortic annulus is weakened or destroyed pledgeted sutures (4/0 Ticron) should be placed in subannular position to hold suture securely, which provides satisfactory buttressing effect and repairs annular ruptures. Because xenografts are not as pliable as homografts and its inversion into the left ventricle followed by being pulled up into the aorta may damage the device, I never use this maneuver. The prosthesis is lowered into the aortic root and sutured with its annulus to the aortic annulus as the baseline line, and all sutures are tied on the skirt. If the prosthesis has three own sinuses, at least the two sinuses facing the native left and right coronary ostia are scalloped out below the level of those recipient coronaries, leaving a 4-5 mm rim of prosthetic tissue behind. To suture sinuses of bioprosthesis to the native aortic sinuses, three continuous suture lines (5/0 polypropylene) are started in the nadir of each sinus below the native coronary ostia and in the nadir of the non-coronary sinus and progress upward to the top of three commissures (supra-annular suture line), taking care not to buckle the stentless tissue or distort the positions of the commissural posts. The sutures are taken outside the aorta, buttressed with a pledget and tied together. The deep bites of continuous sutures on the aortic sinuses can be transverse or horizontal, but they must be full-thickness at the host aortic wall. The broad bites must be taken on the aortic sinuses of bioprosthesis to avoid any space under device. It is also important to pass the needle well away from the margin of the stentless cusp attachment and not to injury the cusps. If the non-coronary sinus of the stentless valve is kept intact (modified subcoronary technique), it is not necessary to use the third suture, and the distal suture line is completed by running along the top to join the first two sutures. A stay suture (pledgeted 2/0 Ticron) may be placed at the top of each commissure to achieve 3D geometric shape of the device. If it is necessary the tops are trimmed down to the level of the native aorta. The aortotomy is closed with double continuous pledgeted sutures (4/0 polypropylene) beginning from each edge.

5.2. Single suture line technique

It is a simple modification of the subcoronary technique and it can be performed according to the design of stentless valve.

Classical subcoronary stentless valves could be implanted with only supra-annular running suture line that places the stentless annulus above and along the native annulus up and around each commissure (Sorin Freedom Solo, CryoLife O'Brien). In this approach, the device should fit the supra-annular area because the aortic trimmed wall of stentless valves is sutured and attached only with proximal supra-annular suture line directly to native aortic sinuses in supra-annular position. Three polypropylene sutures are started at the nadir of each sinus and brought progressively up to each commissural tip with the ends brought outside the aorta for tying (as described above). Because the stentless valve will be placed supra-annular we can choice a 1 or 2 number larger size than the true annular-size and that prevents any transvalvular gradient.

An alternative approach must be preferred in some stentless prostheses designed as having a tubular structure. The outflow orifice is supported by 3 commissural tabs at the distal junction of the leaflets. Inflow implantation is performed with the same running suture line, but the tops of three commissures are equipped at an appropriate location with stay sutures (pledgetless 2/0 Ticron) tied on the outside of the aorta (3f ATS, Shelhigh Superstentless). These tabs are sewn onto the patient's aortic wall, thereby maintaining the tubular integrity of the prosthesis. It is imperative to achieve true-sizing. Should uncertainty arise, the smaller prosthesis should be implanted because larger prosthesis can block a rapid and unobstructed opening, whereas to small prosthesis restricts of fully leaflet-opening. The same problem can also occur with an excessive or insufficient distal traction on the tabs.

5.3. Root inclusion technique

If the original cylindrical shape of the bioprosthetic root devices wants to be preserved without replacement of the native aortic root to avoid bleeding complication, the root inclusion technique can be chosen. A glutaraldehyde-treated porcine aortic root is implanted inside the patient's aortic root. But this technique is more difficult because both native coronary ostia should be anastomosed to the prosthesis like in classic Bentall procedure. After transverse aortotomy a proximal suture line is performed like the subcoronary technique in a circular plane coursing below the commissures. Appropriate opening for coronary ostia are made by excising the sinuses facing the right and left main coronary ostia and then both are sutured continuously (5/0 polypropylene). The only difference between the root inclusion and subcoronary techniques is that the complete sinotubular junction of the stentless valve is preserved. This method is not used nowadays, and if this technique is preferred it should not be used unless the root is large enough to place 23-mm or larger prosthetic root.

5.4. Root replacement technique

Complete replacement of the native aortic root is last preference for those devices. This technique is used mostly during auto- or homograft replacement. A part of the patient's ascending aorta with total aortic root is excised and a new glutaraldehyde-treated porcine aorta with total aortic root is inserted using a single proximal and distal suture lines. Only indication to prefer this approach is an extended pathology through aortic root (endocarditis, annular abscess, porcelain aorta, dissection) if a stentless valve is used. Since the tubular 3D geometry is not altered, its factory-tested performance is not affected by the implantation. All aortic root is excised and both coronary ostia are separated from the root. The valve seizer should fit in the aortic annulus and 1 or 2 number bigger stentless bioprosthesis is chosen. Depending on the anatomical details of the native right coronary artery, the device may be implanted anatomically or rotated to put the porcine left in the patient's right sinus. The proximal suture line is constructed with continuous polypropylene suture or interrupted sutures (4/0). The coronary buttons are re-implanted as the standard fashion (5/0 polypropylene). The distal end of the bioprosthesis is usually smaller than the distal native aorta, but it can be not a problem during distal anastomosis (4/0 polypropylene).

5.5. Direct suture technique of autologous pericardium

Truly stentless AVR using autologous pericardium sutured directly onto the aortic wall without supporting stents is a safe and feasible alternative with excellent hemodynamics of the aortic root [11]. With the use of specially designed instruments, the sinotubular junction is sized, the pericardium is placed on a base, and a cutting blade of the matching size is placed on top of the pericardium, which cuts it to the required size and shape (a trefoil). The cut pericardium is then mounted on a tissue holder to facilitate suturing it to the aortic wall. The prepared autologous pericardium is then sutured directly onto the aortic wall close to the marked annulus using 4–0 polypropylene sutures. Each running suture starting from the base of the leaflet cusp ends at each commissure where it passes through to the outside of the aorta, at which point the knot is tied. The commissures are then securely fixed by passing another mattress suture from inside the commissure to outside the aorta where it is tied. Leaflet symmetry and coaptation are assessed directly at the end of the procedure before closing the aortotomy.

5.6. Sutureless implantation technique

Aortic valve replacement with prosthetic heart valves is the treatment of choice for calcific aortic valve stenosis. Stentless valves are the best option with larger EOA and lower transvalvular gradient, but technically the implantations of these valves are more demanding resulting in longer operation times. However, important comorbid conditions in elderly patients referred for aortic valve replacement require alternative treatment options with possible reductions of the extracorporeal bypass and cross-clamp times and reliable hemodynamic features. In order to comply with these requirements, transcatheter (transfemoral or transapical) valves and sutureless surgical valves have been developed. The transcatheter techniques have the advantage of being performed without circulatory bypass but leaving the aortic calcifications in place, thereby resulting in a high degree of paravalvular insufficiency, atrioventricular block and strokes [37]. The surgical approach has the advantage of removing all calcifications and the valves can be optimally implanted, resulting in minimal paravalvular leak with a low incidence of atrioventricular block and strokes; however, it requires cardiopulmonary bypass. The design of sutureless bioprosthesis stems from the intention to offer an alternative to traditional flexible stentless prostheses using conventional open-heart surgery. Sutureless new designed bioprosthesis is a trileaflet bovine or equine pericardial valve mounted on an expandable metal frame in nitinol (equiatomic alloy of nickel and titanium). New designed stentless bioprostheses have several advantages: reducing cross-clamp and cardiopulmonary bypass times, reducing related risk by placing of proximal sutures, less risk of tearing the aortic annulus and wall, avoiding damage of the bundle of His, preventing foreign particle embolization. The primary benefit of this aortic bioprosthesis is the potential for surgeons to provide the same gold standard outcomes of traditional surgical AVR but without the need for sutures, thereby facilitating less invasive or minimally invasive procedures.

The transverse aortic incision is performed 1 cm above the sinotubular junction to preserve a segment of the ascending aorta above the prosthetic valve. Severe calcific aortic valve is removed and aortic annulus should be decalcified for implantation (it is not necessary a complete decalcification). To ensure the correct positioning and orientation of the prosthesis guide-suture(s) can be used. Avoidance of proximal suture lines makes the procedure easier. The architectural design of this new kind of bioprosthesis allows perfect function after it adapts itself to the aortic root. They have two cylindrical ring segments: 'outflow ring' comprises straight posts designed to support the valve and 'inflow ring' allows the prosthesis to be anchored to the aortic root in the Valsalva sinuses and reaches a final diameter compatible with the aortic root. The configuration of the stentless valve is perfect which allows higher hemodynamic performance. There are two types of sutureless aortic bioprostheses in the market.

The Perceval S Aortic Bioprosthesis (Sorin Biomedia Cardio Srl, Sallugia, Italy) has been introduced for minithoracotomy incision [38]. After the device is introduced and parachuted down into aortic annulus and checking corrected position, a balloon dilatation of the inflow ring is performed in the Perceval S valve. If the device is in malpositioning the valve can be quickly removed using the 'χ movement' and repositioned [39]. Because there are only three number valves (21, 23, 25), paravalvular leakage can be observed in higher incidence (4.4% postoperatively and 4% during follow-up) which can be a result of either inadequate sizing or due to inappropriate decalcification of the annulus [40]. For an enlarged aorta with a ratio greater than 1.3, the predicted diameter according to body surface area represents a contraindication for this device. Early mortality (total 2.4%) and late death (total 2.5%) is acceptable with lower transvalvular gradient (10.8 mmHg) at the first postoperative year [41].

The 3f Enable Aortic Bioprothesis (Model 6000; Medtronic Inc, Minneapolis, USA) is more different and the implantation is more easier: after insertion the device into aortic root in the corrected position, only pour warmer saline (> 30°) onto the device to fully deploy the Nitinol frame into its original shape [42]. If malpositioning occurs after complete deployment, rinsing with chilled saline makes the nitinol stent flexible and enhances repositioning until the valve is correctly placed. Early clinical and hemodynamic performances of the 3f aortic bioprosthesis are similar to those of the regular stentless aortic valves, but both parameters could be inconsistent with the established stentless valves during mid-term follow-up: unfavorable mean gradient especially with smaller number (≤ 23 mm), incomplete left ventricular regression, higher incidence of neurologic complications [43]. However, a multi-center study has shown better early and mid-term results: major paravalvular leakage 2.1%, neurologic events 0.7%, lower mean gradient (10.2 mmHg), lower valve-related early mortality rate (1.4%; total 3.6%); lower late mortality rate (1.5%; total 9.6%), excellent freedom from valve-related mortality at 1-year (96.5%; hazard ratio 1.6%/year), lower paravalvular leakage (0.8%/year) [44].

The analysis of the current outcome of the use of sutureless aortic bioprostheses must take into consideration the preliminary nature of these devices and the relevant implantation learning curve. There are no comparative study analyzing the outcomes of sutureless and stentless bioprostheses, but it can be said that sutureless bioprostheses have better outcome (mortality, neurologic deficit, renal failure, bleeding) than conventional stentless valves in high-risk patients with aortic stenosis (such as older, female, left ventricular dysfunction, calcification in the ascending aorta, previously cardiac operation, pulmonary or renal disease? [45].

5.7. Transcatheter (transfemoral or transapical) aortic valve implantation

The approval of transcatheter aortic valve implantation (AVI) represents a fundamental change in the management of calcific aortic stenosis by offering an alternative to traditional surgical AVR in carefully selected patients. Patient-selection is very strict nowadays, and AVI is a reasonable alternative to surgical AVR in adults with severe symptomatic calcific aortic stenosis if they have suitable aortic and vascular anatomy for transcatheter AVI and a predicted survival > 12 months [46]. Transcatheter AVI can be prefer in patients with severe calcific aortic stenosis if their aortic valve is trileaflet. There are some exclusion criteria in calcific aortic stenosis: en-block calcification (like unicusp), bicuspid aortic valve, severe massive calcification closely coronary ostia, small aortic annulus (< 18 mm) or large aortic orifice (> 25 mm), thoraco-abdominal aortic or peripheral arterial pathologies. Transapical AVI is the another alternative in patients with calcific aortic stenosis associated thoraco-abdominal aortic or peripheral arterial pathologies.

As experience is gained and technology evolves, new areas will be met with this approaches. The most optional area is bioprosthesis dysfunction requiring reoperation and an attractive option is to use a AVI procedure in which the device is deployed within the previously placed bioprosthesis: valve-in-valve. Valve-in-valve procedures require a large enough bioprosthetic valve inserted at the index operation to prevent patient-prosthetic mismatch with the AVI valve.

6. Special situations

Calcific aortic stenosis is a long-term disease and usually associated with other cardiovascular pathologies. Before AVR, all these situations must be reassessmended and case-specific operation procedure and its alternatives must be planned. If we do not think preoperatively that any specific situation needs an intervention intra-operatively, spontaneously home-made resolutions can be also very helpful in the theater when we decide to correct this pathology.

6.1. Proximal ascending aorta aneurysm

Severe aortic stenosis is usually combined with proximal ascending aorta aneurysm causing by turbulent flow. The gold standard treatment is composite aortic valve and root replacement. Several surgical teams have devised strategies to construct their homemade composite conduits intra-operatively. It can be a mechanical valved conduit with excellent long-term results [47]. If any contra-indication for anticoagulation therapy, a composite bioprosthetic valved conduit will be the best alternative. Because severe calcific aortic stenosis is often an elderly disease, improved durability of bioprostheses stimulates also their use in the setting of ascending aorta replacement if proximal ascending aorta requires replacement in this population. The concept of composite bioprosthetic valved conduits has also been taken up by the industry and these conduits are already commercially available in different sizes. There are several technical options to allow replacement of the aortic root and ascending aorta using either stented or stentless bioprosthesis [48]. There are basically two alternatives to built a composite graft with a stentless bioprosthesis: the subcoronary technique and the full-root technique.

The subcoronary implantation technique requires a tubular graft and double suture lines for device implantation is necessary. A stentless valve is placed inside a Dacron tube graft leaving a proximal free margin (3-5 mm) and the proximal suture line of the stentless bioprosthesis is fixed to the graft with a running mattress suture [49]. The free end of the tube graft is then sutured to the native annulus with pledgeted interrupted mattress sutures, and following this, the upper circumference of the stentless valve is reimplanted within the tube graft using a second running mattress suture. To avoid the potential drawbacks of a straight cylindrical tube an aortic graft with pseudo-sinuses can be used [50] or David-V procedure using a stentless bioprosthesis can be applied to build new sinuses [51]. I implant firstly tubular synthetic graft using pledgeted interrupted mattress sutures subannularly, and then a stentless valve is implanted using the single suture line technique as described above. The ready-to-use composite biological valved graft is also available in practice currently [The BioValsalva composite grafts (Sulzer Vascutek, Renfrewshire, Scotland, UK)] [52].

The full-root technique is preferred in order to reduce distortion risk leading valve regurgitation or deterioration, but the commercially available stentless porcine aortic root devices are usually too short to replace the host ascending aorta. There are also four alternatives to suture a stentless conduit directly to the distal ascending aorta with extended tubular devices: extended version of stentless porcine aortic root bioprosthesis, direct anastomosis after extensive mobilization of the host aorta, interposition of a Dacron tube graft, and total xenopericardial valved conduit. The availability of extended root xenograft is extremely limited, but this approach can achieve an anastomosis between xenograft and the distal ascending aorta [53]. Primary end-to-end anastomosis might prevent the need for graft interposition, but extensive mobilization of the aortic arch and its branches can be dangerous and some tension might be left at the distal anastomosis with a risk of late dehiscence and false aneurysm development [54]. The most practical technique appears to be the insertion of a Dacron tube graft between the xenograft root and the native distal ascending aorta [55]. There is a new bioprosthetic conduit, constructed using individual non-coronary porcine cusps, which are fitted on a scalloped shaped tubular bovine pericardium [56]. The 15 cm long pericardial cuff is long enough to facilitate the anastomosis between the conduit and the remaining distal aorta. If mid- or long-term results will confirm excellent results, this option will be an attractive alternative to the others techniques.

6.2. Small aortic annulus

Aortic valve replacement with a small stented prosthetic valve is technically straightforward and frequently performed, but it may result in patient-prosthesis mismatch and a high residual outflow gradient, which is significant risk factor for early mortality [57]. Patient-prosthesis mismatch is associated with an increase in all-cause and cardiac-related mortality over long-term follow-up, and current efforts to prevent prosthesis-patient mismatch should receive more emphasis and a widespread acceptance to improve long-term survival after AVR [58]. When the aortic annulus diameter is less than 20 mm, a relatively high transvalvular velocity has to be expected after valve replacement. In these cases, a stentless bioprosthesis with/without aortic root enlargement would provide better hemodynamic results than stented valves.

For severe small aortic root with small aortic annulus, a xenograft root replacement can be the first alternative and this technique avoids the aortic annulus enlargement, but it can be problematic because of reimplantation of the coronary arteries, calcified aorta and/or coronary ostia, or prolonged operation times. The full-root replacement technique is technically more demanding, but it prevents residual gradient postoperatively, and if one number larger conduit is selected the possible largest orifice area will be gained. Subcoronary techniques with/without intact non-coronary sinus can be also used in these patients with excellent hemodynamics in smaller valve sizes and appropriate device can be implanted safely and easily [59].

Another alternative technique is aortic annulus enlargement to prevent patient-prosthesis mismatch and a two-size-larger prosthesis could be inserted. The most commonly used technique is enlargement of the aortic annulus with a biologic or synthetic patch which can be performed in different approach [60]. A modification of the Manouguian technique has been introduced for aortic annulus enlargement without using a patch [61]. A tubular aortic bioprosthesis of one or two sizes larger than the size of the native annulus is prepared for modified subcoronary implantation technique and non-coronary sinus wall be kept intact. The prosthesis is sutured directly on the enlarged annulus after the aortic incision is extended through the commissure, and the aorta is closed directly with the mural wall of the tubular xenograft.

6.3. Porcelain aorta

The scope of porcelain aorta ranges from isolated plaques to the circumferential calcification of the ascending aorta. Typically, a heavily calcified ascending aorta with calcific aortic stenosis involves aortic annulus, aortic valve, aortic root and ascending aorta (± distal aortic segments). This scenario is associated with higher operative mortality and morbidity than isolated severe calcific aortic stenosis. A more recent study have been demonstrated a link between arterio-sclerotic changes in aortic valve and ascending aorta [62]. This study compared healthy patients with severe aortic stenosis patients shows that the prevalence of aortic root calcification (26% versus 54%; $p = 0.008$) and of atheroma in the ascending aorta (7% versus 24%; $p < 0.001$) are higher in aortic valve disease patients and patients coexisting coronary artery disease have more extensive arteriosclerotic changes in the thoracic aorta compared with those with aortic stenosis alone and control subjects.

The operative management of severe calcific aortic stenosis with porcelain aorta can be difficult and complex because of difficulty of clamping the ascending aorta, aortotomy, supra-annular sutures, or aortic root replacement, and the risk of calcific embolization of major branches (coronary, carotid, or other arteries), aortic dissection. Digital palpation with a lowered systemic blood pressure or epiaortic sonographic evaluation can be used to confirm that there is a softer spot in the aortic arch for cannulation intra-operatively. If there is no any healthy site on the distal ascending aorta or aortic arch for regular arterial cannulation (34%), alternative arterial cannulation should be performed through innominate (8%), axillary (24%) or femoral (34%) artery [63]. There are several alternatives to perform AVR: standard replacement, endarterectomy for calcified porcelain aorta, no touch technique under circulatory arrest (no cross-clamp, no endarterectomy, no ascending aorta replacement), total replacement of the ascending aorta replacement (with/without circulatory arrest), apico-aortic valved conduit, transcatheter AVI. I prefer standard AVR if it is possible, if not I perform David-V total ascending aortic replacement with a stentless bioprosthesis [47]. Last decade, ascending aortic replacement is the most preferred method for the treatment of porcelain aorta, but transfemoral [64] or transapical [65] AVI will replace the first choice of the treatment in this decade. These alternatives demonstrate significant advantages (especially very low incidence of neurological events, avoidance of cardiopulmonary bypass and circulatory arrest) in comparison to other conventional techniques in the setting of severe aortic calcification.

6.4. Concomitant severe coronary artery disease

Many patients with moderate or severe calcific aortic stenosis have significant coronary disease, suggesting that the degenerative changes of the aortic valve leading to aortic stenosis may be part of a similar arteriosclerotic process. Coronary lesion can be also in different coronary arteries or massif calcification involves into coronary ostia. Combined surgical treatment is the main modality, but percutaneous coronary intervention is safer in patients undergoing transcatheter AVI, or in patients with high risk (high comorbidities, reoperation, pericardial adhesion). Because hypercholesterolemia is related to increased risk of aortic valve calcification in patients with aortic stenosis, preventive treatment of hypercholesterolemia could play an important role to decrease or inhibit development of aortic valve calcification [66].

6.5. Concomitant hematologic disease

The best opportunity to improve the treatment of any hematologic disease or to prevent any complication aggravating by hematologic pathologies is avoidance from prosthetic foreign devices. Autologous tissue is the only biologic material preparing prosthetic valve, but that can be limited because of pericardial pathologies, inadequate surgical experience or technical problems. Mechanical valves have life-long durability with some possible hematologic complications such as thrombo-embolism, warfarin related hemorrhage, heparin induced thrombocytopenia, hemolysis. Prosthetic foreign material can also aggravate hematologic diseases. To decide which prosthesis can be the acceptable choice for AVR in patients with hematologic pathology is depend on patient's characteristics and patient-by-patient analysis is required. Biomaterials seem better than mechanical prostheses, and stentless aortic bioprostheses are the best alternatives because of absence of a rigid stent, biodynamic characteristics, larger EOA with lowest transvalvular obstruction, unnecessariness of anticoagulation, which might decrease hematologic complications. I prefer stentless xenografts for AVR in patients with severe hematologic pathologies [67].

Postoperative thrombocytopenia is a transient phenomenon, self–recovering after a few days without any treatment and without any observed recurrence in late follow-up. Microhemodynamic effects of the prosthesis structure or depending on the implantation technique and/or specific chemical preparations of biological prosthesis tissue could act as a trigger for the post-replacement thrombocytopenia. It seems to be possible that transient unspecific activation of platelets result in diffuse consumption and lower platelet levels. The reason for this phenomenon is unknown and the use of consistent monitoring is necessary to prevent severe falls in platelet count. It seems unrelated to the type of aortic bioprosthesis and I have not observed this phenomenon only in stentless pericardial valves, but also in different bioprostheses [68]. However, thrombocytopenia after implantation of the stentless pericardial xenografts can develop more common and becomes dangerous for the patient [69,70].

7. Surgical–technical complications

In spite of all implantation techniques of different stentless bioprostheses are demanding and require an aortic valve surgical experience, some situations can make trouble AVR intra-operatively or impair operative outcomes in the early postoperative period. Every surgeon must be aware of these troubles and keep in mind case specific technical solutions in the theater.

7.1. Severe annular calcification

To replace the diseased aortic valve in patients with calcific aortic stenosis is a serious intervention because of extensive calcification. Debridement of all calcium deposits back to soft tissue improves seating of stentless prostheses in supra-annular position and provides better performance, and may be, protects devices early calcification. I always prefer deep debridement and decalcification of all around structures. If there is no any damage on the annulus, I implant a stentless valve with the single suture technique (supra-annular implantation); if not, I prefer the classic subcoronary technique and use pledgeted sutures in subannular position to repair defects. Calcification after stentless valve implantation is complicated if a stentless bioprosthesis is implanted in young patient: faster calcification in homografts has been reported compared with xenografts [71].

7.2. Conduction disturbances

Permanent of transient conduction defects are well-known complications of aortic valve surgery [72]. Higher degree atrioventricular blocks are often reversible and disappear before discharge from the hospital. Approximately 5% of patients undergone isolated AVR require permanent pacemaker implantation. Risk factors can be patient-specific: bicuspid aorta, annular calcification, hypertension, preexisting conduction disturbances, coronary artery disease. Surgeon-specific risk factors cause mostly mechanical injury of the atrioventricular conduction pathways during aortic valve surgery: annular decalcification, deep suture placement, suturing techniques, pressure on the conduction tissue. Atrioventricular block generally results from trauma to the atrioventricular node or His bundle in the region of membranous septum and right trigone beneath the non-coronary - right coronary cusps commissure. The continuous inflow suture line is the most common cause for atrioventricular block because this suture line is placed below each commissure in a horizontal plane based on the level of the nadir of the attachments of the native aortic valve leaflets to the native aortic valve annulus. Raising the continuous inflow suture line below non-coronary - right coronary commissure prevents such conduction complication. Interrupted inflow sutures are also safer than continuous technique. The best approach is the single suture line technique which does not need any inflow suture line.

7.3. Coronary insufficiency

Coronary flow complications are uncommon after stentless AVR, in spite of calcific aortic valve stenosis appears often with coronary ostia calcification with/without coronary artery disease. Myocardial ischemia developing after AVR can develop due to several reasons. Uniform adequate myocardial preservation during operation is the main preventive strategy. Coronary artery bypass grafting should be added aortic valve surgery if any coronary artery stenosis is proved angiographically before surgery. Technical or pathologic factors must also keep in mind. Extensive calcific involvement of coronary ostia or any calcific particle embolization can block antegrade coronary blood flow postoperatively. Endarterectomy or coronary artery bypass grafting should be performed if not any coronary lesion is proved. Decalcification of the aortic root may be well without any aggressive manipulation on coronary ostia, but rupture around coronary ostia can be fatal. Implantation techniques can damage coronary blood flow due to technical errors. Besides a learning curve for these more complex procedures, other factors that could potentially contribute to excess myocardial ischemia or bleeding causing coronary ostia complications. Technical problems can occur mostly during the aortic root replacement with stentless xenografts. This type of coronary insufficiency is uncommon and more often affects the right coronary artery [73]. Coronary buttons are prepared for suturing to xenografts, but they can be damaged because of extensive cutting, dissection, or aggressive decalcification of buttons. Severe tension on the button anastomoses can cause bleeding, rupture, kinking or obstruction. Preventive maneuvers are recognition of coronary orientation, routine xenograft rotation, adequate coronary button mobilization, oversizing xenograft. The subcoronary implantation is more secure procedure than the root replacement technique and technical complication causing coronary problems can occur very seldom if running sutures bite very close to the coronary ostia.

7.4. Dehiscence

Partial or severe dehiscence of aortic prosthetic valves is a serious, but very rare complication. Complete dehiscence occurs with sudden death and it is not seen during practice life. Demand on the severity of dehiscence, the clinic scenario can be variable. Limited dehiscence can be silent and stable, more serious dehiscence shows some signs and unstable. If the aortic root replacement technique is preferred dehiscence can be very small at the proximal or distal suture line which presents bleeding, hematoma or massif hemorrhage. Dehiscence observed after the subcoronary implantation technique is associated with aortic regurgitation, but using obliterating sutures prevent usually this complication. In the aortic root inclusion technique, the dead space between native and donor aortas might be prevented adequate fusion of the walls and healing of the anastomoses, which is observed mostly in non-coronary sinus [74]. Any symptomatic dehiscence investigated by echocardiography intra- or early postoperatively should be repaired and a reoperation should be performed immediately. In the absence of valve dysfunction, progressive dehiscence, or the development of thrombus a reoperation can be not necessary and conservative management will be safe during early- and long-term follow-up [75].

http://dx.doi.org/10.5772/55373

7.5. Progressive sinotubular junction dilatation

This late postoperative complication is observed in some stentless xenografts when they are implanted with the subcoronary technique. Currently, little is known of the diastolic properties of stentless valves that affect stress and strain on leaflets and, hence, their durability. Despite similar systolic performances, stentless prostheses behave differently during diastole. The commissures of the stentless bioprostheses have to follow the dimensional changes of the native aortic root not only in a cyclic mode but also the increase of the aortic diameter [76]. This change pulls apart the commissures leading to reduction of coaptation area of the cusps and late aortic insufficiency develops. Aortic regurgitation is often mild or moderate depending on bioprosthesis type, especially in old generation, but re-operation rate is low. In a pressurized aortic root model, a series of in-vitro tests is conducted to determine how stentless valves behave in diastole, and how they adapt to different annulus-to-sinotubular junction (STJ) ratios [77]. Pericardial prostheses built to mimic a cylinder (ATS 3F and Sorin Solo) showed the greatest tolerance to STJ dilatation and a larger coaptation surface, but also a tendency to roll in on themselves in an italic S-shape if oversized. Valves built to mimic native aortic leaflets (porcine Prima Plus and Medtronic Freestyle) showed a reduced tolerance to STJ dilatation, resulting in regurgitation and a smaller coaptation surface, but also a reduced tendency to roll if oversized.

A significant difference of tolerance against aortic regurgitation with respect to dilatation of the sinotubular junction was found in an in vitro study: fresh porcine aortic root (higher) > fresh porcine pulmonary root > stentless porcine bioprosthesis (lower) [78]. This loss of adaptability may be related to the glutaraldehyde fixation leading stiffness and shrinkage of the bioprosthetic leaflets which leaves inadequate coaptation reserve. An increase of sinotubular junction diameter of more than 32% for the Toronto SPV and 43% for Medtronic Freestyle stentless valves results in a distinct loss of leaflet coaptation and causes aortic regurgitation.

New generation of pericardial stentless valves developed for subcoronary implantation have larger coaptation area than those old generation or porcine stentless valves, which may provide better adaptability to adverse changes in root dimensions [79]. With massif progressive stepwise dilatation at sinotubular junction level, the free edges of the leaflets are stretched wider and a triangle-shaped central coaptation defect will occur. For the 3F Aortic valve regurgitation started at approximately 156% of the labeled valve size and 145% for the Sorin Solo valve. The increased tolerance of pericardial bioprostheses may improve long-term valve performance, but durability of these valves may be affected by the redundant leaflet tissue leading increase of leaflet stress and degeneration.

To overcome this disadvantage of stentless valves, a slight oversizing of the devices may result better valve competence and hemodynamic efficiency compared to size-for-size implantation. Sizing with a supra-annular seizer is helpful to find the largest stentless valve number which is minimum equal to the sinotubular junction diameter in patients with healthy aortic root. The single suture line technique is fixed prosthetic sinuses onto the native aortic wall to prevent any leakage or stretching.

7.6. Reoperation of a stentless aortic bioprosthesis

Stentless aortic valve reoperations may become more common as these bioprostheses reach the limits of their durability, which are a challenging procedure with an increased risk of death [80].The current generation of stentless valves have been implanted since the early 1990s and are therefore starting to reach the limits of their durability. Reoperation for stentless valves is a complex procedure, especially root inclusion or full-root replacement was preferred. The risk of trauma to the coronary ostia, aortic wall, aortic annulus, anterior mitral valve, and membranous septum can all occur when severe adhesions or calcification are present around the stentless valve. Reoperation after a stentless valve is more complex than after a stented tissue or mechanical valve if root replacement techniques is used in the first operation. However, reoperation of subcoronary implanted stentless bioprosthesis is easier than any stented prosthesis because cutting only the suture line is enough to remove the degenerated bioprosthesis. Valve-in-valve replacement with transfemoral [81] or transapical [82] AVI is a more conservative alternative strategy for re-replacement of degenerated xenograft in high risk patients.

8. Clinical results

8.1. Survival

Risk of death is highest immediately after AVR in patients with severe aortic stenosis, decreased to its nadir approximately 1 year postoperatively (early hazard period), and then gradually increased (late hazard period) [83]. From approximately 2 years after operation, survival is similar to that of matched population estimates. Early outcome of patients with aortic stenosis after AVR is primarily influenced by severity of the stenosis, left ventricular hypertrophy and dysfunction at operation. Severity of aortic stenosis, severe left ventricular hypertrophy, left ventricular dysfunction, older age and patient-prosthesis mismatch worsen also long-term survival. Furthermore, stentless AVR requires longer cross-clamp and cardiopulmonary bypass times.

Several meta-analysis studies confirm that stentless AVR does not worsen the early and late outcome when compared to stented bioprostheses. Also, longer operation times do not have any adverse effect on the intra-operatively mortal complications and postoperative outcomes. Contrarily, early recovery of hemodynamic malfunctions caused by calcific stenotic native aortic valve brings better early and late outcomes.

Hospital mortality rate of stentless bioprostheses is lower than those of stented xenografts [84,85]. Early hospital or 30-day mortality is similar between stentless and stented bioprosthesis replacement in a meta-analysis (3.2% versus 2.4%; $p = 0.39$), and further analysis of 30-days mortality is subgroups included predominantly patients with aortic stenosis shows still no significant difference between two types of aortic bioprosthesis (3.7% versus 2.6%; $p = 0.44$) [86]. Only one retrospective multicenter study has shown if stentless valves are used only in selected patients (older age, female, full-root replacement) the 30-day mortality is increased when compared with stented valves (7.5% versus 3.3%; p = 0.026), but if stentless valves are used widely there is no significant difference in operative mortality between stentless and stented groups [87].Using autologous pericardium does not worse the early hospital outcome and early mortality is not seen [11].

Several studies showed an improved mid-term (< 10 years) survival after stentless AVR compared to stented valves [88,89]. A meta-analysis shows that mortality at the first year is lower after stentless aortic bioprosthesis replacement than stented bioprosthesis, but not significant: 7.5% versus 8.9%; p = 0.73 [15]. Another meta analysis also confirm no significant difference for valve-related mortality between stentless and stented xenograft replacement in the first postoperative year [86]. Lehmann and associates [89] showed in a randomized trial that 8-year survival was 78.1% ± 3.8% stentless versus 66.7% ± 4.9% stented (p = 0.03). They concluded that there was no difference in survival when compared stentless patients with an age-matched German control population.

The long-term results (≥ 10 years) with stentless valves are excellent [90]. The overall 10- and 15-year survival rates of Freestyle bioprosthesis are 60.7% and 35%, respectively [91]. The 10-year actuarial survival (44.1% ± 4.3% in subcoronary, 47.3% ± 8.15 in full-root, and 45.4% ± 13.7% in root inclusion groups; p = 0.89) and freedom from valve-related death (94.5% ± 2.9% in subcoronary, 92.9% ± 5.8% in full-root, and 87.8% ± 12.5% in root inclusion groups; p = 0.17) are similar between implants techniques with the Freestyle stentless bioprosthesis [92]. Longer follow-up (> 15 years) of stentless valves is also necessary to compare the excellent results of stented valves to establish that stentless xenografts are significantly superior than stented devices.

8.2. Durability

The rate of structural valve deterioration increases over time, especially after the initial 7 to 8 years after implantation. Structural degeneration increases long-term events and the rate of failure is < 1% at 10 years in patients older than 65 years [93]. Pericardial valves might be better than porcine valves, but all newer-generation bioprostheses are more durable. In spite of the rate of failure of any bioprosthesis decreases with the age of the patient at the time of implantation (< 10% at 10 years in patients older > 70 years), the number of implanted stentless xenografts has increased due to improved hemodynamic performance and long-term durability during last decade. Theoretically, xenogenic stentless aortic valves have better durability than stented valves. But in real life, the freedom rate from structural valve deterioration is similar in stentless and stented bioprostheses (> 90% at 10 years). CryoLife O'Brien and St Jude Toronto SPV valves have worst durability compared the other stentless valves (Medtronic Freestyle, Edwards Prima, St Jude Biocor, Sorin Pericarbon and Solo, ATS 3f).

When we focus on the implantation techniques, there are very rare papers in the literature. The overall freedom from reoperation with Freestyle stentless bioprosthesis is 91.0% and 75.0% at 10 and 15 years, whereas freedom from reoperation for structural valve deterioration was 95.9% and 82.3%, respectively. At 10 and 15 years, freedom from reoperation for structural valve deterioration is 94.0% and 62.6% for patients < 60 years of age and 96.3% and 88.4% for patients ≥ 60 years of age (p = 0.002) [90]. The actuarial freedom from reoperation (91.7% ± 3.5%

in subcoronary, 92.3% ± 6.0% in full-root, and 92.0% ± 10.7% in root inclusion groups; $p = 0.82$) and from structural valve deterioration (97.0% ± 2.2% in subcoronary, 96.0% ± 4.5% in full-root, and 90.9% ± 11.2% in root inclusion groups; $p = 0.54$) are similar between implants techniques with the Freestyle stentless valves [91].

The truly stentless autologous pericardial aortic valve may be better choice in patients who cannot or do not want to take anticoagulation, especially young population, because excellent long-term durability and easier reoperation, which is technically undemanding compared to other stentless bioprostheses. The use of autologous pericardium avoids any immune reaction between the host and the implanted valve, and minimizes tissue calcification and pannus formation, which are important causes of structural valve deterioration. The absence of a stent and sewing ring is also helpful for long-term durability with a freedom from structural valve deterioration of 100% at 7.5 years [11]. Long-term durability seems better than the other bioprostheses because it has been reported that there is no calcification, no structural dysfunction on the autologous pericardium used for aortic leaflet extension at 13 years [94]. Reoperation must be easier because there is no calcification on the aorta and pericardial aortic valve.

8.3. Echocardiographic outcomes

The advantage of stentless xenografts is providing a greater EOA index for a given valve size, which results lower transvalvular gradients compared with stented valves. These improvements have been reported in a meta analysis: lower mean aortic valve gradient (-3.57 mmHg; $p < 0.01$), lower peak gradient (-5.8 mmHg; $p < 0.01$), but higher EOA index in stentless group compared with the stented [15]. It has been shown in an experimental porcine model that the annular cross-sectional area of stentless valves is significantly larger than stented valves [23]. The EOA will increase after first postoperative year in stentless valves and significant differences in mean and/or peak pressure differences between stentless and stented valves will continue during long-term follow-up [95,96].

The Freedom SOLO stentless bioprosthesis with all size-number has a lower mean (10.6 ± 3.6 mmHg) and peak (15.9 ± 9.1 mmHg) transvalvular gradient at discharged, and below 10 mmHg in all sizes (21-27 mm) at the first postoperative year [97]. The similar results have been shown by other groups: lower mean gradient (6.7 +/- 4.1 mmHg) and a significant regression of left ventricular hypertrophy (23%) at 12 months [98].

3f aortic bioprosthesis has a satisfactory hemodynamic performance with substitutes larger than 23 mm (< 10 mmHg), but smaller valves have a significant higher mean transvalvular gradient at the 4-postoperative year (18 mmHg for 21 mm and 14 mmHg for 23 mm devices) [36]. The left ventricular mass index decreases during follow-up (showed 18% regression), but cannot reach the normal range, especially with small devices. In another study with a mean valve size 26.0 ± 1.9 mm has shown that the mean transvalvular gradient of 3f bioprostheses has increased at 5 years (15.2 ± 5.3 mmHg) [99].

The Edwards Prima Plus stentless valve bioprosthesis is a porcine aortic root cylinder and is associated with high early peak and mean transprosthetic gradients (37 ± 16 and 18 ±8 mmHg, respectively), which regress with significant improvement at 1 year (25 ±7 and 12 ±4 mmHg, respectively) and concomitant regression of left ventricular hypertrophy [100]. The Edwards Prima Plus stentless xenograft implanted with intact non-coronary sinus technique prevents the geometry of the device and has excellent long-term result (mean gradient < 10 mmHg) in all sizes (21-29 mm) [101].

There are some studies showing different results regarding transaortic gradient, which might be a result of different stentless xenografts or implantation methods. There is no any significantly difference among implantation techniques when the same stentless xenograft is used with different implantation techniques, but full root (4.8 mmHg) or root inclusion technique (5.1 mmHg) has lower mean transvalvular gradient than the subcoronary technique (7.2 mmHg) [102]. Transvalvular gradient and EOA are significantly worse in subcoronary groups in the first postoperative period, but this difference will be insignificant due to decreasing EOA and root inclusion approach will have the worst hemodynamics at 10th postoperative year [90].

Stentless valves are the best choice in patients with small aortic annuli than large annuli, because the lower transaortic pressure difference of stentless valves has no any significant advantage over stented bioprostheses if a valve larger than 23 mm will be used [103]. The difference will be significantly when a stentless valve sized 23 mm is used (Freestyle inclusion 11 mmHg versus Perimount 25 mmHg) [21]. The Freedom SOLO stentless bioprosthesis seems to have better hemodynamics even in patients received a small aortic bioprosthesis with a lower mean transvalvular gradient (9 ± 2.9 mmHg for 21 mm, and 7.6 ± 5 mmHg for 23 mm) [97].

Physically active patients might benefit from stentless valves. Several studies showed that the gradient difference between different aortic stentless and stented bioprostheses of similar size with different implantation techniques increased significantly at each exercise level in favour of stentless valves [104-105106].

9. Conclusion

Aortic valve replacement means that native valve disease is replaced with prosthetic valve inadequacy affected by prosthetic valve hemodynamics, durability, and thrombogenicity. Stentless bioprostheses have better hemodynamic properties because of larger effective orifice area, better coronary flow, lower transvalvular gradient and better left ventricular mass regression than stented bioprostheses. They have also better biomechanical properties and the preserved distensibility may diminish stress considerably. Valve-related morbidity and structural valve degeneration are not worse than stented valves, but their implantation is demanding and required experience in this field. Although experienced centers give excellent results with stentless xenografts, most surgeons also prefer a stented xenograft to keep the procedure quick, safe, and simple. But, there is a trend to favor stentless valves nowadays because these valves provide larger effective orifice area, lower transvalvular gradients and excellent hemodynamics which stimulate rapid and effective reduction in left ventricular hypertrophy. It seems that the usage of stentless valves has more advantages in patients with impaired left ventricular function, small aortic, or aortic root abscess or more active patients. In future, using of stentless valves will increase with simpler implantation techniques, increased surgical experience, new design of prostheses, may be, using sutureless valves.

Author details

Kaan Kirali*

Address all correspondence to: imkbkirali@yahoo.com

Depertment of cardiovascular surgery, kosuyolu heart and research hospital, Istanbul, Turkey

References

[1] Ross DN. Homograft Replacement of the Aortic Valve. Lancet 1962;2:487.

[2] Barrat-Boyes BG. Homograft Aortic Valve Replacement in Aortic Incompetence and Stenosis. Thorax 1964;19:131-150.

[3] Binet JP, Duran CCT, Carpentier A, Langlois J. Heterologous Aortic Valve Transplantation. Lancet 1965;2:1275-1276.

[4] Sievers HH, Lange PE, Bernhard A. Implantation of a xenogenic Stentless Aortic Bioprosthesis. First Experience. Thoracic Cardiovascular Surgeon 1985;33(4):225-226.

[5] David TE, Pollick C, Bos J. Aortic Valve Replacement with Stentless Porcine Aortic Bioprosthesis. Journal of Thoracic Cardiovascular Surgery 1990;99(1):113-118.

[6] Pelletier LC, Carrier M. Bioprosthetice Heart Valves: 25 Years of Development and Clinical Experience. In: Acar J and Bodnar E (eds). Textbook of Acquired Heart Valve Disease. ICR Publishers: London; 1995. p920-956.

[7] David TE. Stentless Bioprosthetic Valves. In: Acar J and Bodnar E (eds). Textbook of Acquired Heart Valve Disease. ICR Publishers: London; 1995. p957-964.

[8] Takkenberg JJM, Klieverik LMA, Schoof PH, van Suylen R-J, van Herwerden LA, Zondervan PE, Roos-Hesselink JW, Eijkemans MJ, Yacoub MH, Bogers AJ. The Ross Procedure. A Systematic Rewiev and Meta-Analysis. Circulation. 2009;119(2): 222-228.

[9] El-Hamamsy I, Clark L, Stevens LM, Sarang Z, Melina G, Takkenberg JJ, Yacoub MH. Late Outcomes Following Freestyle versus Homograft Aortic Root Replace-

ment. Results from a Prospective Randomized Trial. Journal of American College of Cardiology 2010;55(4):368-376.

[10] Love JW. Autologous Pericardial Reconstruction of Semilunar Valves. Journal of Heart Valve Disease 1998;7(1):40–47.

[11] Chan KMJ, Rahman-Haley S, Mittal TK, Gavino JA, Dreyfus GD. Truly StentlessAutologous Pericardial Aortic Valve Replacement: An Alternative to Standard Aortic Valve Replacement. Journal of Thoracic Cardiovascular Surgery 2011;141(1):276-283.

[12] Frost MW, Funderl JA, Klaaborg KE, Wierup P, Sloth E, Nygaard H, Hasenkam JM. Leaflet Opening and Closing Dynamics of Aortic Bioprostheses. Journal of Heart Valve Disease 2010;19(4):492-498.

[13] Revanna P, Fisher J, Watterson KG. The Influence of Free Hand Sturing Technique and Zero Pressure Fixation on the Hemodynamic Function of Aortic Root and Aortic Valve Leaflets. European Journal of Cardiovascular Surgery 1997;11(2):280-286.

[14] Cohen G, Christakis GT, Joyner CD, Morgan CD, Tamariz M, Hanayama N, Mallidi H, Szalai JP, Katic M, Rao V, Fremes SE, Goldman BS. Are Stentless Valves Hemodynamically Superior to Stented Valves? A Prospective Randomized Trial. Annals of Thoracic Surgery 2002;73(3):767-775.

[15] Kunadian B, Vijayalakshmi K, Thornley AR, de Belder MA, Hunter S, Kendall S, Graham R, Stewart M, Thambyrajah J, Dunning J. Meta-analysis of Valve Hemodynamics and Left Ventricular Mass Rregression for Stentless versus Stented Aortic Valves. Annals of Thoracic Surgery 2007;84(1):73-78.

[16] Perez de Arenaza D, Lees B, Flather M, Nugara F, Huseybe T, Jasinski M, CisowskiM, KhanM, HeneinM, GaerJ, GuvendikL, BochenekA, WosS, LieM, VanNootenG, PennellD, PepperJ. Randomized comparison of Stentless versus Stented Valves for Aortic Stenosis: Effects on the Left Ventricular Mass. Circulation 2005;112(17): 2696-702.

[17] Dunning J, Graham RJ, Thambyrajah J, Stewart MJ, Kendall SW, Hunter S. Stentless vs Stented Aortic valve Bioprostheses: A Prospective Randomized Controlled Trial. European Heart Journal 2007;28(19):2369-2374.

[18] Gulbins H, Reichenspurner H. Which Patients Benefit from Stentless Aortic Valve Replacement? Annals of Thoracic Surgery 2009;88(6):2061-2068.

[19] Rabus MB, Kirali K, Kayalar N, Tuncer EY, Toker ME, Yakut C. Aortic Valve Replacement in Isolated Severe Aortic Stenosis with Left Ventricular Dysfunction: Long-term Survival and ventricular Recovery. AnatolianJournalofCardiology2009;9(1):41-46.

[20] Borger MA, Carson SM, Ivanov J, Rao V, Scully HE, Feindell CM, David TE. Stentless Aortic Valve are Hemodynamically Superior to Stented Valves During Mid-term Fol-

low-up: A Large Retrospective Study. Annals of Thoracic Surgery 2005;80(6): 2180-2185.

[21] Williams RJ, Muir DF, Pathi V, MacArthur K, Berg GA. Randomized Controlled Trial of Stented and Stentless Aortic Bioprostheses: Hemodynamic Performance at 3 Years. Seminars Thoracic Cardiovascular Surgery1999;11(4 Suppl 1):93-97.

[22] Narang S, Satsangi DK, Banerjee A, Geelani MA. Stentless Valves versus Stented Bioprotheses at the Aortic Position: Midterm Results. Journal of Thoracic Cardiovascular Surgery 2008;136(4):943-947.

[23] Ali A, Halstead JC, Cafferty F, Sharples L, Rose F, Coulden R, LeeE, DunningJ, ArganoV, TsuiS. Are Stentless Valves Superior to Modern Stented valves? A prospective Randomized Trial. Circulation 2006;114(1 Suppl):I535-I540.

[24] Funder JA, Ringgaard S, Frost MW, Wierup P, Klaaborg KE, Hjortdal V, NygaardH, HasenkamJM. Aortic Root Distensibility and Cross-sectional Areas in Stented and Subcoronary Stentless Bioprostheses in Pigs. Interactive Cardiovascular Thoracic Surgery 2010;10(6):976-980.

[25] Ennker JAC, Albert AA, Rosendahl UP, Ennker IC, Dalladaku F, Florath I. Ten-Year Experience With Stentless Aortic Valves: Full-Root Versus Subcoronary Implantation. Annals of Thoracic Surgery 2008;85(2):445-453.

[26] Schoof PH. Stentless Valve Dehiscence. Journal of Thoracic Cardiovascular Surgery 2008;136(1):231.

[27] Al Kindi AH, Huu AL, Shum-Tim D. Early Stenosis of Stentless Aortic Valve Prosthesis: A Word of Caution. Annals of Thoracic Surgery 2012;

[28] Tuncer A,Tuncer EY,Polat A, Mataracı İ, Keleş C, Aulasaleh S, Boyacıoğlu K, Kara İ, Kırali K. Axillary Artery Cannulation in Ascending Aortic Pathologies. Turkish Journal of Thoracic Cardiovascular Surgery 2011;19(4):539-544.

[29] Güler M, Akıncı E, Dağlar B, Kırali K, Eren E, Balkanay M, Berki T, Gürbüz A, Yakut C. Continuous Retrograde Coronary Sinus Isothermic Blood Cardioplegia with no Antegrade Combination in Aortic Valve Surgery. Turkish Journal of Thoracic Cardiovascular Surgery 1998;6(3):292-300.

[30] Kırali K, Göksedef D, Yakut C. Reverse "U" Aortotomy for Aortic Valve Replacement After Previous Coronary Artery Bypass Grafting. Journal of Cardiac Surgery 2005;20(3):269-270.

[31] Kobayashi J. Stentless Aortic Valve Replacement: An Update. Vascular Healt Risk Management 2011;7:345-351.

[32] Beholz S, Dushe S, Konertz W. Continuous Suture Technique for Freedom Stentless Valve: Reduced Crossclamp Time. Asian Cardiovascular Thoracic Annals 2006;14(2): 128-133.

[33] Song Z, lehr EJ, Wang S. An Alternative Subcoronary Implantation Technique Decreases the Risk of Complete Heart Block After Stentless Aortic Valve Replacement. Journal of Cardiovascular Disease Research 2012;3(1):46-51.

[34] Aymard T, Eckstein F, Englberger L, Stalder M, Kadner A, Carrel T. TheSorinFreedomSOLOStentlessAorticValve:TechniqueofImplantationandOperativeResultsin109Patients.Journal of Thoracic Cardiovascular Surgery 2010;139(3):775-777.

[35] Repossini A, Kotelnikov I, Bouchikhi R, Torre T, Passaretti B, Parodi O, Arena V. Single-suture Line Placement of a Pericardial Stentless Valve. JournalofThoracicCardiovascularSurgery 2005;130(5):1265-1269.

[36] Pillai R, Ratnatunga C, Soon JL, Kattach H, Khalil A, Jin XY. 3f Prosthesis Aortic Cusp Replacement: Implantation Technique and Early Results. Asian Cardiovascular Thoracic Annals 2010;18(1):13-16.

[37] D'OnofrioA, MessinaA, LorussoR, AlfieriOR, FusariM, RubinoP, RinaldiM, DiBartolomeoR, GlauberM, TroiseG, GerosaG. Sutureless Aortic Valve Replacement as an Alternative Treatment for Patients Belonging to the "Gray Zone" Between Transcatheter Aortic ValveImplantation and Conventional Surgery: A Propensity-matched, Multicenter Analysis. JournalofThoracicCardiovascularSurgery 2012 Sep 10. pii: S0022-5223(12)00883-5. doi: 10.1016/j.jtcvs.2012.07.040. [Epub ahead of print]

[38] Shrestha M, KhaladjN, BaraC, HoefflerK, HaglC, HaverichA. A Ataged Approach Towards Interventional Aortic Valve Implantation with a Sutureless Valve: Initial Human Implants. ThoracicCardiovascularSurgeon 2008;56(7):398-400.

[39] Santarpino G, Pfeiffer S, Concistrè G, Fischlein T. ASupra-annularMalpositionofthePercevalSSuturelessAorticValve:The'χ-movement'RemovalTechniqueandSubsequentReimplantation.Interactive Cardiovascular Thoracic Surgery 2012;15(2):280-281.

[40] Folliguet TA, Laborde F, Zannis K, Ghorayeb G, haverich A, Shrestha M. Sutureless Percaval Aortic Valve Replacement: Results of Two European Centers. Annals of Thoracic Surgery 2012;93(5):1483-1488.

[41] Santarpino G, Pfeiffer S, Schmidt J, Concistrè G, Fischlein T. SuturelessAorticValveReplacement:First-yearSingle-centerExperience.Annals of Thoracic Surgery2012;94(2): 504-508.

[42] Cox JL, Ad N, Myers K, Gharib M, Quijano RC. Tubular Heart Valves: A New Tissue Prosthesis Design - Preclinical evaluation of the 3f Aortic Bioprosthesis. Journal of Thoracic Cardiovascular Surgery 2005;130(2):520-527.

[43] Risteski P, Adami C, Papadopoulos N, Sirat SA, Moritz A, Doss M. Leaflet Replacement for Aortic Stenosis Using the 3f Stentless Aortic Bioprosthesis: Midterm Results. Annals of Thoracic Surgery 2012;93(4):1134-1140.

[44] Martens S, Sadowski J, Eckstein FS, Bartus K, Kapelak B, Sievers HH, Schlensak C, Carrel T. ClinicalExperiencewiththeATS3fEnable®SuturelessBioprosthesis.European Journal of Cardiothoracic Surgery 2011;40(3):749-755.

[45] Sepehripour AH, Harling L, Athanasiou T. What Are the Current Results of Sutureless Valves In High-risk Aortic Valve Disease Patients? Interactive Cardiovascular Thoracic Surgery 2012;14(5):615-621.

[46] HolmesDRJr, MackMJ, KaulS, AgnihotriA, AlexanderKP, BaileySR, CalhoonJH, CarabelloBA, DesaiMY, EdwardsFH, FrancisGS, GardnerTJ, KappeteinAP, LinderbaumJA, MukherjeeC, MukherjeeD, OttoCM, RuizCE, SaccoRL, SmithD, ThomasJD. 2012 ACCF/AATS/SCAI/STS Expert Consensus Document on Transcatheter Aortic Valve Replacement: Developed in Collaboration with the American Heart Association, American Society of Echocardiography, European Association for Cardio-Thoracic Surgery, Heart Failure Society of America, Mended Hearts, Society of Cardiovascular Anesthesiologists, Society of Cardiovascular Computed Tomography, and Society for Cardiovascular Magnetic Resonance. AnnalsofThoracicSurgery 2012;93(4): 1340-1395.

[47] Kirali K, Mansuroğlu D, Omeroğlu SN, Erentuğ V, Mataraci I, Ipek G, Akıncı E, Işık Ö, Yakut C. Five-year Experience in Aortic Root Replacement with the Flanged Composite Graft. Annals of Thoracic Surgery 2002;73(4):1130-1137.

[48] Kirsh MEW, Ooka T, Zannis K, deux JF, Loisance DY. Bioprosthetic Replacement of The Ascending Thoracic Aorta: What Are The Options? European Journal of Cardiothoracic Surgery 2009;35(1):77-82.

[49] Urbansky PP, Hacker RW. Replacement of the Aortic Valve and Ascending Aorta with a Valved Stentless Composite Graft: Technical Considerations and Early Clinical Results. Annals of Thoracic Surgery 2000;70(1):17-20.

[50] De Paulis R, Nardi P, De Matteis GM, Polisca P, Chiariello L. Bentall Procedure with a Stentless Valve and a New Aortic Root prosthesis. Annals of Thoracic Surgery 2001;71(4):1375-1376.

[51] Kırali K, Sarıkaya S, Elibol A, Göçer S, Özer T, Altaş Ö, Ünal ÜS, Şişmanoğlu M. Aortic Root Replacement with the Reimplantation Procedure: Simplifiying the Sizing of Tubular Graft. 20th Annual Meeting for Asian Society for Cardiovascular and Thoracic Surgery, 7-11 March 2012; Bali, Indonesia.

[52] Kaya A, Heijmen RH, Kelder JC, Morshuis WJ. First 102 Patients With the Biovalsalva Conduit for Aortic Root Replacement. Annals of Thoracic Surgery 2012;94(1): 72-77.

[53] Hemmer WB, Botha CA, Böhm JO, Herrmann T, Starck C, Rein JG. replacement of the Aortic Valve and Ascending Aorta with an Extended Root Stentless Xenograft. Annals of Thoracic Surgery 2004;78(6):2150-2153.

[54] Massetti M, Veron S, Neri E, Coffin O, le Page O, Babatasi G, Buklas D, Maiza D, Gerard JL, Khayat A. Long-term Durability of Resection and End-To-End Anastomosis for Ascending Aortic Aneurysms. Journal of Thoracic Cardiovascular Surgery 2003;127(5):1381-1387.

[55] Akpınar B, Güden M, Aytekin S, Sanisoğlu I, Sagbas E, Ozbek U, Caynak B, Bayramoglu Z. The Use of Stentless Valves for Root Replacement During Repair of Ascending Aortic Aneurysms with Aortic Valve Regurgitation. Heart Surgery Forum 2002;5(1):52-56.

[56] Carrel TP, Berdat P, Englberger L, Eckstein F, Immer F, Seiler C, Kipfer B, Schmidt J. Aortic Root Replacement with a New Stentless Aortic Valve Xenograft Conduit: Preliminary Hemodynamic and Clinical Results. Journal of Heart Valve Disease 2003;12(6):752-757.

[57] Rabus MB, Kirali K, KayalarN, Mataracil, YanartasM, Ulusoy-BozbugaN, YakutC. Effects of Patient-Prosthesis Mismatch on Postoperative Early Mortality in Isolated Aortic Stenosis. Journal of Heart Valve Disease2009;18(1):18-27.

[58] Head SJ, Mokhles MM, Osnabrugge RLJ, Pibarot P, Mack MJ, Takkenberg JJM, Bogers JJCA, Kappetein AP. The Impact of Prosthesis–Patient Mismatch on Long-term Survival After Aortic Valve Replacement: A Systematic Review and Meta-Analysis of 34 Observational Studies Comprising 27 186 Patients with 133 141 Patient-years. European Heart Journal 2012;33():1518–1529.

[59] Shiono N, Watanabe Y, Kawasaki M, Yokomuro H, Fujii T, Koyama N. Evaluation of Bioprosthetic Valve for Small Aortic Root in Elderly Patients. Asian Cardiovascular Thoracic Annals 2007;15(1):102-105.

[60] Ardal H, Toker ME, Rabuş MB, Uyar İ, Antal A, Şişmanoğlu M, Mansuroğlu D, Kırali K, Yakut C. Does Aortic Root Enlargement Impair theOoutcome of Patients With Small Aortic Root? Journal of Cardiac Surgery 2006;21(5):449-453.

[61] Bical OM, Nutu O, D2eleuze P. A Technique of Aortic Annulus Enlargement with a Freestyle Stentless Bioprosthesis. Annals of Thoracic Surgery 2012;93(3):680-681.

[62] Goland S, Trento A, Czer LSC, Eshaghian S, Tolstrup K, Naqvi TZ, De Robertis MA, Mirocha J, Iida K, Siegel RJ. Thoracic Aortic Arteriosclerosis in Patients With Degenerative Aortic Stenosis With and Without Coexisting Coronary Artery Disease. Annals of Thoracic Surgery 2008;85(1):113-119.

[63] GillinovAM, LytleBW, HoangV, CosgroveDM, BanburyMK, McCarthyPM, SabikJF, PetterssonGB, SmediraNG, BlackstoneEH. The Atherosclerotic Aorta at Aortic Valve Replacement: Surgical Strategies and Results. Journal of Thoracic Cardiovascular Surgery 2000;120(5):957-963.

[64] Rode´s-Cabau J,Webb JG, Cheung A, Ye J, Dumont E, Feindel CM, Osten M, Natarajan MK, Velianou JL, Martucci G, DeVarennes B, Chisholm R, Peterson MD, Lichtenstein SV, Nietlispach F, Doyle D, DeLarochellie`re R, Teoh K, Chu V, Dancea A,

Lachapelle K, Cheema A, Latter D, Horlick E. Transcatheter Aortic Valve Implantation for theTtreatment of Severe Symptomatic Aortic Stenosis in Patients at Very High or Prohibitive Surgical Risk: Acute and Late Outcomes of the Multicenter Canadian Experience. Journal of American Collage Cardiology 2010;55(11):1080-1090.

[65] Buz S, Pasic M, Unbehaun A, Drews T, Dreysse S, kukucka M, Mladenow A, Hetzer R. Trans-apical Aortic Valve Implantation in Patients with Severe Calcification of the Ascending Aorta. European Journal of Cardiothoracic Surgery 2011;40(2):463-468.

[66] RabuşMB, KayalarN, SareyyüpoğluB, ErkinA, Kirali K, YakutC. Hypercholesterolemia Association with Aortic Stenosis of Various Etiologies. JournalofCardiacSurgery 2009;24(2):146-150.

[67] Taş S, Dönmez AA, Kırali K, Alp M, Yakut C. Aortic Valve Replacement for a Patient with Glucose-6-Phosphate Dehydrogenase Deficiency and Autoimmune Hemolytic Anemia. Jornal of Cardiac Surgery 2005;20(4):380-381.

[68] Kirali K, Aksoy E, Buyukbayrak F, Yanartas M, Elibol A, Ozer T, Boyacioglu K, Kis M, Sismanoglu M, Mataraci I. Does Thrombocytopenia Aggravate early Outcome After Aortic Valve Replacement with a Bioprosthesis. 16th World Congress on Heart Disease for Intenational Academy of Cardiology, 23-26 July 2011; Vancouver, Canada.

[69] RepossiniA, BlochD, MunerettoC, PiccoliP, BisleriG, BeholzS. Platelet Reduction After Stentless Pericardial Aortic Valve Replacement. InteractiveCardiovascularThoracicSurgery 2012;14(4):434-438.

[70] GersakB, GartnerU, AntonicM. ThrombocytopeniaFollowingImplantationoftheSstentlessBiologicalSorinFreedomSOLOValve.Journal of Heart Valve Disease 2011;20(4): 401-406.

[71] El-Hamamsy I, Zaki M, Stevens LM, ClarkLA, RubensM, MelinaG, YacoubMH. Rate of Progression and Functional Significance of Aortic Root Calcification After homograft versus Freestyle AorticRrootRreplacement. Circulation 2009;120(Suppl 1):S269-S275.

[72] Erdoğan HB, Kayalar N, Ardal H, Ömeroğlu SN, Kırali K, Güler M, Akıncı E, Yakut C. Risk Factors for Requirement of Permanent Pacemaker Implantation After Aortic Valve Replacement. Journal of Cardiac Surgery2006;21(3):211-215.

[73] Kincaid EH, Cordell R, Hammon JW, Adair SM, Kon ND. Coronary Insufficiency After Stentless Aortic Root Replacement: Risk Factors and Solutions. Annals of Thoracic Surgery 2007;83(3):964-968.

[74] Schoof P, Baur L, Kappetein A, Hazekamp M, vanRijk-Zwikker G, Huysmans H. Dehiscence of the Freestyle Stentless Bioprosthesis. Seminars in Thoracic Cardiovascular Surgery 1999;11(suppl 1):133-138.

[75] Hopkins R, Gitter H, Stave J, Bert A, Atalay M. Stable Partial Dehiscence of Aortic Homograft Inserted Freehand by Using the Subcoronary Intra-aortic Root Noncoro-

nary Sinus Ross Scallop Inclusion technique. Journal of Thoracic Cardiovascular Surgery 2008;135(1):214-216.

[76] David TE, Ivanov J, eriksson MJ, Feindel CM, Rakowski H. Dilatation of the Sinotubular Junction Causes Aortic Insufficiency After Aortic Valve Replacement with the Toronto SPV Bioprosthesis. Journal Thoracic Cardiovascular Surgery 2001;122(5): 929-934.

[77] WeltertL, NardellaS, GirolaF, ScaffaR, BellisarioA, MaselliD, DePaulisR. Diastolic Properties of the SorinSolo, ATS 3F, Edwards Prima Plus and Medtronic Freestyle Stentless Valves: An Independent in-vitro Comparison. JournalHeartValveDis-ease. 2012;21(1):99-105.

[78] Nötzold A, Scharfschwerdt M, Thiede L, Hüppe M, Sievers HH. In-vitro Study on the Relationship Between Progressive Sinotubular Junction Dilatation and Aortic Regurgitation for Several Stentless Aortic Valve Substitutes. European Journal of Cardiothoracic Surgery 2005;27(1):90-93.

[79] Scharfschwerdt M, Sievers HH, Hussein A, Kraatz EG, Misfeld M. Impact of Progressive Sinotubular Junction Dilatation on Valve Competence of the 3F Aortic and Sorin Solo Stentless Bioprosthetic Heart Valves. European Journal of Cardiothoracic Surgery 2010;37(3):631-634.

[80] Borger MA, Prasongsukarn K, Armstrong S, Feindel CM, David TE. Stentless Aortic Valve Reoperations: A Surgical Challenge. Annals of Thoracic Surgery 2007;84(3): 737-744.

[81] Finch J, Roussin I, Pepper J. Failing Stentless Aortic Valves: Redo Aortic Root Replacement or Valve in a Valve. European Journal of Cardiothoracic Surgery 2012;42():

[82] Ferrari E. Transapical Aortic 'valve-in-valve' Procedure for Degenerated Stented Bioprosthesis. European Journal of Cardiothoracic Surgery 2012;41(3):485-490.

[83] Mihaljevic T, Nowicki ER, Rajeswaran J, Blackstone EH, Lagazzi L, Thomas J, Lytle BW, Cosgrove DM. Survival After Valve Replacement For Aortic Stenosis: Implications for Decision Making. Journal of Thoracic Cardiovascular Surgery 2008;135(6): 1270-1279.

[84] Luciani GB, Casali G, Auriemma S, SantiniF, MazzuccoA. Survival After Stentless and Stented Xenograft Aortic Valve Replacement: A Concurrent, Controlled Trial. Annals of Thoracic Surgery 2002;7485):1443-1449.

[85] Dunning J, Graham RJ, Thambyrajah J, StewartMJ, KendallSW, HunterS. Stentless vs Stented Aortic Valve Bioprostheses: A Prospective Randomized Controlled Trial. European Heart Journal 2007;28(19):2369-2374.

[86] Murtaza B, Pepper JR, Jones C, Nihoyannopoulos P, Darzi A, Athanasiou T. Does Stentless Aortic Valve Implantation Increase perioperative Risk? A Critical Appraisal

of the Literature and Risk of Bias Analysis. European Journal of Cardiothoracic Surgery 2011;39(5):643-652.

[87] Westaby S, JönsonA, PayneN, SaitoS, JinXY, DelRizzoDF, GrunkemeierG. Does The Use of a Stentless Bioprosthesis Increase Surgical Risk?SeminarsThoracicCardiovascularSurgery 2001;13(4, Suppl 1):143-147.

[88] Borger MA, Carson SM, Ivanov J, RaoV, ScullyHE, FeindelCM, DavidTE. Stentless Aortic Valve Are Hemodynamically Superior to Stented valves during Mid-term follow-up: A Large Retrospective Study. Annals of Thoracic Surgery 2005;80(6): 2180-2185.

[89] Lehmann S, Walther T, Kempfert J, Leontjev A, Ardawan R, Falk V, Mohr FW. Stentless Versus Conventional Xenograft Aortic Valve Replacement: Midterm Results of a Prospectively Randomized Trial. Annals of Thoracic Surgery 2007;84(2):467-472.

[90] Bach DS, Kon ND, Dumesnil JG, Sintek CF, Ross DB. Ten-Year Outcome after Aortic Valve Replacement with the Freestyle Stentless Bioprosthesis. Annals of Thoracic Surgery 2005;80(2):480-487.

[91] Mohammadi S, Tchana-Sato V, Kalavrouziotis D, Voisine P, Doyle D, Baillot R, Sponga S, Metras J, Perron J, Dagenais F. Long-termClinicalandEchocardiographicFollow-upoftheFreestyleStentlessAorticBioprosthesis.Circulation 2012;126(11 Suppl 1):S198-S204.

[92] Bach DS, Kon ND, DumesnilJG, SintekCF, DotyDB. Ten-year Outcome After Aortic Valve Replacement With the Freestyle Stentless Bioprosthesis. AnnalsofThoracicSurgery 2005;80(2):480-486.

[93] Borger MA, Prasongsukarn K, Armstrong S, Feindel CM, David TE. Stentless Aortic Valve Reoperations: A Surgical Challenge. Annals of Thoracic Surgery 2007;84(3): 737-744.

[94] Jeong DS, Kim K-H, Ahn H. Long-term Results of the Leaflet Extension Technique in Aortic Regurgitation: Thirteen Years of Experience in a Single Centre. Annals of Thoracic Surgery 2009;88(1):83-89.

[95] Cohen G, Zagorski B, Christakis GT, Joyner CD, Vincent J, Sever J, HarbiS, Feder-ElituvR, MoussaF, GoldmanBS, FremesSE. Are Stentless Valves Hemodynamically Superior to Stented valves? Long-term Follow-up of a randomized trial Comparing Carpentier-Edwards Pericardial Valve With The Toronto Stentless porcine Valves? Journal of Thoracic Cardiovascular Surgery 2010;139(4):848-859.

[96] Chamber JB, Rimington HM, Hodson F, Rajani R, Blauth CI. The Subcoronary Toronto Stentless Versus Supra-annular Perimount Stented Replacement Aortic Valve: Early Clinical and Hemodynamic results of a Randomized Comparison in 160 Patients. Journal of Thoracic Cardiovascular Surgery 2006;131(4):878-882.

[97] Iliopoulos DC, Deveja AR, Androutsopoulou V, Filias V, Kastelanos E, Satratzemis V, Khalpey Z, Koudoumas D. Single-centerExperienceUsingtheFreedomSOLOAor-

ticBioprosthesis. Journal of Thoracic Cardiovascular Surgery 2012;(:http://dx.doi.org/10.1016/j.jtcvs.2012.06.041)

[98] BeholzS, RepossiniA, LiviU, SchepensM, ElGabryM, MatschkeK, TrivediU, EckelL, DapuntO, ZamoranoJL. The Freedom SOLO Valve for Aortic Valve Replacement: Clinical and Hemodynamic Results from a Prospective Multicenter Trial. Journal-HeartValveDisease 2010;19(1):115-123.

[99] Linneweber J, Heinbokel T, Christ T, Claus B, Kossagk C, Konertz W. Clinical Experience with the ATS 3F Stentless Aortic Bioprosthesis: Five Years' Follow Up. Journal Heart Valve Disease 2010;19(6):772-777.

[100] TanakaK, KinoshitaT, FujinagaK, KanemitsuS, TanakaJ, SuzukiH, TokuiT. HemodynamicPerformanceoftheEdwardsPrimaPlusStentlessValveat1Year. GeneralThoracicCardiovascularSurgery2008;56(9):441-445.

[101] Luciani GB, Viscardi F, Cresce GD, Faggian G, Mazzucco A.Seven-Year Performance of the Edwards Prima Plus Stentless Valve with the Intact Non-Coronary Sinus Technique.Journal of Cardiac Surgery 2008;23(3):221-226.

[102] Kappetein AP, Braun J, Baur LHB, Prat A, Peels K, Hazekamp MG, Schoof PH, Huysmans HA. Outcome and Follow-up of Aortic Valve Replacement with The Freestyle Stentless Bioprosthesis. Annals of Thoracic Surgery 2001;71(2):601-607.

[103] Van Nooten G, Caes F, Francois K, Van BY, Taeymans Y. Stentless or Stented Aortic Valve Implants in Elderly Patients? European Journal of Cardiothoracic Surgery 1999;15(1):31-36.

[104] Eriksson MJ, Rosfors S, Radegran K, Brodin LA. Effects of Exercise on Doppler-derived Pressure Difference, Valve Resistance, and Effective Orifice Area in Different Aortic Valve Prostheses of Similar Size. American Journal of Cardiology 1999;83(4):619-622.

[105] Bleiziffer S, Eichinger WB, Wagner I, Guenzinger R, Bauernschmitt R, Lange R. The Toronto Root Stentless Valve in the Subcoronary Position is Hemodynamically Superior to the Mosaic Stented Completely Supra-annular Bioprosthesis. Journal of Heart Valve Disease 2005;14(6):814-821.

[106] Fries R, Wendler O, Schieffer H, Schaefers HJ. Comparative Rest and Exercise Hemodynamics of 23-mm Stentless Versus 23-mm Stented Aortic Bioprostheses. Annals of Thoracic Surgery 2000;69(3):817-822.

Chapter 15

New Therapeutic Approaches to Conventional Surgery for Aortic Stenosis in High-Risk Patients

Omer Leal, Juan Bustamante, Sergio Cánovas and
Ángel G. Pinto

Additional information is available at the end of the chapter

http://dx.doi.org/10.5772/54333

1. Introduction

Aortic stenosis (AS) is the most frequent type of valvular heart disease in Europe and North America. It mainly presents as calcified aortic stenosis in older adults (2-7% of the population> 65 years), which is the most common cause of valve replacement in the western world. Its incidence increases with age [1]. With the increasing age and life expectancy of the population, an increase in the prevalence of aortic stenosis had been observed. Furthermore, the elderly patient usually presents multiple comorbidities associated with increased surgical risk. Aortic valve replacement (AVR) is currently the treatment of choice in patients with symptomatic aortic stenosis and/or left ventricular systolic dysfunction (see Indications for surgery), even though some cases present high or extremely high surgical risk.

Our goal is to update the treatment of severe aortic stenosis in high-risk patients, mainly the elderly and those cases where risk assessment scales indicate a high- or very high-risk patient. Here we analyse the role of new therapeutic approaches in the treatment of these patients and their short and long-term results, as well as the use of new devices and prosthesis.

2. Etiology

AS without accompanying mitral valve disease is more common in men than in women [2] and rheumatic etiology is currently rare. Age-related degenerative calcific AS is currently the most common cause of AS in adults and the most frequent reason for aortic valve replacement (AVR) in patients with AS. Sclerosis of the aortic valve is observed in up to 30%

of elderly people: 25% of people aged 65 to 74, and 48% of people older than 84 years [3,4]. This calcific disease progresses from the base of the cusps to the leaflets, eventually causing a reduction in leaflet motion and effective valve area without commissural fusion. Calcific AS is an active disease process characterized by lipid accumulation, inflammation, and calcification, with many similarities to atherosclerosis. In approximately half of cases there is a bicuspid aortic valve basis. Bicuspid aortic valve valvulopathy affects 2% of the population, making it the most frequent congenital anomaly, representing the more common cause among young adults [5].

3. Evaluation and grading the degree of stenosis

Patient history and physical examination remain essential. Careful exploration for the presence of symptoms (shortness of breath on exertion, angina, dizziness, or syncope) is critical for proper patient management. It is important to be aware that patients may not notice symptoms but they significantly reduce their activities. The characteristic systolic murmur draws attention and guides further diagnostic work in the right direction. However, on occasion the murmur may, be faint and the primary presentation may be heart failure of unknown cause. The disappearance of the second aortic sound is specific to severe AS, however, it is not a sensitive sign.

Several studies [6-9] reports that biomarkers such as B-type natriuretic peptide (BNP) has been shown to be related to functional class and prognosis, particularly in AS and MR. In fact, Lancellotti et al. [9] reports in their study that a left atrial area index of > or = 12.4 cm2/m2, systolic annular velocity of < or = 4.5 cm/s, E/Ea ratio >13.8, late diastolic annular velocity of < or = 9 cm/s, and BNP of > or = 61 pg/ml were identified as the best cutoff values to predict events (death, symptoms, or surgery). They found, in asymptomatic AS, tissue Doppler imaging and BNP measurements provide prognostic information beyond that from clinical and conventional echocardiographic parameters. However, Natriuretic peptides have been shown to predict symptom free survival and outcome in normal- and low-flow severe AS and may be useful in asymptomatic patients, helping to discriminates those patients who can benefits from an early intervention [7-9]. Nevertheless, evidence regarding its incremental value in risk stratification remains limited so far.

Echocardiography is indicated when there is a systolic murmur of grade III/VI or higher, a single S2, or symptoms that might be due to AS [10]. A 2-dimensional (2D) echocardiogram is valuable for assessing valve anatomy and function and determining the LV response to pressure overload. In nearly all patients, the severity of the stenotic lesion can be defined with Doppler echocardiographic measurements. Echocardiography is also used to assess LV size and function, degree of hypertrophy, and presence of other associated valvular disease. Transoesophageal echocardiography (TOE) is rarely helpful for the quantification of AS, as valve area planimetry becomes difficult in calcified valves [11] however, it is useful when transthoracic visualization is poor and leaflets only moderately calcified [12]. TOE may, however, provide additional evaluation of mitral valve abnormalities and has gained impor-

http://dx.doi.org/10.5772/54333

tance in assessing annulus diameter before TAVI and in guiding the procedure. Intraprocedural TOE enables us to monitor the results of percutaneous procedures [11]. Three-dimensional TOE offers a more detailed examination of valve anatomy than two-dimensional echocardiography and is useful for the assessment of complex valve problems or for monitoring surgery and percutaneous intervention [11]. Three-dimensional echocardiography (3DE) is useful for assessing anatomical features which may have an impact on the type of intervention chosen, if it is needed. AS severity could be graded on the basis of a variety of hemodynamic and natural history data, using definitions of aortic jet velocity, mean pressure gradient, valve area and velocity ratio as shown in Table 1.

		Aortic Stenosis	
Indicator	*Mild*	*Moderate*	***Severe***
Aortic jet velocity (m/s)	2.6-3	3-4	≥4
Mean gradient (mmHg)	≤30(25)	30-50(25-40)	≥50(40)
Indexed AVA (cm^2/m^2)	≥0.9	0.6-0.9	≤0.6
AVA (cm^2)	≥1.5	1-1.5	≤1
Velocity ratio	≥0.50	0.25-0.50	≤0.25

Table 1. Classification of the Severity of Aortic Valve Disease in Adults

Based on the European Society of Cardiology (ESC) Guidelines on the management of valvular heart disease [12], American College of Cardiology/American Heart Association (ACC/AHA) Guidelines for the Management of Patients With valvular heart disease [10] and ASE/EAE Recommendations for Quantitation of Stenosis Severity, [13] ACC/AHA guidelines use lower mean gradient cutoffs as indicated in parentheses. The ESC definitions apply only in the presence of normal flow conditions. The velocity ratio is included in the ASE/EAE guidelines only.

Multi-slice computed tomography (MSCT) and cardiac magnetic resonance (CMR) provide additional information on the assessment of the ascending aorta when it is enlarged. MSCT may be useful in quantifying the valve area and coronary calcification, which aids in assessing prognosis. MSCT may contribute to the evaluation of the severity of valve disease, particularly in AS, either indirectly by quantifying valvular calcification, or directly through the measurement of valve planimetry. Also, MSCT has become an important diagnostic tool for evaluation of the aortic root, the distribution of calcium, the number of leaflets, the ascending aorta, and peripheral artery pathology and dimensions before undertaking TAVI [11]. In patients with inadequate echocardiographic quality or discrepant results, CMR should be used to assess the severity of valvular lesions—particularly regurgitant lesions—and to assess ventricular volumes and systolic function, as CMR assesses these parameters with higher reproducibility than echocardiography [11]. In practice, the routine use of CMR is limited because of its limited availability, compared with echocardiography. Due to its high negative predictive value, MSCT may be useful in excluding CAD in patients who are at low risk of atherosclerosis [11]. MSCT plays an important role in the work-up of high-risk patients with AS considered for TAVI. The risk of radiation exposure—and of renal failure due to contrast injection—should, however, be taken into consideration.

There are contraindications for exercise testing in symptomatic patients with AS, however it is useful for unmasking symptoms and in the risk stratification of asymptomatic patients with severe AS [12]. Stress tests are currently under-used in patients with asymptomatic AS. In some patients, it may be necessary to proceed with cardiac catheterisation and coronary angiography at the time of initial evaluation [10]. This could be appropriate if there is a discrepancy between clinical and echocardiographic examinations or if symptoms might be due to coronary artery disease (CAD).

4. Indications for surgery

Early valve replacement should be strongly recommended in all symptomatic patients with severe AS, because it is the only effective treatment. Thus, the development of symptoms identifies a critical point in the natural history of AS. The interval from the onset of symptoms to the time of death is approximately 2 years in patients with heart failure, 3 years in those with syncope, and 5 years in those with angina, with a high risk of sudden death (Figure 1).

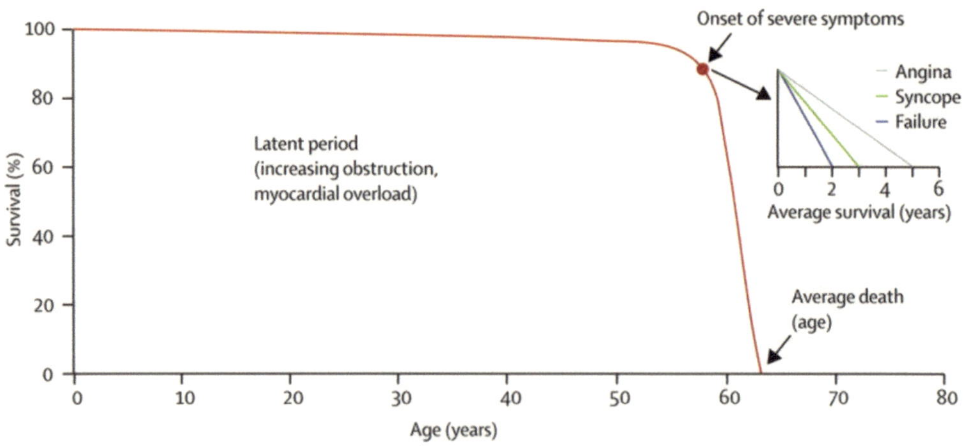

Figure 1. Natural History. Ross J Jr. & Braunwald E, 1968 [14]

There is some disagreement about the optimal timing of surgery in asymptomatic patients, and the decision to operate on this kind of patient requires careful weighing of the benefits against the risks. Early elective surgery, at the asymptomatic stage, can only be recommended in selected patients, with low operative risk [12]. A proposed management strategy for patients with severe AS based on the ESC Guidelines on the management of valvular heart disease [12] and ACC/ AHA Guidelines for the Management of Patients with valvular heart disease [10] is shown in Figure 2.

Although there are no prospective randomized trials, data from retrospective analysis indicates that patients with moderate AS (mean gradient in the presence of normal flow 30–50 mmHg, valve area 1.0–1.5 cm^2) will generally benefit from valve replacement at the time of coronary surgery. However, individual judgement must be recommended [12], based on the evolution of the echocardiography severity parameters and the patient's clinical evaluation.

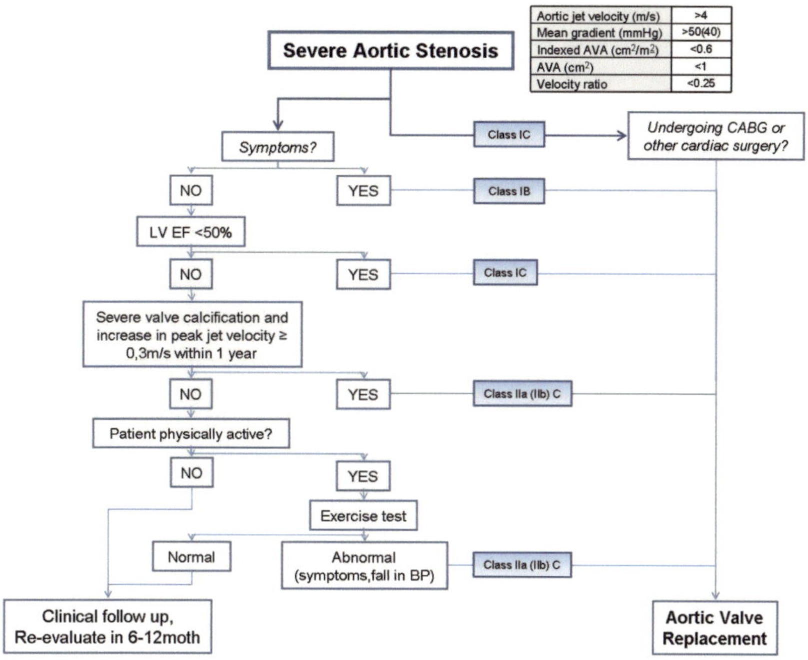

Figure 2. Management of Severe Aortic Stenosis.

Based on the ESC Guidelines on the management of valvular heart disease [12] and ACC/ AHA Guidelines for the Management of Patients with valvular heart diseaseb [10]. ACC/AHA recommendations has been shown ın parentheses.

5. Risk stratification

Patient selection for AVR for AS is well outlined by ACCF/AHA and ESC guidelines. Problems arise when the patients present significant symptoms and significant structural disease, complicated by the presence of significant comorbidity. A number of risk algorithms for cardiac surgery have been developed. Experience accrued since the development of the Parsonnet scale reveals that this scale assigns too much weight to age. Nowadays the STS score and logistic EuroSCORE are the most commonly used. These provide information concerning short term operative risks, however, they are not able to predict symptom resolution, quality-of-life improvement, or return to independent living.

As discussed above (see also Evaluation and Grading the Degree of Stenosis), several studies have reported the usefulness of BNP in risk stratification of asymptomatic or mildly symptomatic patients, which could help to discriminate which patients would benefit from an early surgical management. However, there is not enough evidence to recommend the routine use of these biomarkers.

Although both are accurate in low-risk patients, accuracy is reduced in higher-risk subsets [15]. The logistic EuroSCORE is based on 12 covariates derived from 14,799 patients undergoing all types of cardiac operations in 8 European countries in 1995. On the other hand, the STS risk predictor is based on 24 covariates derived from 67,292 patients undergoing isolated AVR only in the United States between 2002 and 2006. Both use an algorithm based on the presence of coexisting illnesses in order to estimate 30-day operative mortality. There is a much simpler variation of the EuroSCORE logistic model, which can be calculated at the patient's bedside, adding points manually. This model is called the additive EuroSCORE. It assigns a specific value to each risk factor, and the points are simply added to obtain the estimated operative mortality rate.

With improved outcomes after cardiac surgery in more recent years, EuroSCORE has become less well calibrated. EuroSCORE II has been developed using data from 22.381 patients who underwent cardiac surgery during 2010, and represents a necessary and timely update of the original EuroSCORE models. EuroSCORE II improves on the original logistic EuroSCORE, though mainly for combined AVR and CABG cases. However, concerns still exist, about its use for isolated AVR procedures, aortic surgery and miscellaneous procedures. There is still room for improvement in risk modelling and several studies are currently being carried out to validate EuroScore II. Nevertheless, Grant et al [16] report that EuroSCORE II performs well overall in contemporary UK adult cardiac surgery, with good discrimination for all kinds of cardiac surgery; in fact, they report that the logistic EuroSCORE is now obsolete and their study demonstrates that it is appropriate to use EuroSCORE II as a generic risk model for contemporary UK cardiac surgery.

There is growing debate about the definition of high-risk patients and the validity of risk assessment using different risk-scoring systems for prediction of mortality (see also **High-Risk Patient**). Current models do not include some risk factors that may be particularly important in the prediction of outcomes for high- or very high-risk populations including frailty, pulmonary hypertension (PH), porcelain aorta, and the presence of hepatic dysfunction, although all these have been included in EuroSCORE II.

Nevertheless, the sample of elderly patients considered for the design of these scales represents a small proportion of the population, resulting in less accurate risk assessment, and interpretation should be made with caution. In this regard, a recent study which included 1245 elderly patients (mean age 77.2 years) who underwent AVR with or without CABG reports that only STS-PROM correlated with mortality rates [17]. Thielmann et al [18] also report that the logistic EuroSCORE and the Parsonnet score clearly overestimated the risk of mortality, whereas the STS score and the additive EuroSCORE were much more accurate in predicting the risk of mortality.

Certain authors, such as Rosenhek [19] and others, suggest the need to include other variables such as cognitive function and functional capacity in surgical risk stratification, mainly in the elderly group. There are physiological characteristics inherent to elderly patients that make them different in risk estimation; an example of this is the amount of creatinine considered in the EuroSCORE scale as a predictor of mortality. This scale assigned a particular score (2 points) to patients with creatinine levels greater than 2.26 mg / dl, which through a logistic regression analysis could estimate risk in percentage terms. However creatinine is not the best parameter to define renal function and its value can be influenced by various factors such as age, race, muscle mass and metabolic state, as has been demonstrated in several studies, hence glomerular filtration rate provides a much more accurate estimation [20]. Obviously in the elderly there is a physiological involution of organs and systems that should be taken into account since surgery represents a stressful situation that can reveal or tip the balance for certain pathologies. However, numerous reports have demonstrated excellent results in terms of morbidity and mortality in most patients. Hospital mortality is significantly related to the preoperative presence of depressed left ventricular systolic function, pulmonary hypertension, symptoms of heart failure, kidney failure, long-standing mitral valve disease, and nutritional deficiencies. When these risk factors are absent in the preoperative period, mortality is similar to that of the youngest patients. It should be emphasized that risk models serve as one aspect of patient selection, but need to be considered alongside clinical judgement and other methods of risk assessment.

6. High risk and elderly patients, are they the same?

6.1. Elderly patient

The ageing of the population is an important social and sanitary phenomenon. Consensus about allowing access to health care unconstrained by age limits, together with increased life expectancy and advances in highly specialised medicine have brought us to the point where surgical treatment is indicated in progressively older sectors of the population [21]. The diagnosis and management of valvular heart disease in the elderly has been affected by the dramatic increase in life expectancy that began in the last half of the 20th century. In the United States, for example, the number of persons aged 80 years or older is expected to increase from 6.9 million in 1990 to approximately 25 million by the year 2050. As a result, degenerative valve disease is likely to become an increasing problem. In the Helsinki Ageing Study [22], 501 randomly selected men and women aged 75 to 86 underwent imaging and Doppler echocardiography. The prevalence of at least moderate aortic stenosis, defined as an aortic valve area (AVA) ≤ 1.2 cm^2 and velocity ratio ≤ 0.35, was 5 percent; the prevalence of critical aortic stenosis (AVA ≤ 0.8 cm^2, and velocity ratio ≤ 0.35) increased with age from 1 to 2 percent in persons aged 75 to 76 up to almost 6 percent in those aged 86. With the rapidly increasing geriatric population, it is common in current practice to have elderly patients referred for surgical treatment of AS. In 2006, in the United States, approximately 40% of patients undergoing AVR were at least 75 years old Nevertheless, even though valve replacement is the procedure of choice in this population, currently a large percentage of suitable candidates are, unfortunately, not referred for surgery, mostly because of their age.

As in [21], increased risk in these patients is related to:

- Ageing, which causes structural changes in the heart and reduces the physiological reserves of most organs, thus impairing the capacity to recover from surgical aggression;
- An increase in associated diseases, as studied by Rodríguez et al [23], especially diabetes, kidney failure, arterial hypertension, chronic obstructive pulmonary disease, and cerebrovascular disease;
- The advanced phase of heart disease, as indicated by the greater incidence of heart failure, depressed left ventricular function, and preoperative pulmonary hypertension;
- Reduction of the inflammatory response to surgical aggression,
- Undernourishment, measured by anthropometric and biochemical parameters, which is a frequent preoperative finding before cardiac surgery; its incidence is even greater in older persons and is associated with an increment in postoperative complications due to an impaired response to surgical aggression.
- The increased complexity of surgical techniques for these patients, due to the presence of severe calcification of the aortic ring and the greater incidence of associated coronary and valvular surgery, which require longer aortic clamping times.

Age has been considered an independent predictive factor for mortality, but the way to estimate its influence on the calculation of the risk of surgery has evolved since the introduction of the Parsonnet risk scale, which gave excessive weight to age. Currently the most accepted risk assessment tools are the STS-PROM score and EuroSCORE (with the EuroSCORE II currently being validated).Although they are widely used, there is a possibility of overestimating the operative mortality rates by using these risk-prediction models, and an inescapable discrepancy between the estimated and observed mortality rate has been acknowledged. In a study published in Ann Thorac Surg in 2009 Thielmann et al [18] report that the logistic EuroSCORE clearly overestimates the risk of mortality, whereas the STS score seems to be more accurate in predicting the risk of mortality. Moat et al. [24] also report the relative lack of utility of EuroSCORE in risk/outcome prediction for their group of patients and confirm the need for more sophisticated and procedure-specific (rather than generic) scoring systems. There is no perfect method for weighing all of the relevant factors and identifying specifically high- and low-risk elderly patients, but this risk can be estimated well in individual patients, and the decision to proceed with surgery should depend on many factors, including the patient's wishes and expectations.

Although the proportion of elderly patients with multiple comorbidities is increasing, operative outcomes following AVR have improved over the past decade. Likosky et al [25] pub-

http://dx.doi.org/10.5772/54333

lished the outcomes of the very elderly undergoing aortic valve surgery in a study comprising 7584 patients, including 815 over the age of 80. They found that short- and long-term survival was favourable across all age groups. Specifically, more than half of the patients undergoing aortic valve procedures were alive 6 years after surgery. Among patients under 80 years of age, survival favoured those undergoing isolated AVR procedures, but among octogenarians, concomitant CABG surgery did not result in reduced survival. Yamane K et al [26] published the outcome of a single-centre study of conventional AVR in patients aged 70 or older. In their analysis, patients aged 80–92 who underwent isolated AVR or AVR with CABG showed an acceptable mortality rate of 4.0%, comparable to the 3.8% mortality rate in patients aged 70–79. Brown et al [27] published the outcomes of isolated AVR in North America by analysing the STS National Database, comprising 108,687 patients, and compared the mortality rates in 1997 with those in 2006. In their analysis, patients aged 70–75 had a mortality rate of 3.2% in 1997 and 2.9% in 2006; for patients aged 80–85, the mortality rate was 6.3% in 1997 and 4.9% in 2006. These improvements in operative outcome over the past decade could be related to multiple factors, including patient selection and perioperative management. A better understanding of the role of preoperative respiratory preparation, improved myocardial protection of otherwise severely hypertrophic myocardium, as well as normothermic cardiopulmonary bypass may have contributed to the improved early postoperative results in recent studies as compared to those several decades ago. Yamane K et al [26] propose that with the elderly, especially those aged 80 years or older, goal-oriented strategies such as early extubation, judicious sedation management, medication dosage based on renal or liver function, early involvement of physical or occupational therapists, and speech/swallow specialists are all indispensable.

From a patient's perspective, functionality after surgery may be more important than simple survival. Using the Seattle Angina Questionnaire, Huber et al [28] interviewed 136 patients who were 80 years of age at the time of cardiac surgery (isolated CABG, AVR, or AVR +CABG). They found that 95% lived in their own homes, and 93% reported that they had experienced no reduction in their quality of life. Kolh et al [29] interviewed 61 long-term survivors of AVR and found that 92% of patients believed that having heart surgery at age 80 was a "good choice," with 88% of patients feeling "as good or better" than they had before surgery. Also, Maillet et al [30] reported results from 84 octogenarians undergoing either AVR or AVR+CABG between 1998 and 2001. The majority (91.1%) lived in their own homes (compared with 75% of the general French population aged 80 years), whereas 26.7% of patients required help with activities of daily living (compared with 35% to 40% of the general population). Sundt et al [31] reported functional status and survivorship up to 5 years among 133 patients undergoing AVR with or without CABG. Patient-reported functional status was comparable to the general population.

Because there is no effective medical therapy and balloon valvotomy is not an acceptable alternative to surgery, AVR is the gold standard for the treatment of severe stenosis and must be considered in all elderly patients who have symptoms caused by AS [10]. Age, per se, should not be considered a contraindication for surgery. Decisions should be made on an individual basis, taking into account patients' wishes and cardiac and non-cardiac factors

[12]. In this population, the need for an emergency operation, or, at the other end of the clinical spectrum, very early intervention at an asymptomatic stage, should be avoided.

The surgical community worked vigorously over the past two decades to reduce the trauma of the conventional aortic valve operation. Ongoing studies of transcatheter aortic valve implantation (TAVI) have demonstrated feasible short- and mid-term results in patients who were not considered suitable candidates for conventional AVR. Minimally invasive approaches like partial upper sternotomy have replaced the conventional complete median sternotomy when performing AVR in many centres. By aiming for smaller incisions, without compromising the quality of the operation and the effectiveness of myocardial protection, improved early outcomes have been achieved.

In a prospective randomised trial, Dogan et al [32] show that minimally invasive AVR can be performed with only slightly longer operative times, good cosmetic results and improved rib cage stability as well as significantly less blood loss. Furthermore, limited surgical access had no negative effects on the patients' neurological outcome nor the efficacy of myocardial protection. More recently, the implantation technique for AVR has also been modified, without compromising the hemodynamic performance of the valve substitute, all in order to reduce implantation times, and therefore reduce ischemia in the myocardium and cardiopulmonary bypass times. In 2009 Martens et al [33] reported on initial clinical experiences with the sutureless, nitinol-stented Enable (Medtronic Inc., Minnesota, USA) aortic valve prosthesis in 32 patients. Implantation time could be significantly reduced, down to 9±5 minutes, the first report of multi-centre experience with this particular valve substitute and implantation technique in 140 patients was published in the European Journal of Cardiothoracic Surgery in 2011. Reproducibility as well as feasibility and safety were demonstrated with the ATS 3f Enable® Bioprosthesis. Valve implantation resulted in excellent hemodynamics and significant clinical improvement. Further comparative studies are under way to prove the clinical benefit using this less-time-consuming implantation technique versus the conventional one.

6.2. High risk patient

How could we define a cardiac high-risk patient? Which parameters must we consider in order to assess risk? Which is the most accurate assessment tool to calculate a patient's risk?

We could define high risk cardiac patients as those who present several factors that significantly affect their outcome after surgery and could compromise their survival. Multiple series have documented that patients were deemed to have a high risk of operative complications or death on the basis of coexisting conditions such as advanced age, diabetes mellitus, existence of preoperative shock, LVEF ≤40%(≤30%), preoperative NYHA class III or IV, concomitant CAD, concomitant surgical procedure (CABG, valve surgery or surgery on thoracic aorta), renal failure and chronic obstructive pulmonary disease (COPD). Although attempts have been made to identify the high-risk population for AVR, there is currently no ideal model for precisely identifying high-risk patients. STS-PROM score and the European System for Cardiac Operative Risk Evaluation (EuroSCORE) have been used as part of the inclusion/exclusion criteria for the TAVI trials and to quantify the operative risk of conven-

http://dx.doi.org/10.5772/54333

tional AVR. Nevertheless, several previous reports on TAVI defined high-risk patients as patients with a logistic EuroSCORE between 10% and 30% [18]. Smith et al [34] in a TAVI versus AVR paper published in the New England Journal of Medicine in 2011 used as a guideline a score of at least 10% on the risk model developed by the STS to define high-risk patients. However, there are multiple additional risk factors, which are not currently considered by existing risk scoring systems; for example the presence of a porcelain aorta and considerations such as social integration, mobility, frailty, and the individual's overall health status must be taken into account, as well as the patient's wishes and expectations. A further definition that must be taken into account for evaluation of those patients who underwent TAVI is that very or extremely high-risk patients are those with a logistic EuroSCORE above 30% or STS score higher than 15% (see Table 2). The 2012 ACCF/AATS/SCAI/STS Expert Consensus Document on Transcatheter Aortic Valve Replacement [15] used the term *prohibitive risk*. This includes some patients for whom surgery might be deemed unsuitable based on the physician's assessment of the patient's risk for surgery; whereas in others, the surgeon may decide that the operation cannot be performed successfully because of technical considerations.

	Risk assessment tool	
	EuroSCORE	**STS score**
High risk	10-30%	"/>10%
Very or extremely high risk	"/>30%	"/>15%

Based on the 2012 ACCF/AATS/SCAI/STS Expert Consensus Document on Transcatheter Aortic Valve Replacement [15].

Table 2. Risk Assessment

In the absence of evidence in the literature and recommended guidelines, the determination of inoperability in any given patient depends on the judgement of the Heart team. It is generally agreed that patients with limited life expectancy due to concurrent conditions such as malignant tumours, dementia, primary liver disease or COPD, among others, are not appropriate for AVR. Frailty and poor physical condition are known to result in an inability to recover from major heart surgery such as AVR. These conditions can potentially contribute to increased surgical mortality and morbidity in the elderly. The surgeon may judge a patient inoperable as a result of technical considerations that preclude safe performance of AVR, such as prior mediastinal irradiation, porcelain aorta or severe periannular calcification, severe atheromatous disease, prior cardiac operations, and other conditions such as the internal mammary artery crossing the midline. In summary, a substantial percentage of patients with AS are judged to be inoperable for surgery based primarily on the physician's or surgeon's determination of operative risk and probability of survival [15]. Although some patients may be found to be inoperable for technical and surgical reasons, most inoperable patients are considered to be too ill due to associated comorbid conditions. In conclusion, the decision to proceed with AVR or TAVI requires careful weighing of the potential for improved symptoms and survival and the morbidity and mortality of surgery.

7. Surgical approach

7.1. Conventional AVR

Aortic valve replacement has permitted thousands of lives to be saved since it was first successfully carried out by Harken and Starr in 1960 [35, 36]. Since then, advances in prosthetic technology including improved hemodynamics, durability and thromboresistance, and techniques in cardiac surgery such as cardioplegia, management of the small aortic root, and replacement of associated aortic aneurysm have resulted in improvements in both operative and long-term results.

The conventional approach to AVR is the following: A mid-line incision and sternotomy is made and a pericardial well created. The patient is cannulated via the aorta and a single atrial venous cannula. After cross-clamping of the aorta, a transverse aortotomy is made approximately 1 cm above the take-off of the right coronary artery, slightly above the level of the sinotubular ridge (Figure. 3).

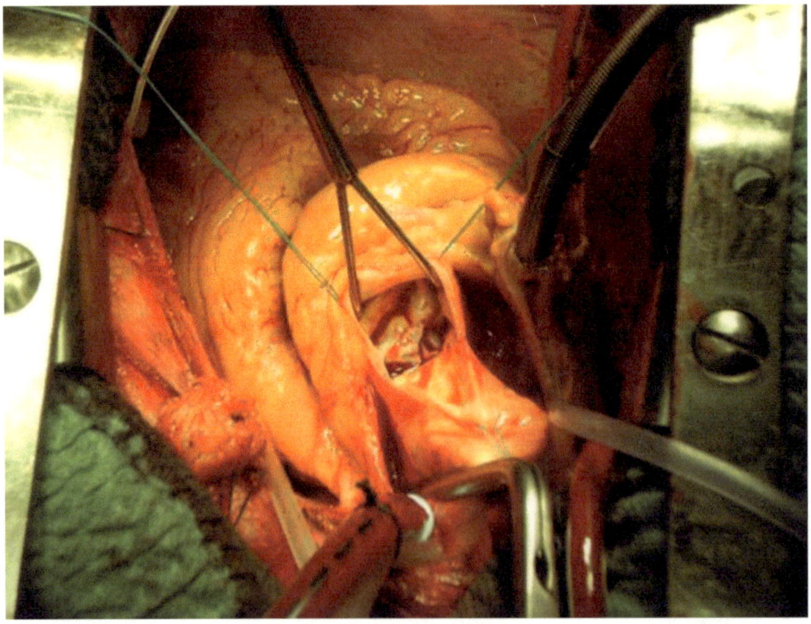

Figure 3. Transverse aortotomy

The incision is extended three-quarters of the way around the aorta, leaving the posterior one-quarter of the aorta intact allowing excellent visualization of the native aortic valve and

http://dx.doi.org/10.5772/54333

annulus. The leaflets of the aortic valve are excised to the level of the annulus and the annulus is thoroughly debrided of any calcium. Braided 2-0 sutures with pledgets are applied. Beginning at the non-coronary commissure, the annulus is encircled with interrupted mattress sutures (Figure 4) extending from the ventricular to the aortic surface.

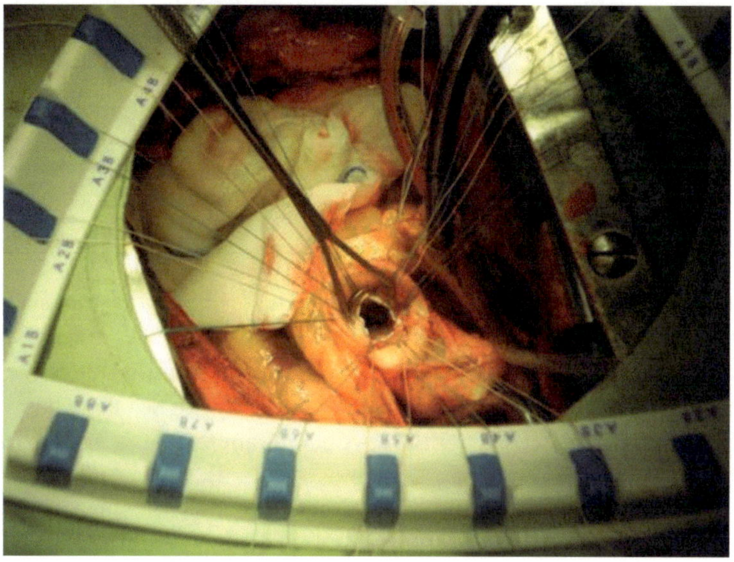

Figure 4. Aortic annulus encircled with interrupted mattress sutures

Next, each half of the suture bundles are implanted in the sewing ring and the prosthesis seated. The sutures are tied first at the left coronary cusp extending to the mid-portion of the right coronary cusp. Lastly, the sutures of the non-coronary cusp are secured, seating the valve appropriately. In case of mechanical valve prosthesis leaflet motion should always be checked and the surgeon must be assured that the coronary arteries are not obstructed. The aortotomy is closed with a double layer of polypropylene suture consisting of an underlying mattress suture and a more superficial over-and-over suture.

7.1.1. Conventional AVR results

Regardless of surgical approach, elected AVR is the gold standard for the treatment of severe AS. Several studies have shown acceptable short- and long-term outcomes, as well as improved quality of life in elderly patients. Although the proportion of elderly patients with multiple comorbidities is expanding, operative outcomes following AVR were still improving in the past decade. Recent series such as Likosky et al [25], report 30-day mortality among patients who underwent isolated AVR of 3.7% for patients <80, 6.7% in the 80 to 84 age group, and 11.7% in those ages >85 (P<0.001). Among patients undergoing AVR+CABG, 6.2% of patients <80 years died within 30 days, 9.4% among those 80 to 84, and 8.5% of patients ≥85 years (P=0.01). Also M. Di Eusanio et al [37] published a multi-centre study including 638 octogenarians who underwent AVR from an Italian regional cardiac surgery registry (2003-2009), They report hospital mortality of 4.5%, which favourably compares with those reported in other series (ranging from 4.3% to 13.7%). Recent surgical series [3, 38] report operative mortality rates for aortic valve replacement as low as 1%, increasing to 9% in higher-risk patients. Long-term survival after valve replacement is 80% at 3 years, with an age-corrected postoperative survival that is nearly normalized. Significant postoperative morbidity, such as thromboembolism, haemorrhagic complications from anticoagulation, prosthetic valve dysfunction, and endocarditis, are rare and occur at a rate of 2% to 3% per year [38]. These improvements in operative outcome could be related to multiple factors, including patient selection and perioperative management.

A number of studies have also examined outcomes of AVR conducted with concomitant CABG surgery. With few exceptions, concomitant CABG surgery does not increase a patient's operative risk. Considering the mounting evidence for the acceptable perioperative outcomes after AVR with or without concomitant CABG in the elderly, perhaps the fact that as many as one-third of patients >80 years of age with severe aortic stenosis are still denied surgery because of their age is due at least in part to the lack of evidence for long-term outcomes. Likosky et al [25] published the outcome of the very elderly undergoing aortic valve surgery comprising 7584 patients, including 815 over the age of 80. They have demonstrated that aortic valve replacement with or without concomitant CABG is a safe and effective option for elderly patients with severe aortic stenosis. Specifically, more than half of the patients undergoing aortic valve procedures were alive 6 years after surgery. Although concomitant CABG adds a slight mortality risk in the immediate postoperative period, it does not appreciably affect long-term survival among patients older than 80 years.

Survival has been also improved in elderly patients who underwent AVR. Asimakopoulos et al [39] reviewed United Kingdom Heart Valve Registry data from 1100 patients >80 years of age who underwent AVR from January 1986 to December 1995. They reported 30-day mortality as 6.6% with actuarial survival of 89%, 79.3%, 68.7%, and 45.8% at 1, 3, 5, and 8 years, respectively. Likosky et al [25] report a 6-year survival of 54.7% in patients aged 80 to 84 following AVR and 53.3% in patients aged 80 to 84 following AVR+CABG. Yamane et al [26] published their single centre study in 2011, reporting Survival at 1, 3, 5, and 10 years in patients aged 70–79 as 91.6%, 85.1%, 77.2%, and 38.0%, respectively, as compared with 84.1%, 75.7%, 63.0%, and 21.7% in patients aged 80– 92 (P=0.002). More recently M. Di Eusanio et al [37] report a 1, 3 and 6 year survival of 91.3%, 80.6% and 67.5% respectively in octogenarian patients who underwent isolated AVR.

In several studies, estimates of quality of life, as measured by NYHA functional class improvement, autonomy or satisfaction after receiving surgery have shown excellent functional recovery after AVR in patients >80 years (also see Elderly patient). Wu et al [40] in a recent study, determining the economic value of the additional life given to patients undergoing AVR, concluded that AVR is cost-effective for all ages, and still worthwhile in octogenarian and nonagenarian patients.

In conclusion, conventional AVR in selected octogenarians has similar outcomes to those in "younger" elderly patients, with good mid-term survival and excellent functional recovery

http://dx.doi.org/10.5772/54333

with a marked improvement in quality of life; in fact, their level of function and quality of life are the same as a general population of age-matched subjects.

7.2. Minimally Invasive Surgical (MIS) approaches

MIS approaches appear to improve the results observed in conventional surgery. The latter shows good results with acceptable morbidity and mortality rates in most cases, including in patients with aortic valve disease, however, in some subgroups of patients these outcomes tend to be worse. Minimally invasive surgery aims to minimise the degree of surgical intrusiveness. Currently there are several surgical approaches. A partial upper sternotomy is the most frequently used incision for a minimally invasive approach to the aortic valve and this is usually carried out via a parasternal incision over the second and third intercostal space, depending on the patient's anatomy as observed in preoperative imaging studies such as CT. The partial sternotomy is also frequently used, and there are several possible approaches. The table below summarises the various possible techniques (Table 3).

Partial sternotomy
Para-sternal incision [41,42]
Trans-sternal incision [41]
Upper sternotomy (Byrne et al., 2000) [38]
T mini-sternotomy [44]
V-shaped incision [45]
Inverted L incision [44]
Reversed L incision [46]
J incision [41,47]
Reversed C incision
Inverted T incision [48]
Thoracotomy
Right anterior thoracotomy 2° or 3° inter-costal space [49]
Right anterior thoracotomy 4° or 5° inter-costal space [50]
Video-assisted vision
Port access [51]
Video-direct vision
AESOP 3000 (Computer Motion, Goleta, CA) [52]
Da Vinci System (Intuitive Surgical, Sunnyvale, CA) [53]
Zeus (Computer Motion, Goleta, CA) [41]

Bustamante et al., 2012 [54]

Table 3. Minimally Invasive Approaches.

The "J" incision is the most widely used approach among the partial sternotomy approaches (Figure 5 & 6).

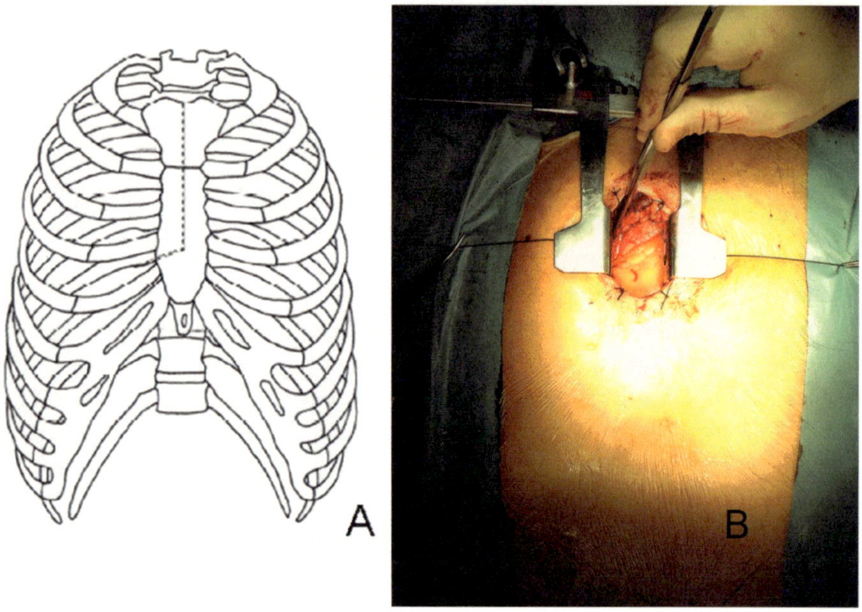

Figure 5. A & B: Reversed L incision.

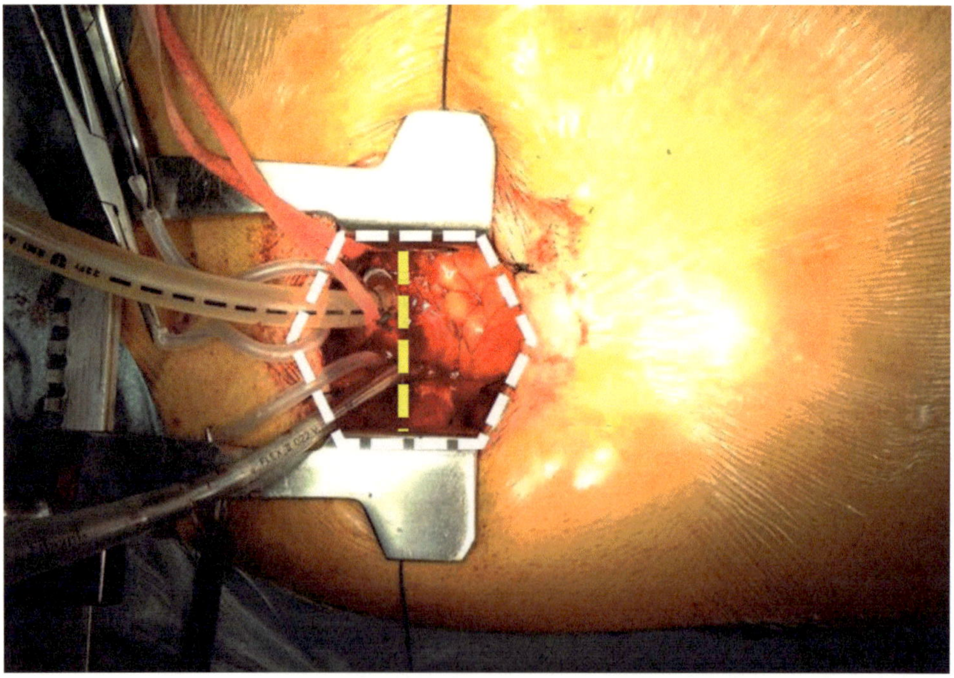

Figure 6. Operative field distribution from surgeon view.

However there are other approaches that are gaining popularity and some groups are beginning to use it quite often, so is the case of the right anterior thoracotomy through 2º or 3º inter-costal space (Figure 7).

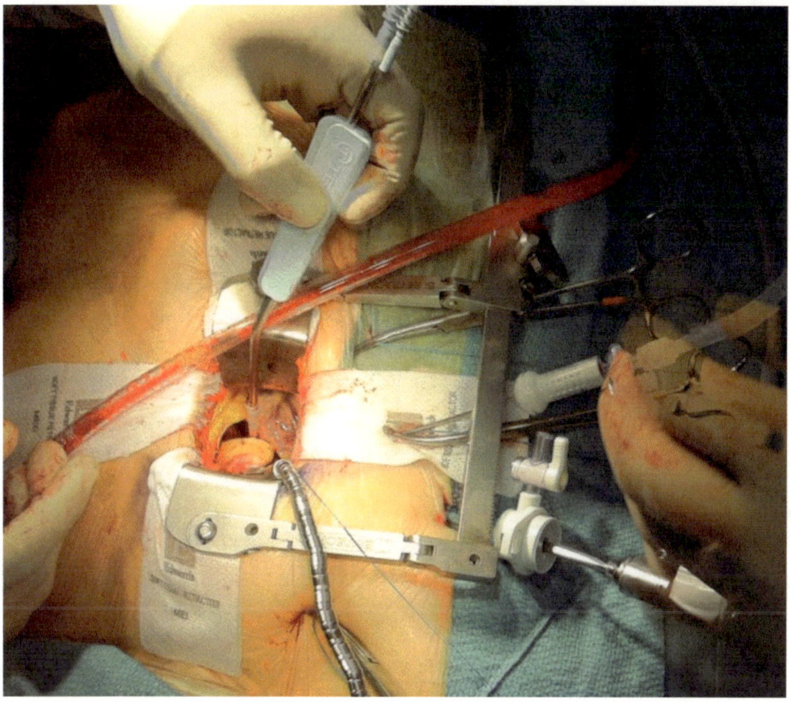

Figure 7. Right anterior thoracotomy through 2º or 3º inter-costal space.

Some controversy exists as to the benefits of these approaches. There are currently very few randomized studies able to answer this question and those that do exist have certain limitations [55, 56]. However, in the medical literature we do find numerous articles that report broad series of patients in which the effects can be observed and several aspects of these approaches can be compared to conventional approaches.

A series of advantages traditionally exist in the application of MIS for aortic valve replacement. There is no methodological uniformity across the studies that have been carried out, which sometimes complicates comparison between studies and makes it difficult to draw conclusions about the impact of these approaches on patient treatment. This is due to the fact that the aspects considered by the different studies differ in some cases. For example, some focus on length of hospitalization and specific complications and others give more relevance to surgical aspects such time spent with extracorporeal circulation or clamping. In summary, we can say that there is a group of patients about which there is a certain consensus as to the benefits of the MIS approaches. This group includes the elderly [50], and patients who have previously undergone interventions involving myocardial revascularisation [43]. In the first case the benefit fundamentally lies in the reduction of surgical aggression in cases where patients are more susceptible to developing post-operative complications, leading to a much faster functional recovery time compared to patients subjected to conventional interventions. In the second case the benefit lies in the fact that it is not necessary to dissect the mediastinal structures, thus avoiding the risk of damaging coronary implants, and the complications that would entail [57, 58].

7.2.1. Advantages and disadvantages of MIS approaches in aortic stenosis

In other patients there are arguments in favour of MIS. Benefits have been observed in certain aspects such as:

- Reduction in bleeding in surgery and therefore in the use of hemoderivatives. There are also discrepancies in this aspect, as while some studies indicate the benefit [55, 59-61], others, such as Stamou et al [44] do not observe this effect. A possible explanation for this disparity of results is that in the assessment of reduced post-operative bleeding, no prior adjustments for risk factors for post-operative bleeding were made. The debate is further complicated by the fact that Dogan et al [32], observed differences in the reduction of post-surgical bleeding in a randomised study. In our group we did observe a statistically significant reduction in blood loss during surgery and in the need for hemoderivatives.

- Reduction in the pain perceived by the patient. Numerous studies indicate this benefit [55, 62, 63] which is based on a reduction in the distension of costovertebral ligaments and traction of the brachial plexus. This results in reduced consumption of analgesic pharmaceuticals by the patient.

- Less reduction in tidal lung volume, thus reducing the appearance of respiratory complications such as atelectasis by maintaining the integrity of the thorax [56].

- Better aesthetic results. This is one of the clear benefits of the technique, due to the reduced size of the surgical incisions and their relocation to less visible areas.

- There are other benefits, such as the reduction in complications in the surgical wound/ infections. Grossi et al [64] observe an incidence of infection of 0.9% for minimally invasive approaches as against 5.7% in cases of patients with the approach by sternotomy, $p=0.05$. It has been observed that this difference increases in elderly patients (1.8 and 7.7% respectively). Other authors observe that in comparison with the classical approach there is a lesser incidence of infectious complications [65, 66].

A certain consensus exists around the benefits mentioned above. There is also the question of the impact of MIS on duration of surgery. There is disparity in the results found in the literature. Along with other research groups, we observed that, once the learning curve has been overcome, these times tend to equal out and there is no significant difference to be observed between the different approaches. Studies that support an increase in the time for cardiopulmonary bypass and aortic clamping are Farhat et al, Detter et al, de Vaumas et al, and Stamou et al. [44, 46, 48, 67]; contradictory results can be found in Corbi et al., Sharony et al or the randomised study by Bonachi et al. [45, 50, 55]. Another aspect that is highly valued in MIS surgery is the impact it has on the duration of hospitalisation and time spent in

http://dx.doi.org/10.5772/54333

intensive care units. This has been taken into consideration in reducing the cost of the process, in a context of increased life expectancy and rising healthcare costs. In terms of patient treatment it is relevant in that the reduction of both is accompanied by a lesser incidence of other complications, basically infections, particularly respiratory infections, surgical wound infections and urinary tract infections.

7.3. Transcatheter Aortic Valve Replacement (TAVR)

Transcatheter aortic valve implantation (TAVI) was developed as an alternative to AVR in the very or extremely high-risk patient population. The first implant in man was performed by Cribier [68] in 2002, using a balloon expandable frame and equine valve. Since the introduction of minimally invasive and catheter-based therapies, patients want less invasive options for all types of medical procedures including general surgical, orthopaedic, spinal, and urological operations with the goal of decreasing morbidity and mortality and shortening recovery time. Other issues with traditional aortic and mitral valve surgery include the fact that patients may not even be offered operation; in multiple series from different centres and in different countries, up to 40% of patients with severe aortic stenosis are treated medically [69, 70]. Some of these patients may be deemed to be too sick for surgery because of associated medical comorbidities, and some may be considered too old. Finally, some who may benefit the most from an operation may decline surgery even though they develop irreversible damage from the valve lesion that could have been treated. These factors have led to the continuous development of less invasive strategies with lower mortality, lower morbidity, and less invasiveness [71]. Transcatheter aortic valve replacement seems to offer a new window of treatment for those patients with severe aortic valve stenosis that are either extremely high-risk or inoperable for conventional aortic valve replacement. Today around 40000 patients have received a transcatheter aortic valve implantation (TAVI) worldwide. Multiple single- and multi-centre registries, and a single randomized trial, the PARTNER trial (Placement of AoRTic TraNscathetER Valve Trial), have documented favourable outcomes using a wide spectrum of endpoints, including survival, symptom status, quality of life, and need for repeat hospitalization.

7.3.1. Implantation techniques

TAVI is currently carried out using two main approaches (retrograde transfemoral and antegrade transapical), which share the same main principles. Trans-axillary artery or transaortic are other approaches that are gaining popularity when the transfemoral approach is not feasible. Specific anatomic issues must be considered in device design. These include the rigid structure and pattern of the valvular calcification and the aortic annulus, and the need for as full an apposition as possible to the annulus in an attempt to minimize periprosthetic leaks. In the case of eccentric, bulky calcifications, this may be difficult. The close proximity to the coronary ostia, the width and height of the sinuses, the membranous ventricular septum with the His bundle and the anterior leaflet of the mitral valve are also important anatomical considerations. In addition, the size and degree of severity of peripheral arterial disease are all factors that could limit catheter size [15]. It is therefore highly recommended to perform an adequate preoperative assessment of the degree of peripheral arterial disease through imaging studies such as CT (Figure 8).

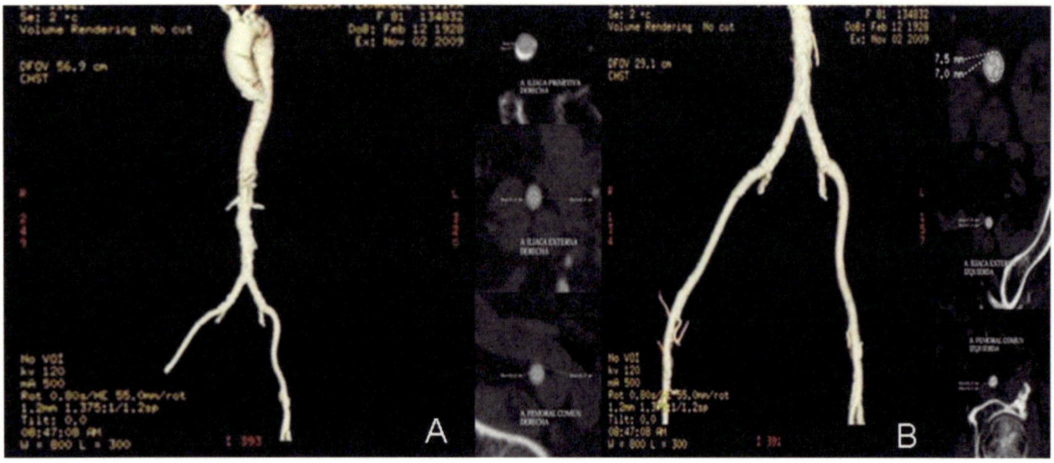

Figure 8. (A) CT reconstruction of the aorta. (B) CT reconstruction of iliofemoral arteries

Most teams perform the procedure under general anaesthesia, although sedation and analgesia may suffice for the transfemoral approach. Peri-procedural transoesophageal echocardiography (TEE) monitoring is desirable to correctly position the valve as well as to detect complications. After crossing the aortic valve, Balloon aortic valvuloplasty is performed to pre-dilate the native valve and serve as a rehearsal for TAVI. Simultaneous rapid pacing decreases cardiac output, stabilizing the balloon during inflation. Normal blood pressure must be completely recovered between sequences of rapid pacing. In order to position the prosthesis at the level of the aortic valve annulus different methods can be used, such as fluoroscopy to assess the level of valve calcification (Figure 9); aortography, using different views, performed at the beginning of the procedure and repeated with the undeployed prosthesis in place, to determine the position of the valve and the plane of alignment of the aortic cusps; and echocardiography. TEE is particularly helpful in cases with moderate calcification.

Three dimensional real-time TEE seems to provide extra information to the teams that use it. When positioning is considered correct, the prosthesis is released. Rapid pacing is used at this stage for balloon-expandable devices but not for self-expanding ones. Immediately after TAVI, aortography and, whenever available, TEE or, in the absence of TEE, Transthoracic echocardiogram(TTE) are performed to assess the location and degree of aortic regurgitation and the patency of the coronary arteries, and to rule out complications such as haemopericardium, and aortic dissection. The hemodynamic results are assessed using pressure recordings and/or echocardiography. After the procedure, the patients should stay in intensive care for at least 24 hours and be closely monitored for several days, particularly as regards hemodynamics, vascular access, rhythm disturbances (especially late atrioventricular block), and renal function.

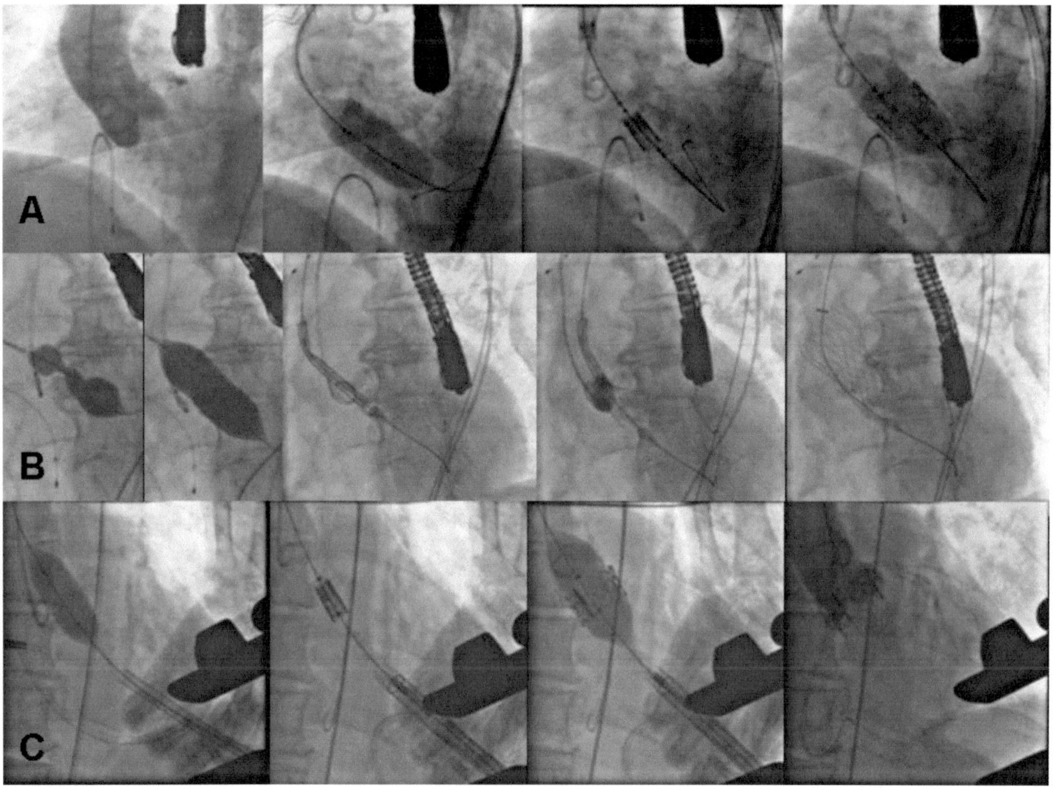

Figure 9. First row (A). Edwards Sapiens transfemoral implantation. Second row (B). Transfemoral Corevalve implantation. Third row (C). Edwards Sapiens transapical implantation.

The specific issues related to the different approaches include the following: In the transfemoral approach, close attention should be paid to the vascular access. The common femoral artery can be either prepared surgically or approached percutaneously. Echo-guided femoral access could be useful. Manipulation of the introductory sheaths should be careful and fluoroscopically guided. Depending on the size of the device, closure of the vascular access can be effected surgically or using a percutaneous closure device. Femoral access and cardiopulmonary bypass should be on standby for patients for whom surgical conversion is an option in case of complications.

The transapical approach requires an antero-lateral mini-thoracotomy (Figure 10), pericardiotomy, identification of the apex, and then puncture of the left ventricle using a needle through purse-string sutures. Subsequently, an introductory sheath is positioned in the LV, and the prosthesis is implanted using the antegrade route.

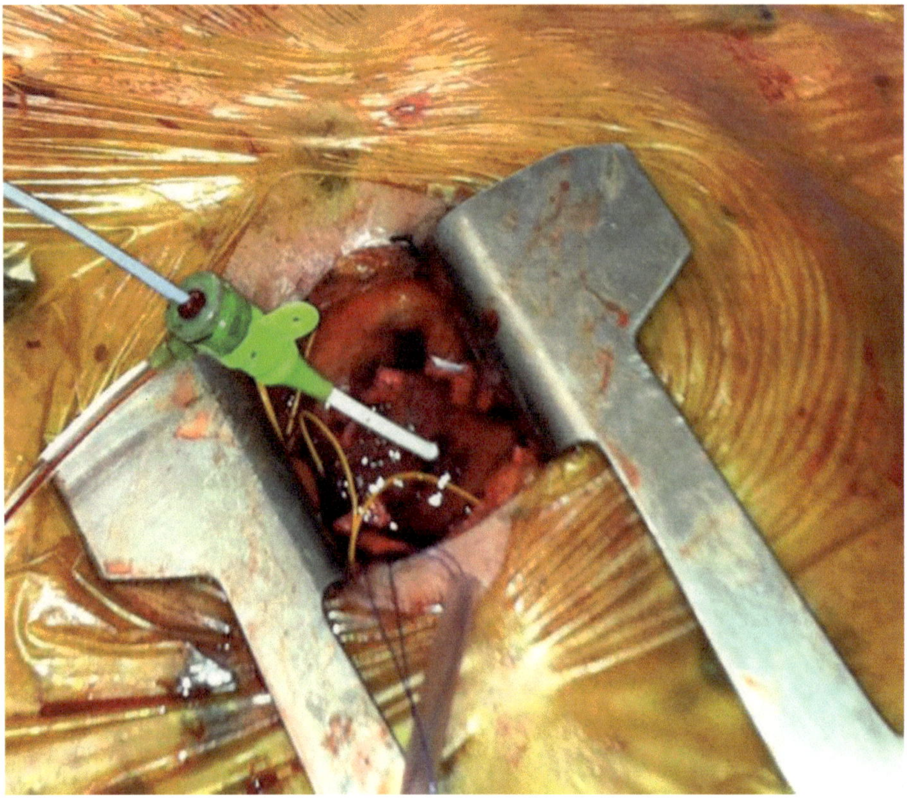

Figure 10. Anterior minitoracotomy for transapical approach of a TAVI procedure.

7.3.2. TAVR results

The PARTNER trial has been followed with great interest. The PARTNER trial was basically 2 parallel trials: 1) PARTNER Cohort A, which randomized high-risk surgical patients to either traditional aortic valve replacement or to TAVI by either a transfemoral or transapical approach; and 2) PARTNER Cohort B in which patients who were inoperable were randomized to either a TAVR by a transfemoral approach or to conventional medical therapy, which typically consisted of balloon aortic valvuloplasty.

Screening required evaluation by 2 experienced cardiac surgeons to agree on the surgical risk using the STS Predicted Risk of Mortality score and was rigorous, with approximately one-quarter to one-third of screened patients subsequently enrolled. The primary endpoint was death from any cause at 1 year. The results of PARTNER Cohort B included 358 patients deemed unsuitable for conventional aortic valve replacement because of predicted probability of≥ 50% mortality or the risk of a serious irreversible complication within 30 days. At 1 year, all-cause mortality with TAVR was 30.7% versus 50.7% with medical therapy (hazard ratio: 0.55, 95% confidence interval: 0.40 to 0.74). Despite the marked improvement in survival and event-free survival, there were some significant safety hazards, particularly a higher incidence of major strokes (5.0% versus 1.1%) as well as increased major vascular complications (16.2% versus 1.1%) with TAVR, both of which may adversely impact early and longer-term outcome. Longer-term outcomes will be required. These results were received enthusiastically; however, they have important limitations. Firstly, they can be applied only in patients similar to those in the study (i.e., those patients deemed to be inoperable). Secondly, they are the result of treatment by very experienced operators working as a heart team in a hybrid operating room or similar facility with a specific device and do not necessarily apply to other devices.

The results of the PARTNER Cohort A trial also have important implications. The primary endpoint of the trial was met, with TAVR found not to be inferior to aortic valve replacement for all-cause mortality at 1 year (TAVR versus aortic valve replacement, 24.2% versus 26.8%, respectively, $p=0.001$ for non-inferiority). Death at 30 days was lower than expected in both arms of the trial: TAVR mortality (3.4%) was the lowest reported in any series, despite an early generation device and limited previous operator experience. Aortic valve replacement mortality (6.5%) was lower than the expected operative mortality (11.8%). Furthermore, both TAVR and aortic valve replacement were associated with important but different peri-procedural hazards: major strokes at 30 days (3.8% versus 2.1%, $p=0.20$) and 1 year (5.1% versus 2.4%, $p=0.07$), and major vascular complications were more frequent with TAVR (11.0% versus 3.2%, $p<0.001$). Major bleeding (9.3% versus 19.5%, $p<0.001$) and new onset atrial fibrillation (8.6% versus 16.0%, $p<0.001$) were more frequent with aortic valve replacement.

Rates of stroke were similar whether the access was transfemoral or transapical. Bioprosthetic-valve gradients and orifice areas were slightly better after transcatheter replacement than after surgical replacement, probably because of the less bulky support frame with transcatheter replacement [34]. However, transcatheter replacement resulted in much more frequent paravalvular aortic regurgitation. Although this condition was stable at 1 year, repeat intervention was required in some cases. A reduction in the incidence and severity of paravalvular AR represents an obvious target for technical improvements in the design of transcatheter valves and of implantation techniques [24]. Clinical benefits of transcatheter replacement included significantly shorter stays in the intensive care unit and in hospital. In addition, the NYHA functional class and 6-minute walk distance were strikingly improved at 1 year [34]. Transcatheter aortic valve implantation by means of either the transfemoral or the transapical approach is a reasonable and promising treatment option for patients who are at high risk or had been refused for conventional AVR. Recommendations made to individual patients must balance the appeal of avoiding the known risks of open-heart surgery against the less invasive transcatheter approach, which has different and less well understood risks, particularly with respect to stroke and paravalvular aortic regurgitation.

8. New prostheses in mini-invasive approaches

These prostheses were designed by industry with a view to facilitating the implantation of the prosthesis through conventional surgery; that is to say, using a cardio-pulmonary bypass and aortic clamping. The gold standard for the use of these prostheses is in association with MIS approaches, providing a reduction in surgical aggression in addition to the reduction in ECC and aortic clamping time, the consequences of which we have already examined. These designs have the common feature of being expandable, anchoring themselves to the aortic ring in a similar way to the devices used in TAVI.

To date there are three commercially available models: 3f Enable ® (Medtronic Inc, Minneapolis, MN), Perceval S (Sorin Group Cardio Srl, Sallugia, Italy) and Intuity (Edwards Lifesciences, Irvine, California). These differ from each other in a few characteristics.

3f Enable ® aortic bioprosthesis (Figure 11): This prosthesis is especially indicated in patients with small aortic annulus where the possibility of having a severe mismatch is high with the use of conventional prosthesis. Several studies report an acceptable hemodynamic behavior with this type of prosthesis. Furthermore, there is no need to match the measure between the annulus and the sinotubular junction, because the prosthesis is anchored only to the annulus. Of the three prostheses this is the oldest and different models have been developed since its initial commercialisation with a view to improving hemodynamics, durability and facilitating surgeons in its implantation [72-74]

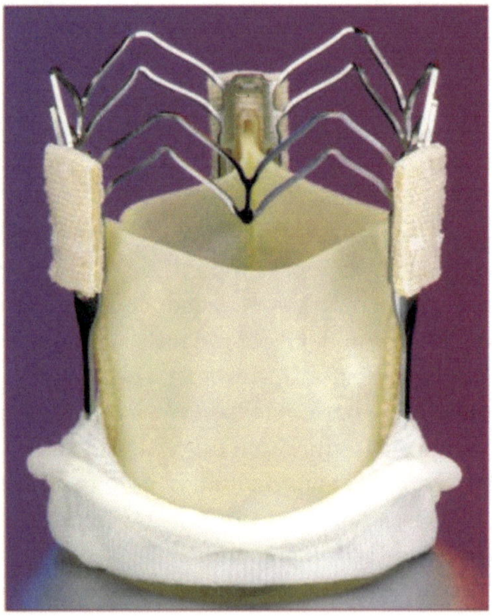

Figure 11. Enable ® (Medtronic Inc, Minneapolis, MN)

Perceval S (Sorin Biomedica Cardio Srl, Sallugia, Italy) (Figure 12): Prosthesis aimed at patients with a high surgical risk in which a reduction in surgery time may have a significant impact, for patients where it is necessary to carry out mixed procedures, and patients undergoing re-intervention, and patients with a small aortic ring, because of the hemodynamic characteristics of the prosthesis [75, 76]

http://dx.doi.org/10.5772/54333

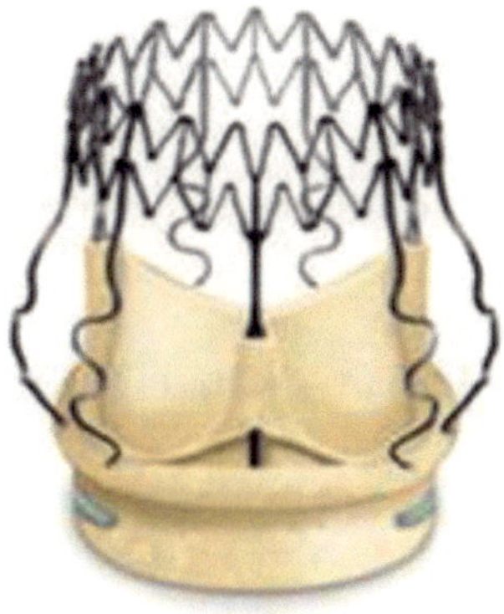

Figure 12. Perceval S (Sorin Biomedica Cardio Srl, Sallugia, Italy)

Intuity (Edwards Lifesciences, Irvine, California) (Figure 13): Of these three prostheses this is the most recently commercialised and results as to its hemodynamic profile and durability in clinical practice are not available. Arguments in its favour, as put forward by the company, are the conjunction between the Edwards Perimount bioprosthesis, the clinical and hemodynamic results of which are widely known, and the experience in the development of new prostheses such as the Sapien transcatheter. The mode of implantation for this prosthesis allows the aortic clamping and extracorporeal circulation times to be reduced. For a number of reasons, one of the most important being ischemic reperfusion, these two variables are known to be directly related to the surgical morbidity and mortality of procedures, which is why this model may be attractive, in addition to the comfort of implantation, as it does not require stitches in the aortic ring.

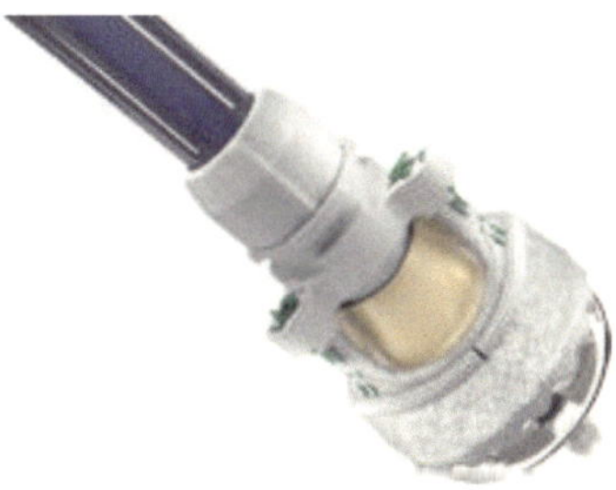

Figure 13. Intuity (Edwards Lifesciences, Irvine, California)

The disadvantage of these prostheses is their cost, as they ultimately increase resource consumption. Results for hemodynamics and durability are becoming better understood as preliminary studies are published. From the beginning we find data in the literature relating to safety and effectiveness in the implantation of aortic valve replacements. Some of the complications associated with their use, such as perivalvular leaks are understood to be intimately related to the decalcification of the ring; in some cases, it has been possible to correct other complications, such as bad positioning, with new designs being applied to the already existing prosthetics [77]

9. Conclusions

Medical science is progressing faster than ever and the field of cardiovascular disease is one of its greatest exponents. Patient care and treatment must adapt to changing patient characteristics as well as to new technologies and treatment options. In the case of aortic valve disease, whose prevalence is booming in the western world, we must be capable of a comprehensive approach to ensure optimal results and efficient use of resources. Currently, age, *per se*, is not a contraindication for the treatment of aortic valve disease; hence a thorough assessment should be undertaken to design the best therapeutic approach for high-risk patients. Understanding of treatment options of this disease has increased. New devices have been developed and advances have been made in perioperative management of cardiac surgical patients. Nevertheless, there is still room for improvement in this interesting field of cardiac surgery.

Author details

Omer Leal[1], Juan Bustamante[1*], Sergio Cánovas[2] and Ángel G. Pinto[3]

*Address all correspondence to: jbustamantemunguira@gmail.com

1 Department of Cardiovascular Surgery, Hospital Universitario La Princesa, Madrid, Spain

2 Department of Cardiac Surgery, Hospital General Universitario de Valencia, Valencia, Spain

3 Department of Cardiac Surgery, Hospital Universitario Gragorio Marañon, Madrid, Spain

References

[1] Schmitto J.D., Mohr F.W., Cohn L.H. Minimally invasive aortic valve replacement: how does this perform in high-risk patients? Curr Opin Cardiol. 2011; 26(2):118-122.

[2] Chambers J.B. Aortic stenosis. Eur J Echocardiogr. 2009; 10(1):i11-9.

[3] Freeman RV, Otto CM. Spectrum of calcific aortic valve disease: pathogenesis, disease progression, and treatment strategies. Circulation. 2005 Jun 21;111(24): 3316-3326.

[4] Otto CM, Lind BK, Kitzman DW, Gersh BJ, Siscovick DS. Association of aortic-valve sclerosis with cardiovascular mortality and morbidity in the elderly. N Engl J Med. 1999 15;341(3):142-147.

[5] Kurtz CE, Otto CM. Aortic stenosis: clinical aspects of diagnosis and management, with 10 illustrative case reports from a 25-year experience. Medicine (Baltimore). 2010;89(6):349-379.

[6] Steadman CD, Ray S, Ng LL, McCann GP. Natriuretic peptides in common valvular heart disease. J Am Coll Cardiol 2010;55:2034–2048.

[7] Bergler-Klein J, Klaar U, Heger M, Rosenhek R, Mundigler G, Gabriel H, et al. Natriuretic peptides predict symptom-free survival and postoperative outcome in severe aortic stenosis. Circulation 2004; 109:2302–2308.

[8] Monin JL, Lancellotti P, Monchi M, Lim P, Weiss E, Pie´rard L, et al., Risk score for predicting outcome in patients with asymptomatic aortic stenosis. Circulation 2009;120:69–75.

[9] Lancellotti P, Moonen M, Magne J, O'Connor K, Cosyns B, Attena E, et al., Prognostic effect of long-axis left ventricular dysfunction and B-type natriuretic peptide levels in asymptomatic aortic stenosis. Am J Cardiol 2010; 105:383–388.

[10] Bonow RO, Carabello BA, Chatterjee K, de Leon AC Jr, Faxon DP, Freed MD, et al. 2008 focused update incorporated into the ACC/AHA 2006 guidelines for the management of patients with valvular heart disease: a report of the American College of Cardiology/American Heart Association Task Force on Practice Guidelines (Writing Committee to revise the 1998 guidelines for the management of patients with valvular heart disease). Endorsed by the Society of Cardiovascular Anesthesiologists, Society for Cardiovascular Angiography and Interventions, and Society of Thoracic Surgeons. J Am Coll Cardiol. 2008 23;52(13):e1-142.

[11] Vahanian A, Alfieri O, Andreotti F, Antunes MJ, Barón-Esquivias G, Baumgartner H, et al. Guidelines on the management of valvular heart disease (version 2012): The Joint Task Force on the Management of Valvular Heart Disease of the European Society of Cardiology (ESC) and the European Association for Cardio-Thoracic Surgery (EACTS). Eur J Cardiothorac Surg. 2012 27. doi:10.1093/eurheartj/ehs109.

[12] Vahanian A, Baumgartner H, Bax J, Butchart E, Dion R, Filippatos G, et al. Guidelines on the management of valvular heart disease: The Task Force on the Management of Valvular Heart Disease of the European Society of Cardiology. Eur Heart J. 2007;28(2):230-268.

[13] Baumgartner H, Hung J, Bermejo J, Chambers JB, Evangelista A, Griffin BP, et al. American Society of Echocardiography; European Association of Echocardiography. Echocardiographic assessment of valve stenosis: EAE/ASE recommendations for practice. J Am Soc Echocardiogr. 2009;22(1):1-23.

[14] Ross J Jr, Braunwald E. Aortic stenosis. Circulation. 1968;38(1 Suppl):61-67.

[15] Holmes DR Jr, Mack MJ, Kaul S, Agnihotri A, Alexander KP, Bailey SR, et al. 2012 ACCF/AATS/SCAI/STS expert consensus document on transcatheter aortic valve replacement: developed in collaboration with the American Heart Association, American Society of Echocardiography, European Association for Cardio Thoracic Surgery, Heart Failure Society of America, Mended Hearts, Society of Cardiovascular Anesthesiologists, Society of Cardiovascular Computed Tomography, and Society for Cardiovascular Magnetic Resonance. Ann Thorac Surg. 2012;93(4):1340-1395.

[16] Grant SW, Hickey GL, Dimarakis I, Trivedi U, Bryan A, Treasure T, et al. How does EuroSCORE II perform in UK cardiac surgery; an analysis of 23 740 patients from the Society for Cardiothoracic Surgery in Great Britain and Ireland National Database. Heart. 2012 Aug 21. doi:10.1136/heartjnl-2012-302483.

[17] Frilling B, von Renteln Kruse W, Riess FC. Evaluation of operative risk in elderly patients undergoing aortic valve replacement: the predictive value of operative risk scores. Cardiology. 2010;116(3):213-218.

[18] Thielmann M, Wendt D, Eggebrecht H, Kahlert P, Massoudy P, Kamler M, et al. Transcatheter aortic valve implantation in patients with very high risk for conventional aortic valve replacement. Ann Thorac Surg. 2009;88(5):1468-1474.

[19] Rosenhek R, Iung B, Tornos P, Antunes MJ, Prendergast BD, Otto CM, et al. ESC Working Group on Valvular Heart Disease Position Paper: assessing the risk of interventions in patients with valvular heart disease. Eur Heart J. 2012;33(7):822-828.

[20] Bustamante J, Gómez-Martínez ML, Bustamante E, Tamayo E. Occult chronic kidney disease in the ederly with coronary heart disease. Med Clin (Barc). 2009;133(13):524.

[21] Herreros JM. Cardiac surgery in elderly patients. Rev Esp Cardiol. 2002;55(11): 1114-1116.

[22] Lindroos M, Kupari M, Heikkilä J, Tilvis R. Prevalence of aortic valve abnormalities in the elderly: an echocardiographic study of a random population sample. J Am Coll Cardiol. 1993;21(5):1220-1225.

[23] Rodríguez R, Torrents A, García P, Ribera A, Permanyer G, Moradi M, et al. Cardiac surgery in elderly patients. Rev Esp Cardiol. 2002;55(11):1159-1168.

[24] Moat NE, Ludman P, de Belder MA, Bridgewater B, Cunningham AD, Young CP, et al. Long-term outcomes after transcatheter aortic valve implantation in high-risk patients with severe aortic stenosis: the U.K. TAVI (United Kingdom Transcatheter Aortic Valve Implantation) Registry. J Am Coll Cardiol. 2011;58(20):2130-2138.

[25] Likosky DS, Sorensen MJ, Dacey LJ, Baribeau YR, Leavitt BJ, DiScipio AW, et al. Long-term survival of the very elderly undergoing aortic valve surgery. Circulation. 2009;120(11 Suppl):S127-133.

[26] Yamane K, Hirose H, Youdelman BA, Bogar LJ, Diehl JT. Conventional aortic valve replacement for elderly patients in the current era. Circ J. 2011;75(11):2692-2698.

[27] Brown JM, O'Brien SM, Wu C, Sikora JA, Griffith BP, Gammie JS. Isolated aortic valve replacement in North America comprising 108,687 patients in 10 years: changes in risks, valve types, and outcomes in the Society of Thoracic Surgeons National Database. J Thorac Cardiovasc Surg. 2009;137(1):82-90.

[28] Huber CH, Goeber V, Berdat P, Carrel T, Eckstein F. Benefits of cardiac surgery in octogenarians a postoperative quality of life assessment. Eur J Cardiothorac Surg. 2007;31(6):1099-1105.

[29] Kolh P, Lahaye L, Gerard P, Limet R. Aortic valve replacement in the octogenarians: perioperative outcome and clinical follow-up. Eur J Cardiothorac Surg. 1999;16(1): 68-73.

[30] Maillet JM, Somme D, Hennel E, Lessana A, Saint-Jean O, Brodaty D. Frailty after aortic valve replacement (AVR) in octogenarians. Arch Gerontol Geriatr. 2009;48(3): 391-396.

[31] Sundt TM, Bailey MS, Moon MR, Mendeloff EN, Huddleston CB, Pasque MK, et al. Quality of life after aortic valve replacement at the age of >80 years. Circulation. 2000;102(19 Suppl 3):III70-74.

[32] Dogan S, Dzemali O, Wimmer-Greinecker G, Derra P, Doss M, Khan MF, et al. Minimally invasive versus conventional aortic valve replacement: a prospective randomized trial. J Heart Valve Dis. 2003;12(1):76-80.

[33] Martens S, Sadowski J, Eckstein FS, Bartus K, Kapelak B, Sievers HH, et al. Clinical experience with the ATS 3f Enable® Sutureless Bioprosthesis. Eur J Cardiothorac Surg. 2011;40(3):749-755.

[34] Smith CR, Leon MB, Mack MJ, Miller DC, Moses JW, Svensson LG, et al. Transcatheter versus surgical aortic-valve replacement in high-risk patients. N Engl J Med. 2011;364(23):2187-2198.

[35] Harken, D.E., Soroff, H.S., Taylor, W.H. Aortic valve replacement, in Merendino KA (ed): Prosthetic Valves for Cardiac Surgery. Springfield, IL, Thomas; 1961, p 508-526

[36] Starr A, Edwards ML. Mitral replacement: clinical experience with a ball-valve prosthesis. Ann Surg. 1961; 154:726-740.

[37] Di Eusanio M, Fortuna D, Cristell D, Pugliese P, Nicolini F, Pacini D, et al. Contemporary outcomes of conventional aortic valve replacement in 638 octogenarians: insights from an Italian Regional Cardiac Surgery Registry (RERIC). Eur J Cardiothorac Surg. 2012;41(6):1247-1252.

[38] Rahimtoola SH. Choice of prosthetic heart valve in adults an update. J Am Coll Cardiol. 2010;55(22):2413-2426.

[39] Asimakopoulos G, Edwards MB, Taylor KM. Aortic valve replacement in patients 80 years of age and older: survival and cause of death based on 1100 cases: collective results from the UK Heart Valve Registry. Circulation. 1997;96(10):3403-3408.

[40] Wu Y, Jin R, Gao G, Grunkemeier GL, Starr A. Cost-effectiveness of aortic valve replacement in the elderly: an introductory study. J Thorac Cardiovasc Surg. 2007;133(3):608-613.

[41] Cohn LH, Adams DH, Couper GS, Bichell DP, Rosborough DM, Sears SP, Aranki SF. Minimally invasive cardiac valve surgery improves patient satisfaction while reducing costs of cardiac valve replacement and repair. Ann Surg. 1997;226(4):421-426.

[42] Navia JL, Cosgrove DM 3rd. Minimally invasive mitral valve operations. Ann Thorac Surg. 1996;62(5):1542-1544

[43] Byrne JG, Karavas AN, Adams DH, Aklog L, Aranki SF, Couper GS, Rizzo RJ, Cohn LH, et al. Partial upper re-sternotomy for aortic valve replacement or re-replacement after previous cardiac surgery. Eur J Cardiothorac Surg. 2000;18(3):282-286.

[44] Stamou SC, Kapetanakis EI, Lowery R, Jablonski KA, Frankel TL, Corso PJ. Allogeneic blood transfusion requirements after minimally invasive versus conventional aortic valve replacement: a risk-adjusted analysis. Ann Thorac Surg. 2003;76(4): 1101-1106.

[45] Corbi P, Rahmati M, Donal E, Lanquetot H, Jayle C, Menu P, et al. Prospective comparison of minimally invasive and standard techniques for aortic valve replacement: initial experience in the first hundred patients. J Card Surg. 2003;18(2):133-139.

[46] Detter C, Deuse T, Boehm DH, Reichenspurner H, Reichart B. Midterm results and quality of life after minimally invasive vs. conventional aortic valve replacement. Thorac Cardiovasc Surg. 2002;50(6):337-341.

[47] Doll N, Borger MA, Hain J, Bucerius J, Walther T, Gummert JF, et al. Minimal access aortic valve replacement: effects on morbidity and resource utilization. Ann Thorac Surg. 2002;74(4):S1318-1322.

[48] Farhat F, Lu Z, Lefevre M, Montagna P, Mikaeloff P, Jegaden O. Prospective comparison between total sternotomy and ministernotomy for aortic valve replacement. J Card Surg. 2003;18(5):396-401.

[49] Burfeind WR, Glower DD, Davis RD, Landolfo KP, Lowe JE, Wolfe WG. Mitral surgery after prior cardiac operation: port-access versus sternotomy or thoracotomy. Ann Thorac Surg. 2002;74(4):S1323-1325.

[50] Sharony R, Grossi EA, Saunders PC, Schwartz CF, Ribakove GH, Culliford AT, et al. Minimally invasive aortic valve surgery in the elderly: a case control study. Circulation. 2003;108 Suppl 1:II43-47.

[51] Galloway AC, Shemin RJ, Glower DD, Boyer JH Jr, Groh MA, Kuntz RE, et al. First report of the Port Access International Registry. Ann Thorac Surg. 1999;67(1):51-56.

[52] Falk V, Walther T, Autschbach R, Diegeler A, Battellini R, Mohr FW. Robot-assisted minimally invasive solo mitral valve operation. J Thorac Cardiovasc Surg. 1998;115(2):470-471.

[53] Carpentier A, Loulmet D, Aupècle B, Kieffer JP, Tournay D, Guibourt P, et al. Computer assisted open heart surgery. First case operated on with success. C R Acad Sci III. 1998;321(5):437-442.

[54] Bustamante J, Cánovas S, Fernández AL, Minimally Invasive Aortic Valve Surgery - New Solutions to Old Problems In Hirota M (Ed) Aortic Stenosis - Etiology, Pathophysiology and Treatment. Rijeka: InTech; 2012. p 91-114.

[55] Bonacchi M, Prifti E, Giunti G, Frati G, Sani G. Does ministernotomy improve postoperative outcome in aortic valve operation? A prospective randomized study. Ann Thorac Surg. 2002;73(2):460-465.

[56] Moustafa MA, Abdelsamad AA, Zakaria G, Omarah MM. Minimal vs median sternotomy for aortic valve replacement. Asian Cardiovasc Thorac Ann. 2007;15(6): 472-475.

[57] Yap CH, Sposato L, Akowuah E, Theodore S, Dinh DT, Shardey GC, et al. Contemporary results show repeat coronary artery bypass grafting remains a risk factor for operative mortality. Ann Thorac Surg. 2009;87(5):1386-1391.

[58] Yau TM, Borger MA, Weisel RD, Ivanov J. The changing pattern of reoperative coronary surgery: trends in 1230 consecutive reoperations. J Thorac Cardiovasc Surg. 2000;120(1):156-163.

[59] Cosgrove DM 3rd, Sabik JF, Navia JL. Minimally invasive valve operations. Ann Thorac Surg. 1998;65(6):1535-1538.

[60] Tam RK, Almeida AA. Minimally invasive aortic valve replacement via partial sternotomy. Ann Thorac Surg. 1998;65(1):275-276.

[61] Mächler HE, Bergmann P, Anelli-Monti M, Dacar D, Rehak P, Knez I, et al. Minimally invasive versus conventional aortic valve operations: a prospective study in 120 patients. Ann Thorac Surg. 1999;67(4):1001-1005.

[62] Candaele S, Herijgers P, Demeyere R, Flameng W, Evers G. Chest pain after partial upper versus complete sternotomy for aortic valve surgery. Acta Cardiol. 2003;58(1): 17-21.

[63] Liu J, Sidiropoulos A, Konertz W. Minimally invasive aortic valve replacement (AVR) compared to standard AVR. Eur J Cardiothorac Surg. 1999;16 Suppl 2:S80-83.

[64] Grossi EA, Galloway AC, Ribakove GH, Zakow PK, Derivaux CC, Baumann FG,et al. Impact of minimally invasive valvular heart surgery: a case control study. Ann Thorac Surg. 2001;71(3):807-810.

[65] Lee JW, Lee SK, Choo SJ, Song H, Song MG. Routine minimally invasive aortic valve procedures. Cardiovasc Surg. 2000;8(6):484-490.

[66] Tabata M, Umakanthan R, Cohn LH, Bolman RM 3rd, Shekar PS, Chen FY, et al. Early and late outcomes of 1000 minimally invasive aortic valve operations. Eur J Cardiothorac Surg. 2008;33(4):537-541.

[67] de Vaumas C, Philip I, Daccache G, Depoix JP, Lecharny JB, Enguerand D, et al. Comparison of minithoracotomy and conventional sternotomy approaches for valve surgery. J Cardiothorac Vasc Anesth. 2003;17(3):325-328.

[68] Cribier A, Eltchaninoff H, Bash A, Borenstein N, Tron C, Bauer F, et al. Percutaneous transcatheter implantation of an aortic valve prosthesis for calcific aortic stenosis: first human case description. Circulation. 2002;106(24):3006-3008.

[69] Charlson E, Legedza AT, Hamel MB. Decision-making and outcomes in severe symptomatic aortic stenosis. J Heart Valve Dis. 2006;15(3):312-321.

[70] Pellikka PA, Sarano ME, Nishimura RA, Malouf JF, Bailey KR, Scott CG, et al. Outcome of 622 adults with asymptomatic, hemodynamically significant aortic stenosis during prolonged follow-up. Circulation. 2005;111(24):3290-3295.

[71] Holmes DR Jr, Mack MJ. Transcatheter valve therapy a professional society overview from the American college of cardiology foundation and the society of thoracic surgeons. J Am Coll Cardiol. 2011;58(4):445-455.

[72] Cox JL, Ad N, Myers K, Gharib M, Quijano RC. Tubular heart valves: a new tissue prosthesis design- preclinical evaluation of the 3F aortic bioprosthesis. J Thorac Cardiovasc Surg. 2005;130(2):520-527.

[73] Pillai R, Ratnatunga C, Soon JL, Kattach H, Khalil A, Jin XY. 3f prosthesis aortic cusp replacement: implantation technique and early results. Asian Cardiovasc Thorac Ann. 2010;18(1):13-16.

[74] Wendt D, Thielmann M, Buck T, Jánosi RA, Bossert T, Pizanis N, et al. First clinical experience and 1-year follow-up with the sutureless 3F-Enable aortic valve prosthesis. Eur J Cardiothorac Surg. 2008;33(4):542-547.

[75] Flameng W, Herregods MC, Hermans H, Van der Mieren G, Vercalsteren M, Poortmans G, et al. Effect of sutureless implantation of the Perceval S aortic valve bioprosthesis on intraoperative and early postoperative outcomes. J Thorac Cardiovasc Surg. 2011;142(6):1453-1457.

[76] Shrestha M, Folliguet T, Meuris B, Dibie A, Bara C, Herregods MC, et al. Sutureless Perceval S aortic valve replacement: a multicenter, prospective pilot trial. J Heart Valve Dis. 2009;18(6):698-702.

[77] Aymard T, Kadner A, Walpoth N, Göber V, Englberger L, Stalder M, et al. Clinical experience with the second-generation 3f Enable sutureless aortic valve prosthesis. J Thorac Cardiovasc Surg. 2010;140(2):313-316.

Chapter 16

Indications for Transcatheter Aortic Valve Implantation

Ibrahim Akin, Stephan Kische, Henrik Schneider,
Tim C. Rehders, Christoph A. Nienaber and
Hüseyin Ince

Additional information is available at the end of the chapter

http://dx.doi.org/10.5772/53437

1. Introduction

Rising life expectancy results in an increase of degenerative and neoplastic diseases. Population-based observational studies report that 1% to 2% of patients older than 65 years have moderate-to-severe aortic stenosis (AS) [1]. Surgical aortic valve replacement (AVR) dates back to 1960 and is currently the only treatment option for severe AS that has been shown to improve survival, regardless of age [2]. In the ideal candidate, surgical AVR has an estimated operative mortality of 4% [2]. Unfortunately, up to one-third of patients with severe AS are ineligible for corrective valve surgery, either because of advanced age or the presence of multiple comorbidities [3]. Current treatment options for those patients not offered surgery include medical treatment or percutaneous balloon aortic valvuloplasty, although neither has been shown to reduce mortality. Medically treated patients with symptomatic AS have 1- and 5-year survival of 60% and 32%, respectively [4,5]. With the introduction of percutaneous aortic valve implantation in 2002, there seems to be an alternative for these patients.

2. Selection of patient

Due to the existence of tried and tested surgical AVR with good long-term results, the selection of patients for transcatheter aortic valve implantation (TAVI), which should done in a multidisciplinary consultation between cardiologists, surgeons, imaging specialists, and anesthesiologists, involves several critical steps [6]. Candidates considered for TAVI must have severe symptomatic AS in addition to a formal contraindication to surgery or other characteristics that would limit their surgical candidacy because of excessive mortality or morbidity (Figure 2). The procedure should be offered to patients who have a potential for functional improvement after valve replacement. It is not recommended for patients who simply refuse surgery on the basis of personal preference.

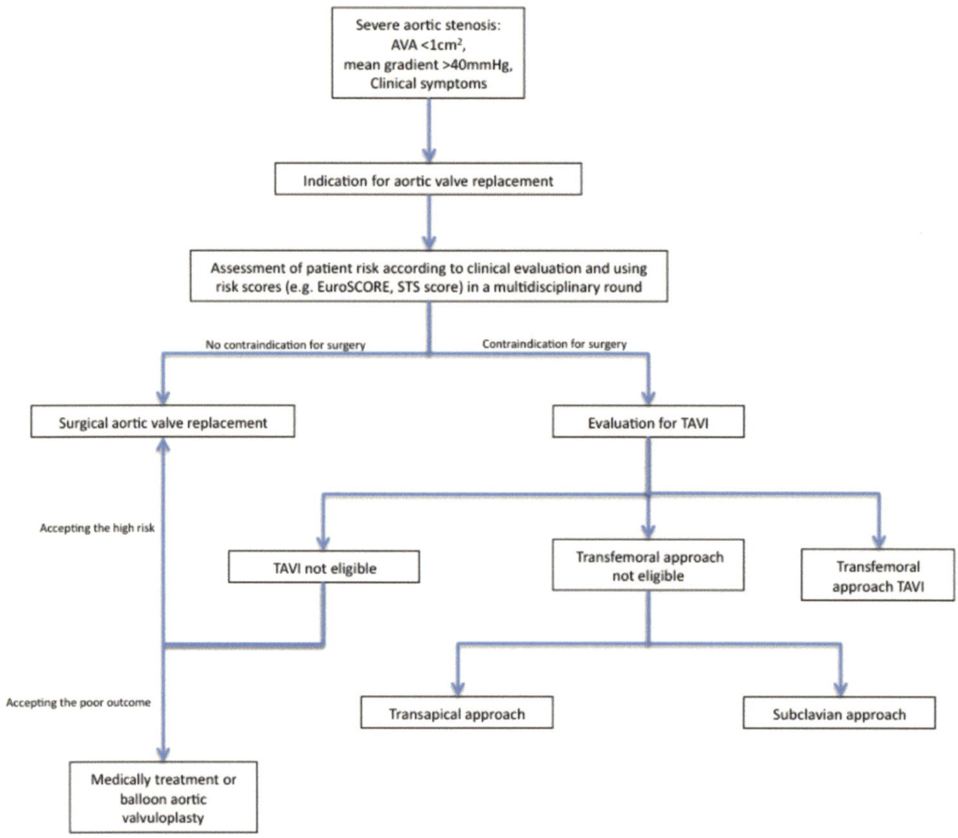

Figure 1. Algorithm to determine the treatment options of patients with severe AS (AVA: aortic valve area; TAVI: transcatheter aortic valve implantation)

3. Confirming the severity of aortic stenosis

Actually, TAVI is indicated only for patients with calcified pure or predominant symptomatic AS. The different imaging modalities can assist in the selection process by providing important information on the aortic valve, coronary arteries, and vascular structures. First,

http://dx.doi.org/10.5772/53437

the severity of AS should be assessed. Both transthoracic (TTE) and transesophageal (TEE) Doppler echocardiography are the preferred tools (Figure 2).

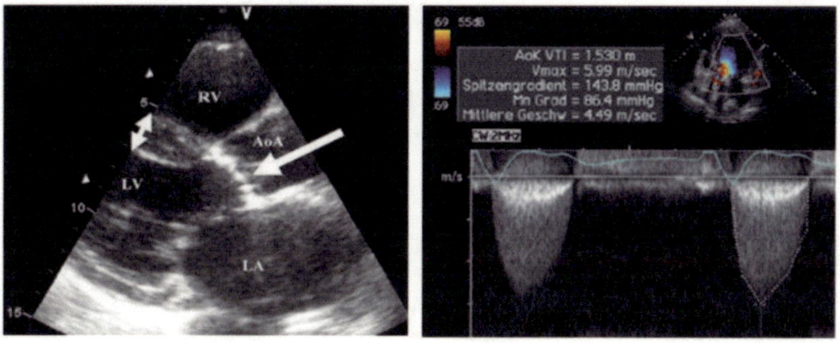

Figure 2. TTE in the assessment of severe AS

In addition, the exact anatomy of the aortic valve should be assessed. Echocardiography, multislice CT (MSCT), and magnetic resonance imaging (MRI) can all help to distinguish between a bicuspid and a tricuspid aortic valve. It is important to point out that implantation of available percutaneous prostheses is contraindicated in the case of a bicuspid aortic valve, because of the risk of incomplete deployment, significant paravalvular regurgitation, and displacement of the prosthesis [6,7] (Figure 3).

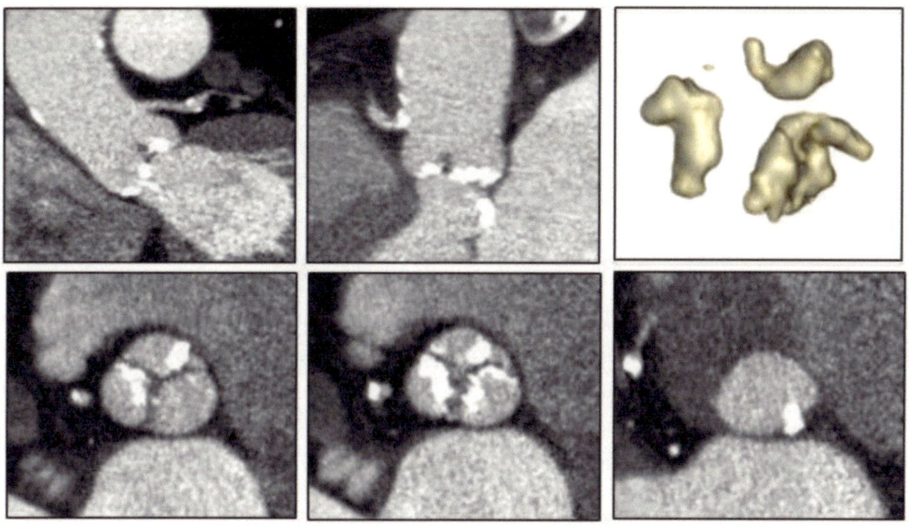

Figure 3. ECG-gated CT-scan in a patient with severe aortic valve stenosis (the upper right panel shows the isolated calcification of the tricuspid aortic valve)

A severely calcified aortic valve may result in the inability to cross the native valve with the catheter. Bulky leaflets and calcifications on the free edge of the leaflets may increase the risk of occlusion of the coronary ostia during aortic valve implantation. Therefore, the extent and exact location of calcifications should be carefully assessed before the implantation procedure. Assessing coronary anatomy is also important in the selection process. Conventional coronary angiography, which remains the "gold standard", should be done to exclude the presence of significant coronary artery disease (Figure 4).

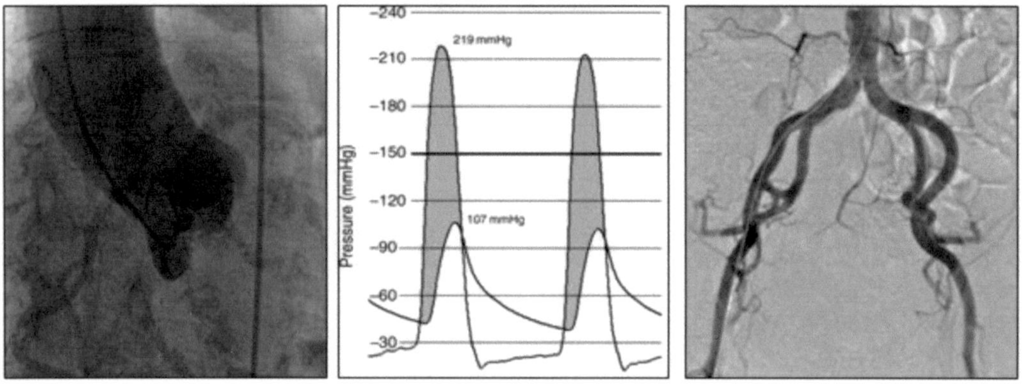

Figure 4. Invasive diagnostic prior TAVI, including aortography and access vessels as well as transvalvular gradient

4. Analysis of surgical risk and evaluation of life expectancy and quality of life

The precise evaluation of surgical risk in a specific patient is not easy and involves an attempt at individualization based on statistical data from databases containing a large number of procedures. The most accepted and validated algorithms that are widely available today are the EuroSCORE, the STS (Society of Thoracic Score) score,and the Parsonnet score. These algorithms predict the surgical risk by assigning weight to various factors that affect the clinical result, but it is clear that they can underestimate or overestimate the risk in certain groups of patients who are not represented satisfactorily in the population used to generate the algorithm [8]. There is some evidence in the literature of the incorrect prediction of aortic AVR outcome using the EuroSCORE model [9]. The key element for establishing whether patients are at high risk for surgery is multidisciplinary clinical judgment, which should be used in association with a more quantitative assessment, based on the combination of several scores (for example, expected mortality >20% with the EuroSCORE and >10% with STS score). This approach allows the team to take into account risk factors that are not covered in scores but often seen in practice, such as chest radiation, previous aortocoronary bypass with patent grafts, porcelain aorta, liver cirrhosis.

http://dx.doi.org/10.5772/53437

5. Assessment of feasibility and exclusion of contraindications for TAVI

After criteria of severe symptomatic aortic valve stenosis and high surgical risk are evaluated, the technical evaluation of the patient's suitability for the percutaneous implantation technique begins (Table 1).

Indication for Transcatheter aortic valve implantation
Severe aortic stenosis (AVA: <1cm^2,mean gradient "/>40mmHg, severe symptoms)
Contraindication for surgical valve replacement
Contraindication for Transcatheter aortic valve implantation
Mild to moderate aortic stenosis
Asymptomatic patients
Life expectancy <1 year
Surgical aortic valve replacement possible, but patient refused
Aortic anulus <18 or "/>25mm (balloon-expandable) and <20 or "/>27mm (self-expandable)
Bicuspid aortic valve
Asymetric heavy valvular calcification
Aortic root "/>45mm at the aortotubular junction
Presence of left ventricular apical thrombus
Contraindication for transfemoral approach
Severe calcification, tortuosity, small diameter of the iliac arteries
Previous aortofemoral bypass
Severe angulation, severe atheroma of the aorta
Coarctation of the aorta
Aneurysm of the aorta with protruding mural thrombus
Contraindication for transapical approach
Previous surgery of the left ventricle using a patch
Calcified pericardium
Severe respiratory insufficiency
Non-reachable left ventricular apex

Table 1. Actually proposed indications and contraindications for TAVI

The two most basic parameters are the suitability of the peripheral arteries and the size of the aortic valve annulus. Contrast angiography is needed to assess the former, while the latter requires an initial assessment of the diameter of the aortic annulus on a TTE. In general terms, a large artery with dominant elastic elements should have a diameter up to 1 mm smaller than the external diameter of the sheath that has to be introduced for the valve implantation. Thus, current systems with an external sheath diameter of 28 F (SAPIEN 26 mm, Edwards Lifescience LLC, Irvine, CA), 25 F (SAPIEN 23 mm, Edwards) and 22 F (CoreValve, Medtronic, Inc., Minneapolis, MN) require minimum diameters of 8, 7, and 6 mm, respectively. Apart from the minimum diameter, the existence of significant vessel tortuosity (>90°), especially when combined with wall calcifications, makes advancing the large sheath problematic, with a high risk of vascular complications that could potentially affect the final outcome. In addition, the existence of extensive circumferential calcifications limits the elastic dilation of the artery; thus, the minimum diameters referred to above are underestimated. Patients who do not meet the criteria of suitable peripheral arterial access may still be candidates for transapical implantation. For the assessment of aortic annulus diameter, we should keep in mind that TTE underestimates its size by a mean of 1.4 mm compared with TEE [6,10], while the latter method also underestimates the size by 1.2 mm compared with intraoperative measurement [10]. Therefore, in order to avoid undesirable and often catastrophic displacement of the prosthesis, there should be a margin of at least 1-2 mm between the diameter of the valve and the size of the aortic annulus estimated using TEE, so that the former may be successfully and safely anchored within the latter. Computed tomography scan aortography and angiography of the ascending aorta are the most appropriate examinations for investigating these aspects. Those examinations will also be used for the measurement of the dimensions of the ascending aorta and the aortic arch, which are essential for checking eligibility for the CoreValve (the most important being the diameter of the ascending aorta, which should be <4.3 cm) (Figure 5).

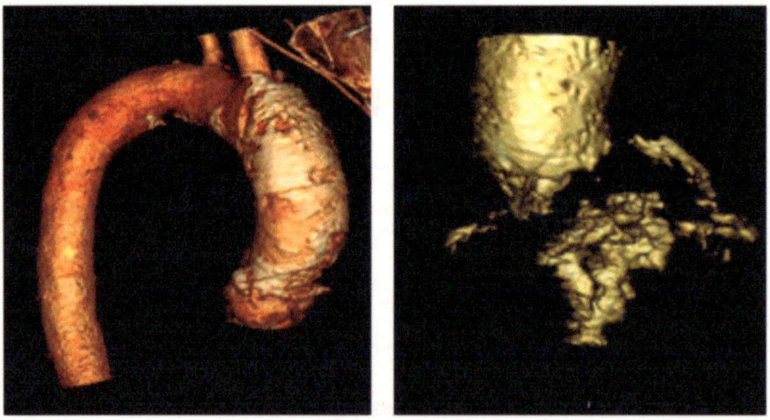

Figure 5. ECG-gated CT-scan of a patient with severe aortic valve stenosis and porcelain aorta after radiation exposure

The anatomy of the thoracic aorta (any chance of porcelain aorta) and the abdominal aorta should be studied by some imaging method for the existence of extensive atheromatosis, mural thrombi and aneurysm (Figure 6).

http://dx.doi.org/10.5772/53437

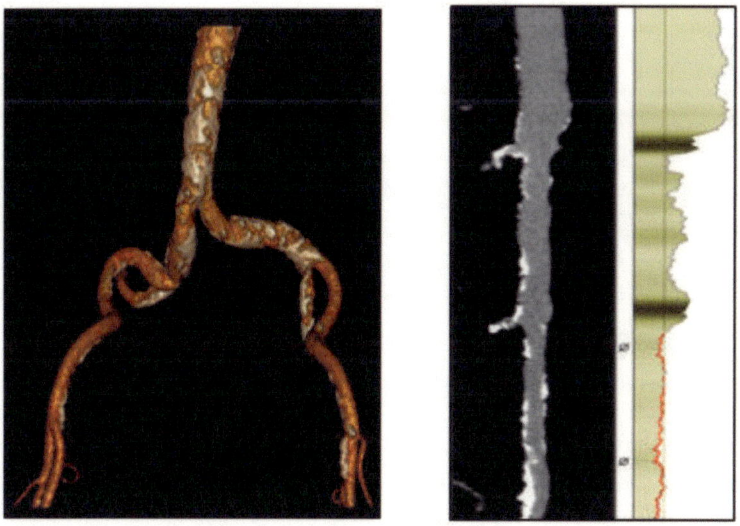

Figure 6. Three-dimensional reconstruction of contrast-enhanced CT angiography to assess morphology of femoral arteries (left) and centerline stretched view (right)

6. Different transcatheter aortic valves

On the basis of first results from clinical trials, CoreValve Revalving System and Edwards Lifescience SAPIEN obtained CE mark approval in 2007 with the specification that these valves are intended for patients with a high or prohibitive risk for surgical valve replacement or who cannot undergo AVR. The first generation balloon-expandable valve was entitled Cribier-Edwards valve (Edwards Lifesciences), whereas at present the Edwards SAPIEN valve (Edwards) is commercially available (Figure 7). The Edwards Lifesciences SAPIEN THV device is a balloon-expandable valve. It consists of bovine pericardium that is firmly mounted within a tubular, slotted, stainless steel balloon-expandable stent. Two valve sizes have been developed (23mm and 26mm). At present, available prosthesis sizes are 23 and 26 mm for aortic annulus diameters between 18–22 mm and 21–25 mm, respectively. The CoreValve Revalving device is a self-expanding frame-valve prosthesis (Figure 7). It consists of a porcine pericardial tissue valve that is mounted and sutured in a multilevel self-expanding nitinol frame. It is available in 26, 29 and 31 mm sizes. The device has a broader upper segment (outflow aspect), which yields proper orientation to the blood flow. The first-generation valve used bovine pericardial tissue and was constrained within a 25 French (F) delivery catheter. The second-generation valve was built with porcine pericardial tissue within a 21 F catheter to allow access through smaller-diameter vascular beds. The third-generation of the device features a catheter with a valve delivery sheath size of 18 F and a follow-on shaft of 12 F.

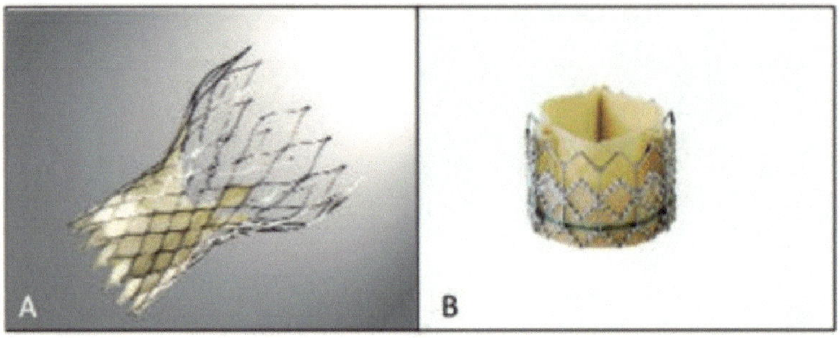

Figure 7. Profile of the CoreValve Revaving System (A) and Edwards SAPIEN Transcatheter Heart Valve (B)

Newer devices that have first-in-man application include Paniagua (Endoluminal Technology Research, Miami, FL), Enable (ATS, Minneapolis, MN), AoTx (Hansen Medical, Mountain View, CA), Perceval (Sorin Group, Arvada, CO), Jena (JenaValve Technology, Wilmington, DE), Lotus Valve (Sadra Medical, Campbell, CA), and Direct Flow percutaneous aortic valve (Direct Flow Medical, Inc., Santa Rosa, CA). TAVI represents a unique challenge for anesthesiologists. As with other invasive procedures, a careful preoperative assessment, appropriate intraoperative monitoring and imaging, meticulous management of hemodynamics, and early treatment of expected side effects and complications is of utmost importance. An unexpected decrease or increase in systemic vascular resistance resulting in decreased coronary perfusion pressure or acute heart failure by elevated left ventricular end-diastolic pressure should be avoided by maintaining a normotensive blood pressure and heart rate between 60 bpm and 100 bpm. The choice of anesthetic technique, either local anesthesia with mild sedation promoting spontaneous respiration, deep intravenous sedation with insertion of a laryngeal mask, or general anesthesia, varies among centers and is probably not associated with a significant difference in outcome. Post valvuloplasty and implantation, which were done under rapid right ventricular pacing due to reduce left ventricular ejection and cardiac motion, may require some additional inotropic support. Tracheal extubation can usually be done at the end of the procedure. Close postoperative monitoring is necessary, and admission to an intensive care unit is required. However, at present a retrograde approach through the femoral artery is used. During the procedure, a balloon valvuloplasty is first done to facilitate passage of the native aortic valve. During rapid right ventricular pacing, the prosthesis is positioned and deployed under fluoroscopy and echocardiographic guidance. Alternatively, in patients with difficult vascular access because of extensive calcifications or tortuosity of the femoral artery or aorta, a transapical approach can be used. After a partial thoracotomy, direct puncture of the apical portion of the left ventricular free wall is done to gain catheter access to the left ventricle and aortic valve. The prosthesis is subsequently positioned and deployed, similar to the antegrade approach.

http://dx.doi.org/10.5772/53437

7. Implantation approaches

With regard to the delivery systems and their introduction into ascending aorta, two specific pathways have been explored so far: the antegrade pathway, which uses direct transapical access, and the retrograde pathway, which uses either transfemoral or trans-subclavian or trans-axillary access [11].

7.1. The transapical approach

The main advantages of using transapical procedures are: [1] the feasibility does not rely on the absence of a concomitant peripheral vascular disease or previous aortic surgery; [2] the delivery system seems to be more "steady" and the procedure itself more "straightforward"; and [3] this access potentially reduces the risk of calcium dislodgement due to the passage of a stiff transfemoral device into a diseased aortic arch. A transapical approach can be used in the operating room, in a hybrid room, or in a catheterization laboratory with a patient under general anesthesia. Regardless of where the transapical approach is done, it is a prerequisite that high-quality fluoroscopic imaging must be guaranteed. Apical bleeding is very rare, mostly related to patient tissue fragility or to the team learning curve, and represents the most dangerous complication related to transapical access itself. In transapical TAVI, the cardiac apex is prepared through a small left anterolateral mini-thoracotomy using a purse-string or a crossing suture reinforced by pledgets and, after the procedure, a chest tube is routinely inserted into the left pleura with pain releasers injected in the intercostal tissue (Figure 8).

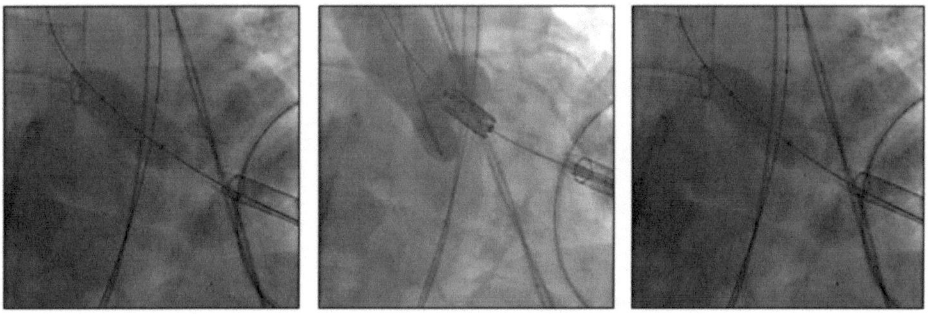

Figure 8. TAVI using the transapical approach

7.2. The transfemoral approach

The transfemoral approach is used mostly in cardiac catheterization laboratory or a hybrid room. One of the main advantages of this technique is that it allows fully percutaneous implantation in conscious patients, as long as the peripheral vessels are of an adequate caliber (more than 6mm diameter), there are no very tortuous vessels, and vascular closure devices are available (Figure 9). Alternatively, the standard technique requires surgical preparation of the common femoral artery under local or general anesthesia. Major and minor postoperative vascular complications have been reported quite often in recent series [12,13] and some critical events (vessel dissections, ruptures or avulsions) might be catastrophic when not promptly and adequately treated.

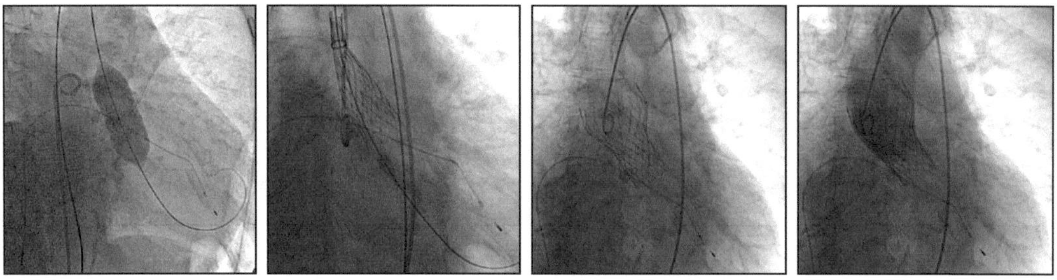

Figure 9. TAVI using the transfemoral approach

7.3. The trans-subclavian approach

Trans-subclavian access is an alternative retrograde pathway that has been recently explored. It requires a surgical exposure of the left subclavian artery and an adequate minimal vessel inner diameter for 18F delivery systems (Figure 10). There are some advantages in using this approach: firstly, the distance between the site of introduction and the aortic valve is short, compared with the transfemoral option, and it results in a steadier pathway. Secondly, as long as the subclavian artery is intact, the trans-subclavian procedure can be done in case of a concomitant vascular disease involving the abdominal aorta or the legs, and it does not require a thoracotomy. Unfortunately, the presence of a patent internal mammary artery, such as a diseased subclavian artery, in redo coronary surgery contraindicates this approach. However, at this moment, this interesting approach remains "off-label" and is not yet formally recommended by the industry.

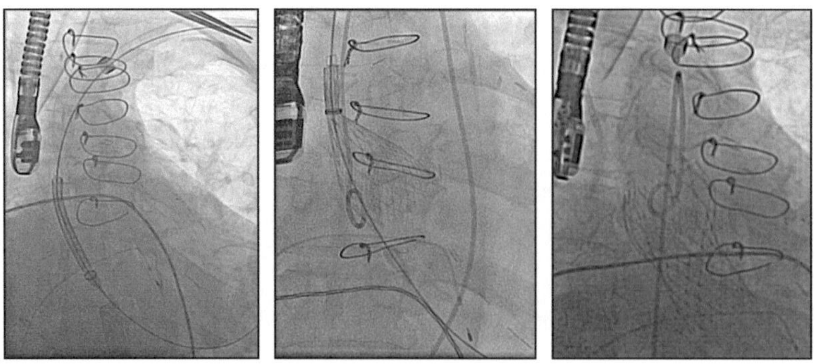

Figure 10. TAVI using the subclavian approach

7.4. The trans-aortic approach

In case of severe vascular disease and a concomitant contraindication to transapical procedures, an alternative, interesting, retrograde approach has been proposed: through an upper "J-shape" mini-sternotomy, the guidewire and the delivery system are inserted, retrogradely, into the ascending aorta and are secured with a double-string suture. TAVI is then done as a transfemoral procedure. The presence of "porcelain" aorta and the risk of postoperative massive bleeding limit this approach to selected patients.

8. Results from the literature

8.1. Cribrier-Edwards valve

Cribier *et al.* did the first human implantation in 2002 [14]. The Edwards SAPIEN valve was approved for use in the European Union in November 2007 (for the transfemoral approach) and in January 2008 (for transapical delivery). In the Initial Registry of EndoVascular Implantation of Valves in Europe (I-REVIVE) trial, followed by the Registry of Endovascular Critical Aortic Stenosis Treatment (RECAST) trial, a total of 36 patients (mean (SD) EuroSCORE 12 (2)) were included [15]. Twenty-seven patients underwent successful percutaneous aortic valve implantation (23 antegrade, 4 retrograde). The 30-day mortality was 22% (6 of 27 patients), and the mean AVA increased from 0.60 ± 0.11cm2 to 1.70 ± 0.10cm2 (p<0.001). Importantly, this improvement in AVA was maintained up to 24 months follow-up [16]. Since these first trials, the Cribrier-Edwards prosthesis and the Edwards SAPIEN prosthesis have been used in numerous studies. Overall, acute procedural success is achieved in 75–100% of the procedures, and 30-day mortality ranges between 8–50% in the published studies. Using the transapical technique and the Sapien valve, Walther et al. [17] has reported their initial multicenter results of 59 consecutive patients, which is the largest feasibility study published thus far. Procedural success using the transapical technique was achieved in 53 patients. Thirty-day mortality was 13.6% and none of these were thought to be valve related as there was good valve function at autopsy. The overall procedural success of 1038 SAPIEN implants from 32 centers within the European SOURCE registry was 93.8%. The 30-day survival within SOURCE was 93.7% (transfemoral) and 89.7% (transapical) [18]. The 1-year survival of the cohort was 81.1% (transfemoral) and 72.1% (transapical), respectively. In cohort B of the PARTNER randomized trial, 179 patients receiving transfemoral SAPIEN aortic valve with 179 patients receiving standard medical therapy (including balloon aortic valvuloplasty), confirmed the superiority of transfemoral TAVI with regard to overall survival and cardiac functional status [19]. The Kaplan-Meier 1-year mortality from any cause was 30.7% (TAVI) versus 50.7% (standard medical therapy), corresponding to a 0.55 hazard ratio with TAVI (p<0.001). The fraction of surviving patients at 1-year, in New York Heart Association functional class III-IV, was lower in the TAVI group (25.2% versus 58%; p<0.001). Nevertheless, the TAVI group had a higher 30-day incidence of major stroke (5.0% versus 1.1%; p=0.06) and major vascular complications (16.2% versus 1.1%; p<0.001). Early and 1-year outcomes from the REVIVAL trial, which consisted of 55 patients with a mean AVA of 0.57±0.14cm2 and a mean logistic EuroSCORE of 33.5±17%, have been reported [20]. TAVI was successful in 87%. Mean echocardiographic AVA improved from 0.56±14 to 1.6±0.48cm2 after the procedure (p<0.0001). Thirty-day all-cause mortality and major adverse cardiac events (MACE) were 7.3% and 20%, respectively. These rates increased to 23.6% and 32.7%, respectively, at 1 year, with most late events related to underlying comorbidities. The mean NYHA functional class improved from 3.22±0.66 at baseline to 1.50±0.85 at 1-year follow-up (p<0.001).

8.2. CoreValve ReValving

Since the first implantation of the CoreValve prosthesis in a patient in 2005 [12], a large number of patients have been treated with this device. The feasibility and safety of this valve was studied in a prospective, multicenter trial [12]. A total of 25 symptomatic patients with an AVA < 1cm^2 were enrolled in the study. The device was successfully implanted using the retrograde technique in 22 of 25 patients. Procedural success and aortic mean pressure gradients were markedly improved immediately following implantations with pre-procedure gradients 44.24 ± 10.79 mmHg to 12.38 ± 3.03 mmHg post-procedure, and were about the same at 30-day follow-up (11.82 ± 3.42 mm Hg). NYHA functional class improved by 1 to 2 grades in all patients. MACE, defined as death from any cause, major arrhythmia, myocardial infarction, cardiac tamponade, stroke, urgent or emergent conversion to surgery or balloon valvuloplasty, emergent percutaneous coronary intervention, cardiogenic shock, endocarditis, or aortic dissection, occurred in 8 of the 25 hospitalized patients. Recently, Grube *et al.* [21] reported the results with the three different generations of the CoreValve Revalving system in a non-randomized, prospective study of 136 patients. Ten patients were treated with first-generation devices, 24 patients with second-generation, and 102 patients with third-generation devices. At baseline, mean AVA was 0.67cm^2 and mean logistic EuroSCORE was 23.1% in the overall study population. With the new-generation devices, the overall procedural success rate significantly increased from 70.0% and 70.8% to 91.2% for the first-, second-, and third-generation prostheses, respectively (p = 0.003). Interestingly, using newer devices, periprocedural mortality decreased from 10% (first-generation) to 8.3% (second-generation) to 0% (third-generation). Overall 30-day mortality for the three generations was 40%, 8.3% and 10.8%, respectively. Pooled data demonstrated a significant improvement in mean NYHA functional class (from 3.3 to 1.7, p<0.001), without a difference between the three generations. Importantly, NYHA functional class and mean pressure gradient remained stable up to 12 months follow-up in all three generations. In addition, the results of a multicenter registry with the third-generation CoreValve Revalving system have recently been reported [22]. A total of 646 patients from 51 centers were included in the registry. It was a high-risk elderly population (mean age: 81 years) with a poor functional class (85% of the patients in NYHA class III or IV), and a high logistic EuroSCORE (mean: 23.1%). Procedural success was achieved in 628 of the 646 patients (97.2%). All-cause 30-day mortality was 8%, and the combined end point of procedural related death, stroke, or myocardial infarction was reached in 60 patients (9.3%). After successful implantation, mean pressure gradient decreased from 49 mmHg to 3 mmHg [22]. The FRANCE real-world registry of 244 consecutive high-risk patients with symptomatic severe AS, enrolled from 16 centers over a period of 5 months in 2009, reported 98.3% procedural success for both Edwars SAPIEN and Medtronic CoreValve (66% transfemoral, 5% subclavian, and 29% transapical) prostheses [13]. The 30-day mortality was 12.7%, and, at 1 month, 88% of patients were in NYHA class I-II. Buellesfeld *et al.* [23] reported on a 2-year follow-up of 126 patients who underwent TA-VI. Thirty-day all-cause mortality was 15.2%. At 2-years, all-cause mortality was 38.1%, with a significant difference between the moderate-risk group and the combined high-risk groups (27.8% versus 45.8%; p=0.04). This difference was attributable to an increased risk of noncardiac mortality in high-risk groups. Hemodynamic results remained unchanged during follow-up (mean gradient: 8.5±2.5mmHg at 30 days and 9.0±3.5mmHg at 2 years) without any incidence of structural valve deterioration.

The larger CoreValve prostheses (26, 29 and 31 mm) were the only device for annulus between 26 and 29 mm, before the currently available 29-mm SAPIEN XT valve for transapical implantation. The CoreValve prosthesis had previously been the only device suitable for transarterial implant in patients with limited iliofemoral artery access, but this has changed with the SAPIEN NovaFlex delivery system. The growing experience with the subclavian artery approach, however, allows the CoreValve prosthesis to be implanted in patients with unusable iliofemoral arteries. Because of these results, the indications for TAVI expanded (e.g. in patients with porcelain aorta, with previous cardiac surgery, etc.) [24] (Figure 11,12).

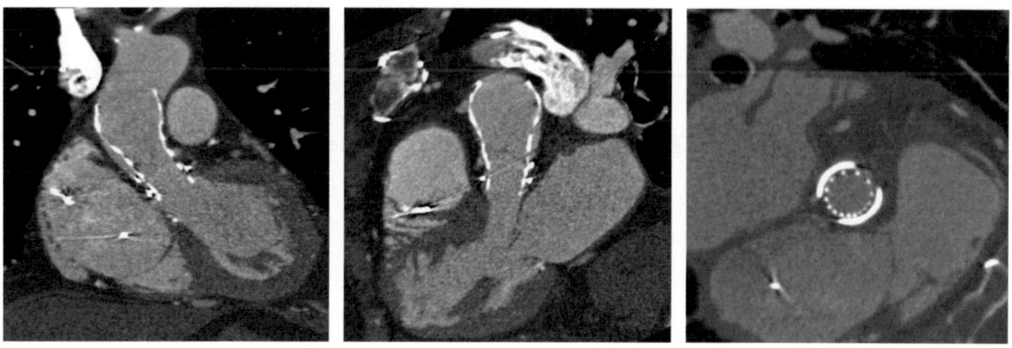

Figure 11. TAVI in a patient with a history of AVR

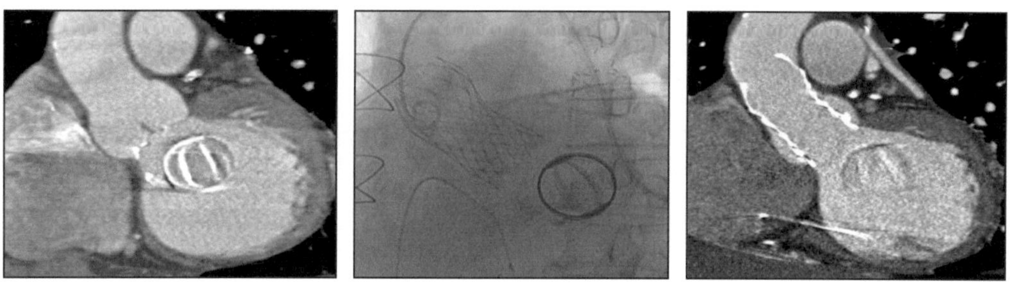

Figure 12. TAVI in a patient with a history of mitral valve replacement

9. Conclusion

Transcatheter aortic valve implantation was developed to provide an alternative and less invasive method of treating aortic valve stenosis. Actually, it has been proved that the method is feasible, with results that have been reproduced by many physicians in many centers (approximately 10,000 implantations to date). Today there are at least 10 new transcatheter aortic valves that have had their first implantation in humans, many more that have reached the level of animal experiments, and even more that are still in the initial design stage. As a new treatment tool, it has to be evaluated in randomized controlled trials with long-term follow-up in order to assess safety and efficacy. Therefore, TAVI should be restricted to a limited number of high-volume centers, that have both cardiology and cardiac surgery departments as well as expertise in structural heart disease intervention and high-risk valvular surgery. Because of excellent results with surgical valve replacement, patient selection, which should be done in multidisciplinary conferences, is of utmost importance. Like other interventional procedures, there is a learning curve with significant improvements in the success rate and the clinical results after the first 25 procedures, which implies that the TAVI procedure should initially be done by and thereafter supervised by a special team [25,26]. In addition to patient selection and intervention of TAVI, a close follow-up with assessment of clinical and objective parameters is mandatory for defining the indications of this technique.

Author details

Ibrahim Akin, Stephan Kische, Henrik Schneider, Tim C. Rehders,
Christoph A. Nienaber and Hüseyin Ince

University of Rostock, Germany

References

[1] Nkomo VT, Gardin JM, Skelton TN, et al. Burden of valvular heart disease: a population-based study. Lancet 2006;368(9540): 1005-11.

[2] Kvidal P, Bergstrom R, Horte LG, et al. Observed and relative survival after aortic valve replacement. J Am Coll Cardiol 2000;35(3): 747-56.

[3] Iung B, Cachier A, Baron G, et al. Decision-making in elderly patients with severe aortic stenosis: why are so many denied surgery. Eur Heart J 2005;26(24): 2714-20.

[4] Varadarajan P, Kapoor N, Bansal RC, et al. Clinical profile and natural history of 453 nonsurgical managed patients with severe aortic stenosis. Ann Thorac Surg 2006;82(6): 2111-5.

[5] Ross J Jr, Braunwald E. Aortic stenosis. Circulation 1965;38(2): V61-7.

[6] Vahanian A, Alfieri O, Al-Attar N, et al. Transcatheter valve implantation for patients with aortic stenosis: a position statement from the European Association of Cardio-Thoracic Surgery (EACTS) and the European Society of Cardiology (ESC), in collaboration with the European Association of Percutaneous Cardiovascular Interventions (EAPCI). Eur Heart J 2008;29(11): 1463-70.

[7] Zegdi R, Ciobotaru V, Noghin M, et al. Is it reasonable to treat all calcified stenotic aortic valves with a valved stent? Results from a human anatomic study in adults. J Am Coll Cardiol 2008;51(5): 579-84.

[8] Roques F, Nashef SA, Michel P, et al. Risk factors for early mortality after valve surgery in Europe in the 1990's: lesson from the EuroSCORE pilot program. J Heart Valve Dis 2001;10(5): 572-8.

[9] Grossi EA, Schwartz CF, Yu PJ, et al. High-risk aortic valve replacement: are the outcomes as bad as predicted. Ann Thorac Surg 2008; 85(1): 102-6.

[10] Babaliaros VC, Liff D, Chen EP, et al. Can balloon aortic valvuloplasty help determine appropriate transcatheter aortic valve size. JACC Intv 2008;1(5): 580-6.

[11] De Robertis F, Asgar A, Davies S, et al. The left exillary arter-a new approach for transcatheter aortic valve implantation. Eur J Cardiothorac Surg 2009;36(5):807-12.

[12] Grube E, Laborde JC, Gerckens U, et al. Percutaneous implantation of the CoreValve self-expanding valve prosthesis in high-risk patients with aortic valve disease: Siegburg first-in-man study, Circulation 2006;114(15): 1616-24.

[13] Eltchaninoff H, Prat A, Gilard M, et al. Transcatheter aortic valve implantation: early results of the France (French Aortic National CoreValve and Edwards) registry. Eur Heart J 2011; 32(2): 191-7.

[14] Cribrier A, Eltchaninoff H, Bash A, et al. Percutaneous transcatheter implantation of an aortic valve prosthesis for calcific aortic stenosis: first human case description. Circulation 2002;106(24): 3006-8.

[15] Cribrier A, Elchaninoff H, Tron C, et al. Early experience with percutaneous transcatheter implantation of heart valve prosthesis for the treatment of end-stage inoperable patients with calcific aortic stenosis. J Am Coll Cardiol 2004;43(4): 698-703.

[16] Cribrier A, Elchaninoff H, Tron C, et al. Treatment of calcific aortic stenosis with the percutaneous heart valve: mid-term follow-up from the initial feasibility studies: the French experience. J Am Coll Cardiol 2006;47(6): 1214-23.

[17] Walther T, Simon P, Dewey T, et al. Transapical minimally invasive aortic valve implantation: multicenter experience. Circulation 2007;116(Suppl 11): I240-5.

[18] Thomas M, Schymik G, Walther T, et al. Thirty-day results of the SAPIEN aortic Bioprosthesis Outcomes (SOURCE) Registry: A European registry of transcatheter aortic valve implantation using the Edwards SAPIEN valve. Circulation 2010;122(1): 62-9.

[19] Leon MB, Smith CR, Mack M, et al. Transcatheter aortic-valve implantation for aortic stenosis in patients who cannot undergo surgery. N Engl J Med 2010;363(17): 1597-607.

[20] Kodali SK, O'Neill WW, Moses JW, et al. Early and late (one year) outcomes following transcatheter aortic valve implantation in patients with severe aortic stenosis (from the United States REVIVAL Trial). Am J Cardiol 2011;107(7): 1058-64.

[21] Grube E, Buellesfeld L, Mueller R, et al. Progress and current status of percutaneous aortic valve replacement: results of three device generation of the CoreValve Revalving system. Circ Cardiovasc Intervent 2008;1(3): 167-75.

[22] Piazza N, Grube E, Gerckens U, et al. Procedural and 30-day outcomes following transcatheter aortic valve implantation using the third generation (18 Fr) CoreValve revalving system: results from the multicentre, expanded evaluation registry 1-year following CE mark approval. EuroIntervention 2008;4(2): 242-9.

[23] Buellesfeld L, Gerckens U, Schuler G, et al. 2-year follow-up of patients undergoing transcatheter aortic valve implantation using a self-expanding valve prosthesis. J Am Coll Cardiol 2011;57(16): 1650-7.

[24] Wenaweser P, Buellesfeld L, Gerckens U, Grube E. Percutaneous aortic valve replacement for sévère aortic régurgitation in degenerated bioprosthesis : the first valve in valve procédure using Corevlave Revalving system. Catheter Cardiovasc Interv 2007 ;70(5) :760-4.

[25] Walther T, Dewey T, Borger MA, et al. Transapical aortic valve implantation: step by step. Ann Thorac Surg 2009;87(1): 276-83.

[26] Webb JG, Pasupati S, Humphries K, et al. Percutaneous transarterial aortic valve replacement in selected high-risk patients with aortic stenosis. Circulation 2007 ;116(7): 755-63.

Aortic Valve Replacement for Calcified Aortic Valves

Kazumasa Orihashi

Additional information is available at the end of the chapter

http://dx.doi.org/10.5772/53418

1. Introduction

Valve replacement has been the standard treatment for aortic stenosis until the development of transcatheter aortic valve implantation (TAVI). Although TAVI provides a treatment with fairly acceptable outcomes for patients with high surgical risk, aortic valve replacement remains essential even in the TAVI era, because surgical treatment is indicated when TAVI cannot be performed due to a small aortic annulus or inappropriate access route. In addition, surgical treatment may be necessary when complications develop during TAVI procedures. Therefore, a more meticulous procedure is required for surgeons. With an increasing number of elderly patients who need surgical treatment and are at high risk due to aging, comorbidities, or medications such as steroids or antiplatelet drugs, trivial pitfalls during surgery can lead to catastrophic results. Furthermore, many patients with hemodialysis and marked systemic calcification require aortic valve surgery in Japan [1].

Complications encountered during surgery for aortic stenosis can be associated with catastrophic events such as myocardial infarction, cerebral embolism or aortic dissection. This is because a calcified aortic valve rarely exists alone, but is often associated with marked and diffuse calcification in the aorta, coronary arteries, mitral valve or even cerebral vessels [2]. The goal of surgical treatment is to implant a prosthetic valve of adequate size in each individual patient without perivalvular leak, while avoiding undesirable complications such as stroke, cardiac events or bleeding. This chapter is devoted to the tips and pitfalls in aortic valve replacement of calcified aortic valves with a discussion of preoperative and intraoperative strategies to achieve the best possible outcomes.

2. Calcified aortic valve

2.1. Etiologies of calcification

There are three main etiologies of aortic stenosis. The location and extent of calcification in the aortic valve varies depending on its etiology (Fig. 1). In rheumatic valvular disease, there is initial thickening and fusion of the cusps with later involvement of the annulus. The fusion of cusps results in the formation of a valve orifice that looks like a fish mouth. There is also severe mitral valve calcification in patients with combined valvular disease. In arteriosclerotic aortic stenosis, calcification is most prominent in the annulus, sinus of Valsalva and ascending aorta. Calcification of the cusps and calcium deposits on them markedly limit cusp opening. In bicuspid aortic stenosis, disease on the annulus is rather mild but fusion of the commissures reduces the valve orifice area and forms a slit-like orifice. Calcification is often present in bicuspid aortic stenosis, but is rather mild compared with that in arteriosclerotic aortic stenosis.

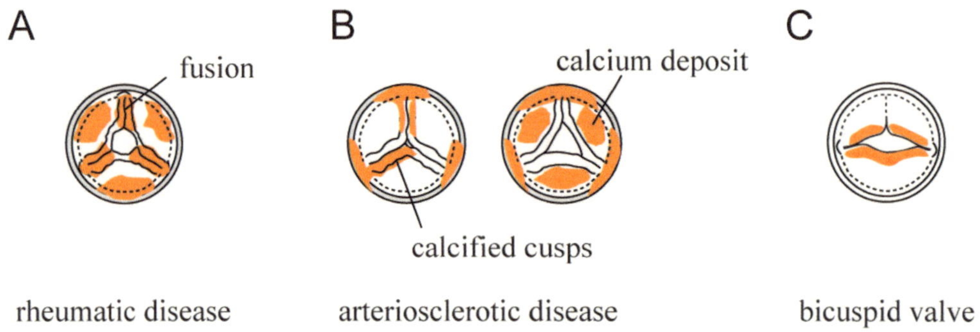

Figure 1. Etiologies of aortic stenosis. A: Rheumatic disease initialy occurs on the cusps and extends toward the annulus. Fusion of the cusps causes a stenotic orifice like a fish mouth. B: Arteriosclerotic disease extends from the aorta toward the cusps. Opening of the cusps is often disturbed by rigidity of the cusps and calcium deposits on them. C: In bicuspid valve, calcification takes place mainly on the cusps.

2.2. Removal of calcium

A calcified aortic valve can be a cause of arterial embolism resulting in stroke or myocardial infarction [3-5]. A mobile mass is occasionally found attached to the calcified portion of the aortic valve. A calcified aortic valve as well as the presence of a mobile mass can be assessed by transthoracic echocardiography. Computed tomography (CT) is suitable for precisely assessing the presence and extent of calcification in the annulus and the entire aorta [6,7]. As the calcified cusps are resected, calcium in the annulus needs to be adequately removed to allow subsequent sutures for valve implantation. Calcium deposits are hard but easily crumble into pieces. They can be crushed by clamps and removed or can be fragmented by a Cavitron Ultrasound Surgical Aspirator (CUSA). Either way, loosened calcium needs to be carefully eliminated to prevent it from entering the left ventricle and causing stroke, or entering the left coronary artery and causing myocardial infarction. Digital palpation for irregularity and

http://dx.doi.org/10.5772/53418

rigidity is helpful for evaluating the adequacy of calcium removal. To minimize the chance of perivalvular leakage following valve implantation, the inner aspect of the annulus should be smooth with the sewing cuff of the prosthetic valve sealing the small gaps between the sutures.

However, excessive removal of calcium may result in perforation of the aortic root or damage of the mitral valve [8]. Fig. 2 summarizes intraoperative transesophageal echocardiography (TEE) assessment and several measurements on the calcified aortic valve [9].

The extent of calcification should be carefully checked in the annulus and the aorta (described later). It is important to measure the dimensions of the annulus and sinotubular junction. When the latter is equal to or smaller than the former, difficult insertion of the prosthesis may be encountered. Although the valve can be narrowly inserted by distorting the bioprosthetic valve or the aorta, calcification in the aorta or sinotubular junction makes the latter difficult.

Acoustic shadow indicates the presence and extent of calcification. Fig. 3 shows three different degrees of calcification in the annulus of the noncoronary cusp. When it is transmural or continues to the anterior mitral leaflet as shown in Fig. 3C, excessive removal of calcium should be avoided and limited to a reasonable depth.

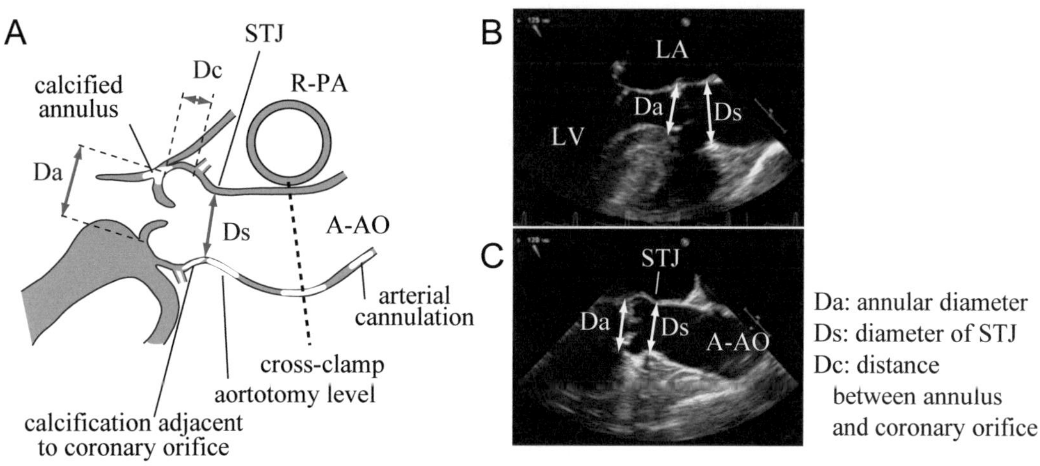

Figure 2. Intraoperative transesophageal echocardiography (TEE) assessment. A: Calcification in the annulus, sinus of Valsalva, and A-AO is assessed. Important measurements are shown. Annular diameter (Da) is usually smaller than the diameter of STJ (Ds) (B). When Ds is equal or smaller than Da (C), difficult insertion of prosthetic valve may be encountered. (modied from reference 9)

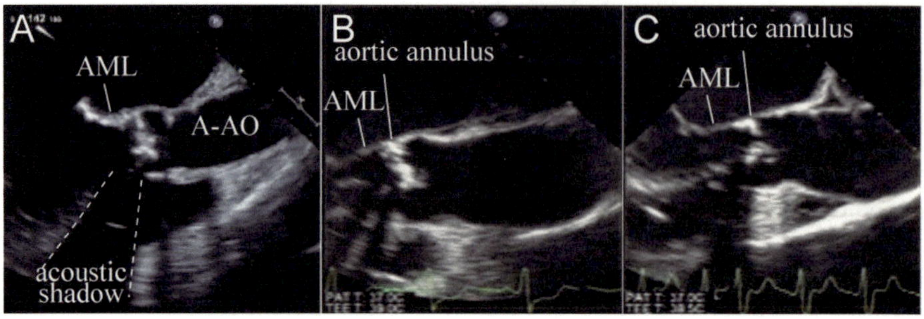

Figure 3. Calcification in the aortic annulus. A: Calcification is present on the cusps, accompanied by acoustic shadow but not in the annulus. B: Calcification in the annulus. C: Calcification extends to the AML.

2.3. Optimizing valve size

A calcified aortic valve limits the size of the prosthetic valve that can be implanted. When the aortic annulus is too small, patient-prosthesis mismatch can arise that may lead to sustained pressure overload of the left ventricle and subsequent chronic heart failure. A bioprosthetic valve is desirable for elderly patients with poor anticoagulation compliance to minimize the risk of cerebral infarction, or in patients that need antiplatelet therapy (patients with stroke or coronary stents); however, there are occasions where only a small-sized mechanical valve can be inserted due to a small aortic annulus [19]. Several solutions are illustrated in Fig. 4.

2.3.1. Annular dilatation

To enlarge the annulus, the aortotomy incision line is extended proximally toward the commissure between the left and non-coronary cusps or toward the noncoronary sinus of Valsalva (Fig. 4A) [11]. However, a markedly calcified annulus and/or sinus of Valsalva makes this procedure difficult or even increases the risk of uncontrollable bleeding at the suture line. Preoperative CT assessment or intraoperative TEE is helpful for making a decision.

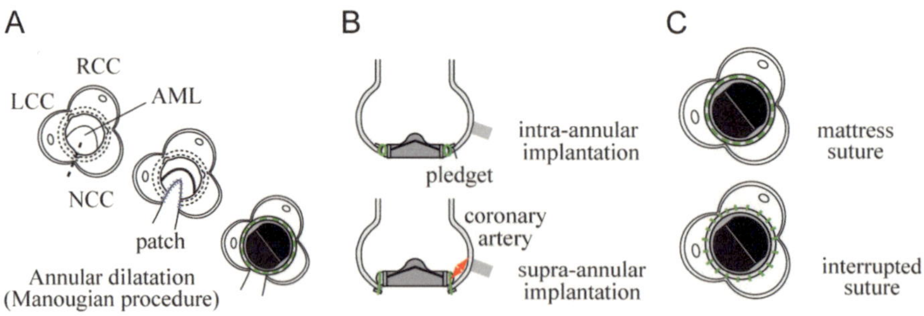

Figure 4. Solutions for small aortic annulus. A: Annular dilation by Manougian procedure. The commissure between LCC and NCC is incised and a patch is placed. B: Supra-annular implant. Care should be taken to avoid an obstruction of coronary artery. C: Interrupted suture. Cutting of annular tissue while tying is a pitfall.

http://dx.doi.org/10.5772/53418

2.3.2. Supra-annular implantation

This allows implantation of a prosthetic valve that is one size larger and is commonly used in many institutes (Fig. 4B). A non-everting suture is placed along the annulus. However, this generates a risk of occlusion of the coronary ostium when it is located at an unusually low level. It can be evaluated by CT, but may be missed by coronary angiography. Intraoperative TEE is helpful for making a decision (Fig. 2A).

2.3.3. Interrupted suture

Although mattress sutures slightly reduce the circumference of the aortic annulus, interrupted sutures allow insertion of a prosthetic valve with the same size as the annulus (Fig. 4C). This slightly increases the number of sutures required. Since appropriate seating of the sewing ring on the annulus cannot be confirmed by the pledget adjacent to the sewing cuff, it needs to be inspected through the valve by manually opening the leaflet. When the annulus is severely calcified, it is important to prevent a gap between the annulus and sewing ring. Furthermore, cutting of annular tissue should be avoided while the suture is tied. Two other solutions are stentless aortic valve implant [12,13] and apicoaortic conduit [14-16]. The reader should consult the literature for further details on these two methods.

3. Calcified aorta

Calcification in the aorta occasionally necessitates modification of the surgical strategy because of the safety of arterial cannulation, aortic cross-clamping, insertion of a root cannula, aortotomy and suture closure of the aorta. Calcification can be precisely assessed by preoperative CT. The principal strategy can be selected based on the CT findings. Intraoperative TEE and/or epiaortic echo may be used to identify the precise location and extent of calcification and atheromatous plaque in the surgical field. Echo-guided marking of calcification on the aorta can be helpful for subsequent surgical procedures. Three-dimensional (3D) TEE is capable of visualizing the entire ascending aorta (Fig. 5). The xPlane mode allows serial sections of the aorta to be scanned from the aortic valve to the aortic arch. The diseased portion of the aorta can be located by digital compression of the aorta during visualization by TEE.

Fig. 6 demonstrates several TEE images of calcified aortas. Fig. 6A shows a calcified aortic wall just distal to the sinotubular junction, accompanied by acoustic shadow. The aortotomy line needs to be shifted distally. Calcification can take place at the level of the aortic cross-clamp, where the right pulmonary artery crosses behind the ascending aorta (Fig. 6B). Fig. 6C shows calcification at the level of arterial cannulation. The use of epiaortic echo is desirable to accurately locate the site of calcification. Fig. 6D is a TEE image of rather mild calcification. In this case, the aorta could be clamped without cerebral complications. Fig. 6E shows atheromatous plaque on the anterior wall of the ascending aorta at the level of cross-clamping and insertion of the root cannula. Since enhanced CT is not often employed for preoperative assessment before aortic valve replacement, care should be taken to avoid missing such findings. Palpation of the aorta cannot detect the presence of atheroma. TEE or epiaortic echo is needed to avoid an embolic event.

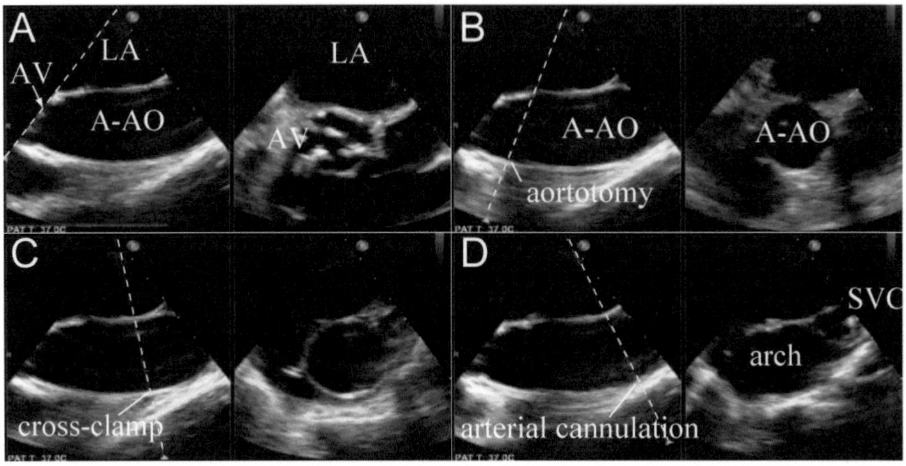

Figure 5. Scanning the entire A-AO using xPlane mode. In the midesophageal A-AO long-axis view, the scanning plane orthogonal to the reference plane is tilted from the AV up to the arch level. Short-axis view of A-AO can be visualized.

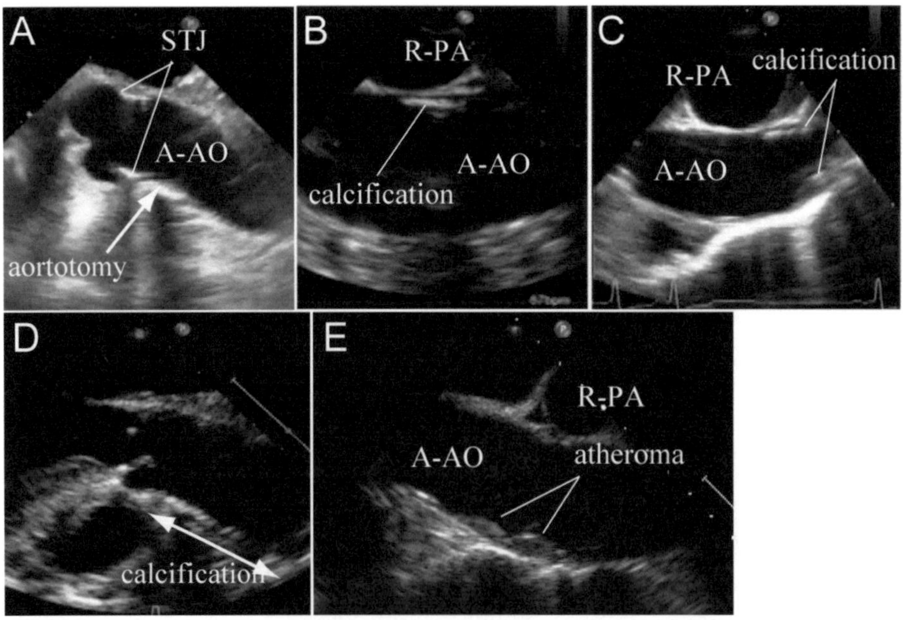

Figure 6. Examples of TEE images of calcified A-AO. A: Calcification of anterior wall just distal to STJ. B: Calcification at the level of cross-clamping (R-PA level). C: Calcification at the arterial cannulation level. D: Mild calcification of A-AO. E: Atheromatous plaque in the A-AO.

3.1. Arterial cannulation and insertion of a root cannula

Calcification often involves the distal portion of the ascending aorta and makes arterial cannulation difficult (Fig. 6C). Since an adequate space for aortotomy needs to be spared for procedures on the aortic valve, the cannulation site should not be too proximal. Arterial cannulation of a calcified aorta might cause aortic dissection at the time of cannulation and/or difficult hemostasis following decannulation. When aortic cannulation is not desirable, the axillary or femoral artery can be used as an alternative perfusion route. However, in patients with a calcified aorta, there can also be stenosis or atheromatous lesions in the innominate or iliac artery; thus, it is mandatory to check for these lesions before surgery. The insertion site of the root cannula should be carefully determined. Epiaortic echo is helpful for examining the presence and location of calcification and atheroma. A safe placement of the root cannula requires a certain length of nearly normal wall, which allows secure closure of the puncture site. When an adequate area is not available, an elastic needle may be used instead.

3.2. Aortic cross-clamp

In cases with severe and diffuse calcification of the aorta (porcelain aorta), concomitant replacement of the ascending aorta should be considered [17-19]. However, in the majority of calcified aortic valve cases, calcification is present but not severe; it is often scattered without apparent atheromatous plaque on the intima. It is important to determine the safety of aorta cross-clamp in all cases, since cross-clamp of a calcified aorta potentially causes fracture of the calcified layer that can lead to aortic dissection or embolism of fragmented calcium.

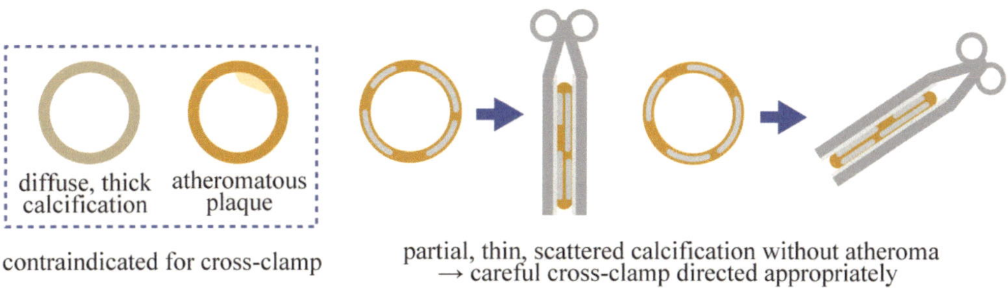

Figure 7. Strategies for clamping in cases of calcified aorta. When calcification is diffuse and thick or atheromathous plaque is present, cross-clamp is avoided. If calcification is partial and thin without atheroma, the aorta can be clamped according to the distribution of calcified portion.

Fig. 7 shows the strategy of the author. When calcification is diffuse and thick or atheromatous plaque is present, aortic cross-clamp is avoided. If the calcified layer is partial and not thick, the aorta may be clamped with some fracture of the calcified portion, but without incompetent clamp or the development of dissection. The clamp may be applied as parallel to the calcified wall as possible to minimize fracture of the calcified section and the shear force on the intima. Initially, the ratchet is locked slowly and less deeply. The blood flow in the proximal aorta is checked with TEE before antegrade cardioplegia is given. When there is some leak through the clamp site, the ratchet is advanced. If full clamp is not effective, another straight clamp is added adjacent to the first clamp or conversion to aortic repair is considered, depending on the risk of aortic repair in each individual case. It should be kept in mind that a clamp on the calcified aorta flattens the proximal aorta and narrows the surgical field following aortotomy. In the case shown in Fig. 6D, the aorta was carefully clamped and valve replacement was performed without neurologic sequelae. For porcelain aorta, endovascular clamping may be another option [20].

3.3. Aortotomy

An incision line is determined based on the distribution of calcification. It may be modified from the standard J-shaped incision line to a rather transectional or more oblique and distal incision. In the case shown in Fig. 6A, aortotomy at a more distal level or meticulous removal of calcification is needed. If there is an insufficient margin for suture closure of the aortotomy (at least 1 cm in width), the surgeon should be prepared for difficult suturing. When the calcified portion of the aorta is to be incised and sutured, calcium needs to be carefully removed following aortotomy, but before implanting a prosthetic valve. The use of CUSA is helpful for reducing the amount of calcium, enabling an adequate attachment of the aortic walls during suture closure. A new device for this purpose may be helpful [21].

4. Coronary arteries

Myocardial protection is one of the most important issues in aortic valve replacement. Left ventricular hypertrophy and/or coronary artery disease is often associated with aortic stenosis. In addition, surgical procedures may potentially cause new myocardial ischemia. Therefore, careful observation of coronary perfusion is essential. Fig. 8 shows visualization of the coronary arteries with TEE. The coronary arteries can be visualized bilaterally in the majority of cases and coronary artery assessment is done routinely in our institute. The ostia of the right and left coronary arteries are depicted in the short-axis view at the level of sinus of Valsalva (Fig. 8 A,B). The right coronary artery travels in the groove between the right atrium and right ventricle, whereas the left coronary artery crosses behind the pulmonary artery. The left main truncus divides into the left anterior descending and left circumflex arteries. The right coronary ostium can also be depicted in the midesophageal aortic valve long-axis view, giving an idea of its distance from the annulus (Fig. 8C).

To further visualize the distal portion of the left coronary artery, the scanning plane is rotated counterclockwise from the midesophageal aortic valve long-axis view (Fig. 8D). The left coronary sinus takes the place of the noncoronary sinus, and the short-axis view of left main truncus appears. The left anterior descending artery courses toward the 6 to 7 o'clock direction. The distal portion of the left circumflex artery is visualized in the atrioventricular groove. With the 3D en face view, the height of coronary take-off can be observed (Fig. 8E). The author meticulously uses TEE for intraoperative assessment of coronary perfusion, because it is the

http://dx.doi.org/10.5772/53418

most important factor that affects the outcomes of aortic valve replacement, especially for calcified aortic valves. Several pitfalls related to myocardial ischemia are shown in Fig. 9.

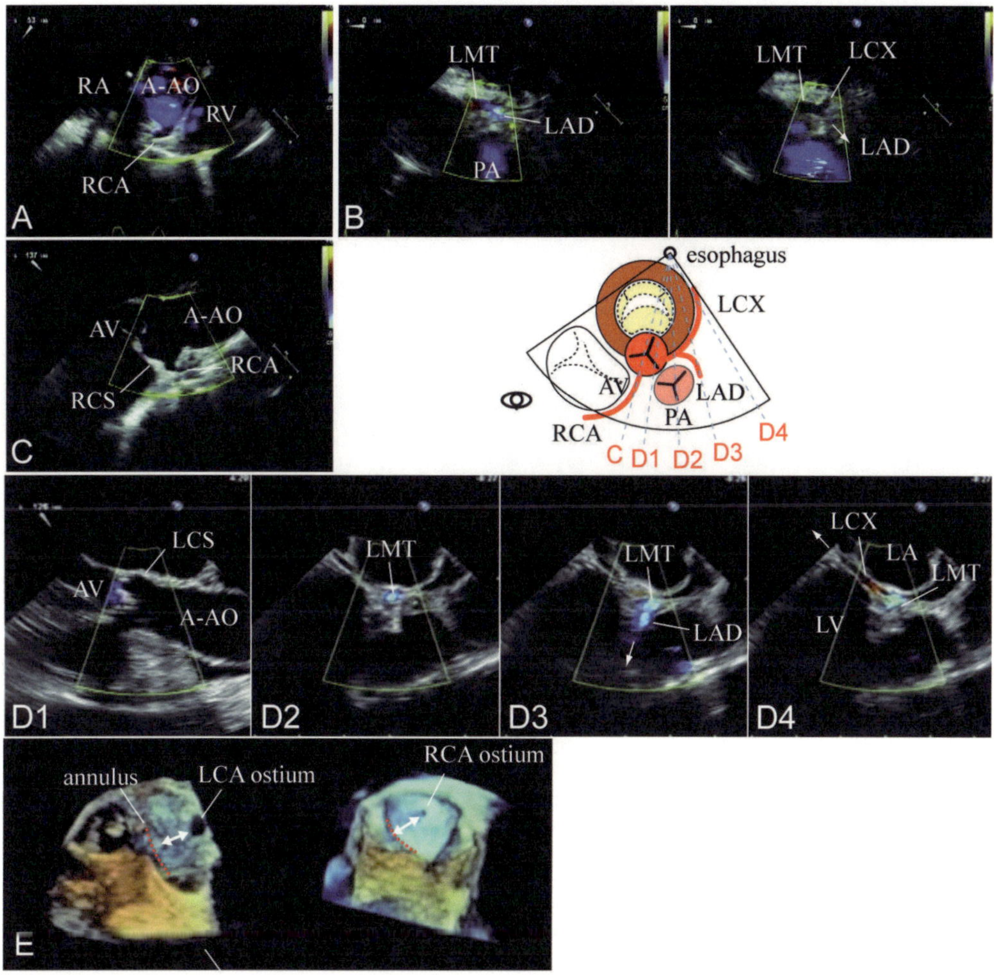

Figure 8. Visualization of coronary arteries with TEE. A: In short-axis view at the level of sinus of Valsalva, RCA arises from RCS at 6 o'clock position directed to the groove between RA and RV. B: The LCA takes off from LCS at 3 o'clock position. LMT courses behind PA and divides to LAD and LCX. C: In midesophageal AV long-axis view, RCA arises from RCS (C). D: As the probe is rotated counterclockwise, LCA arises from LCS and LMT divides to LAD and LCX. LAD is directed toward the LV apex and LCX courses posteriorly along the atrioventicular groove between LA and LV. E: In 3D en-face view, distance from AV annulus to the ostia is recognized.

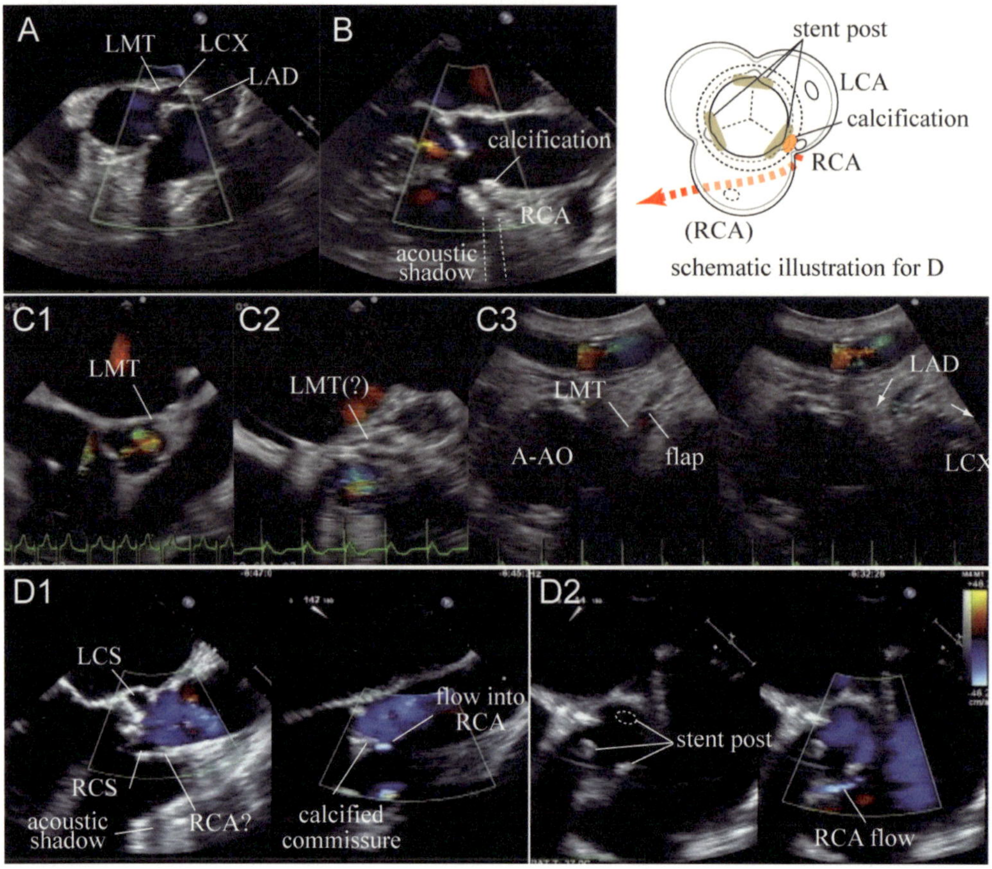

Figure 9. Pitfalls related to coronary artery in aortic valve replacement. A: Short LMT divides to LAD and LCX near the ostium. B: Calcification adjacent to RCA ostium. C: New dissection in the LMT. LMT was intact before bypass (C1), but no flow was detectable during wearing from bypass (C2) associated with akinetic LV. Epicardial echo following coronary bypass to the LAD shows a flap obstructing the LMT and blood flow from LAD toward LCX (C3). D: Anomalous origin of RCA. RCA was not found in the RCS, but at the commissure between RCC and LCC (D1). Following valve replacement, RCA was seen originating from the commissure in front of the stent post (D2). Schematic illustration of D is shown.

4.1. Short left main truncus

The left main truncus is occasionally found to be short (Fig. 9A). As the cannula is forcefully thrust into the ostium, the cannula tip may enter either the left anterior descending or left circumflex artery. Any unperfused region of the left ventricle may be poorly protected during the procedure.

4.2. Calcified ostium

The coronary ostium as well as the surrounding wall of the coronary sinus of Valsalva may be rigid or irregular, occasionally making it difficult to selectively infuse cardioplegic solution into the coronary artery, because the cannula tip does not fit properly and there is significant leakage. When calcification accompanied by acoustic shadow is present adjacent to the coronary ostium (Fig. 9B), this pitfall may occur. A highly echogenic projection accompanied by acoustic shadow, usually on the side of the sinotubular junction, is a typical TEE finding. Calcification in the aortic root also makes it difficult to locate the right coronary ostium, especially when the sinus wall of Valsalva is rigid and cannot be folded back. Unsuccessful infusion of cardioplegic solution potentially leads to right heart failure, since the right coronary region cannot be adequately perfused via the retrograde approach. Although a large-bore cannula tip does not adequately fit the calcified ostium, a small-caliper cannula causes little leakage but the velocity of jet stream ejected out of the cannula can exceed 2 m/sec, potentially causing intimal damage or dissection. Fig. 9C shows the TEE findings of dissection that occurred in the left coronary artery following cardiopulmonary bypass in a case of difficult coronary perfusion. Although the left coronary artery was intact before bypass, no blood flow was detected during weaning from bypass in the area that was thought to contain the left main truncus. Since the anterior and posterior walls of the left ventricle were akinetic, immediate coronary bypass grafting to the left anterior descending artery was performed. Subsequent epicardial echo revealed a flap in the left main truncus and retrograde blood flow in the left anterior descending artery from the coronary bypass graft that perfused the left circumflex artery.

4.3. Anomalous origin of the right coronary artery

Anomalous origin of the right coronary artery is rather rare (Fig. 9D), but is difficult to diagnose based on preoperative coronary angiography. In a case of aortic stenosis with an intact right coronary artery in preoperative coronary angiography, the right coronary ostium could not be found in the right coronary sinus of Valsalva. Selective perfusion of the left coronary artery caused backflow from the right coronary ostium, which was identified at the commissure between the right and left coronary cusps. Calcified protrusion was continuous from the commissure to the ostium. The right coronary artery was successfully perfused, and the calcium at the orifice was left unresected. However, when calcium is exposed without being covered by the sewing ring, there is the potential for thrombus formation adjacent to the right coronary ostium. Following aortic valve replacement, TEE demonstrated that the stent post was located in front of the right coronary ostium, because the stent posts were oriented so that the left coronary ostium was not covered by the stent post. The right coronary artery coursed along the right coronary sinus and could have been inadvertently injured by the surgical procedures.

4.4. Myocardial perfusion during cardioplegia

Retrograde cardioplegia is a solution for difficult antegrade coronary perfusion. However, the region perfused by the right coronary artery is poorly protected because the cardioplegic solution predominantly enters the coronary veins along the left coronary artery (great cardiac vein) but not the middle or small cardiac veins. Although the latter may be perfused via collaterals between the veins, this is not certain. Also, in cases where it is difficult to fit the coronary perfusion cannula and there is considerable leakage, perfusion of the myocardium is a concern. A myocardial thermometer was conventionally used, but may not be useful in warm heart surgery. Real-time assessment of myocardial perfusion is desired, especially in cases with deteriorated cardiac function. Here, a novel method for noninvasively assessing myocardial perfusion is demonstrated (Fig. 10). The transgastric basal or midventricular short-axis view is visualized. In pulsed-wave Doppler mode, the sample volume is placed on the myocardium. When this portion of myocardium is perfused, a flow signal is detected. Under selective perfusion of the left coronary artery, blood flow is detected in the anterior wall but not in the inferior wall. As coronary perfusion is discontinued, the flow signal instantaneously disappears. The perfused region is identified by mapping the myocardium. This can be helpful for examining the extent of retrograde delivery of cardioplegic solution.

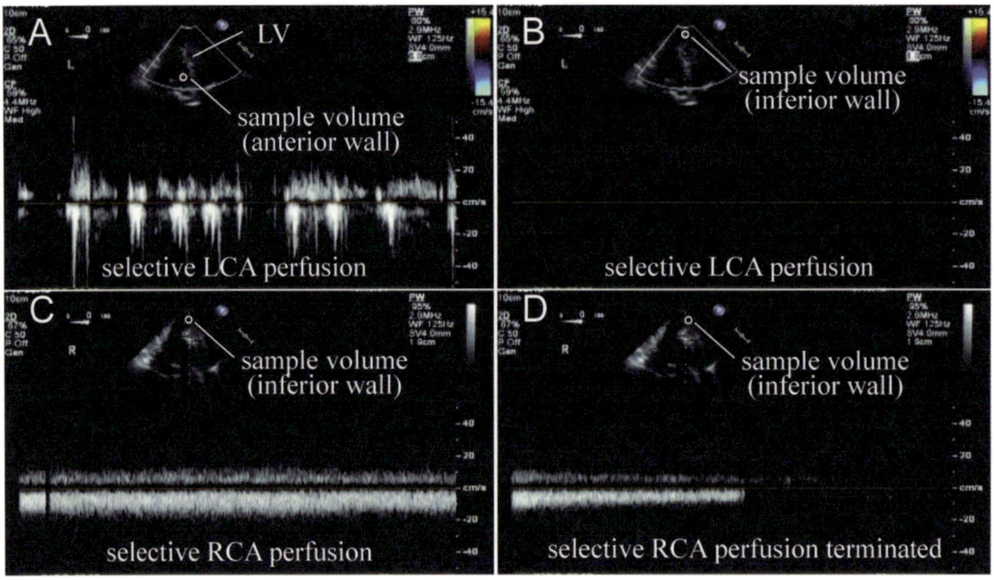

Figure 10. TEE assessment of myocardial blood flow during cardioplegia. Under selective perfusion to LCA, blood flow is detectable in the anterior wall (A) but not in the inferior wall (B). As selective RCA perfusion is terminated, blood flow detected in the inferior wall (c) instantaneously disappears (D)

5. Assessment following implantation

After the aortotomy is closed, several pitfalls need to be checked (Fig. 11,12). If an unexpected event is detected, a prompt decision for additional intervention should be made.

5.1. Perivalvular or transvalvular leakage

During weaning from bypass, the surgeon should check for perivalvular leakage. A calcified aortic valve can result in inadequate contact between the annulus and the suture ring of the

http://dx.doi.org/10.5772/53418

prosthetic valve. It is readily examined by TEE in the midesophageal long-axis view (Fig. 11A). A minor leak that originates inside of the ring and deviates inwards is transvalvular leak and is not significant (Fig. 11B). When significant leakage is detected in the left ventricular outflow tract that originates outside of the suture ring, perivalvular leakage is probable (Fig. 11C). The assessment of leakage is difficult in cases with concomitant mitral valve replacement. The ring of the prosthetic valve implanted in the mitral position casts an acoustic shadow on the left ventricular outflow tract (Fig. 11D). In such an instance, leakage is assessed in the deep transgastric long-axis view via the left ventricular apex (Fig. 11E).

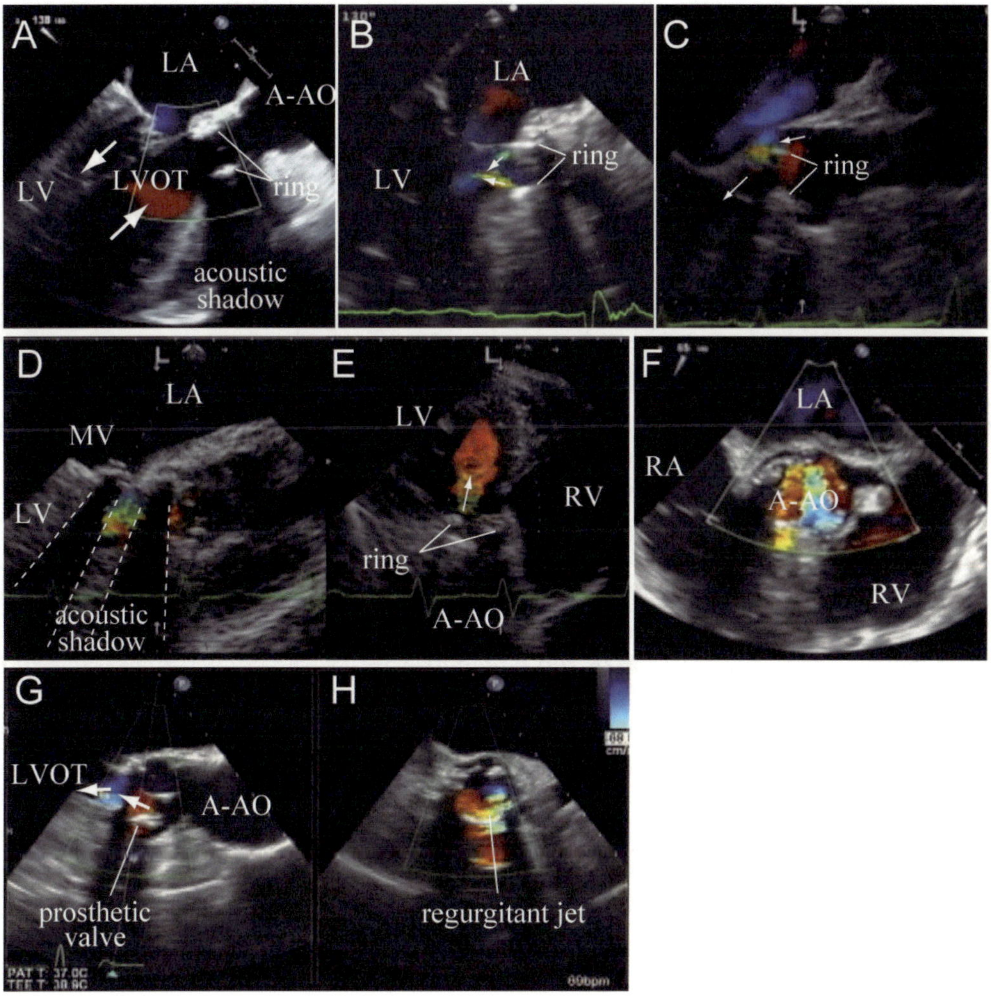

Figure 11. TEE assessment of prostethic valve following aortic valve replacement. A: Midesophageal long-axis view without abnormal leak from the prosthetic valve. B: Minor transvalvular leak. C: Significant perivalvular leak around the valve. D: Leakage is suspected but visualization is disturbed by the valve in mitral position. E: Deep transgastric view shows mild transvalvular leak F: Blood flow in the entire area of ascending aorta just distal to the prosthetic valve indicates good opening of discs. G,H: Massive transvalvular leak from the bioprosthesis due to everted leaflet.

Valve dysfunction should be checked during weaning from bypass. Dysfunction of a mechanical valve includes an immobilized disc at the open or closed positions. Since the disc itself is hardly depicted by TEE, dysfunction is examined in the color Doppler mode. In the short-axis view of the ascending aorta at the level just above the valve, opening of both discs can be confirmed by the flow signal, which fills the entire area of the aorta (Fig. 11F). Incompetence of the valve is caused by an immobilized disc of a mechanical valve at the open position probably due to debris or calcium between the disc and ring or by jammed leaflets of a bioprosthetic valve. It can be recognized by massive aortic regurgitation, demonstrated by a regurgitant jet in the left ventricular outflow tract originating from inside of the ring in midesophageal or deep transgastric view (Fig. 11G,H). In this case, exploration revealed that there was unintended eversion of a leaflet on the noncoronary side without jamming or leaflet damage. The leaflet was returned to the normal position and the aortotomy was closed [22].

5.2. Coronary ostium and ventricular contraction

Obstruction of coronary ostium is checked during weaning from bypass to minimize myocardial damage under warm ischemia. This event is important especially for the valve implanted in the supra-annular position. In the early timing following aortic declamping, patency and blood flow in both coronary arteries is checked. Both ostia can be visualized in the short-axis view just above the valve (Fig. 12A). In the midesophageal aortic valve long-axis view, the right coronary ostium is seen above the sewing ring (Fig. 12B). The presence of flow and distance from the ring of the prosthetic valve is checked.

Blood flow in the left coronary artery is examined proximal to its bifurcation into the LAD and LCX as shown in Fig. 8. Fig. 12D shows TEE views in a case of a low origin of the LMT. Before cardiopulmonary bypass, the midesophageal long-axis view showed a short distance between the aortic annulus and left main truncus. Following valve replacement at the intra-annular position, knots were found to be in front of the left coronary ostium and accelerated flow was seen. In the midesophageal long-axis view, the left coronary ostium was just above the ring. Surprisingly, the left main truncus was just behind the annulus. A deep suture could have injured the left main truncus. Fig. 12E and F demonstrate a case with a normal origin of the main left coronary artery. Before cardiopulmonary bypass, the coronary orifice was approximately 1 cm above the aortic annulus (Fig. 12E1,2). The 3D en face view clearly demonstrated an adequate distance (Fig. 12 E3). After replacement, TEE showed that there was no obstacle in front of the left main truncus in the short-axis view (Fig. 12F1). In the long-axis view, there was adequate distance between the ring and left main truncus (Fig. 12F2). 3D TEE also clearly showed safe implant of the prosthetic valve (Fig. 12F3). As ventricular contraction recovers, regional wall motion abnormalities can be assessed in the midesophageal, 2-chamber and 4-chamber views, or the transgastric basal or mid-short-axis views.

If coronary obstruction is suspected as in Fig. 9, early coronary revascularization is to be considered for minimizing myocardial damage. Ischemia can develop not only by obstruction of coronary ostium but by poor myocardial protection or embolism of dislodged calcium or even intracardiac air. Sustained circulatory support may be advantageous or retrograde cardioplegia may potentially help to displace any calcium or air embolus toward the coronary ostium.

http://dx.doi.org/10.5772/53418

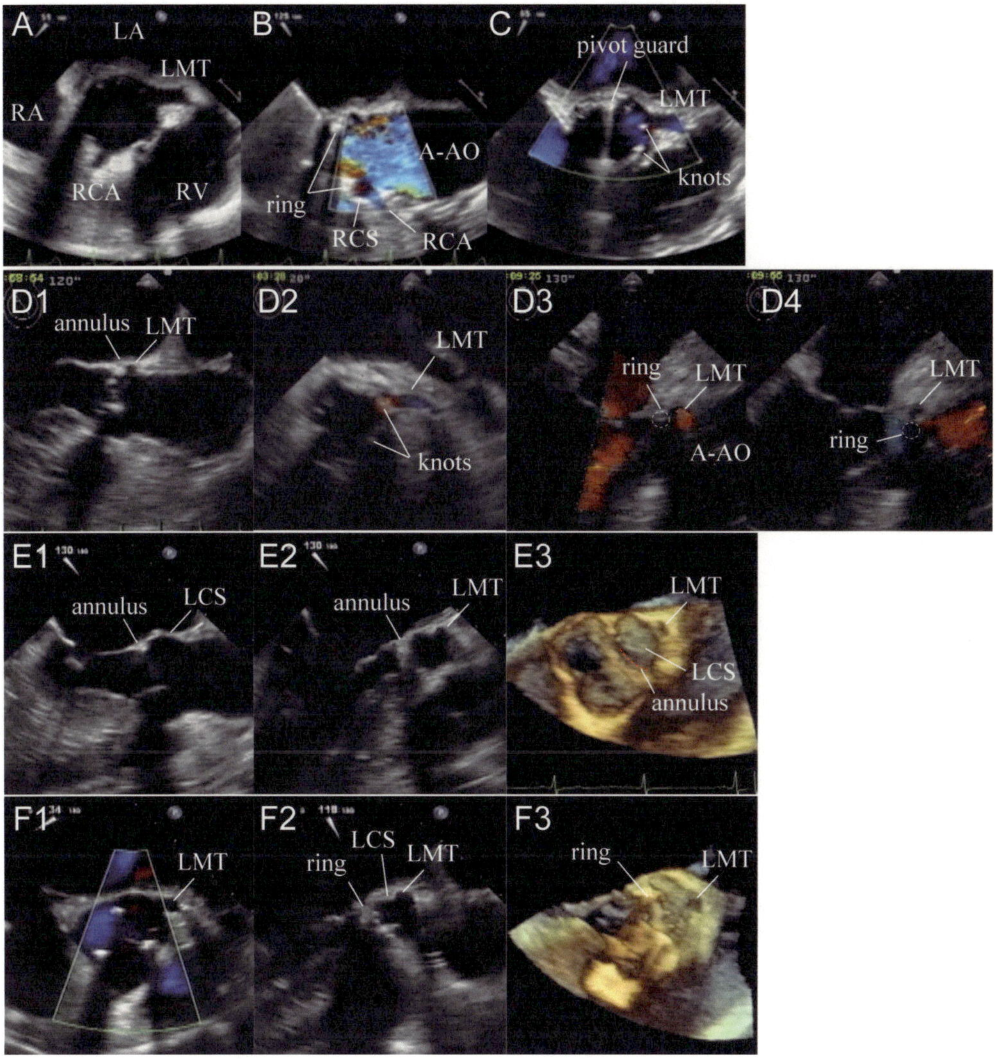

Figure 12. TEE assessment of coronary arteries in aortic valve replacement. A; Short-axis view at the level of the sinus of Valsalva that shows patent ostia of the RCA and LMT. B: RCA flow in midesophageal AV long-axis view. Distance from the ring to RCA ostium is checked. C: LMT flow in short-axis view of sinus of Valsalva. Knots are seen without obstruction. D: Low take-off of LMT (D1). Following valve replacement, the knots are in front of LMT ostium. A mild acceleration of blood flow is seen (D2). In midesophageal long-axis view, the LMT orifice is just above the ring (D3). LMT was found to course very close to the suture (D4). E: Normal take-off of LMT. LMT originates from the LCS at approximately 1 cm above the aortic annulus (E1 to E2). 3D en face view clearly demonstrates the distance of LMT from the annulus (E3). F: TEE views following valve replacement. There is no obstruction in front of the LMT (F1). There is adequate distance from the ring to the LMT orifice, depicted in midesophageal long-axis view (F2) and 3D en face view (F3)

5.3. New mitral regurgitation

Mitral regurgitation may appear following aortic valve replacement. One reason is perforation of the mitral annulus caused by excessive decalcification of the aortic annulus. Another mechanism is systolic anterior motion of the mitral leaflet, which is caused by reduced left ventricular dimensions and/or a sigmoid septum due to left ventricular hypertrophy. When several measures are not effective, emergent mitral valve replacement should be considered.

5.4. Aortic dissection

Following aortic declamping, the aorta distal to the clamp site should be checked for new dissection. It may potentially develop due to detachment of the calcified aortic wall, and inner or outer layer. Dissection can also originate from the arterial cannulation site, root cannula site or aortotomy site.

In conclusion, it is essential to watch for pitfalls in aortic valve replacement for calcified aortic valve, because it is commonly associated with various pathologies that can affect the surgical outcomes. Meticulous monitoring and intraoperative diagnostic imaging are helpful for achieving the best possible results in cases with increased risk factors.

Abbreviations for figures

A-AO ascending aorta

AML anterior mitral leaflet

AV aortic valve

LA left atrium

LAD left anterior descending artery

LCA left coronary artery

LCC left coronary cusp

LCS left coronary sinus

LMT left main truncus

LVOT left ventricular outflow tract

MV mitral valve

NCC noncoronary cusp

PA pulmonary artery

RA right atrium

RCA right coronary artery

RCC right coronary cusp

RCS right coronary sinus

R-PA right pulmonary artery

RV right ventricle

STJ sinotubular junction

SVC superior vena cava

Author details

Kazumasa Orihashi

Department of Cardiovascular Surgery, Kochi Medical School, Kochi, Japan

References

[1] Tanaka, K, Tajima, K, Takami, Y, et al. Early and late outcomes of aortic valve replacement in dialysis patients. Ann Thorac Surg (2010). , 89, 65-70.

[2] Kaden, J. J, Eckert, J. P, Poerner, T, et al. Prevalence of atherosclerosis of the coronary and extracranial cerebral arteries in patients undergoing aortic valve replacement for calcified stenosis. J Heart Valve Dis (2006). , 15, 165-8.

[3] Staico, R, Armaganijan, L, & Lopes, R. D. Coronary embolism and calcified aortic valve: is there a correlation? J Thromb Thrombolysis (2012). , 34, 425-7.

[4] Mannino, G, Romano, M, Calanchini, M, Mannino, C, & Cascone, N. C. Branch retinal artery embolization due to calcific aortic valve stenosis. Eur J Ophthalmol (2010). , 20, 625-8.

[5] Mahajan, N, Khetarpal, V, & Afonso, L. Stroke secondary to calcific bicuspid aortic valve: case report and literature review. J Cardiol (2009). , 54, 158-61.

[6] Rivard, A. L, Bartel, T, Bianco, R. W, et al. Evaluation of aortic root and valve calcifications by multi-detector computed tomography. J Heart Valve Dis (2009). , 18, 662-70.

[7] Aviram, G, Sharony, R, Kramer, A, et al. Modification of surgical planning based on cardiac multidetector computed tomography in reoperative heart surgery. Ann Thorac Surg (2005). , 79, 589-95.

[8] Islamoglu, F, Apaydin, A. Z, Degirmenciler, K, et al. Detachment of the mitral valve anterior leaflet as a complication of aortic valve replacement. Tex Heart Inst J (2006). , 33, 54-6.

[9] Orihashi, K. Intraoperative imaging in aortic valve surgery as a safety net (Chapter 1). IN: Motomura N, ed. Aortic Valve Surgery. InTech Co., Croatia, (2011). , 3-18.

[10] Taniguchi, S, Noguchi, M, Onohara, D, et al. Aortic valve replacement with 17-mm St. Jude Medical Regent prosthetic valves for a small calcified aortic annulus in elderly patients. Gen Thorac Cardiovasc Surg (2010). , 58, 506-10.

[11] Coutinho, G. F, Correia, P. M, Paupério, G, et al. Aortic root enlargement does not increase the surgical risk and short-term patient outcome? Eur J Cardiothorac Surg (2011). , 40, 441-7.

[12] Karimov, J. H, Cerillo, A. G, Solinas, M, et al. Stentless aortic valve implantation in heavily calcified aorta. J Cardiovasc Med (Hagerstown) (2009). , 10, 813-4.

[13] Di Matteo G Masala N, Swanevelder J, et al. Clinical outcome of a simplified technique for aortic valve replacement with stentless bioprostheses. J Heart Valve Dis (2009). , 18, 111-8.

[14] Shin, H, Mori, M, Suzuki, R, et al. Apicoaortic valved conduit with an apical connector for aortic stenosis with a calcified aorta. Gen Thorac Cardiovasc Surg (2009). , 57, 467-70.

[15] Chahine, J. H, Rassi, I, & Jebara, V. Apico-aortic valved conduit as an alternative for aortic valve re-replacement in severe prosthesis-patient mismatch. Interact Cardiovasc Thorac Surg (2009). , 9, 680-2.

[16] Crestanello, J. A, Zehr, K. J, Daly, R. C, et al. Is there a role for the left ventricle apical-aortic conduit for acquired aortic stenosis? J Heart Valve Dis (2004). , 13, 57-62.

[17] Chung, S, Park, P. W, Choi, M. S, et al. Surgical experience of ascending aorta and aortic valve replacement in patient with calcified aorta. Korean J Thorac Cardiovasc Surg (2012). , 45, 24-9.

[18] Iliopoulos, D. C, Deveja, A. R, Satratzemis, V, et al. Deep hypothermic arrest for aortic valve replacement in case of porcelain aorta. Asian Cardiovasc Thorac Ann (2009). , 17, 415-6.

[19] Okamoto, H, Fujimoto, K, Tamenishi, A, et al. Aortic valve replacement in a heavily calcified "porcelain" aorta. Jpn J Thorac Cardiovasc Surg (2001). , 49, 453-6.

[20] Ooi, A, Iyenger, S, Langley, S. M, et al. Endovascular clamping of porcelain aorta in aortic valve surgery using Foley Catheter. Heart Lung Circ (2006). , 15, 194-6.

[21] Kudo, M, Misumi, T, & Koizumi, K. Aortotomy and endarterectomy of the ascending aorta for aortic valve replacement in a patient with porcelain aorta. Surg Today (2005). , 35, 1000-3.

[22] Orihashi, K, Kurosaki, T, & Sueda, T. Everted leaflet of a bovine pericardial aortic valve. Interact Cardiovasc Thorac Surg (2010). , 10, 1059-60.

Chapter 18

Congenital Aortic Stenosis in Children

Hirofumi Saiki and Hideaki Senzaki

Additional information is available at the end of the chapter

http://dx.doi.org/10.5772/54806

1. Introduction

Congenital aortic stenosis (AS) is caused by abnormal morphological development of the aortic valve. [1, 2] Valvular abnormalities may be accompanied by supra- or sub-valvular stenosis. The embryogenic process that forms aortic valves begins approximately 31–32 days of gestation. Cavity formation in the basal portion of the truncus arteriosus is a key process in the development of the leaflet and sinus of Valsalva, which are important components of the aortic valve. Therefore, incomplete formation of the cavity causes various morphological abnormalities of the aortic valve, including bicuspid valve with or without commissural fusion, tricuspid valve with commissural fusion, monocuspid valve, and myxomatoid leaflet valve (dysplastic valve). The most frequent type of congenital AS is a bicuspid aortic valve, [3] accounting for approximately 90% of AS cases.

Although the morphological features of the aortic valve are closely associated with the AS severity, the pathophysiology and resultant clinical manifestation of AS are fundamentally determined by the severity of the stenosis (effective orifice area). In this sense, congenital AS in children is classified into 2 major types: severe AS that becomes symptomatic and necessitates interventions during the neonatal period or early infancy and a milder form of AS with signs and/or symptoms that develop later in childhood.

In this chapter, we will outline the pathophysiology, clinical characteristics, and management of congenital AS observed in children (from fetus to adolescence) for each type of AS mentioned above. We will also briefly discuss the differences in ventricular adaptation, which are strongly linked to the clinical manifestation of AS, to the increased afterload caused by AS between children and adults.

2. Pathophysiology of congenital AS

The mechanism underlying the increase in severity of AS in children is similar to that seen in adults. The orifice size can decrease because of increased thickness and rigidity of the valve leaflets, independent of the morphological anomalies of the aortic valve, although native abnormal morphological features have greater impact on the progression of stenosis in children than in adults. The mechanisms underlying the exacerbation of stenosis also need to be determined. Valvular fibrosis, lipid accumulation, [4,5] inflammatory changes, [6] and acquired fibrotic fusion of commissures, which increase cusp thickness/stiffness, [5,7] could also be associated with the development of valvular stenosis, even in childhood AS. Metabolic syndrome is an emerging issue even in children and may be associated with these exacerbating mechanisms, [8] resulting in calcification, which reduces the possibility of valvular plastic surgery. In addition, bicuspid aortic valves possibly develop aortic calcification earlier than tricuspid aortic valves. [9,10] In this section, we will discuss the hemodynamic aspects of aortic stenosis in fetuses, neonates, and children.

2.1. AS with signs and symptoms that develop during the fetal or neonatal period

The fundamental underlying pathophysiology of AS involves an increase in afterload to the left ventricle (LV). The mechanism by which the LV copes with this increase in afterload is an increase of myocardial mass (hypertrophy) to generate a higher force to confront the increased afterload. If the aortic valve stenosis is too severe to allow the LV to become adaptive, LV contractility is depressed and the LV becomes markedly dilated. In this critical condition, the fetal circulation can maintain, to some extent, the systemic output using the right ventricle (RV), because there are interatrial communication (foramen ovale) and ductus arteriosus in the fetal ciculation. The ascending aortic flow and sometimes even the coronary arterial flow rely on retrograde blood flow from the ductus arteriosus. However, an LV exposed to massive afterload with relatively reduced coronary blood flow supply is at high risk of progressive ventricular failure, and is associated with an increased risk of sudden cardiac death. If the patient can survive this condition for a certain period, a marked increase in LV end-diastolic pressure (EDP) hinders the blood flow from the left atrium entering into the LV, leading to a gradual reduction of LV cavity volume. This process is postulated as one mechanism of evolving hypoplastic left heart syndrome (HLHS). Degeneration of the endocardium may accompany this process, representing a condition known as endocardial fibroelastosis. [11]

In other cases, an increase in LV afterload may allow the LV to exert its adaptive mechanism of hypertrophy, which also inhibits LV inflow due to increased LV stiffness and resultant EDP rise. [12] This is another form of evolving HLHS physiology (Figure 1A).

Of course, the above pathophysiological mechanisms should be understood as a continuum, [13, 14] and some patients may be born with a markedly dilated LV and depressed contractility, known as critical AS (Figure 1B). Such patients suffer from severe circulatory failure and pulmonary congestion, which is often life threatening and requires emergency intervention, either by catheters or surgery, as discussed below.

http://dx.doi.org/10.5772/54806

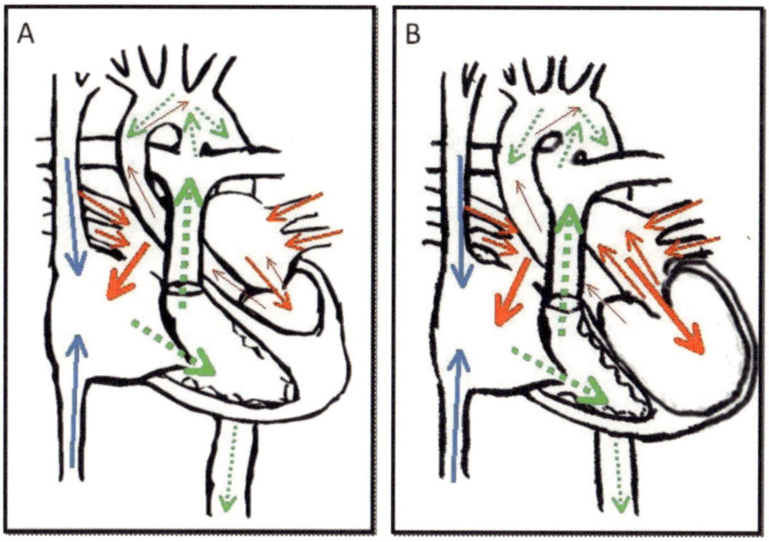

Figure 1. A schema of hypoplastic left heart syndrome (A) and that of critical aortic stenosis (B).

2.2. AS with signs and/or symptoms that develop during late infancy and school age

When the severity of AS is mild such that the LV can cope with the increased afterload, patients present with clinical symptoms during late infancy or school age. Although their LV exhibits hypertrophy, AS may be mild enough in patients such that they will be asymptomatic. There are also a group of patients who had no signs and symptoms other than heart murmur. In general, the aortic valves of this group of patients can supply the systemic blood flow during the neonatal period. This is verified by the fact that the ductus flow during the neonatal period shows left-to-right shunting. The timing of the onset of AS symptoms in this group is dependent on the severity of stenosis that is associated with the LV's capability to exert its adaptive mechanism to increased afterload. Of note, unlike adult onset AS, the severity of AS in children is also influenced by somatic growth, which induces a relative increase in the blood flow through the aortic valve and thereby causes augmentation of LV afterload. In addition, it was reported that an increased pressure gradient across the aortic valve is related to earlier progression of stenosis and a higher frequency of complicating aortic regurgitation. [15, 16] Therefore, the pathophysiology of AS in this age group may be dependent on preload change due to aortic regurgitation as well as the increasing afterload. In the clinical setting, it is important to follow-up with these patients periodically to detect such changes and to determine the appropriate timing and method of treatment. Therefore, we will discuss methods for monitoring the dynamic changes in AS in this particular group of patients in the following section.

2.2.1. Monitoring methods for AS

Clinical symptom evaluation, physical examination, electrocardiogram (ECG), and echocardiography are essential sources for obtaining comprehensive information for appropriate management of AS in this patient group. If fainting, convulsion, or resuscitated cardiac arrest are observed, relieving AS is indicated for preventing further adverse events. [17, 18] Although angina and syncope are reported to be observed only in <10% of patients whose peak-to-peak pressure gradient is greater than 80 mmHg, chest pain is an important clinical sign indicating the need for intervention, as adverse events are likely to occur within a few years after the complaint of initial chest pain.

ECG examinations are informative if ST-segment changes are observed. Usually, severe AS shows a 0–90°QRS-axis with high voltages in the left precordial leads. However, it is important to note that the above ECG findings of LV hypertrophy do not necessarily reflect the severity of the stenosis. Wagner et al. reported that one-third of AS patients with peak-to-peak pressure gradients greater than 80 mmHg do not exhibit the above LV hypertrophic findings on ECG. [17] In contrast, the ST strain pattern in the left precordial leads is thought to be more specific to LV hypertrophy and reflects the severity of AS (Figure 2).

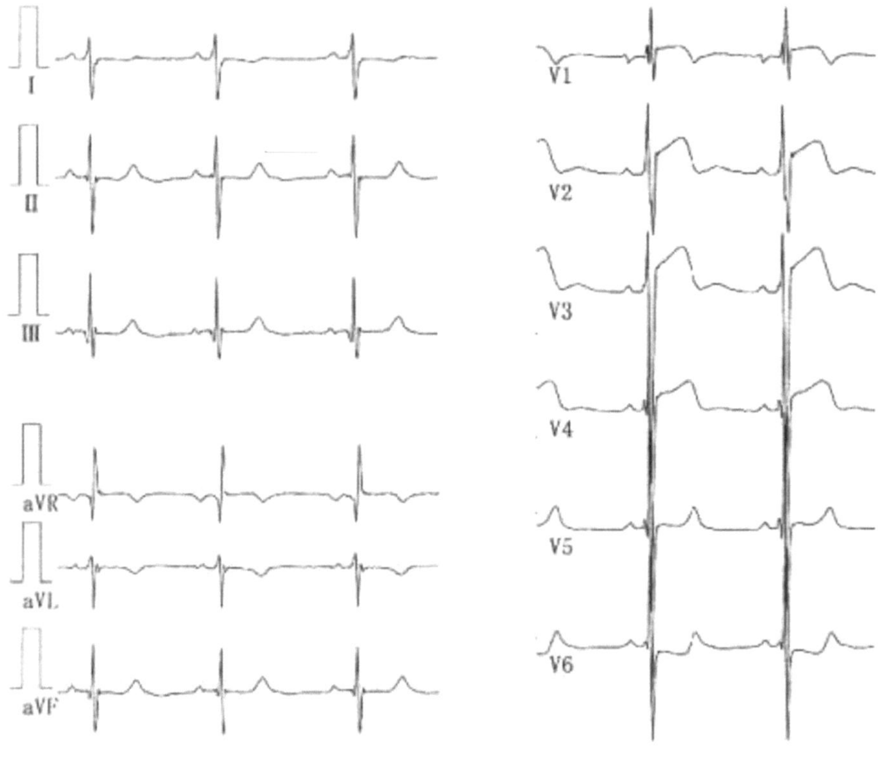

Figure 2. Electrocardiogram of severe aortic stenosis. This is an electrocardiogram (ECG) of a patient with severe aortic stenosis with an estimated pressure gradient of 140mmHg. Surprisingly, ECG shows no prominent finding of left ventricular hypertrophy other than changes in ST-T segment.

Holter ECG is also useful for predicting sudden deaths, even in asymptomatic AS patients. Wolfe et al. reported that multiform ventricular premature contraction, couplet, and ventricular tachycardia are serious arrhythmias that are associated with sudden cardiac death. [19]

http://dx.doi.org/10.5772/54806

Exercise testing may provide more accurate information about the risk of cardiac events than other examinations. Lewis et al. demonstrated the usefulness of exercise testing to identify subclinical ischemia in patients with severe AS. [26] Thus, exercise testing and Holter ECG may play a key role in clinician decision making for the management of AS patients.

Echocardiography is a direct method for evaluating the anatomical features and severity of AS. Valvular anatomy can be assessed for leaflet number, balance, thickening, or doming. The annulus diameter is also important, particularly when intervention is indicated. M-mode study in short-axis view provides information regarding LV pressure calculated by Glanz's equation: LV systolic pressure=225*LVPWs/LVIDs, where LVPWs and LVIDs represent LV systolic posterior wall thickness and LV systolic diameter, respectively. [20] This equation is clinically useful, because the peak-to-peak pressure gradient can be evaluated when coupled with the arterial pressure measurement. The LV dimension and wall thickness values provide information regarding the risk of cardiac events and ischemia. In addition, combining an echocardiography study with exercise testing may be useful for predicting a higher risk of cardiac events, even in asymptomatic patients. [21] Velocity measurement by spectral pulse wave and continuous wave Doppler reflects the severity of AS if cardiac function is not impaired. The pressure gradient calculated by applying the Bernoulli equation in the outflow tract is one of the guides for determining the need for intervention, although it has some limitations. [22, 23] Spectral pulse wave Doppler could also be a powerful tool for confirming the localization of obstruction and estimating the valvular area.

The indication for the catheter examination is limited, but this modality provides accurate information regarding coronary arteries and severity of AS. Because the LV outflow tract is truncated, the severity of AS tends to be over-estimated by velocity-derived pressure gradient. In contrast, a precise PIPG as well as a peak-to-peak gradient can be evaluated by the catheter examination (Figure 3). The aortic valve area is also calculated by Gorlin's method. [24]

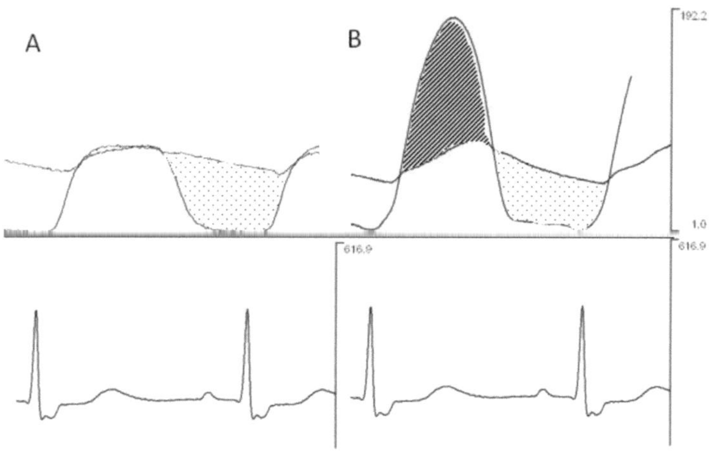

Figure 3. Simultaneous measurements of ascending aortic pressure and left ventricular pressure by the catheter examination. Both instantaneous and peak to peak pressure gradient can be clearly monitored. A; normal, B; aortic stenosis

3. Treatment of AS

3.1. Fetal and neonatal AS

If the patients have an established HLHS circulation with an underdeveloped LV, all the treatment options are directed to the future completion of the Fontan circulation, a final goal for patients with single ventricular circulation. However, if the LV size and components are to be sufficient to generate systemic output when the excessive afterload due to AS is relieved, interventions for the aortic valve per se are indicated, including either catheters or surgery. [25] The most attractive merit of catheter intervention (percutaneous transluminal aortic valvuloplasty [PTAV]) is that it is less invasive. In this procedure, cardiopulmonary bypass, which is a prerequisite for surgical procedures, can be avoided. PTAV is known to accelerate annular growth even in small sized aortic valve [26] if mitral valve stenosis is not complicated [27] .In performing PTAV, the carotid artery is generally used for blood access because lower body hypoperfusion makes it difficult to achieve access from the femoral artery and has a high risk of arterial obstruction with a prolonged sheath insertion, and because the curvature of aortic arch makes it difficult to manipulate the catheter and successfully pass it through the tiny aortic orifice (Figure 4). Therefore, central nervous system damage can be a potential adverse event associated with PTAV. More importantly, PTAV is a procedure used to enlarge the aortic orifice area by tearing the weak portions of the valve, not necessarily in the anatomically proper portion (commissures). Therefore, PTAV cannot be applied to valves with pre-existing aortic regurgitation because the procedure generally worsens this condition, which could be fatal. It was reported that 15% of 113 patients younger than 60 days old who had undergone PTAV developed significant aortic regurgitation. [26] Surgical interventions in this patient group include aortic valve plasty (AVP) and aortic valve replacement (AVR) with the autologous pulmonary artery valve (Ross procedure). The advantage of open AVP is that surgeons can perform the procedure on the basis of a detailed examination of the valve anatomy, which may reduce the risk of aortic regurgitation. Bhabra et al. [28] reported that if the aortic valve is tricuspid, the rate of freedom from reintervention after open AVP was 92% and that of AVR was 100% at a 10-year follow-up. These rates for bicuspid valves were only 33% and 57%, respectively. This report emphasizes the importance of valve morphology as a determinant of outcome following AVP. The other surgical option is the Ross procedure, which is particularly useful when sub/suprastenosis coexists with valvular stenosis (Ross-Konno procedure). The survival rate for the Ross procedure was 77% and rate of freedom from reintervention was 50%, comparable to the results of the Norwood procedure. [29-31] To apply the Ross procedure, autologous graft (pulmonary valve) function is important. Concha et al. reported that the rate of freedom from autograft failure at a 5-year follow-up was 95%, demonstrating a low incidence of autograft failure. [32] However, future pulmonary insufficiency remains as a matter of concern in long-term follow-ups.

We often encounter intermediate cases between established HLHS with underdeveloped LV and potentially normal-sized LV under excessive afterload. In such situations, accurate diagnosis about whether the LV has the potential to generate systemic output after relieving afterload is of primary importance. If the LV is judged to be incapable of generating systemic output, then the systemic circulation should rely on the RV. In such a case, the Fontan procedure becomes a goal of treatment. Multicenter studies have elucidated that the outcome of biventricular repair with a small LV is much worse than that of the Fontan procedure [13, 14], although the survival rate of Fontan completion for patients with a small LV or severely reduced LV function is only approximately 50-70%, even in the recent reports. [33-35]

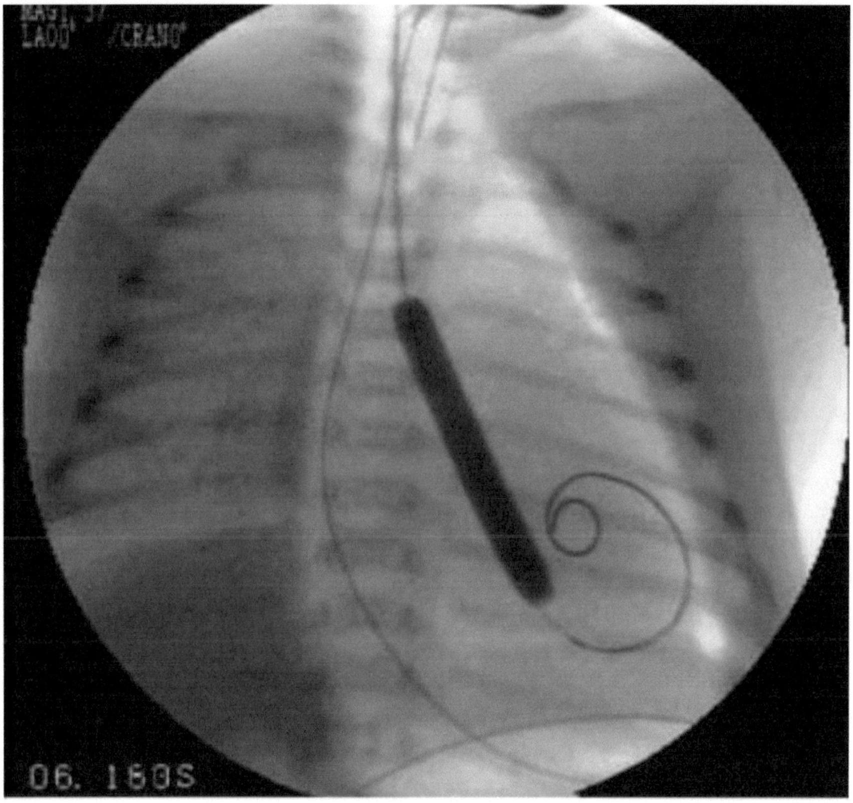

Figure 4. Percutaneous transluminal aortic valvuloplasty performed for a patient with critical aortic stenosis

Based on the pathophysiology of evolving HLHS as previously discussed and the poor survival rate of HLHS patients, fetal intervention has been attempted, aimed at relieving AS at earlier stages before the LV cavity is reduced. For the first time, Maxwell et al. reported their experience of intrauterine balloon dilatation of the fetal aortic valve in 1991. [36] Thereafter, a case series of 12 fetuses that underwent balloon valvuloplasty in the third trimester were reported, with no improvement was observed in their LV growth. [37] Tworetzky et al. also reported the results of fetal intervention for 24 AS patients (ranging from 21 to 29 weeks of gestation) who were thought to have a high probability of developing HLHS. [38] Technical success was achieved in 14 patients, but only 3 patients were able to undergo two-ventricular repair. Therefore, fetal intervention should be regarded as experimental at present, as many issues remain to be solved.

3.2. AS with signs and symptoms that develop during late infancy and school age

The treatment strategy for AS in which signs and/or symptoms develop later in childhood is different from that for neonatal AS. The American College of Cardiology/American Heart Association Guidelines for the management of AS of this group [31] recommended that patients with a peak instantaneous pressure gradient (PIPG) measured by Doppler echocardiography ≥70 mmHg be considered for cardiac catheterization and treatment in asymptomatic children and young adults. If the patients desire to participate in competitive sports or become pregnant, a PIPG of 50–70 mmHg is an indication for further evaluation and interventions. If patients have symptoms (angina, syncope, or dyspnea on exertion), a PIPG ≥50 mmHg is the indication for treatment. If the PIPG is less than 50 mmHg and a symptom is present, another origin of the symptom should be investigated.

There are several treatment options for cases in which intervention is indicated, including PTAV, open AVP, the Ross procedure, and AVR. Procedure selection is primarily dependent upon whether the patient's somatic size (aortic annular size) is large enough to use a prosthetic valve, because AVR is considered as the first-line procedure at present. If the prosthetic valve is not available, procedures other than AVR are selected so that patients can live with their own valve until they can use a prosthetic aortic valve. In such situations, the most important concept for treatment is that the procedure should be regarded as a bridge to AVR. Therefore, the aim of any intervention should be to reduce the afterload without any significant aortic regurgitation so that patients can grow uneventfully until AVR can be performed. In this sense, if these patients do not have heart failure but have exertion-induced ischemic signs, restriction of exercise without invasive intervention may be selected to achieve a better outcome. Application of PTAV in this age group is relatively limited because AVP is thought to be better than PTAV in terms of preserving aortic valve function, [39, 40] and because aortic insufficiency caused by valvuloplasty is known to be progressive in nature. [15, 16] However, some patients may still benefit from PTAV to achieve the therapeutic goal in this AS group. The Ross procedure is also not regarded as a definitive repair surgery, because neoaortic regurgitation and pulmonary insufficiency are frequently observed postoperative complications, which require further interventions in the future. [40, 41] Therefore, the Ross procedure indication is limited to patients who cannot grow due to severe aortic insufficiency.

4. The hemodynamic effects of AS on ventricular function in children

In this last section, we briefly comment on the differences in LV geometric and functional changes between adult- and child-onset of AS. The natural history of LV geometric and functional changes in adult-onset AS is characterized by LV concentric hypertrophy in the early stage, followed by diastolic dysfunction, systolic dysfunction with eccentric hypertrophy, and heart failure at the end-stage. [42] Most of the patients who are candidates for surgical intervention are ranked in the state between diastolic and systolic ventricular dysfunction. Delayed relaxation characterizes early-stage ventricular diastolic dysfunction, and thus is observed in almost all AS patients, [43] while increased diastolic stiffness is observed in more advanced stages in which LV hypertrophy and fibrosis may coexist. The degree of diastolic dysfunction is important for predicting prognosis because it takes years to achieve reverse remodeling of diastolic function after normalization of afterload. [44]

In contrast to the relatively uniform geometric and functional LV changes observed in adult-onset AS, such changes in children's AS are diverse and somewhat different from those of adults. The difference primarily stems from the diversity of the initial impact of afterload on the LV. Because adult onset of AS is largely due to a bicuspid valve or atherosclerotic change with aging, AS gradually increases LV afterload. This allows the LV to confront the increased afterload by inducing hypertrophic changes. However, the severity of AS that initially imposes afterload on the LV is diverse in children, as previously discussed, thus excessive afterload may not allow the LV to become hypertrophic, resulting in LV dilation and systolic dysfunction as observed in critical AS. With increasing age, the LV geometry and function gradually resembles those of adult AS: a hypertrophic LV with diastolic dysfunction. However, it is rare in children to observe a marked increase in LV diastolic stiffness, even in cases of hypertrophic LV (Figure 5). In addition, it is interesting that LV relaxation appears to be relatively preserved in children with AS and hypertrophic LV. These differences in LV functional responses between children and adults may have a clue to a better management of patients with AS.

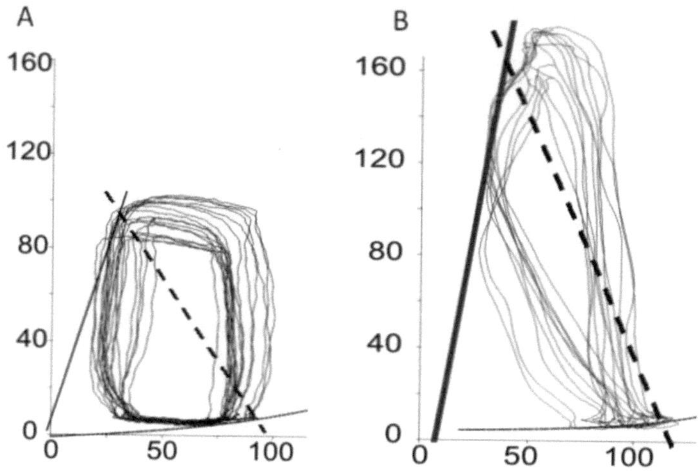

Figure 5. Examples of left ventricular pressure volume relationships in a control patient (A) and a patient with aortic stenosis (B). The steep slope of the end-systolic pressure-volume relationship (solid line) and arterial elastance (dashed line) indicate increased ventricular contractility and afterload. Note that the slope of the end-diastolic pressure-volume relationship in aortic stenosis is comparable to that of control.

5. Conclusions

In adults, AS generally develops slowly, with the progression of valve calcification or leaflet degeneration being independent of the existence of substrates for congenital abnormalities.

This allows the LV to adapt to the increased afterload by becoming concentrically hypertrophied. Therefore, it takes a long time before LV systolic function is severely impaired and critical events occur.[45] Because valvular calcification is a commonly observed morphological change and because a prosthetic valve is generally available for adults, aortic valve replacement is selected as a first-line treatment and plastic surgery is seldom chosen for this population. Thus, the treatment strategy is rather straightforward.

In contrast, as discussed in this chapter, a wide range of clinical phenotypes is seen in pediatric AS. Depending on the severity of the native aortic valve abnormality and associated hemodynamic features, AS could be one of the most severe forms of congenital heart defects in children, leading to a critical condition in neonates or even during fetal life. In the milder form of pediatric AS, no clinical symptoms are seen throughout the patient's life. Therefore, the complexity of the treatment approach depends upon the patient's age, body size, and associated cardiac anomalies. In particular, because of the limited availability of prosthetic aortic valves for small children, the native valve morphological features constitute an extremely important determinant of treatment strategy. A detailed assessment of LV function as well as accurate anatomical diagnosis, including analysis of the potential utility of the native aortic valve, is essential for achieving a better outcome for patients. The use of specific medications [46] and prevention of metabolic syndrome from childhood may help improve outcomes.

Accumulation of information regarding the outcomes of underdeveloped valves, detailed mechanisms underlying disease progression, surgical outcomes, and improvements in surgical techniques should lead to considerably improved outcomes in the pediatric population.

Author details

Hirofumi Saiki and Hideaki Senzaki*

Department of Pediatric Cardiology, Saitama Medical Center, Saitama Medical University, Saitama, Japan

References

[1] Falcone, M. W, Roberts, W. C, & Morrow, A. G. Perloff JK: Congenital aortic stenosis resulting from a unicommisssural valve. Clinical and anatomic features in twenty-one adult patients. *Circulation* (1971).

[2] Aortic StenosisIn Moss's Heart disease in infants, Children, and adolescents, Baltimore The Lippincott Wiliams and Wilkins Co. (2001).

[3] Michelena, H. I, Desjardins, V. A, & Avierinos, J. F. Natural history of asymptomatic patients with normally functioning or minimally dysfunctional bicuspid aortic valve in the community. *Circulation* (2008).

[4] Palta, S, Pai, A. M, & Gill, K. S. Pai RG: New insights into the progression of aortic stenosis: implications for secondary prevention. *Circulation* (2000).

[5] Pohle, K, Maffert, R, & Ropers, D. Progression of aortic valve calcification: association with coronary atherosclerosis and cardiovascular risk factors. *Circulation* (2001).

[6] Olsson, M, Dalsgaard, C. J, Haegerstrand, A, Rosenqvist, M, & Ryden, L. Nilsson J: Accumulation of T lymphocytes and expression of interleukin-2 receptors in nonrheumatic stenotic aortic valves. *J Am Coll Cardiol* (1994).

[7] Parolari, A, Loardi, C, & Mussoni, L. Nonrheumatic calcific aortic stenosis: an overview from basic science to pharmacological prevention. *Eur J Cardiothorac Surg* (2009).

[8] Capoulade, R, Clavel, M. A, & Dumesnil, J. G. Impact of metabolic syndrome on progression of aortic stenosis: influence of age and statin therapy. *J Am Coll Cardiol* (2012).

[9] Pomerance A: Pathogenesis of aortic stenosis and its relation to age. (1972). *Br Heart J.*

[10] Hope, M. D, Urbania, T. H, Yu, J. P, & Chitsaz, S. Tseng E: Incidental aortic valve calcification on CT scans: significance for bicuspid and tricuspid valve disease. *Academic radiology* (2012).

[11] Mcelhinney, D. B, Vogel, M, & Benson, C. B. Assessment of left ventricular endocardial fibroelastosis in fetuses with aortic stenosis and evolving hypoplastic left heart syndrome. *Am J Cardiol* (2010).

[12] Mcelhinney, D. B, Marshall, A. C, & Wilkins-haug, L. E. Predictors of technical success and postnatal biventricular outcome after in utero aortic valvuloplasty for aortic stenosis with evolving hypoplastic left heart syndrome. *Circulation* (2009).

[13] Lofland, G. K, Mccrindle, B. W, & Williams, W. G. Critical aortic stenosis in the neonate: a multi-institutional study of management, outcomes, and risk factors. Congenital Heart Surgeons Society. *J Thorac Cardiovasc Surg* (2001).

[14] Jacobs, J. P, Mavroudis, C, & Jacobs, M. L. Lessons learned from the data analysis of the second harvest ((1998). of the Society of Thoracic Surgeons (STS) Congenital Heart Surgery Database. *Eur J Cardiothorac Surg* 2004, 26(1):18-37.

[15] Eroglu, A. G, Babaoglu, K, & Saltik, L. Echocardiographic follow-up of congenital aortic valvular stenosis. *Pediatr Cardiol* (2006).

[16] Davis, C. K, Cummings, M. W, & Gurka, M. J. Gutgesell HP: Frequency and degree of change of peak transvalvular pressure gradient determined by two Doppler echocardiographic examinations in newborns and children with valvular congenital aortic stenosis. *Am J Cardiol* (2008).

[17] Wagner, H. R, Weidman, W. H, & Ellison, R. C. Miettinen OS: Indirect assessment of severity in aortic stenosis. *Circulation* (1977). Suppl):I, 20-3.

[18] Wagner, H. R, Ellison, R. C, Keane, J. F, & Humphries, O. J. Nadas AS: Clinical course in aortic stenosis. *Circulation* (1977). Suppl):I, 47-56.

[19] Wolfe, R. R, Driscoll, D. J, & Gersony, W. M. Arrhythmias in patients with valvar aortic stenosis, valvar pulmonary stenosis, and ventricular septal defect. Results of hour ECG monitoring. *Circulation* (1993). Suppl):I89-101., 24.

[20] Glanz, S, Hellenbrand, W. E, & Berman, M. A. Talner NS: Echocardiographic assessment of the severity of aortic stenosis in children and adolescents. *Am J Cardiol* (1976).

[21] Lancellotti, P, Lebois, F, Simon, M, Tombeux, C, & Chauvel, C. Pierard LA: Prognostic importance of quantitative exercise Doppler echocardiography in asymptomatic valvular aortic stenosis. *Circulation* (2005). Suppl):I, 377-82.

[22] Little, S. H, & Chan, K. L. Burwash IG: Impact of blood pressure on the Doppler echocardiographic assessment of severity of aortic stenosis. *Heart* (2007).

[23] Giardini, A. Tacy TA: Pressure recovery explains doppler overestimation of invasive pressure gradient across segmental vascular stenosis. *Echocardiography* (2010).

[24] Gorlin, R. Gorlin SG: Hydraulic formula for calculation of the area of the stenotic mitral valve, other cardiac valves, and central circulatory shunts. I. *Am Heart J* (1951).

[25] Mccrindle, B. W, Blackstone, E. H, & Williams, W. G. Are outcomes of surgical versus transcatheter balloon valvotomy equivalent in neonatal critical aortic stenosis? *Circulation* (2001). Suppl 1):I, 152-8.

[26] Mcelhinney, D. B, Lock, J. E, Keane, J. F, & Moran, A. M. Colan SD: Left heart growth, function, and reintervention after balloon aortic valvuloplasty for neonatal aortic stenosis. *Circulation* (2005).

[27] Han, R. K, Gurofsky, R. C, & Lee, K. J. Outcome and growth potential of left heart structures after neonatal intervention for aortic valve stenosis. *J Am Coll Cardiol* (2007).

[28] Bhabra, M. S, Dhillon, R, & Bhudia, S. Surgical aortic valvotomy in infancy: impact of leaflet morphology on long-term outcomes. *Ann Thorac Surg* (2003).

[29] Shinkawa, T, Bove, E. L, Hirsch, J. C, & Devaney, E. J. Ohye RG: Intermediate-term results of the Ross procedure in neonates and infants. *Ann Thorac Surg* (2010). discussion 32.

[30] Hansen, J. H, Petko, C, Bauer, G, Voges, I, & Kramer, H. H. Scheewe J: Fifteen-year single-center experience with the Norwood operation for complex lesions with single-ventricle physiology compared with hypoplastic left heart syndrome. *J Thorac Cardiovasc Surg* (2012).

[31] Feinstein, J. A, Benson, D. W, & Dubin, A. M. Hypoplastic left heart syndrome: current considerations and expectations. *J Am Coll Cardiol* (2012). Suppl):S, 1-42.

[32] Concha, M, Aranda, P. J, & Casares, J. The Ross procedure. *Journal of cardiac surgery* (2004).

[33] Feinstein, J. A, Benson, D. W, & Dubin, A. M. Hypoplastic left heart syndrome: current considerations and expectations. *J Am Coll Cardiol*, 59(1 Suppl):S, 1-42.

[34] Graham, E. M, Zyblewski, S. C, & Phillips, J. W. Comparison of Norwood shunt types: do the outcomes differ 6 years later? *Ann Thorac Surg*, , 90(1), 31-5.

[35] Photiadis, J, Sinzobahamvya, N, & Hraska, V. Asfour B: Does bilateral pulmonary banding in comparison to norwood procedure improve outcome in neonates with hypoplastic left heart syndrome beyond second-stage palliation? A review of the current literature. *Thorac Cardiovasc Surg*, , 60(3), 181-8.

[36] Maxwell, D, & Allan, L. Tynan MJ: Balloon dilatation of the aortic valve in the fetus: a report of two cases. *Br Heart J* (1991).

[37] Kohl, T, Sharland, G, & Allan, L. D. World experience of percutaneous ultrasound-guided balloon valvuloplasty in human fetuses with severe aortic valve obstruction. *Am J Cardiol* (2000).

[38] Tworetzky, W, Wilkins-haug, L, & Jennings, R. W. Balloon dilation of severe aortic stenosis in the fetus: potential for prevention of hypoplastic left heart syndrome: candidate selection, technique, and results of successful intervention. *Circulation* (2004).

[39] Rehnstrom, P, Malm, T, & Jogi, P. Outcome of surgical commissurotomy for aortic valve stenosis in early infancy. *Ann Thorac Surg* (2007).

[40] Miyamoto, T, Sinzobahamvya, N, & Wetter, J. Twenty years experience of surgical aortic valvotomy for critical aortic stenosis in early infancy. *Eur J Cardiothorac Surg* (2006).

[41] Williams, I. A, Quaegebeur, J. M, & Hsu, D. T. Ross procedure in infants and toddlers followed into childhood. *Circulation* (2005). Suppl):I, 390-5.

[42] Lund, O, Flo, C, & Jensen, F. T. Left ventricular systolic and diastolic function in aortic stenosis. Prognostic value after valve replacement and underlying mechanisms. *Eur Heart J* (1997).

[43] Murakami, T, Hess, O. M, Gage, J. E, & Grimm, J. Krayenbuehl HP: Diastolic filling dynamics in patients with aortic stenosis. *Circulation* (1986).

[44] Villari, B, Vassalli, G, Monrad, E. S, Chiariello, M, & Turina, M. Hess OM: Normalization of diastolic dysfunction in aortic stenosis late after valve replacement. *Circulation* (1995).

[45] Rosenhek, R, Binder, T, & Porenta, G. Predictors of outcome in severe, asymptomatic aortic stenosis. *N Engl J Med* (2000).

[46] Leskela, H. V, Vuolteenaho, O, & Koivula, M. K. Tezosentan inhibits uptake of proinflammatory endothelin-1 in stenotic aortic valves. *J Heart Valve Dis* (2012).